# Trounce's Clinical Pharmacology for Nurses

**Ben Greenstein** BA(Hons) BSc(Hons) DHPh PhD FBIH MRPharmS

*Senior Visiting Research Fellow at the Department of Biological Sciences,*
*The Open University, Milton Keynes, UK*
*Visiting Research Professor, Arizona Arthritis Center, University of Arizona, Tucson, USA*

*Nursing Adviser*

**Dinah Gould** BSc MPhil PhD RGN RNT

*Professor of Applied Biology, School of Nursing, City University, London, UK*

*Foreword by*

**John Trounce** MD FRCP

*Professor Emeritus of Clinical Pharmacology, United Medical and Dental Schools, and Physician Emeritus, Guy's Hospital, London, UK*

SEVENTEENTH EDITION

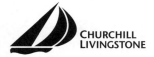

CHURCHILL
LIVINGSTONE

EDINBURGH  LONDON  NEW YORK  OXFORD  PHILADELPHIA  ST LOUIS  SYDNEY  TORONTO  2004

CHURCHILL LIVINGSTONE
An imprint of Elsevier Limited

First edition 1958
Second edition 1961
Third edition 1964
Fourth edition 1967
Fifth edition 1970
Sixth edition 1973
Seventh edition 1977
Eighth edition 1979
Ninth edition 1981

Tenth edition 1983
Eleventh edition 1985
Twelth edition 1988
Thirteenth edition 1990
Fourteenth edition 1994
Fifteenth edition 1997
Sixteenth edition 2000
Seventeenth edition 2004

ISBN 0 443 07208 6

**British Library Cataloguing in Publication Data**
A catalogue record for this book is available from the British Library

**Library of Congress Cataloging in Publication Data**
A catalog record for this book is available from the Library of Congress

**Note**
Medical knowledge is constantly changing. Standard safety precautions must be
followed, but as new research and clinical experience broaden our knowledge,
changes in treatment and drug therapy may become necessary or appropriate.
Readers are advised to check the most current product information provided by
the manufacturer of each drug to be administered to verify the recommended
dose, the method and duration of administration, and contraindications. It is the
responsibility of the practitioner, relying on experience and knowledge of the
patient, to determine dosages and the best treatment for each individual patient.
Neither the Publisher nor the authors assume any liability for any injury and/or
damage to persons or property arising from this publication.

*The Publisher*

**ELSEVIER** your source for books,
journals and multimedia
in the health sciences
**www.elsevierhealth.com**

The
Publisher's
policy is to use
**paper manufactured
from sustainable forests**

Printed in China

# Contents

# Foreword

It gives me great pleasure to write a foreword to the new edition of *Clinical Pharmacology for Nurses* which has been prepared by Ben Greenstein with Professor Dinah Gould acting as nursing advisor.

Although the general principles have been maintained the layout has been restructured to make it more user-friendly, and the text has been extensively revised and updated to bring the contents into line with present day drugs and their therapeutic use. The number of chapters has been increased from twenty-nine to thirty-five which allows for some overlong chapters to be divided, with the insertion of extra material, producing a more logical sequence. Each chapter is preceded by a table of contents, and most usefully, by a list of learning objectives, giving the reader a clear idea of the salient points. At the end of each chapter is a summary which is useful for revision.

There is quite an extensive glossary which will be especially helpful to students who are starting their training and who may not be familiar with some of the terms used in medical textbooks. Overall this refurbishment of the layout and presentation is a great improvement that has made the book considerably easier to use for both learning and reference. Throughout the book various special points have been highlighted. These include Nursing Points which deal with areas of special importance to the nurse; Patient Education, a subject in which nurses are increasingly involved and Safety Points which are relevant to all who use or administer drugs. A list of references which has been updated appears at the end of each chapter.

The text has been considerably, and in some places, radically revised, not only to include new drugs but to indicate where the approach to the treatment of some disorders is changing. A new feature is the inclusion of a number of case histories illustrating how drugs are used in certain clinical situations. They are informative and help to enliven the description of therapeutics. As drugs become more effective and numerous, they are also more difficult to use correctly; incorrect use can lead to a disaster.

Nurses are increasingly involved in drug administration and in prescribing. It is therefore very important that they are familiar not only with the practice of drug therapy but they also need some knowledge of the underlying principles and mode of action of the drugs they are using.

A source of information which is well presented and up-to-date but also strikes a nice balance between basic principles and practical guidance is required. This is admirably provided by the new edition of this book and it will enable members of the nursing profession to face their responsibilities with confidence.

John Trounce

# Preface to the seventeenth edition

This edition marks a change in that authorship switches to Ben Greenstein. Professor Trounce has decided to retire from the book after an almost unprecedented run of 16 editions as author of a textbook. Dinah Gould stays on as Nursing Adviser. In this edition we have strived to retain the original flavour of this classic textbook, *Clinical Pharmacology for Nurses*, while updating information and summarizing text in order to suit the needs of modern teaching methods, so as to fit in with prevailing styles of presentation.

The subject becomes more and more relevant to nurses with the ongoing expansion of the nurse's role and responsibilities in the prescribing, dispensing and monitoring of drugs in patients. Furthermore, drugs are becoming more complex and more sophisticated: for example, the new antibodies for the treatment of rheumatoid arthritis and psoriasis, and some of the cancer chemotherapy drugs, which have to be administered by nurses. This responsibility becomes even more important with the inexorable shift of treatments away from hospitals into the community, where the nurse will be thrown more and more into the front line and into a position of greater responsibility for the prescribing and administration of drugs.

In view of their constant handling of drugs, particularly the immunosuppressive, radioactive and potentially carcinogenic anticancer drugs, nurses need a thorough grounding in the adverse effects of these drugs and in their safe handling. While no text can replace the practical hands-on scenario, this book does attempt to highlight problems of usage and how they are coped with.

Nurses continue to play a pivotal role in the development of new drugs and, particularly, in the supervision of clinical trials, and no training can be complete without giving the student nurse a good grounding in the regulations that underpin the testing and introduction of new drugs. There is now also intense controversy about the funding of drugs and the contentious issue of 'postcode' prescribing. Nurses are well and truly in the thick of it as they very often have to cope with the fears and information needs of patients.

We wish to thank Ninette Premdas, Derek Robertson and Dinah Thom of Elsevier for their patience and support and Dave Burin for superb copy-editing.

It remains only to thank Professor Trounce for introducing this book and for giving us the opportunity to continue with it. We just hope we can live up to the standards he has set. We also wish to thank all those contributors who have enhanced this book; their contributions are acknowledged separately.

London 2004

B.G.
D.G.

# Contributors

Chapter 18. CNS 1: General anaesthesia, local anaesthetics and resuscitation
**Michael Barnett** MB BS FRCA
*Consultant Anaesthetist, Anaesthetic Department, Guy's Hospital, London, UK*

Chapter 28. Drugs and the eye
**Ian Manovel** BPharm MRPharmS
*Pharmacy Department, Moorfields Eye Hospital, London, UK*

Contribution to Chapter 29. Application of drugs to the skin, nose and ears
**Lynette Stone** CBE BA RGN RM(NS) DMS
*Independent Dermatology Nursing Consultant; Chair, Skin Care Campaign, London, UK*

Case studies
**John H R Brook** BSc MB BS DObst DCH MRCGP
*Family Practitioner, Hampstead, London, UK*

**Adam Greenstein** BSc(Hons) MB ChB MRCP
*Registrar, Leeds Infirmary, Leeds, UK*

**Lisa Luger** MSc Dip Paed
*Senior Lecturer, Thames Valley University, London, UK*

# Acknowledgements

We would like to thank the following for permission to reproduce their illustrations:

- Adis International – Tables 35.1, 35.2
- Allen & Hanburys Limited – Figure 4.8
- Becton Dickinson UK Ltd – Figures 2.1, 2.2, 2.3
- Edward Arnold and Professor Ritter – Figure 26.3, from *A Textbook of Clinical Pharmacology*, 3rd edn, Ritter et al
- Graseby Medical Ltd – Figure 10.3
- Kluwer Academic Publishers – Figures 4.6, 7.2, 7.3, 12.1, from *Common Sense Use of Medicines* (1987) by Fry et al
- LAERDAL MEDICAL LTD for ACLS Guidelines – Figure 18.2
- Pharmaceutical Press – Figure 28.2

# Glossary

**ACE inhibitors**: Drugs that inhibit angiotensin-converting enzyme

**Acetylsalicylic acid**: Aspirin

**ACh**: Acetylcholine

**Acidosis**: Abnormal acidity of body fluids and tissues

**Acid reflux**: Backflow of acid from the stomach into the oesophagus

**Acquired specific immune responses**: The responses of the immune system, which is able to recognize as foreign specific proteins of invading organisms or of neoplastic cells and make antibodies against them

**Acromegaly**: Excessive production of growth hormone by a tumour of the pituitary gland in adults

**Acronym**: Word formed from the initial letters of other words, e.g. *BNF* (*British National Formulary*)

**Active immunization**: Promotion of the production by the patient of antibodies or sensitized lymphocytes to certain bacteria or toxins produced by bacteria before infection occurs (see also **passive immunization**)

**Acute confusional states** (called delirium by some practitioners): States of impaired cognition, mood, and self-awareness or attention that are often superimposed on an underlying disease such as dementia or schizophrenia

**Acute inflammatory reaction**: The body's defence mechanism against invading pathogens such as bacteria, cells infected with viruses and neoplastic growth

**Addison's disease**: Disease caused by deficiency of corticosteroid production and release from the adrenal cortex. The main symptoms are loss of energy, muscle weakness and hypotension. Low corticosteroids lower the body's defences against stress and infectious diseases

**Adjuvant therapy**: In cancer treatment, refers to the use of cytotoxic drugs to kill remaining cancer cells after surgery or radiotherapy, particularly if there is a high risk of recurrence of the tumour

**Adrenaline (epinephrine)**: hormone released from the adrenal medulla; one of the **catecholamines**

**Adrenergic**: Describes nerves of the sympathetic nervous system that release norepinephrine, or receptors that respond to noradrenaline (norepinephrine) and sympathomimetic drugs (see also **noradrenergic**)

**Adverse effects**: Unwanted effects; also called side effects

**Aerobes**: Bacteria that require free oxygen

**Afterload**: The arterial pressure that is the resistance against which the heart must pump

**Affinity**: Describes the tightness of the binding reaction between drug and receptor

**Agonist**: Drug that reacts with a receptor, resulting in a cellular response similar to the physiological response of the cell to endogenous activation

**AIDS**: Acquired immune deficiency syndrome

**Akathisia**: Feeling of restlessness with an inability to stand still

**Alzheimer's disease**: Progressive development of dementia characterized by short-term memory loss, and progressive loss of cognitive ability; may be due to loss of certain cholinergic neurones in the brain

**Anabolic**: Promoting tissue growth; forming complex substances such as proteins and laying down glucose as glycogen

**Anaemia**: Clinically significant reduction in haemoglobin in blood

**Analogue**: Drug that is chemically related to a parent substance; e.g. ethinylestradiol is an analogue of the hormone estradiol, and has similar estrogenic properties, but, unlike estradiol, can be taken by mouth

**Anaerobes**: Bacteria that can live and multiply in the absence of free oxygen

**Androgen**: One of a group of compounds, including testosterone, which develops and maintains male sexual function and secondary male characteristics, e.g. hirsutism (hair growth)

**Analgesic**: Drug that relieves pain

**Anaphylactic shock**: Widespread release of histamine as part of an allergic response; can be fatal unless dealt with immediately

**Angina**: A suffocating pain, usually originating in the heart

**Antagonist**: Drug that blocks the action of an agonist

**Anthelmintic**: Chemical used to destroy parasitic worms

**Anti-arrhythmic**: Any drug used to treat heartbeat irregularities

**Antibiotic**: Any substance produced by or derived from an organism, which inhibits the growth of or destroys another organism, usually a bacterial or fungal infection

**Antibody**: Protein produced by a white cell, which binds to and renders harmless a specific antigen such as a bacterium, a foreign blood cell, a virus or pollen

**Anticholinesterase**: A drug that blocks the enzyme acetylcholinesterase, which breaks down the neurotransmitter acetylcholine

**Anticoagulant**: Agent that prevents or slows down the clotting of blood

**Anticonvulsant**: Drug that prevents or reduces the severity of epileptic seizures

**Antidepressant**: Drug that alleviates the symptoms of depression

**Anti-emetic**: Agent that inhibits or reduces vomiting

**Antifertility**: Against allowing reproduction

**Antigen**: Substance seen by the body as foreign, and against which the body makes a specific **antibody**

**Antihistamine**: Agent that blocks the action of histamine, usually by blocking histamine receptors

**Anti-inflammatory**: Reducing or blocking inflammation reactions

**Antimetabolite**: Drug that blocks a metabolic pathway; commonly used in cancer

**Antimuscarinic**: Drug that blocks muscarinic receptors

**Antioxidant**: Any substance that neutralizes oxygen free radicals

**Antipsychotic (neuroleptic)**: Drug used to treat **psychosis**

**Antipyretic**: Lowering of body temperature (e.g. aspirin is antipyretic)

**Antiserum**: Serum containing antibodies directed against specific antigens; used clinically for **passive immunization**

**Antitussive**: Agent to treat coughs

**Antithrombin III**: A protein that is part of the system that regulates clotting. It binds to certain clotting factors and renders them inactive

**Anxiety**: A term used to describe a condition of generalized, all-pervasive fear

**Anxiolytic**: Drug that reduces anxiety

**Aqueous humour**: Fluid that fills the chamber of the eye behind the cornea and in front of the lens (see also **vitreous humour**)

**Ariboflavinosis**: Deficiency of riboflavin (vitamin $B_2$); in humans causes several symptoms, including cracking and fissures at the corner of the mouth and a sore tongue and skin lesions

**Arrhythmia**: Deviation from the normal sinus rhythm of the heart

**Aromatase inhibitor**: Drug that blocks the biosynthesis of estrogens by inhibiting the aromatase enzyme

**Arteriole**: Small branch of artery, important in the control of blood flow and blood pressure, since it is innervated by nerves and responds to drugs that may either dilate or constrict it

**Arthritis**: Inflammation of joints; see also **osteoarthritis** and **rheumatoid arthritis**

**Ascites**: Accumulation of fluid in the peritoneal cavity, which causes the abdomen to swell

**Atheroma**: Degeneration of the inner arterial wall (intima) due to the deposition of fatty plaques and scarring

**Athlete's foot**: Fungal infection of the skin between the toes (tinea pedis)

**Atrial escape rhythm**: a cardiac dysrhythmia occurring when sustained suppression of sinus impulse formation causes other atrial foci to act as cardiac pacemakers

**Atrial fibrillation**: atrial arrhythmia marked by rapid, randomized contraction of small areas of the atrial myocardium, causing an irregular and often rapid ventricular rate

**Atrial flutter**: Atria contract at very high speed, usually about 240–300/minute

**Atrioventricular (AV) node**: body of heart muscle in lower part of right ventricle that receives contractile impulses from the atria and transmits these to the ventricles through the **bundle of His**

**Atrium**: Either of the two upper chambers of the heart

**Atrophy**: Wasting away of tissues or organs due to cellular degeneration

**Auscultation**: Listening to sounds made by fluids or gas in the body, usually with a stethoscope

**Autocrine**: Hormones that act on the cell that produced them

**Autonomic nervous system**: Part of the nervous system that controls functions over which there is little or no conscious control; consists of sympathetic and parasympathetic divisions

**Bactericidal**: Able to kill bacteria, usually rapidly

**Bacteriostatic**: Able to stop bacteria from replicating, but not killing them

**Basal ganglia**: Large masses of grey matter embedded within the white matter of the cerebral hemispheres; they are concerned mainly with control of voluntary movements at a subconscious level

**B cell**: (see **B lymphocyte**)

**Beriberi**: Disease caused by thiamine (vitamin $B_1$) deficiency caused by eating a diet rich in polished rice; leads to nervous degeneration and often death from heart failure unless treated with vitamin $B_1$.

**Bile acid-binding resins**: These drugs combine with bile acids and cholesterol in the gut, thus preventing their absorption and increasing faecal excretion

**Bioavailability**: The drug has reached the circulation and is therefore available to all the tissues

**Biologics**: Therapeutic agents, usually vaccines or genetically engineered proteins, that interact with proteins of bacteria or viruses or with proteins of the body that mediate disease-producing reactions

**B lymphocyte**: White blood cell made in the bone marrow which matures in the lymph nodes and spleen before entering the blood. B lymphocytes make antibodies

**Bronchiole**: A subdivision of the bronchial tree

**Bradycardia**: Slowing of the heart rate; pulse rate falls below 60

**Bronchiectasis**: Suppurating bronchial inflammation

**Bronchospasm**: Narrowing of the bronchial tubes through contraction of bronchial smooth muscle

**Bullous rash**: Rash with blisters

**Bundle of His** (also called atrioventricular bundle): Bundle of modified heart muscle fibres called Purkinje fibres that conduct waves of contraction from the atria to the ventricles

**Calcium antagonist**: Drug that blocks calcium channels; used in hypertension and cardiac arrhythmias

**Carcinogen**: Anything that causes cancer (see also oncogen)

**Cardiac**: Pertaining to the heart; also used to describe the upper end of the stomach

**Cardioversion**: The application of a controlled direct current shock to the heart of an anaesthetized patient using electrodes placed on the chest wall to restore the normal rhythm of the heart. The apparatus used is called a cardiovertor

**Catabolic**: Breakdown of complex substances such as proteins and glycogen to glucose to release energy

**Cataract**: Development of an opaque lens; generally caused by ageing, but can be caused by occupational injuries (infra-red rays) or diseases such as diabetes

**Catecholamine**: An amine which contains the catechol ring; examples are **noradrenaline** (norepinephrine) and **adrenaline** (epinephrine)

**CD4**: A protein on the surface of **helper T cells** that is important in the development of immunity to viral infections

**Cerebral palsy**: Disorder of movement, caused by brain damage before, during or soon after birth; brain damage is permanent, but the disorder is non-progressive

**Chelating agents**: Chemicals that form complexes with some metal ions, thus rendering them harmless; the complex is safely excreted. Chelating agents are useful in cases of, for example, copper poisoning

**Chemoreceptor trigger zone**: Nerve centre in the medulla of the brain that, when stimulated by drugs such as apomorphine, triggers the **vomiting centre**

**Chemotherapy**: Treatment or prevention of disease with chemicals; usually refers to treatment of cancer and infectious diseases with drugs

**Cholecalciferol**: Vitamin D

**Cholinergic**: Usually refers to any function or nerve where acetylcholine is the mediator

**Cirrhosis**: Formation of a network of fibrous tissue and regenerating cells in the liver in response to, for example, alcohol, hepatitis or chronic heart failure

**Claudication**: Lameness, limping

**Clotting factors** (cogulation factors): Components of blood that are part of a cascade of reactions that result in coagulation

**Clotting time** (coagulation time): The time taken for blood or plasma to coagulate under controlled laboratory conditions

**CNS**: Central nervous system

**Coagulation**: In the case of blood, the conversion of liquid blood to a solid fibrous mass

**Coeliac disease**: Disease where the small intestine is unable to digest and absorb food; successfully treated by adopting a strictly gluten-free diet

**Co-enzyme**: Non-protein chemical essential for the function of some proteins; several co-enzymes contain B vitamins as part of their molecular structure

**Colic**: Severe abdominal pain

**Collyrium**: Medicated sterile solution for bathing the eye

**Compliance**: Patient's adherence to a prescribed drug or other programme of treatment

**COMT**: Catechol-O-methyltransferase; an enzyme that breaks down catecholamines

**Congenital**: Any disorder recognized at birth, whether caused genetically or by environmental factors

**Conjunctiva**: Delicate membrane covering the front of the eye and lining the inner surface of the eyelids

**Conjunctivitis** (pink eye): Inflammation of the conjunctiva causing discomfort and discharge; caused by viral or bacterial infection

**Constipation**: Difficult, painful or infrequent evacuation of bowel contents

**Contractility**: Degree of power of the muscle to contract

**Contraindications**: Conditions that mean a drug should not be used

**Coronary**: Relating to the heart

**Coronary angioplasty**: Inflation of part of the coronary artery with a balloon

**Coronary thrombosis**: Thrombus (blood clot) formation in the coronary artery, causing death of some cardiac tissue through a reduction in blood supply

**Corpus striatum**: Part of the **basal ganglia** in the cerebral hemispheres of the brain

**Corticosteroid (corticoid)**: Any steroid hormone synthesized in the adrenal cortex: the two main types are glucocorticoids, e.g. cortisol, and mineralocorticoids, principally aldosterone

**Coupled rhythm**: heartbeats occurring in pairs, the second beat usually being a premature ventricular beat

**COX**: Cyclooxygenase

**Cranial nerves**: 12 pairs of nerves arising directly from the brain, e.g. vagus (X)

**Creatinine**: A chemical derived from creatine in muscle; excreted in the urine

**Crohn's disease** (regional enteritis, regional ileitis): Inflammation of segments of the alimentary tract, which become ulcerated, thickened and inflamed. The cause is unknown

**CSM**: Committee on Safety of Medicines

**Cushing's disease**: Disease caused by excessive production and release of corticosteroid hormones due to an ACTH-secreting tumour in the pituitary or elsewhere in the body. *Cushing's syndrome* is a condition where the patient has the symptoms of Cushing's disease, but is caused, for example, by large amounts of steroid medication

**Cyanacobalamin**: Vitamin $B_{12}$

**Cyanosis**: Skin and mucous membranes turn blue due to inadequate oxygen supply to the tissues

**Cytokine**: Proteins released by cells when they are challenged by antigens, e.g. interleukins; part of the body's protective mechanisms

**Cytomegalovirus** (CMV): One of the herpes group of viruses

**Cytopenia**: Depression of the blood count

**Cytotoxic**: Destroys cells by blocking cell division

**Deep brain stimulation**: A procedure based on that of the cardiac pacemaker. It involves placing electrodes into specific brain areas, specifically the globus pallidus or the thalamus

**Defibrillator**: Apparatus that delivers a controlled electric shock to restore normal heart rhythm in cases of cardiac arrest due to ventricular fibrillation

**Dementia**: Chronic mental disorder of intellectual function and behaviour due to brain degenerative disease or destruction of brain tissue through physical trauma such as stroke. Dementia should not be confused with psychological disorders that produce similar symptoms

**Dependent oedema**: Oedema of ankles caused by sitting, mainly in elderly people

**Depolarization**: Transient change in the membrane potential caused by rapid influx of sodium ions, which may generate a propagated action potential

**Depolarizing blocking drugs**: Neuromuscular blockers that actually excite the muscle fibre by depolarizing the membrane before they block any further membrane depolarization by acetylcholine released from nerve endings at the neuromuscular junction (e.g. suxamethonium)

**Diabetes**: A term to describe a metabolic disorder characterized by production of abnormally large volumes of dilute urine. When used alone, it usually refers to **diabetes mellitus**

**Diabetes insipidus**: This is a rare disease when the patient produces large amounts of dilute urine due to a deficiency of vasopressin

**Diabetes mellitus**: Raised blood sugar due to a deficiency of insulin; there are two types. Type I (juvenile onset; insulin-dependent) diabetes mellitus is an autoimmune disease that involves destruction of the pancreatic beta cells. Type II (non-insulin-dependent) diabetes mellitus occurs when there is a reduced ability of the islets to produce sufficient insulin

**Diarrhoea**: Abnormally high frequency of bowel evacuation, often with soft or liquid stools; it can cause serious loss of water, salts and nutrients

**Diastole**: Period between two contractions of the heart

**Diastolic blood pressure**: The pressure recorded at diastole when the heart is filling; the value obtained reflects predominantly the total peripheral resistance in the vascular beds

**Diuretic**: Drug that increases urine flow

**DMARD**: Disease-modifying antirheumatic drug

**DNA**: Deoxyribonucleic acid

**Dopaminergic**: Refers to nerve cells that use dopamine as neurotransmitter

**Drug absorption**: Movement of the drug into the internal environment

**Drug dependence**: Patient either craves a drug (psychological dependence) or suffers physical symptoms of withdrawal without the drug (physical dependence)

**Drug distribution**: The tissues to which a drug gains access

**Drug elimination**: Movement of the drug out of the body into the external environment (see also **excretion**)

**Drug metabolism**: How the body transforms the drug chemically

**Drug tolerance**: More of a dose of a drug is required in order to achieve the same effect

**Dysmenorrhoea**: Painful menstruation

**Dyspepsia** (indigestion): Disorder of digestion during which there may be pain and discomfort in the abdomen or lower chest, and perhaps nausea and vomiting

**Dyspnoea**: shortness of breath

**Dystonia**: Uncontrolled movements

**Eclampsia**: Convulsions not caused by epilepsy in a pregnant woman after a sudden rise in blood pressure (**pre-eclampsia**) that may be accompanied by **oedema** and **oliguria**

**Ectopic beat**; see **extrasystole**

**Eczema**: Itchy skin disorder; there are several types

**Efficacy**: How effective the drug is (see also **potency**)

**Embolism**: Condition when an **embolus** becomes lodged in an artery and blocks blood flow

**Embolus**: Anything such as air, fat, blood clot, amniotic fluid or a foreign body carried in the blood to lodge elsewhere, e.g. a lung embolism

**Embryo**: In humans, the product of conception up to the 8th week

**EMEA**: The European Agency for the Evaluation of Medicinal Products

**Emetic**: Substance that causes vomiting

**Emphysema** (pulmonary emphysema): Difficulty with breathing caused by damaged alveoli of the lungs. The cause is unknown but smokers may be more prone to emphysema

**Emulsion**: A mixture of two immiscible liquids (e.g. oil and water) in which one is dispersed through the other in a finely divided state, e.g. Milk of Magnesia

**Endocarditis**: Inflammation of the lining of the heart cavity (the endocardium)

**Endocrine gland**: Ductless gland

**Endometriosis**: Occurrence of endometrial tissue in other parts of the pelvis

**Enema**: Fluid infused into the rectum through a tube that has been passed through the anus

**Enzyme**: Protein that catalyses biochemical reactions

**Epidural injection**: The injection of a local anaesthetic into the epidural space in the lumbar region of the spinal cord

**Epinephrine**: see **adrenaline**

**Erythema**: Skin flushing due to capillary dilatation in the dermis

**Erythematous**: Producing erythema

**Erythropoietin**: Hormone secreted by some kidney cells in response to reduced oxygen tension in blood; erythropoietin increases the rate of red blood cell production

**Essential hypertension**: Clinically high blood pressure of unknown cause

**Estrogen**: One of a group of chemicals, including estradiol, which develops and maintains female sexual function and secondary female characteristics such as breast development

**Euphoria**: Elation and optimism for no apparent reason; in extreme form is called **mania**

**Excretion**: Ejection of anything from the body

**Exfoliation**: Flaking off of the upper layers of the skin; separation of the surface epithelium from underlying tissue

**Expectorants**: Drugs that loosen the sputum and thus aid its ejection from the bronchial tree

**Extrasystole**: Also called an **ectopic beat**, it is a heartbeat that originates in the heart away from the sino-atrial node; may be ventricular or supraventricular

**Febrile**: Relating to fever

**Ferritin**: A complex of iron and a protein that is one of the ways in which iron is stored in the tissues

**Fetus**: Unborn child from 8th week of development

**Fibrates**: Fibrates alter the metabolism of lipoproteins, and so lower blood cholesterol and triglycerides

**Fibrillation**: Rapid, chaotic beating of individual cardiac muscle fibres

**Fibrin**: Fibrous insoluble protein of the blood clot

**Fibrinogen**: Soluble protein converted to insoluble fibrin by **thrombin**

**First pass metabolism**: Metabolism of a drug in the liver after its absorption from the gastrointestinal tract (**GIT**)

**Flukes**: Parasitic flatworms; they cause bilharziasis for example

**Focal epilepsy**: The attack arises from a focal electrical discharge in the brain

**GAD** (general anxiety disorder): The patient feels apprehensive and tense for no particular reason, or as a result of some minor problem

**Gallstone** (cholelithiasis): A hard body made of cholesterol, bile pigments and calcium that forms in the gall bladder

**GAS**: General adaptation syndrome

**Gastric**: Relating to or affecting the stomach

**GIT**: Gastrointestinal tract

**Glaucoma**: Loss of vision due to abnormally raised intraocular pressure

**Glomerulus**: Usually refers to the network of blood capillaries in the Bowman's capsule of the kidney; an important function is to filter substances out of the blood into the urine

**Glycogen**: Principal storage form of glucose in the body, consisting of branched chains of glucose

**Gonadotrophins**: Proteinaceous hormones released from the anterior pituitary gland and from the placenta; they are concerned with the growth and structural maintenance of the male and female gonads, and with the synthesis and release of the gonadal sex hormones

**Gonads**: Male or female reproductive organs (testis and ovary, respectively)

**Gout**: Disease in which uric acid metabolism and excretion are impaired, resulting in deposition of uric acid in joints and in cartilage, especially in the ears

**Guttae**: Latin term used in prescriptions meaning 'drops'; also refers to skin lesions that are drop-shaped

**Haemoglobin**: Protein in the red blood cell that carries oxygen

**Haemolytic anaemia**: Anaemia due to destruction of red blood cells (see also **anaemia**)

**Haemorrhage**: Serious escape of blood from blood vessels

**Haptens**: Small molecules that combine with larger molecules such as proteins and turn them 'foreign', e.g. aspirin

**Heart block**: Bundle of His fails to transmit impulses from the atria to the ventricles

**Heart failure**: Inadequate pumping power of the ventricles of the heart

**Helper T cells**: Type of white cell called a lymphocyte that stimulates the production of **killer T cells**, which attack and destroy target cells

**Hepatic**: Relating to the liver

**Heroin**: diacetylmorphine

**Herpes**: Inflammation of mucous membranes or skin caused by the herpes virus. Herpes simplex virus type I causes the cold sore and type II causes genital herpes; herpes zoster causes shingles

**Hirsutism**: Inappropriate and unwanted growth of body hair

**HIV**: Human immunodeficiency virus: **retrovirus** responsible for **AIDS**

**HRT**: Hormone replacement therapy

**Hypercalcaemia**: High blood calcium

**Hypercalcuria**: Clinically raised calcium in the urine

**Hyperglycaemic**: Clinically high blood glucose

**Hyperkalaemia**: High blood potassium

**Hyperlipidaemia** (hyperlipaemia): Abnormally high concentration of fats in the bloodstream

**Hypernatraemia**: Abnormally high blood sodium

**Hyperparathyroidism**: Overactivity of the parathyroid glands

**Hyperplasia**: The increased production and growth of more normal cells in any organ or tissue, e.g. benign prostatic hyperplasia (BPH) in older men.

**Hypertension**: Clinically raised blood pressure that could damage perfused tissues

**Hyperthyroidism**: Over-secretion of thyroid hormone

**Hypertrophy**: The enlargement of the cells themselves without necessarily an increase in cell number; the increase in muscle size following exercise or 'pumping iron' is an example of hypertrophy

**Hypervolaemia**: Overfilling of the vascular system

**Hypnotic**: Drug that induces sleep

**Hypoglycaemic**: Clinically low blood glucose

**Hypokinesia**: Inhibition of voluntary movements

**Hypotension**: Clinically low blood pressure

**Hypothyroidism**: Under-secretion of thyroid hormone

**Idiopathic**: A condition whose cause is unknown and which appears to arise spontaneously

**I.M.**: Intramuscular

**Incontinence**: Involuntary passage of urine

**Inert**: Describes a drug ingredient that has no medicinal properties: e.g. lactose in a tablet

**Inflammatory bowel disease**: Any of a group of inflammatory conditions of the intestine, including Crohn's disease and ulcerative colitis

**Infusion**: Slow injection of a volume into the body, usually into a vein

**Innate response**: The inflammation that is produced at a site of damage

**Insomnia**: Inability to fall asleep or remain asleep for an adequate time

**Insulinoma**: Insulin-producing tumour in the pancreas

**Intercurrent illness**: The occurrence of an illness that may modify the course and treatment of another illness that is present at the same time

**Interferons**: Peptides that are produced by cells infected with viruses

**Intraosseous injection**: Injection into the bone marrow

**Intrathecal injection**: The administration of the drug directly into the central nervous system (CNS), thus bypassing the blood–brain barrier

**Ionization**: Conversion of an electrically neutral chemical into a charged one either by gaining or losing electrons

**Ischaemia**: Inadequate blood flow to a part of the body

**I.V.**: Intravenous

**Kaolin cephalin time**: A method of measuring the clotting time

**Kernicterus**: Staining of the newborn brain by the bile pigment bilirubin, which is displaced from its blood-binding proteins by drugs such as sulphonamides, tolbutamide or aspirin taken by the mother in late pregnancy. It causes brain damage, with subsequent development of symptoms of cerebral palsy about 6 months after birth

**Killer T cells**: Lymphocytes that target and destroy other cells

**Korsakov's psychosis**: Memory defect with failure to learn new information, although already learned information is retained. The usual cause is alcoholism, leading to vitamin $B_1$ deficiency, and it is treated with high doses of vitamin $B_1$.

**LDL**: Low-density lipoprotein that carries cholesterol in the bloodstream

**Lennox–Gastaut syndrome**: Very severe form of childhood epilepsy

**Leukaemia**: Overproduction of leucocytes by the bone marrow and other blood-forming organs due to malignant disease, and suppression of production of platelets, other white cells and of red cells, resulting in immunodeficiency and bleeding; may be acute or chronic

**Lewy body dementia**: Dementia with symptoms overlapping those of Alzheimer's, with loss of cognition, hallucinations and symptoms of Parkinson's disease. Lewy bodies are abnormal lumps seen in degenerating cells of the cortex and substantia nigra

**Libido**: Sexual drive

**Ligand**: Any chemical that binds to another (in pharmacology, usually refers to drugs that bind to receptors)

**Linctus**: A liquid that contains some sweet syrupy substance which is used for its soothing effect on coughs. It may also contain a cough suppressant such as dextromethorphan

**Lipid**: Fat

**Lipoproteins**: Molecules in the blood and lymph consisting of protein and lipids; important in the transport of cholesterol and the uptake of cholesterol into cells

**Livedo reticularis**: Skin discoloration

**Loop diuretics**: Diuretics that act in the ascending limb of the loop of Henle

**Malignant hyperthermia**: Extremely rare familial disorder that is genetically determined. It starts with excessive metabolic activity in muscle cells, which leads to muscle rigidity, a high temperature and widespread severe metabolic disturbances. It used to have a high mortality

**Malignant tumour**: A tumour that invades and destroys a tissue or organ in which it occurs, and which may then spread to other tissues and perhaps prove fatal

**Malnutrition**: Condition arising from improper balance between an individual's diet and what is required in diet for maintenance of health

**Mania**: Wild, extravagant and incoherent speech and behaviour

**MAOI**: Monoamine oxidase inhibitor

**Ménière's disease**: A disease of the inner ear with episodes of buzzing, deafness and vertigo. The medical name is endolymphatic hydrops

**Meningitis**: Inflammation of the meninges, the three membranes that enclose the brain and spinal cord. Symptoms include severe headache, photosensitivity, fever, loss of appetite, muscle rigidity, especially in the neck, and, in severe cases, delirium, convulsions and death

**Menopause**: When cessation of ovulation and menstruation start to occur

**Menorrhagia**: Abnormally heavy bleeding during menstruation

**Miotics**: Drugs that cause contraction of the pupil

**Mixtures**: Liquids that contain several ingredients dissolved or diffused in water or some other solvent, e.g. kaolin mixture for diarrhoea

**MMR vaccine**: Combined vaccine against measles, mumps and German measles (rubella)

**Monoamine oxidase inhibitor (MAOI)**: Drug that inhibits the enzyme monoamine oxidase, that breaks down catecholamines such as norepinephrine and epinephrine; used chiefly to treat depressive illness

**Monoclonal antibody**: Antibody produced from an artificial cell made by fusing a mouse spleen lymphocyte that produces the antibody with a mouse myeloma cell; the resulting artificial cell makes only the one antibody that the lymphocyte originally made

**Monocyte**: Type of white blood cell with kidney-shaped nucleus, whose function is to take in foreign particles such as bacteria and debris

**Morbidity**: Condition or state of being diseased

**Mortality**: Death, i.e. mortality rate = death rate

**MRSA**: Methicillin-resistant *Staphylococcus aureus*

**Mucolytic**: Agent that liquefies phlegm

**Muscarinic**: Describes drugs that bind to and activate muscarinic acetylcholine receptors of the parasympathetic division of the autonomic nervous system or drugs that mimic the effects produced by stimulation of muscarinic receptors

**Mydriasis**: Dilation of the pupil

**Mydriatic**: Drug used to dilate the pupil, e.g. atropine, tropicamide

**Myocardial infarction**: Death of part of the heart muscle, usually in the left ventricle, following interruption of the blood supply

**Myoclonic jerks**: Sudden jerking of the limbs that occurs in patients with epilepsy and in those with degenerative neurological disease

**Myopathy**: Any disease of muscle (e.g. cardiomyopathy)

**Necrosis**: Death of cells within a tissue or organ

**Negative feedback**: A regulatory system whereby the end-product (e.g. testosterone) controls its own synthesis and/or release by inhibiting the system that stimulates its production

**Negative inotropic**: Decreased heart contractility

**Neoplastic growth**: Any new and abnormal growth, which may be either benign or malignant

**Nephrotic syndrome**: Protein loss in the urine and cirrhosis of the liver where there is a failure to make protein

**Nephrotoxic**: Toxic to the kidneys

**Neural transplantation**: Transplanting human fetal tissue containing dopaminergic neurones into the brains of patients with Parkinson's disease

**Neuroleptic**: Antipsychotic drug

**Neutropenia**: Clinically significant reduction in the numbers of neutrophils in the blood

**NICE**: National Institute for Clinical Excellence

**Non-depolarizing blocking drugs**: Drugs that block muscle contraction without themselves causing any depolarization of the muscle fibre membrane (e.g. **tubocurarine**)

**Noradrenergic**: Describes nerves that release noradrenaline (norepinephrine) as neurotransmitter or receptors that respond to noradrenaline (norepinephrine)

**Norepinephrine** (also called **noradrenaline**): A **catecholamine** neurotransmitter released from noradrenergic nerve terminals; small amounts are also released from the adrenal medulla

**NSAID**: Non-steroidal anti-inflammatory drug

**Nucleoside**: A chemical consisting of a pyrimidine or purine base attached to a sugar, e.g. adenosine

**Nucleotide**: A pyrimidine or purine base attached to a sugar, to which is attached a phosphate group; the building blocks of **RNA** and **DNA**

**Obsessive compulsive disorder**: Characterized by repetitive, anxiety-driven behaviour such as the repeated washing of hands or obsessive thoughts and doubts

**Oedema**: Accumulation of excess fluid in body tissues (called dropsy in bygone days)

**Oesophageal varices**: Veins that have dilated in the lower oesophagus because of portal hypertension (high blood pressure in the hepatic portal vein). They can rupture and cause dangerous bleeding

**Oliguria**: Abnormally low urine production

**Oncogen**: Anything that causes a tumour

**Opioid**: Natural substances (e.g. morphine, codeine, endorphins) or synthetic derivatives (e.g. diacetylmorphine) that produce morphine-like effects such as analgesia or sedation

**Oral**: By mouth

**Oral anticoagulants**: Anticoagulants that can be taken by mouth, e.g. warfarin

**Oral contraceptive**: Tablet taken orally that blocks conception

**Osmosis**: Flow of water through a semi-permeable membrane (e.g. the proximal tubule of the kidney) from a region of lower salt concentration to a region of higher salt concentration

**Osteoarthritis** (osteoarthrosis): Degenerative joint disease, involving wear of articular cartilage, which may cause secondary changes in underlying bone. It can be primary, or secondary to abnormal loads to joints or damage to cartilage due to trauma or inflammation

**Osteoporosis**: Loss of bony tissue, resulting in fracture-prone brittle bones

**Ototoxic**: Toxic to the organs of hearing or balance in the inner ear or to the vestibulocochlear nerve

**PABA**: Para-aminobenzoic acid, a precursor of folic acid, which is essential in cell division

**Palliative therapy**: Drug treatment to relieve symptoms, without actually curing a disease; commonly used in cancer

**Pallidotomy (pallidectomy)**: Introduction of electrodes into the brain to destroy a particular part of the brain in an area called the globus pallidus

**Panic attacks** are unexpected attacks of anxiety, often with marked physical symptoms such as tremor, palpitation and dry mouth due to overactivity of the sympathetic nervous system

**Paracrine**: Hormone that acts on cells in the region of those that produced it, rather than on tissues to which it has to be carried in the bloodstream

**Parasympathomimetic**: Drug that mimics the stimulation of the parasympathetic division of the autonomic nervous system

**Parenteral**: Administration of a drug by any route other than orally, e.g. by injection

**Parkinsonism**: A term used to describe the symptoms of Parkinson's disease, which may result, as stated below, not only from the degeneration of the nigrostriatal pathway but also from drugs or infections

**Parkinson's disease**: Degenerative brain disorder in the basal ganglia with the loss of dopaminergic neurones, resulting in rigidity, tremor and progressive difficulty in initiating and stopping movement

**Partial agonist**: A drug that is both an agonist and antagonist under different conditions (usually dose)

**Parturition**: Childbirth

**Passive immunization**: The appropriate antibody against the invading organism or toxin is injected (see also **active immunization**)

**Patch**: Adhesive impregnated with medicine and applied to the skin for slow, continuous release of active agent

**Pediculosis**: Infestation of the skin with lice

**Pepsin**: Stomach enzyme that breaks down proteins

**Peptic**: Relating to pepsin or to digestion

**Peptide**: Molecule consisting of two or more amino acids, e.g. oxytocin

**Pernicious anaemia** (Addison's anaemia): Anaemia caused by deficiency of vitamin $B_{12}$ (**cyanacobalamin**).

**Pessary**: Device usually containing medicine for insertion into the vagina (also called a vaginal suppository)

**Petit mal** (absence) seizure: Brief interference with consciousness

**pH**: Measure of acidity or alkalinity in units from 1 to 14: the pH is the negative logarithm of the hydrogen ion concentration

**Phaeochromocytoma**: A catecholamine-secreting tumour of the adrenal gland

**Pharmacodynamics**: Study of how the body recognizes the drug; how the drug exerts its effect

**Pharmacokinetics**: Study of how the body processes the drug

**Pharynx**: Muscular tube lined with mucous membranes that extends from the base of the skull down to the beginning of the oesophagus; its functions are to carry air from the nose and mouth to the larynx, to act as a resonating chamber for the larynx, and to carry food from the mouth to the oesophagus

**Phlebothrombosis**: Obstruction of a vein by a blood clot

**Phobic states**: The patient fears certain situations. The commonest is agoraphobia in which the subject is frightened to go out

**Phosphodiesterase**: Enzyme that breaks down cyclic AMP

**Phytomenadione**: Vitamin K

**Plasma**: Straw-coloured fluid in which the blood cells are suspended

**Plasma half-life**: The time taken for the plasma concentration of the drug to decline to one half of its value

**Plasmodium**: Genus of **protozoans** that live in human red blood and liver cells; they cause, for example, malaria

**Platelet** (thrombocyte): Disc-shaped body in blood, 1–2 μm in diameter, with functions related to stopping bleeding

**Platelet aggregation**: Sticking together of platelets in the blood

**PMS**: (see **premenstrual syndrome**)

**Pneumocystis pneumonia**: Pneumonia that is caused, usually, in immunosuppressed patients by a protozoan called *Pneumocystis*

**Polyarteritis nodosa** (periarteritis nodosa): Potentially dangerous inflammation of the walls of arteries, producing symptoms of (e.g.) arthritis, asthma, fever and hypertension; kidney failure; and neuritis. It is treated with prednisolone or other corticosteroids

**Positive inotropic**: Increased heart contractility (see **negative inotropic**)

**Post-traumatic stress disorder**: The anxiety that follows traumatic experiences such as rape or warfare

**Potency**: How powerful the drug is: i.e. the lower the dose, the more powerful the drug is

**Pre-eclampsia**: Sudden rise in blood pressure (over 140/90) in a pregnant woman, in whom blood pressure was previously normal

**Preload**: The pressure in the venous system filling the heart and stretching the heart muscle

**Premenstrual syndrome** (premenstrual tension): Irritability, nervousness and depression before menstruation, associated with accumulation of water and salts in the tissues. The condition usually disappears when menstruation begins

**Prodrug**: A drug that is metabolized to the therapeutically active metabolite

**Prosthesis**: Any artificial aid attached to the body, e.g. prosthetic heart valve

**Protease**: Enzyme that catalyses the splitting of proteins

**Proteinuria**: Protein in the urine

**Prothrombin**: Protein that is converted to **thrombin** by **thromboplastin**

**Prothrombin time** (PT): The time taken for clotting to occur in a sample of blood to which thromboplastin and calcium have been added

**Protozoa**: Group of microscopic, single-celled organisms, e.g. *Trypanosoma* (malaria)

**Psoriasis**: Chronic skin disease, relatively common in Britain and often in families, in which scaly, pink patches occur on scalp, elbows, knees and other parts of the body

**Psoriatic arthritis**: Arthritis that is associated with psoriasis

**Psychomotor seizure**: Various involuntary movements, but without loss of consciousness

**Psychosis**: A term used to describe one of a group of psychiatric disorders when the patient loses contact with reality

**Purgatives**: Drugs that loosen the bowel

**Pyridoxine**: Vitamin $B_6$

**RA**: Rheumatoid arthritis

**Receptor**: Protein that recognizes another chemical and binds it, usually transducing the binding reaction into a message to the cell

**Refractory period**: Period between muscle contraction or nerve impulse generation when the muscle or nerve recovers and is unable to respond to an incoming impulse

**Renin**: Enzyme protein released into the circulation by the kidney in response to stresses such as haemorrhage or other causes of low blood pressure

**Retinoids**: Group of drugs derived from vitamin A

**Retrovirus**: RNA-containing virus that converts its RNA into DNA using an enzyme called reverse transcriptase

**Reye's syndrome**: Childhood symptoms of encephalitis with symptoms of liver failure; aspirin is implicated and contraindicated in children below 12

**Rheumatic fever**: Acute rheumatism, this disease affects mainly children and young adults as a delayed complication of haemolytic streptococcal infection of the upper respiratory tract. It may progress to chronic rheumatic heart disease

**Rheumatoid arthritis**: An autoimmune disease, rheumatoid arthritis is a very common form of progressive arthritis, second only to osteoarthritis, and affects soft tissue of joints of fingers, wrists, ankles and feet, and eventually knees, hips, shoulders and neck. Ligaments and bone become damaged. It is more prevalent in women (women:men = 3:1)

**Riboflavin**: Vitamin $B_2$

**Rickets**: Disease caused by vitamin D deficiency in children, whose bones do not develop properly and may be deformed

**RNA**: Ribonucleic acid

**S.C.**: Subcutaneous

**Scabies**: Skin infestation caused by the mite *Sarcoptes scabiei*

**Schizophrenia**: Change of personality with disordered thought processes, which may be associated with hallucinations, delusions and withdrawal

**Scurvy**: Disease caused by vitamin C deficiency

**Second messenger**: Chemical within the cell that carries the message that a hormone, neurotransmitter, etc., has bound to its receptor on the cell membrane; cyclic AMP and inositol triphosphate are examples of second messengers

**Seizure**: Convulsion, fit

**Serum**: Fluid that separates from clotted blood. It is essentially plasma without fibrinogen and other factors involved in coagulation

**Serum sickness**: A delayed hypersensitivity reaction to injection of foreign proteins; symptoms include fever, rashes, lymph node enlargement and joint pain

**Sino-atrial (SA) node**: Tiny modified body of heart muscle in the upper right ventricle near the entry point of the vena cava; called the pacemaker because it has an independent rhythmic beat of about 70/minute

**Sinus rhythm**: The normal heart rhythm that originates in the sino-atrial node

**Skeletal (striated) muscle**: Muscles attached to the skeletal frame, which are under voluntary control

**Smooth muscle**: Muscle of the autonomic nervous system that mediates involuntary contractions, e.g. of arterioles and bronchi

**Specificity**: Describes the selectivity of a receptor for drugs

**Splanchnic**: Refers to the **viscera**, which in turn means the organs within the body cavities, especially those in the abdominal cavities

**Statins (HMG-CoA reductase inhibitors)**: Drugs that block the synthesis of cholesterol in the liver

**Steatorrhoea**: Fatty stools

**Stethoscope**: Instrument used to listen to body sounds

**Stomatitis**: Inflammation of the mucous lining of the mouth

**Stroke**: Weakness or paralysis on one side of the body caused by interruption of blood flow to the brain; in bygone days was called apoplexy

**Sublingual**: Under the tongue

**Suppository**: Formulation for administration of medicine into the rectum

**Supraventricular**: Above the ventricles

**Supraventricular rhythm**: Any cardiac rhythm originating above the ventricles

**Sustained release**: Refers to a medicinal formulation that continuously releases the active agent, e.g. from the GIT. Also called 'retard' preparations

**Sympathomimetic**: Drug that mimics the stimulation of the sympathetic division of the autonomic nervous system

**Systole**: Period of the cardiac cycle when the heart is contracting

**Systolic blood pressure**: The blood pressure at systole, when the ventricles contract and pump blood into the arterial circulation

**Tachycardia**: Very rapid heart rate

**Tachyphylaxis**: The action of a given dose of a drug becomes successively less effective

**Tardive dyskinesia**: Abnormal movements of the mouth and tongue and sometimes the upper limbs

**Teratogenic**: Causes birth defects

**Therapeutic index**: Ratio of a therapeutic dose to one that is actually toxic. The higher the therapeutic index, the safer the drug is

**Thiamine**: Vitamin $B_1$

**Thrombin**: Enzyme that converts soluble **fibrinogen** to insoluble **fibrin** in the clotting process

**Thrombocytopenia**: Reduction in the number of platelets in the blood. It results in bruising of the skin and prolonged bleeding of wounds

**Thrombocytopenic purpura**: Bleeding into the skin

**Thrombolytic**: A drug that dissolves a thrombus

**Thromboplastin** (thrombokinase): Enzyme that converts **prothrombin** to **thrombin**

**Thrombosis**: Solidification of blood in a blood vessel through clot formation

**Thrombus**: Blood clot

**Tincture**: Alcoholic extract from natural tissues such as plants, e.g. tincture of belladonna

**Tinnitus**: Sensation of sounds without any external stimulus

**T lymphocytes**: White blood cells that mature in the thymus gland before they enter the circulation

**Tocolytic agents**: Drugs that inhibit uterine contractions

**Tocopherol**: Vitamin E

**Tonic-clonic (grand mal) seizure**: A focal discharge becomes generalized and the patient falls unconscious and passes through the typical tonic and clonic phases, regaining consciousness after a varying interval

**Total peripheral resistance (TPR)**: Resistance to blood flow caused by resistance only in the peripheral vascular beds, i.e. when the heart is in diastole

**Toxic**: Poisonous to the tissues

**Transient insomnia**: This occurs in people who usually have no sleep problem and is due to altered circumstances, i.e. admission to hospital or travel

**Trophic**: Causing growth

**Tubocurarine**: A non-depolarizing neuromuscular blocker extracted from curare

**Ulcer**: Break in skin through all its layers or break in any mucous membrane

**Ulcerative colitis**: Inflammatory and ulcerative disease of the colon and rectum

**Uric acid**: Chemical excreted in the urine; an end-product of nucleic acid metabolism, which causes gout if deposited in joints

**Uricosuric drugs**: Drugs that increase uric acid excretion in the urine

**Urinary retention**: Difficulty with micturition, e.g. in benign prostatic hyperplasia (BPH)

**Vaccine**: Preparation of material from deactivated bacteria or viruses, which contains antigens against which the body produces antibodies, which confer protection from the live bacteria or viruses

**Vagolytic**: An effect that lessens the influence of the vagus nerve. The vagus slows the heart, so a vagolytic effect is one that speeds up the heart

**Vasoconstriction**: Decrease in diameter of blood vessels, especially arterioles

**Ventricle**: Either of the two lower chambers of the heart: also refers to fluid-filled chambers of the brain

**Ventricular fibrillation**: Cardiac arrhythmia marked by fibrillary contractions of the ventricular muscle due to rapid, repetitive excitation of myocardial fibres without coordinated ventricular contraction and by the absence of atrial activity. It is usually fatal unless treated immediately with a **defibrillator**

**Virus**: Particle visible only with the electron microscope that survives only within living cells. It can infect other microorganisms such as bacteria, plants and animals

**Viscera**: The organs within the body cavities, especially those in the abdominal cavities (see also **splanchnic**)

**Vitamin**: One of a group of chemicals not synthesized in the body but taken in the diet. Vitamins are required in tiny amounts for normal development and cellular function

**Vitreous humour**: Jelly-like transparent substance that fills the chamber of the eye behind the lens

**Vomiting centre**: Nerve centre in the medulla of the brain that when stimulated electrically causes vomiting (see also **chemoreceptor trigger zone**)

**Wernicke's encephalopathy**: Brain disorder with delirium or mental confusion caused by vitamin $B_1$ deficiency, usually associated with alcoholism. It is treated with vitamin $B_1$.

**White coat hypertension**: Rise in blood pressure when having it taken by a health professional

# Introduction

## THE STRUCTURE OF THE BOOK

This introduction explains how the book is laid out and suggests a simple system for keeping notes brief and to the point. Chapters devoted to the general roles and responsibilities of the nurse in the administration of drugs to patients follow this, and the conditions under which drugs are stored, kept and used. As may be imagined, some drugs require strict regulation in terms of their storage and use and the nurse has a very important responsibility in this respect. It is likely that by the time this book is published nurses will be prescribing a wide variety of drugs and so there is a real need to be aware of the conditions of use and the effects of the drugs.

The next chapter sets out the overall picture of the interconnected roles of drug designers, distributors, prescribers and dispensers of drugs, i.e. those who play a part in seeing to it that the drug reaches the patient. There is a brief introduction to the principles that underlie the discovery of drugs, how they produce their desired (and undesired) effects, and how to work out just how much is needed in order to get a beneficial effect without poisoning the patient. Important cellular constituents, such as the *receptor*, that are critical in determining the action of the drug, are introduced early on since they will be often referred to later. Chapter 1 also covers the routes of administration of drugs, some of the main principles that underlie the way they are formulated and the mechanisms of drug action.

The major part of the book is organized into chapters that are devoted to the different systems of the body and, where appropriate, into the different types of drugs. Thus, all the drugs that are used primarily to treat diseases of the heart and blood vessels – such as heart failure, angina or high blood pressure (hypertension) – are described in the section on the cardiovascular system, while those used to treat, for example, urinary retention, are in the section devoted to the urogenital system. Blood itself is treated as a separate system. Some uses of drugs are not associated with specific body systems or organs but with diseases that can strike anywhere, such as cancer and infection. In some cases symptoms rather than the disease itself are treated. There are, for example, many different chemical agents for the treatment of pain, and the subject of pain itself and the effects it has on the patient are described in order to help explain why different drugs may be chosen to treat different types of pain.

Each chapter is designed usually to start with the patients' problems and then work towards the choice of treatment and use of a drug, how it is given, what effects it has in order to achieve its desired effects, the problems that are associated with its use and how the body copes with and gets rid of the drug. The toxic effects of the drug, which may be manifested through overdose, are dealt with as well. Toxicology is a subject in its own right, but no textbook of pharmacology would be complete without some mention of the toxic effects of drugs that are used therapeutically. For each drug or class of drugs the mechanism of action of the drugs at the cellular or molecular level is briefly described.

Some drugs are not used for treating disease but rather for counteracting the effects of other drugs. Drugs are used as antidotes for poisoning through overdose and to help those who use the so-called drugs of abuse. Health care workers need to know what the drugs of abuse are, how they manifest their toxic effects and how to deal with them. Heroin is rapidly addictive and there are drugs that are used to treat this. Drugs such as cocaine, ecstasy, LSD and other drugs of abuse are covered in this book.

A relatively recent phenomenon in the history of medicine is the huge and very widespread use of 'medicines' by healthy people. The most widespread examples are the use of oral contraceptives and HRT (hormone replacement therapy), which are now used virtually worldwide. Nurses, doctors and other health workers are taught what they are, how they work

and the dangers attached to their use. The patient should also be taught about these drugs and there are many books on the market about these drugs that have been written with the user in mind. Another highly popular practice among healthy people is the regular use of vitamins. These are not entirely innocuous and some, such as vitamin A, have killed people who used them excessively in ignorance of their toxic effects.

The book also touches on less conventional but nevertheless very popular chemical methods that are used to treat medical problems. Two of the most widely used methods are homoeopathy and herbal medicine. These are still highly controversial, but since they may be used by up to 30% of the adult population (and rising) they cannot be ignored. In the United States, it has been estimated that upwards of 40% of the annual health expenditure can be attributed to alternative forms of therapy, and most of this is unregulated.

Some herbal preparations are actually dangerous and health workers have to deal with the consequences of their toxic effects. Echinacea, for example, is a potent immunostimulant and can have severe adverse effects in patients with autoimmune diseases such as lupus. This is not to say that these medicines may not be very valuable if used properly and if used under supervision. Many substances that occur naturally in the human body, such as glucosamine and chondroitin, which are thought to help sufferers with osteoarthritis, or 5-hydroxytryptamine (5-HTP; see Ch. 4), which is touted for the treatment of anything from depression to low pain threshold, are sold over the counter in pharmacies and supermarkets in many countries, and are currently under intensive investigation. Homoeopathy has been in use for centuries and although no one knows how such small doses may exert therapeutic effects, many people claim benefit and these preparations are now freely available in pharmacies. Increasing numbers of people, including pharmacists, nurses and doctors, are training as homoeopaths. Acupuncture is now practised in hospitals and is acknowledged in Western societies to be useful for the treatment of pain. This acceptance in the West came about through the efforts of pharmacologists, who identified the body's own version of morphine, namely the enkephalins and the endorphins. This book therefore has a chapter (Ch. 35) that gives a brief and necessarily selective introduction to some alternative forms of medicine.

## NOTE TAKING IN PHARMACOLOGY

Pharmacology teems with drug names that very often bear no relationship to the diseases they are used for. A frequent complaint from students is the sheer volume of drug names and data and the problem of putting data in note form in a way that facilitates learning it. This problem has been addressed, and a method is given below, which many students have found very helpful. It is presented in the hope that some readers may find it useful.

It should be stressed here that students should not and usually are not expected to know the name of every drug that comes up in a course of pharmacology, but readers should be able to mention at least a few representative names of drugs within a section, especially the drugs that are most commonly prescribed, and the best way to find that out is to ask the lecturer, a physician, a nurse or a pharmacist. It is never a bad idea to pop into the hospital pharmacy occasionally and chat to the dispensers, who are necessarily very knowledgeable about which drugs are most frequently prescribed for a given condition. Reputable sites on the Internet, particularly those sponsored by charitable organizations devoted to a specific disease, are also worth having a look at. It is also quite instructive to read what patients suffering from a given disease have to say to each other about the drugs they take on the many Internet chat groups.

## MAKING CONCISE NOTES

The aim when compiling notes is to reduce the volume of notes rather than expand it. The method suggested here is to summarize the data needed about the drug onto both sides of a filing card of dimensions 8 inches by 5 inches (20 cm × 13 cm approximately). These are available from stationery shops and some supermarkets. A suggested format for compiling a list of drugs is given below, although students who adopt this method will doubtless evolve their own systems. The card system can also be used for making tables, diagrams and graphs. The overriding principle is to simplify, summarize and reduce the volumes of notes and it is hoped that some students will find this suggestion helpful (Boxes 1 and 2). An example of their use is given here, using arguably the most famous and widely used medicinal drug in the world: namely, aspirin (Boxes 3 and 4). This system of summarization and learning of pharmacology may not suit everyone but it is offered in the knowledge that very many students have adopted it and found it helpful.

| Box 1    Side 1 of card |
| --- |
| *Drug name and class*: |
| *Source* (if naturally occurring): |
| *Used for*: |
| *Route of administration*: |
| *Action and effects*: |

| Box 2    Side 2 of card |
| --- |
| *Adverse effects and contraindications*: |
| *Mechanism of action*: |

| Box 3    Side 1 of card for aspirin |
| --- |
| *Drug name and class*: aspirin (acetylsalicylic acid); non-steroidal anti-inflammatory drug (NSAID); antipyretic analgesic |
| *Source* (*if naturally occurring*): salicylic acid in willow bark; synthetic |
| *Used for*: pain, e.g. joints, headache; reducing temperature in fever, e.g. rheumatic fever; thrombosis |
| *Route of administration*: oral as tablets |
| *Effects*: anti-inflammatory; reduces pain at source; lowers temperature in fever; inhibits platelet aggregation, thus may reduce danger of thrombosis |

## NOTES MANAGEMENT

Finally, a few tips on note management: it is suggested that cards be made as soon as possible after the lecture. This ensures that a more accurate recollection of the information will be made, and it will also avoid the unpleasant contemplation of a large

> **Box 4    Side 2 of card for aspirin**
>
> *Adverse effects and contraindications (CI):* gastric irritant; causes gastric bleeding, therefore soluble aspirin given but still causes bleeding;
> *CI:* peptic ulcer; liver disease; anaemia; children under 14 danger of Reye's syndrome
> *Drug interactions:* increases effects of anticoagulant, oral hypoglycaemic drugs
>
> *Toxic effects:* overdose; 8th cranial nerve affected; dizziness, tinnitus, deafness, vomiting, acidosis from overbreathing; can increase body temperature
>
> *Mechanism of action:* inhibits prostaglandin synthesis by inhibiting cyclooxygenase enzymes COX 1 and COX 2

mass of notes when examinations suddenly loom as if out of nowhere.

> **Summary**
>
> - Discuss drugs with people who prescribe and who dispense them. This will bring the subject alive
> - Try to summarize details for the drug and for specific mechanisms of drug action onto filing cards
> - Try to keep the cards up to date by doing this as soon as possible after the lectures

## Further reading

Manias E, Bullock S 2002 The educational preparation of undergraduate nursing students in pharmacology: perceptions and experiences of lecturers and students. International Journal of Nursing Studies 39: 757

# Chapter 1

# The use of pharmaceuticals

## Learning objectives

At the end of this chapter, the reader should be able to:

- describe some of the factors that dictate the choice of dose
- list the various routes of administration of drugs
- list the factors that affect absorption and distribution of drugs in the body
- discuss some of the consequences of metabolism and excretion on drug efficacy and duration
- define the terms *agonist*, *antagonist*, *partial agonist* and *ligand*
- explain the basic properties of the $\log_{10}$ dose–response curve

## DRUG DEVELOPMENT

The science of pharmacology is the discovery and characterization of chemicals to the point where they can be used to treat or prevent illness (e.g. aspirin to treat pain or inhibit platelet aggregation). Drugs are also designed to intervene in the normal functions of the body (e.g. contraceptives). The pharmacologist is involved during virtually every stage of this process.

Medicinally useful drugs can be discovered quite by accident, as was the case with penicillin and the oral sulphonylureas for the treatment of adult onset (type II) diabetes (see pp. 302 and 198, respectively). More usually, however, a deliberate attempt is made to introduce a new drug by modifying an existing natural or synthetic drug to increase its potency, improve its absorption and reduce unwanted effects. Once the chemical structure of morphine from the opium poppy was worked out, this led to the use of pethidine for the treatment of pain (see p. 138). Advances in the understanding of physiological processes can also result in new drugs. The discovery that Parkinson's disease results from the selective destruction of certain dopaminergic brain pathways led to the invention of the drug levodopa to try and counteract some of the distressing symptoms of the disease such as tremor, slowness of movement and rigidity (see p. 256). The discovery of the physiological role of the peptide tumour necrosis factor (TNF-α) in the human immune system has led to the use of the very potent and effective anti-TNF-α drugs for the treatment of rheumatoid arthritis (see p. 156).

## THE TESTING OF NEW DRUGS BEFORE USE

Once a potential drug has been identified, it should be rigorously tested to ensure that it is not terato-genic (causes birth defects), carcinogenic (causes cancer) or otherwise harmful to any of the organs and systems of the body (toxicity studies). It should be specific in action and its mechanism of action understood as completely as possible (*pharmaco-dynamic* studies; see below). It is imperative to find the optimal route of administration, dose and fre-quency of dosing in order to maintain effective concentrations in the body.

The *pharmacokinetics* of the drug must be worked out. This entails finding out how the drug is distrib-uted in the body compartments and how long its effective concentrations will be maintained after a dose.

Once all this has been done, it is time to test the drug in human volunteers and patients by means of strictly controlled clinical trials. These are set up through collaboration between pharmaceutical com-panies and the medical professions, and the nurse figures very prominently in these trials. If the drug passes this final test, then government-controlled regulatory bodies will grant a licence for the drug to be routinely prescribed. Even with all these precau-tions some drugs slip through the net. The tragic consequences of the introduction of the drug thali-domide for use by pregnant women remains as an indelible reminder of the risks taken when drugs are allowed into the body.

## BASIC PHARMACOKINETICS

Pharmacokinetics is about how the body deals with the drug. It helps to answer a most important question: What are the factors that determine the maintenance of a therapeutically useful level of the drug in the bloodstream? To answer this question, the following questions must be investigated:

- **The dose:** How much of the drug should be used to get the desired effect without getting unwanted effects?
- **Route of administration:** By what route should the drug be administered?
- **Absorption and distribution:** How is the drug absorbed and compartmentalized in the body, e.g. does most of it dissolve in the aqueous (water) or in the lipid (fatty) compartments? How is it carried in the blood? Is it concentrated in any particular organ? For example, when iodine is administered, most of it is concentrated in the thyroid gland.
- **Metabolism and excretion:** How long does the drug stay in the body? The body's way of dealing with drugs is to try and get them out of it as soon as possible through metabolism and excretion. How often does the patient need to repeat the dose in order to sustain therapeutically effective concentrations of the drug?

## THE DOSE

The aim is to give the patient a dose of the drug that achieves the desired effect without causing harmful side effects. This dose is found experimentally using isolated tissues or cells, experimental animals and human volunteers and patients. The dose–response curve is described below.

### The therapeutic index

The therapeutic index is a measure of the danger of poisoning and the higher it is the safer the drug is. The therapeutic index is a ratio of a therapeutic dose to one that is actually toxic. The therapeutic index for aspirin is around 3.5. For digoxin (from the fox-glove), which is used for cardiac arrhythmias and congestive heart failure, the index is dangerously low (less than 2), and patients taking digoxin need regular and frequent monitoring of blood levels of the drug.

## Choosing and adjusting the dose

In a perfect world, all adults would respond equally to a given dose. In practice, however, there may be considerable interperson variation in plasma concentrations of a given dose of a drug. With some drugs, the therapeutic index is low, and this too demands regular plasma monitoring of the drug and dose adjustment as needed. Some commonly used drugs that usually require close monitoring include:

- ciclosporin, used for suppressing transplant rejection and for rheumatoid arthritis
- digoxin, for treatment of cardiac disease
- gentamicin and other aminoglycoside antibiotics
- lithium, for treatment of manic-depression psychosis
- methotrexate for treatment of rheumatoid arthritis and cancer
- phenytoin, for treatment of epilepsy.

## ROUTE OF ADMINISTRATION – TERMINOLOGY

Before describing the routes of administration it is worth clearing up some points of terminology that can be confusing. These are:

- the internal and external environments
- bioavailability
- topical and parenteral application of drugs.

### Internal and external environments

Where the body is concerned, physiologists talk about the internal and external environments. When anything is swallowed, it remains in the external environment until it or one of its breakdown products passes a cell membrane and gets into a cell of the body. A cherry pip, if swallowed, may be inside the body for a while, but normally it will never get into the internal environment of the body from the gastrointestinal tract.

### Bioavailability

Another important concept is that of bioavailability. The term bioavailability generally means that the drug has reached the circulation and is therefore available to all the tissues. The patient may take 600 mg of aspirin, but after the drug passes into the circulation from the gastrointestinal tract and then emerges from the liver, less than 600 mg of aspirin is available to the body.

## Topical application of drugs

The term topical application of drugs means the application of drugs directly to the surface where its action is wanted. For example:

- Ointments, patches or creams that are applied to the skin.
- Inhalation of drugs to treat asthma directly by dilating airway passages.
- Drops or ointments into the eyes.
- Suppositories and pessaries, which are inserted into the rectum or vagina, respectively (see also below). Some of the drug will get absorbed, but most of the drug will remain at the surface where it is applied unless it has been formulated to penetrate to the bloodstream.

## Parenteral administration of drugs

The term parenteral administration is used to describe the injection of drugs into the tissues, including directly into the blood. Oral administration mainly means the taking of drugs to be absorbed through the gastrointestinal tract, although, as will be mentioned below, some drugs are absorbed into the body directly from the oral mucosa.

When considering the route of administration, several questions need to be addressed:

- Which is the most convenient route for the patient?
- Where is the drug to act e.g. skin, heart, kidneys, brain, etc.?
- How quickly does the prescriber want the drug to reach its site of action?
- For how long does the prescriber want the dose of drug to work, i.e. to stay in the body?
- Which organs is the drug to be kept away from?

The route of administration can have profound effects on:

- the onset of the action of the drug
- the plasma concentrations achieved
- the length of time that the drug will spend in the body (see Fig. 1.1).

## ROUTES OF ADMINISTRATION – DETAILS

The routes of administration are as follows:

- topical
- oral
- transdermal

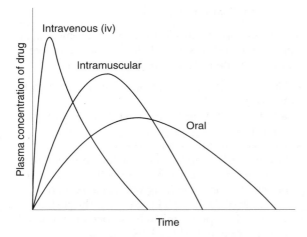

**Figure 1.1** Effects of the route of administration of a single dose of a drug on its plasma levels with time.

- rectal and vaginal
- inhalation
- injection (parenteral)
  - intravenous
  - intramuscular
  - intradermal
  - subcutaneous
  - intrathecal

## Topical

The skin is traditionally the most accessible part of the body for the administration of drugs. Most of the preparations for topical administration to the skin are used for treating skin disorders. There is a huge range of non-pharmaceutical topical products for cosmetic or recreational use and these will not be described in any detail except when their use results in the need for treatment. Skin preparations are formulated mainly into lotions, creams, ointments and powders and are used for a wide variety of purposes, e.g. for the symptomatic relief of an itch or to treat fungal infections such as athlete's foot. They are convenient for the patient, who can use them at home, and, because the drug is generally poorly absorbed, this makes them relatively safe. The one tissue most at risk from the use of these preparations is the skin itself, and a salutary tale is that of the prolonged use of the anti-inflammatory steroid hydrocortisone, which when it was introduced in the 1950s was found to be dramatically effective in reducing inflammation in, for example, eczema. It took some time before it was realized that the prolonged topical use of hydrocortisone causes thinning of skin.

Strictly speaking, the inhalation of drugs for use on lung tissue (see below) is a form of topical application. However, since inhalation is also used as a route for drugs that are to be absorbed (e.g. gaseous anaesthetics), inhalation is treated separately below.

## Oral

The medication is taken by mouth and preparations comprise:

- tablet
- capsule
- powder
- mixture
- emulsion
- linctus.

**Tablets and capsules.** Tablets are prepared by mixing a drug with a base that binds the two together so that the tablets won't disintegrate in the body before they are meant to. They are usually coated and may be coloured. Capsules are made of gelatine or some similar substance and contain a drug that is liberated when the wall of the capsule is digested in the stomach or intestine. The actual formulation of tablets and capsules is very important and determines how satisfactorily the drug is released, which governs their absorption and bioavailability. A great deal of care is taken in the manufacture of tablets to ensure the maximum bioavailability. It is also possible by coating the tablets, modifying the capsule or by binding the drug to some inert substance, to slow down the release of the active ingredient and thus prolong its absorption and effect. These may be called sustained-release or retard preparations.

**Mixtures.** Mixtures are liquids that contain several ingredients dissolved or diffused in water or some other solvent. An example is kaolin mixture for diarrhoea, when insoluble kaolin powder is suspended in the aqueous liquid. An **emulsion** is a mixture of two immiscible liquids (e.g. oil and water) in which one is dispersed through the other in a finely divided state, e.g. Milk of Magnesia. A linctus is a liquid that contains some sweet syrupy substance used for its soothing effect on coughs. It may also contain a cough suppressant such as dextromethorphan.

When liquid drugs are prescribed, they are accompanied by a standard oral syringe, which measures up to 5 ml and is marked with 0.5 ml divisions. This should be used to draw up the fluid to achieve the exact dose. For doses of 5 ml or more, the standard 5 ml plastic spoon can be used. The syringe is issued with a manufacturer's information leaflet advising on use and storage, but verbal explanations are still valuable, especially as liquid medicines are usually given to children and frequently administered by anxious parents. Families appreciate practical demonstrations of the use of the syringe provided by the nurse. Medicines for oral administration to babies are most usually in liquid form.

### Advantages of oral administration

- *Oral administration of drugs is extremely convenient for the patient*. The drug can be taken at home and does not need the attendance of a carer or health professional unless the patient is physically or mentally incapable of self-medication.
- *Oral administration avoids the fear of needles*.
- *The gastrointestinal tract provides a huge surface area for absorption* and drugs are absorbed by diffusion and in some cases by active transport processes, when drugs are pumped from the gastrointestinal tract lumen into the gastric mucosa against concentration gradients (see below).

### Disadvantages of oral administration

- *Absorption can be variable* and depends on the chemical nature of the drug, e.g. its ionization, solubility and stability.
- *Absorption can also depend on the stomach contents*. For example, the absorption of the tetracycline antibiotics (see p. 308) from the gastrointestinal tract is inhibited in the presence of milk. Since these antibiotics have been and in some countries still are used in babies, it is as well to know that they should not be used before or soon after feeding. If a drug is taken with or after a meal it is absorbed more slowly. This is due to delayed emptying of the stomach, where little absorption occurs, and because certain drugs become temporarily bound to food. When a rapid effect is required, the drug should be given on an empty stomach. Drugs such as aspirin, which may irritate the stomach, should be given with food.
- *Rate of gastric emptying and drug interactions*. Drugs may affect gastric emptying (emptying of the stomach) and this may modify absorption. For instance, atropine-like drugs delay gastric emptying, whereas metoclopramide, which is often used for nausea, actually increases the speed of gastric emptying and thus the rate of absorption. If drugs are given together they may bind to each other and prevent absorption. This phenomenon is, however, a rare occurrence and in practice several different types of drug are often given at the same time.

- *All drugs that are taken by mouth will undergo first pass metabolism*, which will reduce the final bioavailability, i.e. blood level. This means that the dose of drug has to be increased to take first pass metabolism in the liver into account. Some drugs that are completely inactivated during first pass metabolism, e.g. glyceryl trinitrate, which is used to treat anginal pain (see p. 94), are nevertheless put in the mouth and placed under the tongue where they are rapidly absorbed from the oral mucosa, thus bypassing the liver.
- *The patient has to remember to take the drug*, and this could be extremely important, for example when oral anticoagulant drugs or antibiotics are prescribed (see pp. 91 and 298, respectively). Confused patients may not remember to take the drug or mix up the doses of the different drugs they take.

## Transdermal

Transdermal administration involves putting an adhesive plastic patch against the skin rather like an adhesive plaster. The patch has a pad impregnated with the drug. The drug is absorbed through the skin into the bloodstream. This avoids first pass metabolism. Absorption is slow and so patches are not used for rapid onset of drug action. There are regional variations in skin permeability, and patches are usually applied to clean, unbroken skin on the trunk or arms, or on the post-auricular area (behind the ears). Patches are used, for example, to help wean smokers off cigarettes, for long-term administration of hormones and for administration of glyceryl trinitrate for angina. Fentanyl is available as a self-adhesive patch, and is changed every 72 hours.

### Advantages
- Long-acting, therefore replacement can be infrequent
- Eliminates the need to remember to take a dose

### Disadvantages
- Absorption may be variable
- Possible adverse skin reactions

## Rectal and vaginal

Drugs can be administered rectally in suppositories and are absorbed into the bloodstream. This, too, bypasses the liver and has been popular for many years in some countries, e.g. France. Suppositories are useful when a local action is wanted. Haemorrhoids ('piles') can be treated with suppositories that contain a local anaesthetic. Constipation can be treated with glycerine suppositories. Bacterial or fungal infections of the vagina can be treated with pessaries (see p. 325).

## Inhalation

Inhalation is used to apply drugs directly to the lungs to treat, for example, asthma. Anti-inflammatory steroids such as beclometasone are inhaled, as are the $\beta_2$-adrenoceptor agonist bronchodilator drugs (see p. 45). The $\beta_2$-receptor agonists work through receptors on the lung cell wall and so do not need to get into the cell to cause bronchodilation. Gaseous general anaesthetics are administered by inhalation during surgical procedures (see p. 229).

## Intravenous (I.V.) injection

The drug is injected directly into a vein, usually in the arm or hand.

### Advantages

- A rapid onset of action is achieved
- The entire injected dose is almost instantly bioavailable, since it bypasses the gastrointestinal tract and first pass metabolism
- A lower dose is administered than if the drug is given orally
- Administration is useful for drugs that are irritant when administered intramuscularly (see below).

### Disadvantages

- The drug has to be administered by a trained person
- Inadvertent injection into an artery can cause arterial spasm with resulting tissue damage
- Accidental overdose can have serious consequences.

Examples of drugs given I.V. are thiopental for induction of general anaesthesia (see p. 231), the anticoagulant heparin (see p. 89) and epinephrine (also called adrenaline) for cardiac arrest (see p. 240). Some drugs are administered continuously or intermittently by I.V. infusion using a motorized syringe-driver. This is an important part of patient-controlled analgesia (PCA; see p. 141). Drugs are sometimes injected directly into arteries – for example the use of radio-opaque chemicals for X-ray purposes – but this is a rare route for the parenteral administration of drugs.

## Intramuscular (I.M.) injection

The drug is injected into a muscle. Absorption is variable, depending on which muscle is used, being most efficient from the deltoids of the arms, and least from the buttocks (Fig. 1.2). Absorption depends on the blood flow through the muscle and is increased by exercising the muscle or rubbing the site of injection. The rate of absorption will be reduced in shock. Drugs used for premedication before surgery are sometimes given via the I.M. route (see p. 230). Certain drugs, for example some steroids used for HRT (see p. 221) are implanted I.M. and released slowly from the implant.

### Advantages

- This injection is technically easier than I.V.
- The gastrointestinal tract and first pass metabolism are avoided
- A long-term effect from a single dose can be achieved.

### Disadvantages

- Injections can be painful
- Self-administration is difficult
- Rarely, abscesses can form at the site of injection
- The needle may puncture a small blood vessel and cause bruising of the skin.

### Safety point

While on the subject of intravenous injections, it is worth highlighting the part of the procedure that helps us prevent giving an *accidental* I.V. dose. When an injection is *not* meant to go I.V., the nurse, doctor or patient should pull back with the plunger before pushing in the contents of the syringe. If blood is withdrawn into the liquid in the syringe, the needle must be withdrawn from the tissues immediately.

## Intradermal injection

The needle is inserted into the skin without penetrating into the subcutaneous space. This is an important route for local anaesthetics, especially in dental surgery. It is an unusual route for drug administration outside dentistry. The aim is to localize the injection as much as possible in order to minimize more general effects and maximize the local effect.

## Subcutaneous (S.C.) injection

The subcutaneous route of injection is widely used. Common sites for injection include the thigh or upper arm. The skin is pinched and the needle inserted so that the drug is administered under the layer of skin.

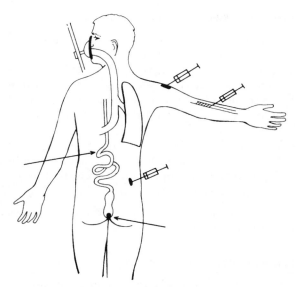

**Figure 1.2**    Methods of administration of drugs.

Insulin is often injected S.C. by the patient (see also p. 196). Some local anaesthetics are administered S.C. and a vasoconstrictor, such as epinephrine may be added to the drug to minimize absorption away from the site of injection and thus maximize the local effect.

### Advantages
- Absorption is slower than after I.M. injection
- The patient can self-administer the drug.

### Disadvantages
- Care has to be taken not to inject I.V.
- Absorption is, as with I.M. injection, dependent on local blood flow, being increased with exercise and decreased in shock
- The needle may puncture a small blood vessel and cause bruising of the skin.

### Intrathecal injection

Intrathecal injection is the administration of the drug directly into the central nervous system (CNS), thus bypassing the blood–brain barrier. The needle is passed through the theca, or connective tissue sheath that surrounds the brain and spinal column, and the drug is injected into the subarachnoid space, through which the cerebrospinal fluid circulates, bathing the surfaces of the brain and spinal cord. This is a hazardous procedure, which is best left to trained, experienced medical personnel, since the spinal cord can be inadvertently damaged. Intrathecal injection is a

route for direct application into the CNS of drugs such as local anaesthetics and antiviral agents.

An epidural injection is the injection of a local anaesthetic into the epidural space in the lumbar region of the spinal cord, and is sometimes used to alleviate the pain of labour. It is an uncomfortable procedure and is not guaranteed to work due to the presence of much connective and other tissue in this space.

## ABSORPTION AND DISTRIBUTION

### Absorption

Absorption of a drug means the transfer of the drug from the external to the internal environment of the body. In order to get into the body the drug needs to get across a cell membrane. These membranes are designed to control the movement of chemicals across them very strictly. Only dissolved substances can cross a membrane. And even then, chemicals that ionize in solution will cross these membranes with difficulty. Cell membranes regulate the ionic composition of the cell very tightly, or else they are unable to function properly. Uncharged molecules such as the steroids and ethyl alcohol move freely across cell membranes. Aspirin, for example, will ionize in the small intestine, which hinders absorption.

Absorption can be effected through:

- passive diffusion
- facilitated transport
- active transport.

**Passive diffusion** is the movement of substances down a concentration gradient and the process does not require energy. **Facilitated transport** (also called facilitated diffusion) is the transport of chemicals across the cell membrane by carrier proteins that do not require energy. The carriers will therefore not work against a concentration gradient and can also be a target for drugs. For example, glucose is carried across the cell membrane by facilitated transfer, and the numbers of glucose carriers in the membrane are increased by insulin. **Active transport** is the pumping of chemicals across the membrane against a concentration gradient and therefore requires energy in the form of adenosine triphosphate (ATP), which is a high energy-yielding chemical. Ions such as $Na^+$ and $K^+$ are actively transported across cell membranes.

### Ionization of the drug and absorption

Aspirin is absorbed far more readily from the stomach than from the small intestine because the stomach is strongly acid. A strongly acid environment will suppress the ionization of a weak acid such as aspirin, and it rapidly crosses the cell membrane and thus enters the internal environment. Many drugs are weak bases and are therefore largely ionized in the stomach and unionized in the small intestine; therefore, they are preferentially absorbed there.

## Distribution of the drug in the body

Those who design and sell drugs need to make very sure that they know where a drug goes to in the body and how long it stays there. They want to be sure it gets to and stays in the tissue where they want it to act so that it can do its job effectively. If it were to act as a diuretic and promote urine flow – e.g. the drug furosemide (frusemide) – they would prefer it to target the kidney selectively. If it were intended to act on the heart to increase contractile power – e.g. digoxin – they would choose one that targets cardiac muscle selectively. They may not want it to get into certain tissues or organs. They will be particularly anxious about whether it gains access to the fetus. Once a drug gets into the bloodstream, however, it is carried to all parts of the body and therefore will come into close proximity with virtually all its tissues and organs, and that fact explains many cases of drug side effects.

**Drugs and the blood–brain barrier.** A physiological barrier, the so-called blood–brain barrier, which actively prohibits many substances from getting across from the bloodstream, protects the brain from certain chemicals. If a drug is to be designed to work in the brain, it must be able to cross the blood–brain barrier. For example, Parkinson's disease is treated by replacing lost dopamine in the brain (see p. 256). Dopamine itself will not cross the blood–brain barrier, and a drug called levodopa is used, which gets into the brain and is there converted to dopamine.

Although a drug may go to all the tissues, it may be preferentially taken up by and concentrated in certain tissues but not others. For example, the female sex hormones used for oral contraception are highly concentrated by the uterus, ovary, pituitary and certain brain areas and held there long after they have gone from the other tissues. This is because those tissues mentioned possess specific receptors that bind the sex hormones (see below).

## First pass metabolism

All substances that are absorbed from the gastrointestinal tract are carried in the portal blood system to the liver, where one of several things can happen:

- The drug escapes from the liver unchanged, e.g. certain oral contraceptive steroids.
- All or some of the drug is converted to an inactive metabolite that is excreted, e.g. 67% of an oral dose of morphine is inactivated in the liver. All of an oral dose of glyceryl trinitrate will be inactivated if it is swallowed.
- The drug is metabolized to an active metabolite that exerts its therapeutic effect, e.g. the antidepressant drug imipramine is converted to the active metabolite desipramine (see also p. 278).

If the drug is given by any other route it escapes first pass metabolism.

## Plasma protein binding of drugs

The blood contains several proteins that bind to hormones and drugs. When these chemicals are bound to plasma proteins they are:

- protected from first pass metabolism
- pharmacologically inert because they cannot get into the cell.

The drug or hormone binds reversibly to the protein such that equilibrium is set up between bound and free hormone or drug. Only the free chemical can be metabolized or interact with target tissues. The more tightly bound the chemical is to the plasma protein, the longer its circulation time, or *half-life* (see below) will be. The sex steroids, for example, are so tightly bound to a plasma protein, not surprisingly called sex hormone-binding globulin (SHBG), that less than 5% of the plasma hormone is available to the tissues at any given moment. Similarly, most of the circulating thyroid hormone thyroxin is tightly bound to a plasma protein that recognizes the hormone specifically.

Plasma protein binding of drugs can have serious clinical implications. Some drugs will displace others from plasma proteins and this can cause unacceptably high free – i.e. pharmacologically active – plasma levels of the drug. The anticoagulant warfarin, for example, displaces many drugs from plasma proteins.

## Elimination of drugs

The rate at which the body eliminates drugs is the most important determinant of their duration of action. Generally, the body tries to get rid of drugs as fast as it can. It does this through enzymes that chemically change – i.e. metabolize – the drug in the liver so that it is eliminated more easily via the lungs, kidneys or the gut.

It is very important to know how and where drugs are metabolized. Take, for example, a diabetic patient whose kidneys have been damaged by the disease. It is necessary to avoid giving this patient drugs such as certain oral sulphonylureas (see p. 198) that are excreted via the kidneys. The liver itself can become damaged, e.g. after paracetamol overdose or in alcohol-induced cirrhosis or cardiac failure. Here, a drug's action may be prolonged beyond its desired duration.

Some drugs actually increase the activity of the liver enzymes that metabolize drugs, which results in faster elimination, and the drug is no longer as effective. It is thus easy to appreciate why drug manufacturers spend so much time and money on pharmacokinetics tests. An important parameter – i.e. measurement of the drug's duration of stay in the body – is the **plasma half-life**. The blood is the only liquid compartment in the internal environment that is easily accessible to the clinician, and in which levels of the drug in the body can be conveniently monitored.

## Plasma half–life of the drug ($t_{1/2}$)

The plasma half-life of the drug is defined as the time taken for the plasma concentration of the drug to decline to one-half of its value. It can be measured by giving a dose of the drug, sampling blood at intervals and plotting the results on a graph. A typical result is shown in Figure 1.3.

The shape of the graph tells us a great deal about how the body eliminates the drug. Ideally, one should like to give a single dose of a drug that maintains steady levels at a therapeutically effective concentration – the so-called **steady state**. In reality this is seldom achieved, and it is required to keep giving doses at intervals to maintain the effective concentrations. After the first dose, blood levels of the drugs start rising, and further doses may be needed to achieve the desired level. Clearly, from Figure 1.3, levels are falling even as more doses are given. From working out the half-life of a drug it has been found that the time taken to reach the steady state is approximately five times the half-life of the drug. For example, the antidysrhythmic drug digoxin (see p. 62) has a half-life of 36 hours; therefore the patient must be given doses regularly for 5 × 36, i.e.

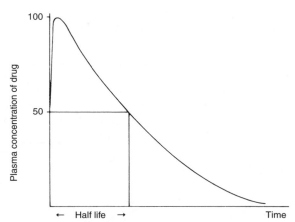

Figure 1.3   Plasma levels and half-life of a drug after a single intravenous injection.

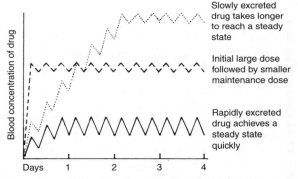

Figure 1.4   Steady-state concentrations of drugs.

180 hours, to attain the steady state. The process can be observed graphically by monitoring drug levels with time (Fig. 1.4).

In practical terms, in order to speed up the process of getting to steady-state levels with a drug that has a longer half-life, it may be necessary to give an initial high 'loading dose' of the drug, followed by smaller maintenance doses. The fate of the administered drug is summarized in Figure 1.5.

**Summary**

Now that all these aspects of pharmacokinetics have been covered, some of the important factors that dictate how much of a drug we need to give, how often and by which route can be summarized. Clearly these are generalities and the choice of drug,

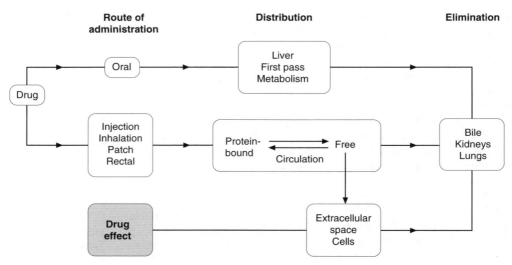

**Figure 1.5** Pathways of systemically acting drugs.

dose and route of administration will vary with the individual patient's needs. The points below are simply a distillation of what has gone before:

- choose a drug that the patient will find most convenient to take, i.e. oral or topical
- for a very rapid effect, give a smaller dose of the drug I.V. if it can be given safely through this route
- for a delayed onset but a longer-lasting effect, give the drug S.C., I.M. or as a patch
- avoid drugs that are eliminated through a damaged organ, e.g. kidney
- for a longer effect, choose a drug that is metabolized more slowly
- drugs with shorter half-lives will need more frequent administration, perhaps even continuously by I.V. infusion
- to speed up attainment of steady-state levels of a drug, give a high loading dose, followed by smaller maintenance doses
- be aware of drug interactions (see p. 410), e.g. drugs that induce liver enzymes will clear other drugs from the body more rapidly.

## FACTORS THAT MAY MODIFY THE EFFICACY AND CHOICE OF DOSE OF THE DRUG IN PATIENTS

The fact of interperson variation in drug response that requires plasma monitoring and dose adjustment has already been mentioned. In some cases, this variation has been traced to specific factors. Even after the drug has been formulated into an injection, mixture, tablet or patch, there are a number of factors that may make the drug more or less effective in some patients. These factors include:

- patient age and size
- genetic factors
- nutritional factors
- ethnicity
- intercurrent illness
- drug interactions
- psychological factors.

## PATIENT AGE AND SIZE

There are considerable variations in response related to patient age and size and these are considered in more detail in Chapter 31, p. 402.

## GENETIC FACTORS

There are a number of inherited variations in drug response that are largely related to differences in drug elimination. Many drugs are broken down by enzymes (usually in the liver) and this terminates their actions. It is now believed that there can be considerable interperson differences in the activity of these enzymes. With certain drugs it is possible to distinguish between two populations of people: one group with a highly active enzyme system that is able to break down the drug rapidly and the other with a less active system and relatively slower breakdown of the drug. This type of genetic variation, where two populations can exist which differ in the metabolism of a drug, is known as **genetic polymorphism**.

## Example

A number of important drugs, including isoniazid (p. 312) and hydralazine (p. 76), are inactivated by acetylation, a process involving enzyme action. In the UK 40% of the population are fast acetylators (with highly active acetylator enzymes) and 60% are slow acetylators. This is an inherited characteristic and the ratio of fast/slow acetylators varies in different parts of the world. The Inuit of North America are without exception rapid acetylators, whereas 80% of Egyptians are slow acetylators.

Differences in acetylator status do not usually matter in the UK, except when high doses of the drugs are being used, when there is a slightly increased risk of toxic effects in subjects who are slow acetylators. In the less-developed world where, for reasons of expense, very minimal doses may be necessary – e.g. isoniazid in the treatment of tuberculosis – those who are rapid acetylators may suffer some falling-off of therapeutic efficacy.

Another example of genetic polymorphism is deficiency (in the enzyme glucose-6-phosphate dehydrogenase (G6PD). This involves largely Africans and Indians, affecting about 100 million people. It is due to an abnormal enzyme in the red blood cells and results in the breakdown of these cells when exposed to, for example:

- quinine
- sulphonamides
- broad beans
- chloroquine
- chloramphenicol.

There are many other examples of inherited differences in response to drugs and some are still being discovered.

## NUTRITIONAL FACTORS

Severe malnutrition can modify responses to drugs. Loss of body mass leads to reduction of body proteins, some of which are the enzymes that metabolize and thus inactivate drugs. Therefore malnutrition will result in prolonged action of drugs, which could be deleterious to the patient.

Malnutrition as such is not usual in the UK, except possibly in certain cases – e.g. illegal immigrants, asylum seekers and those who persist in practising extreme forms of dieting. In the case of prolonged illness, however, perhaps that associated with sepsis and fever, malnutrition can result. Under the last-mentioned circumstances the response to a drug may be greater than expected.

## Example

Warfarin (see p. 91) is an anticoagulant that is broken down in the liver by enzymes. Its effect on coagulation is often greater in patients who have suffered a long illness and who are in a poor nutritional state. They may require a smaller than usual dose or they may suffer haemorrhage.

Even without malnutrition, diet can affect drug response. Vegetarians and heavy smokers both show several differences in enzyme activity, which could modify drug response, although the changes are usually too small to cause serious problems.

## ETHNICITY

The increasingly multicultural nature of societies means that the health worker may be looking after patients of several ethnic groups, and it is becoming apparent that with some drugs different races may show differing sensitivities. For instance, it has been shown in the United States that the β blocker propranolol is less effective in lowering blood pressure in black than in white subjects. These differences could be due to one or more of the following factors:

- genetic differences in drug-metabolizing enzymes, leading to variations in the blood levels achieved
- different lifestyles (e.g. diet), which could also alter the metabolizing enzymes
- differences in the actual response to the drug.

At present very little is known about the problem and with many drugs it is possibly unimportant, but it provides an interesting field for further research.

## INTERCURRENT ILLNESS

Intercurrent illness is the occurrence of an illness that may modify the course and treatment of another illness that is present at the same time. This may both modify drug elimination and affect receptor sensitivity (see p. 16 about receptors) and is an important cause of altered response to a drug. Most drugs are either broken down by the **liver** or excreted by the **kidneys**, so disease of these organs with diminished function can lead to accumulation of the drug with a more intense and prolonged action, which can reach dangerous proportions.

### Example: the liver

An alcoholic patient has cirrhosis of the liver. This disease results in a loss of enzyme-containing liver cells and distortion of liver anatomy such that blood may actually bypass the liver. The patient may be prescribed morphine for pain, and normally morphine is inactivated in the liver. Morphine causes slight depression of respiration, even in therapeutic doses. If its breakdown is impaired, the patient may get an overdose of morphine due to accumulation of the drug with repeated dosing, and may suffer severe depression of respiration.

Drug metabolism may be altered even if the liver is not damaged. For example, in heart failure the blood flow through the liver is reduced, and thus heart failure may indirectly cause a reduction in the rate of drug metabolism by the liver.

### Example: the liver

Lidocaine (lignocaine; see p. 68) is used to treat cardiac arrhythmias, particularly after myocardial infarction; it is broken down by the liver. If it is given to patients with heart failure (a not uncommon occurrence), its elimination is slowed and toxicity will result if the dose is not reduced.

### Example: the kidney

Kidney function may also modify drug response. Gentamicin (see p. 306) is excreted via the kidneys and, when renal function is reduced, serious accumulation occurs with normal dosage. This is why careful monitoring of blood levels with subsequent modification of doses is required when gentamicin is given, particularly in renal disease.

## DRUG INTERACTIONS

One drug can modify the response to another drug in a number of different ways. This is a very important topic and is discussed more fully on p. 410.

## PSYCHOLOGICAL FACTORS

Psychological factors may also be important in the patient's response to a drug. Expectation of a successful outcome may appear to improve the results of treatment. For example, analgesics are more effective if the patient believes they are effective.

Most drugs are given in doses that have been found by experience to be satisfactory, although the dose may be modified by the factors discussed above. As a result, formularies usually give a range of doses. In the light of the clinical response, some alterations may be needed (e.g. the dose of hypotensive drugs is adjusted until a satisfactory fall in blood pressure is achieved).

## BASIC PHARMACODYNAMICS

Pharmacodynamics is the study of how chemicals exert their effects. The practical importance of this knowledge is that it makes possible the design of new and better drugs to treat disease.

## THE RECEPTOR

Receptors are proteins that may occur on the surface of the cell or inside it. They have two important functions:

- to bind the body's own chemical messenger chemicals such as hormones and neurotransmitters
- to convert the binding event into a signal that the cell can recognize and respond to.

Receptors have two important properties:

- specificity
- affinity.

## Specificity

Receptors are designed so that they will recognize specific chemical configurations and bind to them selectively. For example, epinephrine receptors, such as $\alpha$ and $\beta$ adrenoceptors (see p. 41), will bind epinephrine and norepinephrine, but they won't bind, for example, acetylcholine or progesterone. They will also recognize chemicals that are taken into the body. Thus, the epinephrine receptors on bronchiolar smooth muscle cell walls will bind synthetic epinephrine-like chemicals such as **salbutamol**, which is used to treat asthma. Implicit in this is that receptors are critically important tools for the development of drugs for therapeutic use. Any substance that binds to a protein receptor is also called a **ligand**.

## Affinity

Receptors that are designed to recognize and bind certain chemicals will bind these chemicals tightly. We say the receptor has a high affinity for the chemical. This property of affinity is very important, because it means that the receptor will pick up the chemical at very low concentrations of that chemical, and the dose can be kept low.

## AGONISTS AND ANTAGONISTS

### Agonists

When morphine binds to its receptor on a neuronal cell in the brain it may produce nausea, respiratory depression or analgesia, or all three, depending on the dose and which cell it interacts with. This ability of morphine to bind to a receptor with a resulting effect makes the drug an agonist – a drug that produces a response.

### Antagonists

If a patient takes an overdose of morphine, the patient can be rescued by injecting another drug called naloxone (see p. 140). This drug also binds to morphine receptors but produces no response and it doesn't allow morphine to bind to the receptor (Fig. 1.6). Naloxone is called an antagonist. It is the antidote to morphine.

### Partial agonists

Readers will come across the term 'partial agonists' in this book (e.g. p. 139, on opioid analgesics). A partial agonist is a drug that is able to both stimulate and block at a receptor, depending on, for example, the dose used or the duration of the drug's action.

Partial agonists are sometimes not as effective as a full agonist, but are nevertheless used clinically.

## FUNCTIONAL CONSEQUENCES OF AGONIST–RECEPTOR INTERACTION

The functional consequences of agonist ligand–receptor interaction depend very much on the function of the cell. For example:

- when epinephrine binds to its neuronal receptor, this may generate an electrical impulse that travels along the axon of the nerve
- when epinephrine binds to receptors on heart muscle cells, this will generate contraction of the muscle
- when epinephrine binds to its liver cell receptor, it will cause glycogen stored inside the cell to be broken down to glucose
- when hydrocortisone binds to its receptor inside a skin cell, it will stimulate changes in protein synthesis inside the cell that result in an anti-inflammatory response.

## THE $LOG_{10}$ DOSE–RESPONSE CURVE

An important tool in the discovery of new drugs is the $log_{10}$ dose–response curve. This simple little graph can yield much information about a drug's mechanism of action and its potency. For example, it can tell us about the drug's:

- potency
- efficacy
- action as an antagonist.

### Potency

Consider in Figure 1.7 the $log_{10}$ dose–response curves showing the degree of inhibition of gastric acid secretion by two different histamine $H_2$ receptor antagonists. We learn some important information from the graph:

- The curves have identical shapes, especially over the linear rising parts. This suggests that both drugs are acting on the same receptor system in order to lower gastric acid secretion.
- Both drugs are capable of the same maximum effect, i.e. have similar **efficacies** (see below).
- At 50% inhibition of acid secretion, drug B has only one-tenth the **potency** of drug A.

All else being equal, it would be preferable to give drug A to the patient, since ten times less of

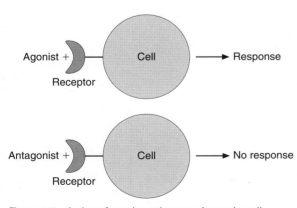

**Figure 1.6**  Action of agonist and antagonist on the cell.

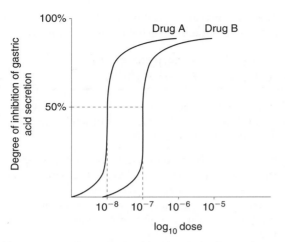

**Figure 1.7** Inhibition of gastric acid secretion by two drugs, A and B. The $\log_{10}$ dose–response curves are for two drugs acting on the same histamine $H_2$ receptors, but drug A is more potent than drug B.

a foreign chemical would be introduced into the body, even if drug B at a high enough dose will suppress acid secretion to the same extent. Drug A is more potent. Both drugs have the same efficacy. This is because both produce the same maximum response. Efficacy depends on factors such as the degree of metabolism of the drug through first pass metabolism before it can get to its site of action.

### Summary

- Receptors are important targets for drugs
- Receptors are targets because they can have high affinity and specificity for drugs
- Receptors are targets because they can be blocked by antagonists of the body's chemical messengers, such as hormones and neurotransmitters
- The dose–response curve is an important tool in the development of new drugs
- High potency means relatively little of the drug is required in order to achieve a powerful effect, and usually means it has a high affinity for the receptor it acts on
- High efficacy means that relatively more of a drug gains access to its target receptors in the body than does another that may be removed by, for example, first pass metabolism.

## Further reading

Holford N H G, Sheiner L B 1981 Clinical Pharmacokinetics 6: 429

# Chapter 2

# The role of nurses in drug administration

## Learning objectives

At the end of this chapter, the reader should be able to:

- appreciate that nurses need to help patients understand the purpose of their treatment and to promote compliance with taking medication
- list the regulations governing the responsibilities in giving drugs, especially for controlled drugs
- ask the patient the important details that need to be taken in order to obtain a reliable drug history
- list the essential details that need to be given on a drug prescription
- outline the responsibilities of the nurse in ensuring that the prescription is interpreted accurately and in understanding and knowing the reason for, action and dose of the drug
- describe the procedure for drug dispensing to patients when two nurses are involved
- list the safety factors for drug supervision on the ward
- describe the procedures for administration to the patient of drugs by oral, rectal, vagina routes and by injection
- explain how to gain the cooperation of children and elderly patients when administering drugs to them
- appreciate the importance of the nurse in educating the patient about compliance
- explain the reasons for medication errors
- give the legal and professional responsibilities of the nurse concerning decisions made by the nurse within the use of hospital protocols

## THE NURSE'S RESPONSIBILITIES

Drug therapy plays a major part in the treatment of patients. Traditionally, medicines have been prescribed by doctors and the nurse's responsibility has been to ensure safe and reliable administration and to monitor side-effects. For nurses in hospitals and those employed by general practitioners (practice nurses) this is still the case. However, in 1994 the law was changed to allow district nurses and health visitors employed in eight pilot sites throughout England to prescribe from a limited formulary. Most of the preparations they are able to prescribe are for over-the-counter preparations but it is likely that this will be extended in future. In 1998 the government announced plans to permit all appropriately qualified community nurses to prescribe. Irrespective of whether or not they are permitted to prescribe and the setting in which they are employed, however, all nurses need to help patients understand the purpose of their treatment and to promote compliance with taking medication.

The nurse must be aware that his or her responsibilities in giving drugs are governed by the Misuse of Drugs Act 1971, for controlled drugs, and the Medicines Act 1968, for prescription only medicines, together with additional regulations formulated by individual health authorities. All Hospital and Community Trusts have their own procedures and policies. The Nursing and Midwifery Council (NMC) code of conduct, in laying down the general responsibilities of the nurse, stipulates that his or her actions should put the patient's safety and well-being first at all times.

In hospital, the custody and administration of drugs is the responsibility of the ward sister/charge nurse, who may delegate this responsibility as instructed by the employing authority's policy. Although it is usual for a qualified nurse to give drugs, with a second nurse checking to prevent error, the UKCC takes the view that registered nurses should be seen as competent to administer drugs on their own and be responsible for their actions. Student nurses will take part in drug administration and senior student nurses who have shown competence may be allowed to act as the senior person giving drugs. Intravenous drugs must also be given by two nurses, the senior of whom must be qualified and certified to do so. Requirements will vary between employing authorities and if a qualified nurse moves she must obtain a certificate for the new district.

The status of the person checking the drug will also be designated by the employing authority. Nurses' actions in relation to drug administration will be legally covered by the employing authority when the rules are followed.

## DRUG HISTORY

A reliable drug history should be obtained from the patient and, if necessary, from relatives or friends. This should include previous exposure to drugs, drugs being taken at the time and, in particular, any adverse effects resulting from their use. If the illness is of a recurrent nature, the efficacy of any drugs used in previous episodes should be noted.

It is important to remember that drugs include local applications, any over-the-counter or herbal remedies that may have been used and recreational drugs.

## THE PRESCRIPTION

In hospital it is normal practice for all drugs to be prescribed. This enables the pharmacist to supply them and instruct the nurse in their administration. The prescription sheet, which is a primary document in the case records, must be headed with the patient's full name, age, number and ward. The prescription must be clearly and indelibly written and must contain the date, the approved name of the drug (preferably in block letters), the dose (using metric dosage), the route and frequency of administration with the validity period and signature of the medical practitioner. If any of these details are omitted the drug should not be given until the prescription has been amended. Frequency of dosage can be ordered by filling in allocated time spaces rather than using Latin abbreviations. Administration is recorded by initialling the relevant box on the prescription sheet. The exact format of this sheet will vary between trusts, and nurses must familiarize themselves with documents in use when moving to a new trust. On no account should a nurse write or alter a prescription in a hospital.

### CONTROLLED DRUGS

In hospital, controlled drugs (see p. 33) must always be given by two people and it is common practice for one to be a qualified nurse. Both nurses must sign the book following each administration at the bedside or in the presence of the patient. The prescription requires the number of doses in words and figures. An additional record is kept in a specially designed book so that every tablet or ampoule is accounted for when used, both nurses signing the book following each administration. The controlled drug record book is retained on the ward for 2 years after the date of the last entry. These are legal requirements for controlled drugs, but some hospitals apply similar rules to other drugs liable to misuse.

## NURSE PRESCRIBING

Nurse prescribing in the UK has a long history. In 1986 the Cumberlege Report proposed that community nurses should prescribe from a limited formulary of medicines, appliances and dressings. This report was followed by the Crown Report in 1989 recommending that nurses with a district nursing or health visiting qualification should be allowed to prescribe from a limited formulary. At the time most other specialist nurses were hospital-based and it was thought that they would not require prescribing powers because they would always be working with medical staff. As a result, the Medicinal Products: Prescription by Nurses Act, which passed through Parliament as a private member's bill in 1992, was limited in scope. It enabled district nurses and health visitors to prescribe only from a very limited range of products, mainly over-the counter medicines, with just a few prescription-only items. These were listed in the Nurses' Formulary which was appended to the *British National Formulary*. The Crown Report also recommended collaboration between nurses and doctors preparing local protocols for drug administration. Qualified nurses were encouraged to administer and supply medicines under protocol – a general prescription that authorized the use of the drug in a community setting. This procedure became commonplace. For example, vaccines were often administered under protocol. However, issues arose relating to legality. The situation was again reviewed in 1992 and this resulted in the publication of two further reports. Currently, there are plans for the government to extend nurse prescribing from the pilot sites and to increase the number of items within the Nurse Prescribers' Formulary. A decision to extend nurse prescribing to all appropriately qualified community nurses was taken by the government in spring 1998.

The Crown Review in 1998 introduced the concept of patient-specific protocols (see below). Group protocols were renamed 'patient group directives' and the legal position was clarified, although some problems remain despite the use of guidelines to control prescription. The Crown Review in 1999 developed a more flexible approach to the powers of prescription. This was taken forward by the Government in May 2001. It announced that nurse prescribers would be able to prescribe all the general sales list medicines and pharmacy medicines that GPs prescribe. They would also be able to prescribe from a list of prescription-only medicines to manage palliative care, minor injuries, minor ailments and health promotion. Patient safety is the key issue and the thrust of the reforms is to benefit patients by permitting more rapid access to medicines. The service benefits because professional time is freed for those with more complex needs. The extension of the nursing role which has resulted from nurse prescribing is in line with health care policy in the UK and extending professional roles. Nurse prescribing policy applies only to qualified nurses and midwives and they must first complete a training course with assessments.

### PROTOCOLS VERSUS NURSE PRESCRIBING

'Protocols', often known as clinical guidelines or standards, have long been used in hospital and community settings to provide written documentation for an agreed method of performing a particular procedure, to achieve continuity and to standardize care. Today it is common practice for drugs to be administered according to protocols in hospital and the community; for example, nurses may administer immunizations or oral contraception under protocol. The use of a protocol is distinct from nurse prescribing as the nurse is unable to make an independent choice of medication or treatment – this will already have been specified within the protocol. The protocol is operating as a substitute prescription authorized and signed by a doctor who remains legally and professionally accountable for the treatment of the patient. Nevertheless, the nurse remains professionally and legally accountable for his or her decisions within the use of the protocol.

Nurse prescribing in law and as a professional task applies only to district nurses, midwives and health visitors in the community. These people may do so only from the limited list of items included

**Table 2.1**   Some items included in the Nurse Prescribers' Formulary

*Gastrointestinal system*
Laxatives
    Senna tablets and granules
Ispaghula granules
    Docusate sodium
Sterculia
    Co-danthramer
Bisacodyl suppositories
Glycerol suppositories
Lactulose
Phosphate enema
Sodium citrate enema

*Stoma care products*
    Adhesives and adhesive removers
    Deodorants
    Skin protectives and cleaners

*Analgesia*
    Aspirin
    Paracetamol

*Anthelmintics*
    Piperazine
    Mebendazole

*Antifungal agents*
    Nystatin oral suspension and pastilles
    Clotrimoxazole cream

*Urinary tract*
    Preparations for maintaining indwelling urinary
    catheters

*Mouthwashes and gargles*
    Thymol

*Skin care*
    Emollient and barrier creams
    Emollient bath additives
    Magnesium sulphate paste (for boils)
    Skin disinfectants
        Aqueous solution of 10% povidone-iodine
        Sodium chloride
    Desloughing agents
        Iodosorb
        Varidase topical (streptokinase, streptodornase)

*Anaesthesia*
    Lidocaine hydrochloride for topical use

*Parasitical preparations*
    All *British National Formulary* items except benzyl
    benzoate

The full list is also given in the *British National Formulary*. It will no doubt be modified with increasing experience.

within the Nurse Prescribers' Formulary (Table 2.1), having undertaken special training. In legal terms 'prescribing' is taken to mean the ability to make a personal, professional and independent assessment of the patient. Based on this, a free choice is made from the Nurse Prescribers' Formulary of the most appropriate drug or treatment. A doctor's opinion is unnecessary. The nurse signs the prescription form and remains professionally and legally accountable for his or her actions.

Research studies have indicated that despite initial lack of confidence, nurses have responded well to the challenge of prescribing and numerous benefits have been reported, including an improvement in patient care, more efficient use of nurses' time, and clarification of professional responsibilities, which have resulted in better communication between members of the primary health care team.

Breakdown of communication is possible after the patient is discharged from hospital and when drugs may be prescribed by more than one person. The new prescribing–dispensing process will mean greater contact between the nurse and pharmacist, especially when problems arise. It has been recommended that prescribing records are stored in the patient's home as district nursing records are already kept. The prescribing record contains details of previous and current drugs, including any additional over-the-counter products and drug allergies. When prescribing, the nurse will need to consider psychosocial as well as physical factors and the need for patient education must be recognized. The record should monitor the response to drugs and reasons for discontinuing their use.

## NURSING ASPECTS OF ADMINISTRATION

In the community most patients, or some member of the family, are responsible for drug administration, although the nurse or health visitor may have a role to play. Many people are now discharged within a few days or hours of surgery and the average length of stay for medical patients has also been reduced. People returning home are often still taking drugs which until recently would have been given only within the confines of a hospital, so monitoring for adverse effects is an increasingly important aspect of the community nurse's role. The nurse must also be aware that some drugs, even if stopped before discharge, may still exert an action or cause side-effects.

The nurse is responsible for interpreting the prescription accurately, recording that the drug has been given and observing the patient's response. Prior to administration the nurse must know the reason for, action and usual dosage of the drug; this should enable him or her to recognize and question mistakes in prescribing. When in doubt about a prescription, advice should be sought and, if necessary, the doctor should be consulted. Observations should be made for therapeutic and adverse effects. The nurse should realize that the patient's condition may alter the effect of a drug and that there may be interactions with concurrent treatment. The nurse is greatly assisted in these circumstances by the pharmacist, with whom a good working relationship will enhance the safety of patient care.

The Committee on Safety of Medicines requests that adverse reactions are reported (yellow cards) and, in addition, may require that a special watch is kept on certain preparations (see p. 414).

## WARD ADMINISTRATION OF DRUGS

Drugs may be given to the whole ward by the same nurses or to a smaller group of patients by those directly involved in their care. The second method is preferable as timing is more accurate and the nurse will know the patients well and can cater for individual needs such as difficulty in swallowing medication. Time can be spent teaching patients about their drugs and student nurses can take part to gain experience in relating drugs to the patient's condition. In some hospitals experimental schemes have involved patients being responsible for their own drugs, particularly if they need to take the same drugs when they go home. On the whole these have been successful and have provided valuable opportunities for patient education. Where members of the family will be giving drugs they can be invited to the ward at the appropriate time to practise a technique (such as giving an injection) or to ask about any anticipated problems. An innovative approach on some wards has been in the timing of drug rounds so that medicines can be given nearer the time patients would take them at home. Many people have taken their drugs at home for years and may be upset by altered timing in hospital. Many schemes have abolished the early morning drug round to give patients longer to sleep.

For a few drugs flexibility is not possible; antibiotics are more effective if doses are spread evenly throughout the day, and insulin must be given before meals. Other drugs such as non-steroidal anti-inflammatory drugs (NSAIDs) are best given with or after food.

## SPECIFIC RULES OF DRUG ADMINISTRATION

Whichever approach is taken, specific rules of drug administration must be followed to obviate errors. The underlying principles – to give the correct dose of the prescribed drug to the right patient, by the right route, at the right time – require the nurse's undivided attention. When two nurses are involved, instructions should be read aloud:

1. Read the patient's full name from the prescription sheet.
2. Read the prescription, checking the validity and time of last administration.
3. Read the name of the drug from the label when removing the container from the shelf.
4. Check the label of the container for the name, strength and dose of the drug, the route of administration where relevant and the expiry date against the prescription.
5. Measure or count the correct dose. Avoid contact with the drug as allergies can develop, particularly if the hands are damp. When measuring liquids, shake the bottle, hold the measure at eye level, placing the thumbnail on the meniscus, and pour from the back of the bottle to keep the label clean. A calibrated measure should be used. When a fractional dose is required, calculations should be made independently before checking the dose.
6. Re-check the label before returning the container to the shelf.
7. Both nurses must verify the patient's identity by checking the details on the prescription sheet with the patient's identity bracelet. If this is absent, ask the patient to state his or her full name. If this is not possible identification must be confirmed by a member of the family or permanent staff.
8. Ensure the patient is in a fit state to receive the drug.
9. Give the dose and see that it has been swallowed.
10. Record the administration. Also record when a drug is not given and the reason.

**Additional points.** Patients who refuse to take a drug or show doubt or anxiety may have a good reason, which will become apparent if the nurse takes time to listen to them.

## SAFETY FACTORS

- Do not leave the drug trolley unattended.
- Do not give drugs from memory; a prescription sheet must always be used.
- Do not give a drug from a container that is not correctly labelled.
- Do not give a drug prepared by anyone else.
- Do not return an unused dose to a stock bottle.
- Unused drugs may be returned to the pharmacy where they will be checked and used for another patient. Drugs returned by outpatients should be destroyed.

## AIDS TO TAKING ORAL DRUGS

- Ensure the patient is sitting up whenever possible to facilitate swallowing.
- Prepare a drink before giving the drug, and see that an adequate amount of fluid is taken with the drug to prevent oesophageal irritation/ulceration.
- Liquid preparations are given via an oral syringe. Soluble tablets should be dissolved completely before presenting them. If a patient has difficulty holding a tablet it should be introduced on a spoon.
- If a patient has difficulty swallowing a tablet, remove it, give a drink and try again. Many drugs can be prepared and given in liquid form if necessary.
- If a drug tastes unpleasant it may be followed by a flavoured drink or mouthwash.

Although many drugs will be given orally, the nurse will also administer them by the rectal and vaginal routes and by injection. In all cases the above rules must be followed.

## RECTAL DRUGS

These are given in suppository form using protective gloves and a small amount of lubricant to ease insertion. It is important that the method is explained to the patient beforehand and that correct positioning is used with the patient lying on their left side with hips and knees flexed. It has been shown that insertion of the blunt end of the suppository aids comfort and retention.

Long-term treatment may be given by this route in which case patients can be taught self-administration most effectively.

## VAGINAL DRUGS

Vaginal pessaries and creams are inserted with the patient lying on her side or back. Clean (rather than sterile) gloves are satisfactory except after delivery. A lubricant is used and the drug inserted into the posterior fornix of the vagina. In some circumstances a pad may be worn after insertion as leakage can occur. Again, patients can be instructed on self-medication by this method. Pessaries are best inserted last thing at night as they tend to become dislodged.

## INJECTIONS

The nurse will be responsible for giving drugs by intradermal, subcutaneous and intramuscular routes. Qualified nurses may give drugs intravenously through an established route. Fractional dosage may be required in these circumstances and careful calculation is vital as errors in dose measurement can occur, the danger of this being compounded by the more rapid action of drugs by injection. When giving injections, sterile equipment must be used and strict aseptic techniques observed. Cleansing of the skin with an alcohol swab is still commonly used, but the benefits of this are questionable: however, where the skin is contaminated or the balance of flora changed, as in debilitated patients, it may be necessary. If used, the alcohol should be allowed to dry before inserting the needle. In most circumstances the site is massaged after removing the needle to aid absorption of the drug.

**Intradermal injection.** The two most common reasons for giving intradermal injections are testing for sensitivity to allergens and immunization. In the former situation there is a risk of an anaphylactic reaction, so epinephrine should be readily available. A very small amount of fluid (0.1 ml or less) is given using a 1 ml syringe, graduated in 0.1 ml divisions, through a short fine needle (26 gauge × ⅜ inch, see Fig. 2.1). This is introduced just under the skin at an angle of 10–15°, which will raise a small weal. The area should not be massaged after removing the needle. The usual site of injection is the lightly pigmented area of the forearm where the reaction can be easily observed.

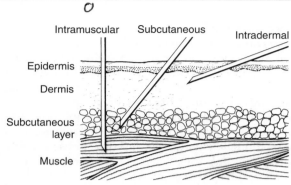

**Figure 2.1**    The position of the needle for intramuscular, subcutaneous and intradermal injections.

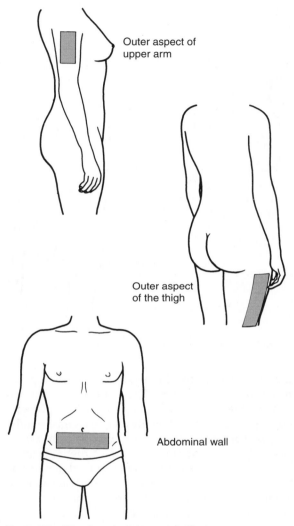

**Figure 2.2**    Sites for subcutaneous injections.

**Subcutaneous injection.**    A subcutaneous injection is given into the fatty layer just under the skin (see Fig. 2.1). Small amounts of fluid are injected (0.5–2 ml) using a 25 gauge × 15/16 inch needle. A fold of skin is raised between the thumb and forefinger and the needle is inserted at an angle of 45° (see Fig. 2.1). After insertion the plunger is withdrawn slightly to ensure a blood vessel has not been entered. If this occurs the needle should be removed, pressure applied to the area and a new injection prepared. For injections of heparin and insulin shorter needles are used. These may be the very short fine needles integral with insulin syringes or 25 gauge × ⅝ inch needles. In these instances the needle enters the skin at 90°. The area is not massaged after withdrawing the needle but firm pressure is used to prevent haematoma formation when heparin is given and to ensure uniform absorption rates in patients with diabetes. Other modifications which may be made when giving insulin are discussed on p. 196.

The usual sites for subcutaneous injections are the outer aspect of the upper arm, the outer aspect of the upper thigh and the skin of the abdominal wall (Fig. 2.2).

**Intramuscular injection.**    This is given into muscle so larger amounts can be injected, e.g. 1–5 ml (Fig. 2.3). The best site is the outer aspect of the thigh, locating the area in the middle third of the space between the knee and greater trochanter of the femur. The upper outer quadrant of the buttock is also used (Fig. 2.3). It is vital to determine the sites carefully to avoid damage to the sciatic nerve and major blood vessels. Alternatively, the upper outer aspect of the arm may be used if the muscle is big enough. To aid relaxation the patient should be positioned comfortably; for buttock injections either lying on the abdomen with the toes turned in or lying on the side with the lower leg extended and the upper leg flexed. For thigh injections the limb should be slightly flexed and supported.

When preparing injections care should be taken to prevent skin contamination, as contact dermatitis can occur. Gloves may be worn in some circumstances and the hands washed thoroughly after completion of the procedure. Drugs which may cause this reaction are penicillin, the aminoglycosides and chlorpromazine. Special precautions are taken when using cytotoxic drugs (see p. 349). When giving an intramuscular injection the skin is held taut and a 21 gauge × 1½ inch needle introduced at 90° (see Fig. 2.1). As in the subcutaneous technique the

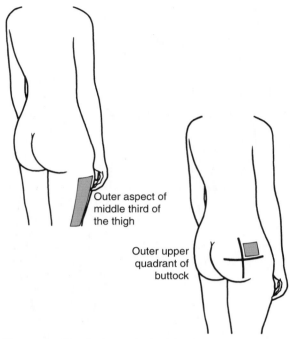

Outer aspect of
middle third of
the thigh

Outer upper
quadrant of
buttock

**Figure 2.3**    Sites for intramuscular injections.

plunger is withdrawn to check for inadvertent punc-
turing of a blood vessel. The fluid is then injected
slowly, the needle withdrawn quickly, pressure
applied initially and then the area massaged gently.

When injecting substances such as iron, which
cause skin discoloration, the Z track method can be
used. In this technique the skin is pulled to one side
before inserting the needle, a few seconds are allowed
to elapse before it is withdrawn, at which point the
skin is released, thus achieving the Z track.

**Intravenous injections and additives.**    It has been
estimated that 12% of patients have an intravenous
infusion at some time during their stay in hospital,
usually for one or more of the following reasons:
fluid replacement treatment, drug treatment, monitoring central venous pressure, hyperalimentation
or to provide emergency access to a vein. Responsibility for drug administration by the intravenous
route is now becoming part of the nurse's extended
role, although in most health districts it is necessary to have attended a special training course and
received a certificate of competence, which may not
be valid in another institution. The intravenous route
is most often used for heparin, cytotoxic drugs and
antibiotics. Individual drugs may be given as a bolus
or added to the infusion fluid, in which case careful
mixing and labelling are vital and it is important to

check that drugs do not interact with each other in the
infusion bottle. Intravenous drugs need very careful monitoring and the nurse requires an adequate
knowledge of potential side-effects. It is therefore
essential that student nurses involved in checking
and observing the effects of drugs given by this
route are closely supervised. When the flow rate
is mechanically controlled it is still necessary to
check independently that the correct dose is being
delivered. Any adjustment to dosage must only be
undertaken by trained nurses.

Infection is a known hazard of intravenous can-
nulation and is increased when drugs or additives
are given because the apparatus will be handled
more often. Patients must therefore be observed for
signs of local infection at the site of the cannula and
their temperature monitored carefully. Continuous
infusion of drugs by an infusion apparatus is not
very accurate, although the use of a paediatric volume control administration device will render the
flow rate more easily controllable.

60 microdrops (Soluset) = 1 ml
20 macrodrops (standard giving set) = 1 ml

For more satisfactory and accurate dosage an
infusion pump should be used.

---

**Nursing point**

Needle stick injuries pose an occupational hazard to
nurses and may result in the transmission of blood-
borne infection – hepatitis B, hepatitis C or, more
rarely, HIV. Risks can be reduced by disposing of the
needle and the syringe immediately after use,
without attempting to recap the needle, as research
studies indicate that recapping is particularly likely
to result in injury. All sharps should be placed in a
designated container, which should be disposed of
when or more than two-thirds full. Sharps should
never be transported in the hands or in pockets and
hands should never, under any circumstances, be
inserted into the sharps container. Injuries, when
they occur, should be recorded in acceptance with
local policy and medical opinion should be sought.

---

## GIVING DRUGS TO CHILDREN

Obtaining cooperation from children is very important and a simple, honest explanation helps to
achieve this. Children are more likely to take drugs

from a familiar person and, where appropriate, parents and relatives can actually give drugs observed by the nurses who have prepared the medication. As paediatric doses are so different from those of adults, it is important for nurses familiar with children's care to be involved in checking drugs, adhering to local policies. Fractional dosage is used and needs careful calculation to avoid error. Most drugs are given in liquid form. For very young children a medicine dispenser is useful. This is a special 1 ml syringe into which the required dosage is drawn via a special bottle adaptor. With the child sitting up, the dispenser is inserted into his or her mouth with the tip pointing to the inside of the cheek and the plunger is depressed slowly, allowing the drug to be swallowed naturally. For older children a special graduated syringe is used. Medicines should not be given in milk or food and it is important to praise the child for taking them.

## GIVING DRUGS TO ELDERLY PATIENTS

Many elderly patients dislike taking oral drugs and, to overcome this, adequate time should be taken for simple explanation. If swallowing tablets proves difficult, it may be possible to prescribe the drug in liquid form or to use semi-solids such as ice cream as a vehicle for introducing medication. If there is doubt as to whether it has been swallowed, inspection of the mouth may be needed.

## COMPLIANCE AND EDUCATION

In the past, giving drugs usually involved only passive participation by the patient, with little information being offered unless it was requested. There is increasing evidence that adequate explanation to the patient increases the likelihood of adherence to a prescribed course of treatment. Indeed, according to the Patients' Charter issued by the Department of Health in 1991, every citizen has the right to a clear explanation of any proposed treatment – clearly this includes any drugs prescribed. In order to comply, an understanding and acceptance of the treatment is vital; failure to do so may be unintentional due to lapse of memory, or deliberate, when timing and dosage may be altered by the patient. Studies show that non-compliance is a major problem, resulting in omission or repetition of drug treatment, which may require readmission to hospital. Unused drugs may be a potential danger to patients and relatives,

increasing the risk of deliberate or accidental self-poisoning.

Education of the patient with regard to drug treatment is the responsibility of the doctor, pharmacist and nurse. However, this also applies to educating other health care professionals such as social workers, occupational therapists, physiotherapists, non-professional carers and the general public to improve overall understanding of the significance of the proper use of drugs as a part of treatment.

In hospital the nurse is in an expedient position to fulfil this role by being the person primarily involved in drug administration and having continued contact with the patient. The aim of teaching is to help the patient to gain insight into the way drugs can be used to treat his or her disorder. Implicit in this is the nurse's knowledge of the disease process and drug action. Answering patients' questions will impart a certain amount of information, but this must be accompanied by a more structured approach.

Teaching begins on the patient's admission when an understanding of his or her present treatment should be established. Poor literacy or language difficulties impede comprehension and any problems elicited will need sensitive discussion. Anxiety about the harmful effects of chemicals and addiction to drugs may concern some patients and will hinder learning if not overcome. It is also important to ascertain whether any regular self-medication is occurring, as this may influence the action of prescribed drugs: e.g. the use of antacids concurrently with tetracycline reduces absorption rates.

At this time drugs brought in by the patient are seen by the doctor and permission gained, if possible, to dispose of them, explaining the dangers of error if a different regimen is prescribed on discharge. Teaching should continue during the hospital stay. It is common practice for the patient to be given brief, rather hurried instructions on drug treatment when being handed the bottles of drugs immediately before leaving the ward. At this time motivation and concentration may be low, as the patient is more concerned with going home.

## TEACHING IN PREPARATION FOR DISCHARGE

Patients vary as to the amount of information they need so this must be tailored to individual requirements, but should include the following:

1. The name and purpose of the drug, stressing its positive effects.

2. Frequency and timing of administration according to home routine, including advice about 'as required' medications.
3. Method of administration with explanation where special equipment will be required for routes other than oral.
4. Proposed length of treatment – short or long term.
5. The importance of not stopping or starting drugs without advice and where to obtain that advice.
6. How to obtain further supplies and safely dispose of unwanted drugs.
7. Adverse effects to be reported and how to carry out special tests and observations to show if they are developing. The aim is to give adequate information without causing unnecessary alarm. Most drugs produce side-effects, some of which are minor, but others are potentially serious. In some cases it may be possible to advise on the relief of side-effects. If sufficient information is not given patients may just stop taking the drugs rather than report the adverse effects, or they may stop treatment when symptoms subside, as perhaps in the case of antibiotic treatment. A well-informed patient able to participate in his or her own care will feel more in control and thus more responsible, contributing to compliance.

Teaching should continue during the stay in hospital and *should include members of the patient's family as appropriate*.

Some wards have experimented with schemes in which patients, under supervision, are responsible for their own drug administration. There is also evidence that a simple explanatory booklet given to patients on discharge reinforces teaching. Patients taking drugs such as steroids or anticoagulants should be given a card with information about dosage, etc.

## MISSED DOSES

The preceding discussion should have emphasized the importance of taking drugs in the correct dose, via the correct route and following particular instructions. It will also have highlighted the problem of non-compliance, which continues to be a major stumbling block in therapeutics. In hospital the nurse is in a strong position to influence patient compliance and to provide explanations and allay anxieties as they occur. Time spent listening to patients' points of view and exploring their concerns is helpful to both nurses and patients.

In the community patients are more likely to be left alone to cope with their drugs and, often, non-compliance occurs through forgetfulness or misunderstanding.

As nurse prescribing becomes a reality, those in a position to influence which drugs and doses patients should take must remember:

1. It is sensible to choose drugs whose efficacy is unlikely to be affected by the occasional missed dose.
2. Drugs should not be used at the limits of their duration of action – a drug with an intermediate duration of action is more efficacious if taken twice daily rather than stretched to once daily by taking a higher dose.
3. Drugs that are eliminated slowly and accumulate in the body are least impaired by poor compliance.

## ADDITIONAL USEFUL POINTS

1. Drugs prescribed for others should not be taken even if the problems appear similar.
2. Drugs may deteriorate from moisture if kept in bathroom cabinets.
3. Different drugs should not be put in the same container as errors may occur. The drugs may interact chemically.
4. All drugs should be kept out of the reach of children, preferably in a locked cupboard. They should never be referred to as 'sweets'.

Special problems of compliance may be found in patients with memory impairment, defects of sight or hearing and those with physical handicaps which interfere with mobility and dexterity. Elderly patients also form a group at particular risk as many of these problems may exist in one patient. Another group with special needs comprises patients with diabetes or other endocrine disorders, psychiatric disorders, hypertension and tuberculosis, for whom long-term treatment is necessary. Some of the drugs may be unpleasant to take, may affect the whole way of life of the patient or give rise to particularly unpleasant side-effects. In these situations ongoing educational support is essential.

In all situations it is useful to have verbal information reinforced by written instructions, as it is well known that anxiety limits retention of information. It is especially important that this is done where there is memory impairment. Instruction should be kept simple; memory aids such as tear-off calendars and recording cards can be of value.

Special dose boxes, e.g. the Dosett pill dispenser, which hold up to 1 week's supply of drugs can be used, but may be too complicated for some patients and still require another person to fill them.

Containers need to be labelled with adequate-sized lettering and/or colour coding. Information on the label as to the purpose of the drug, e.g. 'heart tablets' or 'water tablets', may be helpful for elderly patients. Braille labels can be used for blind patients.

Drug manufacturers could also contribute to compliance by appropriate packaging and presentation of drugs. The container should be easy to open; child-resistant containers are used increasingly, but are very difficult for elderly patients and those with arthritis to handle. Many people are unaware that ordinary screw-top bottles are available. Caps with wings can be supplied where necessary; the occupational therapist will be able to assess the patient's need and offer other helpful suggestions.

Despite these aids there will still be some patients who are unable to cope with drug administration independently. In these situations education of other family members, friends, neighbours or 'home helps' will be necessary. A number of trials of self-administration of drugs in elderly patients have been carried out in some parts of the country in preparation for discharge from hospital and to improve compliance. These programmes aim to identify individual patient problems well before discharge, but require the total commitment of all staff involved and continued counselling and follow-up in the community. It appears that these programmes have proved useful in training elderly patients and it may be that special self-administration programmes could have a wider application.

## MEDICATION ERRORS

Occasionally, medication errors are made by nursing staff. Such episodes not only have the potential to endanger patients but also have a serious effect on the self-esteem and confidence of the nurse and need to be investigated fully and objectively so that any lessons learnt can be used to reduce the risk of future errors.

Reasons for medication errors include:

1. *The patient*: Failure to understand self-administration systems or to recognize adverse effects if they occur: poor compliance; and interactions with self-administered alternative treatment.
2. *The nurse*: failure to take an adequate drug history with particular reference to previous adverse effects; failure to identify the patient correctly; failure to educate the patient adequately; lack of knowledge of the properties and actions of the drug involved; confusion over the names of drugs; and errors in calculation or measurement of the dose or in the mode and site of administration.
3. *Organizational*: inadequate control of ordering and storing of drugs; errors in labelling and inaccurate prescriptions; and failure to guard constantly against errors and to investigate the cause if errors occur and to take steps to prevent their recurrence.

## NON-PRESCRIPTION DRUGS

For years social scientists have been interested in the 'sick role' phenomenon and the factors which cause people to decide they are ill and behave accordingly by taking drugs or going to bed. It has also become apparent that some people visit their doctors more frequently than others, whereas some diagnose themselves as not ill enough to 'trouble' a doctor or nurse but, nevertheless, take some form of drug. Indeed, few households are without some mild form of analgesic or antiseptic. Most people who travel abroad wisely purchase antidiarrhoeal drugs and every year large numbers of people dose themselves for coughs, motion sickness and constipation. Health care professionals need to know what the patient is taking and this extends to over-the-counter as well as prescribed drugs. Aspirin is widely available, but many people do not realize the full range and potency of its therapeutic effects. Paracetamol, another mild analgesic, can cause severe and fatal liver damage in overdose. Both these drugs are incorporated into numerous proprietary medicines. For example, several forms of *Anadin* are marketed containing different amounts of aspirin and in some cases paracetamol, with its implications in overdose or if prescribed drugs are needed. When the nurse assesses the patient on hospital admission or the initial community visit he or she should not only enquire about prescribed drugs but any medication and, if possible, see it. The commercial preparation *Lomotil* for diarrhoea contains atropine, which in overdose may cause atropine toxicity or interact with other drugs. Some expectorants induce drowsiness and a few contain appreciable amounts of alcohol. Patients need to be aware of the likely side-effects and actions of these drugs as much as of those which are prescribed.

With nurse prescribing now a reality, a sound knowledge of non-prescription drugs is essential for all who provide care in hospital or the community.

## Further reading

Bird C 1990 Drug administration; a prescription for self-help. Nursing Times 24(43): 54–57

Britten N 1994 Patients' ideas about medicines – a qualitative study in a general practice population. British Journal of General Practice 44, 387: 465–468

Carlisle D 1996 Errors but no trials. Nursing Times 92(42): 50–51

Carlisle D 2002 Hidden agenda. When patients refuse medication. Nursing Times 98: 24

Collingsworth S, Gould D J, Wainwright S P 1997 Patient self-administration of medication: a review of the literature. International Journal of Nursing Studies 34: 256–269

Department of Health 1989 Report of the Advisory Group on Nurse Prescribing. DoH, London

Department of Health 1991 The Patient's Charter. HMSO, London

Drug Administration 1988 A nursing responsibility, 2nd edn. Royal College of Nursing, London

Editorial 1991 Helping patients to make the best use of medicines. Drug and Therapeutics Bulletin 29(1): 1–2

Elliott-Pennells C J 1997 Nurse prescribing. Professional Nurse 13(2): 114–115

George C 1994 What do patients need to know about prescribed drugs? Pharmaceutical Journal 252: 7–8

Gould D 1988 Called to account. Nursing Times 84(12): 28–31

Howell M 1996 Prescription for disaster. Nursing Times 92(34): 30–31

Lapham R, Agar M 1995 Drug calculations for nurses. Headline, London

Nixon P 1996 Homing in on drug rounds (medicine administration in nursing homes). Nursing Times 92(16): 59–60

United Kingdom Central Council for Nursing, Midwifery and Health Visiting 1992 Standards for the administration of medicines. UKCC, London

Walker R 1982 Suppository insertion. World Medicine 18: 58

Williams A 1996 How to avoid mistakes in medicine administration. Nursing Times 92(13): 40–43

Woodrow P 1998 Numeracy skills. Nursing Standard 12(30): 48–55

Chapter **3**

# Nurses and the pharmaceutical service

## Learning objectives

At the end of this chapter, the reader should be able to:

- understand that the patient to be discharged needs to know exactly how to take any medication that is taken away with him or her
- understand the regulations under the Misuse of Drugs Act and the Medicines Act which affect the nurse
- appreciate the nurse's responsibilities for the handling of drugs
- identify the labelling requirements for controlled drugs
- define who is legally responsible on the ward for possession of controlled drugs and for custody of keys to cupboards that contain controlled drugs
- appreciate that drug trolleys must be locked when not in use
- understand the correct, taught procedures for reconstituting sterile powders for injection
- define the procedures for handling hazardous drugs such as cytotoxic drugs
- appreciate the hospital's regulations for authorization to add drugs to infusions
- appreciate that drugs are administered under the supervision of the sister or staff nurse and that since nurses dispense the vast majority of drugs on the ward that great responsibility rests with the nursing staff to give the correct drugs and doses
- appreciate that nurses have to observe the effects of administered drugs by measuring, for example, the temperature, blood pressure, urine output and protein in

urine; the measures will depend on the drug being taken and the condition being treated

## THE WORKING RELATIONSHIP BETWEEN PHARMACIST AND NURSE

In hospital the overall responsibility for the care and supply of drugs lies with the pharmacist, who will advise on their handling and use. The nurses' responsibilities for the handling of drugs fall into seven areas: they will obtain drugs, possibly prescribe them, store them, prepare and administer them to patients, record the administration, and observe their effects, in accordance with the requirements of the law and with hospital protocols and procedures. In all of these activities they are able to call upon the pharmacist for help and advice.

A close working relationship can be built up between nurses and pharmacists where there is an active clinical pharmacy service attached to the ward. The usual practice is for the pharmacist to visit the ward once or twice a day, to see the prescription sheets, initiate the dispensing of any drugs required, raise any queries on dosage, availability or incompatibility with the doctor, and offer any drug information required by the doctor or nurse. By doing this, the pharmacist very quickly becomes familiar with the requirements of the ward, both in terms of supply and information, and can play a considerable part in ensuring the safe handling and use of drugs. Many pharmacists in hospital attend ward rounds as part of the clinical team to ensure that pharmaceutical care is provided appropriately to patients from admission to discharge.

## DRUG SELECTION AND DOSAGE

### Nursing point

*MIMS for Nurses* started publication quarterly from February 2003. Direct enquiries to MIMS for Nurses, Units 12 and 13, Friendly Gardens Industrial Estate, Cranleigh, Southall, Middlesex UBI 2DV. Tel: (020) 8606 7500

The selection of a drug is the responsibility of the doctor, advised as appropriate by senior colleagues or the pharmacist. Many hospitals now have their own drug formularies, which combine treatment guidelines and recommend a 'best-buy' drug from the often bewildering range available, and give information on dosage, routes of administration, costs, contraindications and side-effects. Hospital pharmacies usually stock only those drugs listed in the formulary.

Nurses are now permitted to prescribe some preparations as further development of their extended role (see p. 21).

## DRUG SUPPLY

Drugs in frequent use in a ward, or likely to be required in an emergency, are usually supplied as ward stock. Traditionally, the nurse has been responsible for ordering stock drugs, either by writing out a list of items required or by using a pre-printed order form, in each case basing requirements on the empty containers in the cupboard or trolley. In most hospitals the pharmacy now operates a top-up system with a pharmacy technician checking and supplying drugs to an agreed stock level on a weekly basis, thus removing the responsibility of ordering from the nurse. Whichever system is used, the aim must be to avoid both wasteful overstocking and running out at times when the pharmacy is closed.

Individual patient dispensing is used for less-frequently required drugs and in cases where the preparation is tailored to the patient's particular requirements. Although most drugs are manufactured by industry, hospital pharmacies are always able to prepare different dose forms or strengths; for example, a mixture for a patient unable to take solids, a paediatric mixture where the child needs a lower dose, or a suppository if the oral route is contraindicated. Some hospitals are able to prepare injections of novel or little-used chemicals, or formulate a chemical substance into preparations suitable for administration by a variety of routes. These more expert services, although concentrated in a few hospitals, are available to all through service contracts. The ward pharmacist can always advise on a suitable preparation and arrange for it to be made available.

The law requires that drugs of addiction, known as controlled drugs, must be supplied only against the signature of a registered nurse, usually the nurse in charge of the ward or deputy, and that the requisitions for these drugs must state precisely the name, form, strength and quantity of the drug required. Controlled drugs most likely to be met by the nurse include morphine, diamorphine (heroin), methadone, dextromoramide, buprenorphine and fentanyl. In addition, some hospitals place similar controls on other drugs liable to misuse, such as night sedatives, tranquillizers and antidepressants, and on spirits such as whisky and brandy.

## DRUG STORAGE

All drugs are potentially dangerous and all must be stored in locked cupboards reserved specifically for drugs. Ward sisters are legally authorized to possess controlled drugs for use on their wards (but not for any other purpose) and these and all other drugs issued to the ward are in their custody. Keys to the drug cupboards must be held by a sister, staff nurse or nurse in charge of the ward at the time. Drugs in current use may be stored in drug trolleys provided that these are locked and immobilized between drug rounds. Topical preparations such as ointments, lotions and disinfectants are also dangerous if misused, and these too must be locked in cupboards. This has been mandatory for many years in children's wards. More specific policies may be developed to suit local situations.

Storage conditions are important for most drugs and it is the pharmacist's responsibility to ensure that the label on the container bears adequate instructions such as 'store in a refrigerator'. Drugs which need cool or cold storage will begin to deteriorate if left at room temperature for more than a few hours, and if this happens the pharmacist's advice must be sought – it is not sufficient to put the drug in the fridge after 2 days and hope for the best.

All injections and many tablets have expiry dates assigned by the manufacturer, and if a drug is nearing this date the nurse should mention the fact to the ward pharmacist, who may be able to arrange for it to be used elsewhere. Drugs should be checked regularly and procedures in place to ensure timely replacement of preparations before reaching their expiry date. A nurse should not administer a drug which has passed its expiry date unless advice has been sought of the pharmacist who, with knowledge of the drug, may authorize its use. Similar constraints apply if the nurse feels that the condition or appearance of the drug is unusual or unsuitable.

## DRUG PREPARATION

Nurses are required to do little in the way of preparation of drugs except for reconstituting injection solutions and making additions to intravenous infusion fluids. The practice of crushing tablets and mixing them with jam or sugar to get a child to take them, or of crushing tablets to put down a nasogastric tube, should be used only on specific pharmaceutical advice, as many tablets are carefully formulated to give a sustained release of the drug, while others have the drug protected by a film, sugar or enteric coating to disguise a bitter taste or prevent gastric irritation; these characteristics will be destroyed if the tablet is crushed. The pharmacist can always prepare a suitable formulation for a particular patient.

Reconstitution of injection solutions from vials of sterile powder is taught as a nursing procedure. Reconstitution of certain drugs, such as the cytotoxic agents, can be hazardous to the nurse, and local precautions, including the use of protective clothing, must be obeyed. Only specially trained nurses undertake this activity, and most cytotoxic injections are reconstituted centrally by pharmacy staff in cabinets designed to protect the product from microbial contamination and the operator from the drug. Such centralized services can save money by avoiding wastage of residues from reconstituted vials. Repeated contact with antibiotics can cause skin sensitization, and care must be taken to avoid skin or mucous membrane contact when these are being handled (see p. 317). Reconstitution of any drug should be carried out immediately before use, using the diluent recommended in the package leaflet or advised by the pharmacist, and in general any reconstituted solution remaining should be discarded. In the case of very expensive preparations it may be possible to store and re-use the residue, but great care must be paid to storage conditions and expiry, both of which will differ from those of the dry powder. Local policies and procedures must be followed. Limitations on re-use are that the reconstituted solution must never be stored in a syringe, must not be used for intravenous or intrathecal injection and must be used within 6 hours. In cases of doubt, the pharmacist will advise.

The majority of drugs for single parenteral use are for intramuscular or subcutaneous injection, but where a very rapid effect is required, or the drug is too irritant for intramuscular injection, or if it is desired to give the drug at a constant rate over several hours, the intravenous route may be used, either by direct intravenous injection, by injection as a bolus into the intravenous giving set, by addition to an intravenous infusion fluid or the use of a syringe pump.

The addition of drugs to intravenous infusion fluids has become an acceptable procedure for nurses who have been specially trained and authorized. Authorization is restricted to first-level nurses with practical experience, but requirements will differ between hospitals. Problems which may arise in this procedure are microbial contamination of the infusion fluid, incomplete mixing of the drug and the fluid, and chemical incompatibilities (not always visible) between the drug and the fluid or between two drugs added to the same fluid. The first two problems are a result of faulty technique, whereas the third problem may be prevented by reference to incompatibility data that will be available through a pharmacist. Most hospitals provide a 24-hour advisory service from the pharmacy, and many have a resident pharmacist.

## DRUG LABELS

The style and content of labels will vary from hospital to hospital, but some typical labels for drugs dispensed for inpatients and outpatients are shown in Figure 3.1. In each case the name and strength of the drug appears at the top with directions on the frequency and method of administration for the patient on the outpatient label. Inpatient labels do not normally include directions for use, as the dosage frequency and administration often changes in hospitalized patients. Warnings on storage conditions and precautions are shown on all labels. The patient's name, quantity dispensed and date of dispensing also appear on each label. Patient information leaflets are also dispensed with the medication for patients to take home and read.

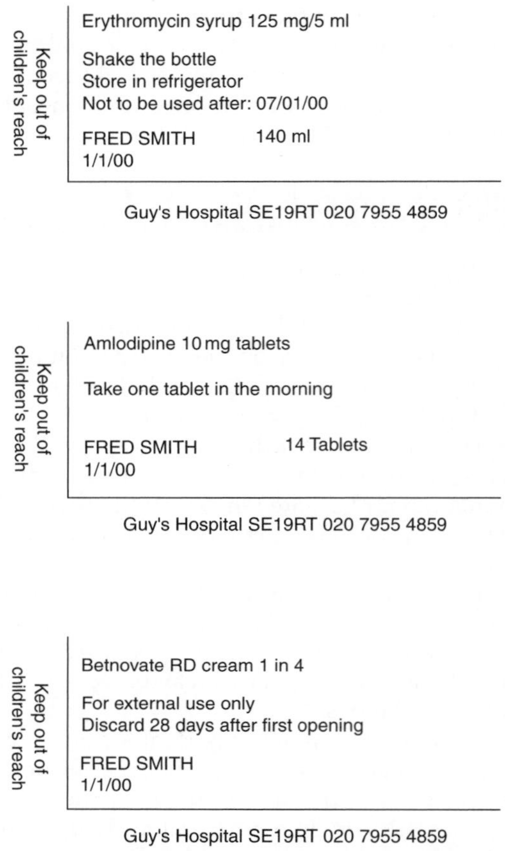

## DRUG ADMINISTRATION

Drugs are administered under the supervision of the ward sister or staff nurse, and great responsibility rests on the nursing staff to ensure that there is no error. The principles behind the rules are that the right patient must receive the right dose of the right drug in the right form by the right route at the right time, and that the fact is duly recorded. Local policies and procedures must be followed. A full discussion of the nurse's role may be found on p. 22.

It is important that the precise directions for dose, time and frequency are followed. With some potent drugs, variations in times of dosing may lead to a loss of efficacy. Taking medication before, during

Keep out of children's reach

Erythromycin syrup 125 mg/5 ml

Shake the bottle
Store in refrigerator
Not to be used after: 07/01/00

FRED SMITH          140 ml
1/1/00

Guy's Hospital SE19RT 020 7955 4859

Keep out of children's reach

Amlodipine 10 mg tablets

Take one tablet in the morning

FRED SMITH          14 Tablets
1/1/00

Guy's Hospital SE19RT 020 7955 4859

Keep out of children's reach

Betnovate RD cream 1 in 4

For external use only
Discard 28 days after first opening

FRED SMITH
1/1/00

Guy's Hospital SE19RT 020 7955 4859

**Figure 3.1**   Typical labels for drugs dispensed for patients.

or after food can also significantly alter its clinical effect.

Many hospitals are rewriting their drug policies to permit administration of drugs by a nurse without this being checked. Hospitals are developing computer systems on which the doctor will prescribe and the nurse record the administration of drugs, avoiding the traditional medicine sheets. This will provide an excellent tool for audit and costing purposes.

Schemes for self-administration of drugs by patients prior to discharge are being implemented in many hospital wards and involve training and assessment by pharmacists and nurses together. If a nurse thinks a prescribed dose is unusually high (or low), the nurse in charge should be informed, the dosage checked in the *British National Formulary* and hospital formulary and the doctor contacted if necessary. When in doubt, the nurse must seek advice before giving the dose; it may be too late afterwards.

It is often assumed that once a patient leaves the ward he or she will continue to take the drugs provided in accordance with the directions, but this is frequently not the case. There should be an ongoing preparation of the patient for discharge, including an explanation of how drugs should be taken or used, the importance of following the dosage instructions, and details of any precautions which should be observed. This can result in a significant improvement in patient adherence to a medication regime. Written instructions and background information reinforce verbal explanations, particularly for patients and their carers.

Patients receiving steroids, insulin or anticoagulant treatment or being treated for depression with monoamine oxidase inhibitors must be issued with cards describing precautions to be taken, and instructed to show the card to their doctor, dentist or pharmacist when receiving treatment or purchasing proprietary medicines. Such cards are usually available on the wards or from the pharmacy.

Some hospitals now issue patients with cards detailing their drugs, which are shown to the patient's GP and amended by him or her if the treatment changes. In this way, any practitioner treating the patient will be presented with an up-to-date drug profile.

## OBSERVING THE EFFECTS OF DRUGS

Having given the drug, nurses are required to observe its effect by taking measurements, such as recording temperature, monitoring pulse rate or blood pressure, measuring urine output or testing urine for glucose, proteins, etc. Such observations are part of the ward routine and contribute to building up a picture of the patient's condition and progress. Nurses are in an ideal position to observe their patient's progress throughout the day so they should know the desired effect of the drug, its side-effects, its possible interaction with other drugs and how its effect might be modified by the patient's condition; it is in this area that the pharmacist can play an important part advising nurses.

## INFORMATION NEEDS OF NURSES

During training nurses will acquire a basic knowledge of therapeutics and pharmacology which will probably have been extended by reading textbooks. It is possible, however, that they will be very familiar with only a limited number of drugs, usually those in widespread use in the hospital wards where they are allocated during clinical placements. It is certain that during their professional career they will meet new drugs – either those which have been recently introduced, or those which are only occasionally used for common disease, or those which are used to treat rare disorders. The ward pharmacist is an ideal source of information about the handling and administration of new and rarely used drugs.

Most large hospital pharmacies have drug information units, which provide information on request to doctors, nurses and other health workers.

The ward pharmacist should provide a link between nurses and the drug information unit, supplying appropriate information. Some hospitals also provide information cards or files that are kept on the wards and contain concise nurse-oriented information on drugs likely to be encountered, although the range of drugs covered in this way will not be complete. Computer databases are sometimes available on the wards, although care must be taken to select concise and appropriate information for inclusion. In addition, ward pharmacists will willingly talk to groups of nurses about any aspects of drugs and their use. Students who are given projects involving drugs are also encouraged to seek the help of the drug information unit.

## LEGAL RESPONSIBILITY OF NURSES AS REGARDS DRUGS

The laws affecting drug supply and use are the Misuse of Drugs Act 1971 and the Medicines Act 1968, together with Regulations made under these Acts. The Misuse of Drugs Act governs the drugs of addiction, termed 'controlled drugs', whereas the Medicines Act governs the manufacture, marketing and supply of all drugs. The Secretary of State for Health is empowered under the National Health Services Act to make regulations concerning aspects of practice, including the prescribing and administration of drugs.

Under the Misuse of Drugs Act and Regulations, the sister or acting sister in charge of a ward, theatre, or other department in a hospital or nursing home may possess controlled drugs supplied to him or her by the pharmacist, and may administer them in accordance with the directions of a doctor or dentist. Midwives have additional authority under the Act to obtain, possess and administer pethidine in the practice of their profession. A doctor may not prescribe diamorphine (heroin) or cocaine for the treatment or relief of addiction unless licensed to do so by the Home Office.

Drugs may not be marketed without a product licence, which is granted by the Secretary of State on the advice of the Committee on Safety of Medicines, an expert body which considers evidence on the safety and efficacy of each new product.

Since April 1985, doctors, whether in hospital or general practice, have not been able to prescribe certain blacklisted drugs and drug preparations on a National Health Prescription. This restriction was imposed by the Secretary of State for Health to reduce public expenditure on drugs which were considered by their advisers to be unnecessary, or for which a cheaper alternative was available. The drugs banned included some antacids, laxatives, vitamins and cough and cold remedies, and are listed in the *Drug Tariff* (HMSO, published monthly).

The Medicines Act and its Regulations permit a hospital nurse to obtain and possess 'prescription only' medicines, i.e. those which are only available to patients on the prescription of a practitioner, for use on their ward, and to administer them in accordance with the directions of a doctor or dentist. Hospital rules usually extend this control to all drugs whether they are legally 'prescription only' or not. Midwives are permitted under the Act to administer a specified range of drugs in the practice of their profession. Nurses in hospitals have no authority to administer drugs except on the directions of a doctor or dentist, whether these are in the form of a specific prescription for a patient or as part of a written procedure accepted by the hospital authority. Any nurse doing so may face disciplinary action and, if harm comes to the patient, may be liable to civil action. Hospital policies are based on *Guidelines for the safe and secure handling of medicines* (The Duthie Report, Department of Health, 1988) and the *UKCC Standards for the Administration of Medicines* (October 1992).

Certain procedures in the administration of drugs which were formerly performed by doctors only are now regarded as part of the extended role of the nurse. Policy varies from hospital to hospital, but two examples are the addition of drugs to intravenous infusion fluids and the intravenous injection of drugs as a bolus via an intravenous line, which are sometimes undertaken by nurses who have been specially trained and authorized. This applies particularly to trained nurses working in Accident and Emergency Departments, Theatres, Intensive Care and Cardiac Units where an extended role may be practised.

## IN THE COMMUNITY

Nurses now have considerable experience in the community before they qualify. The new roles of the district nurses and health visitors are discussed on p. 21. In the community, the local pharmacist has the same role as in a hospital, supplying prescribed drugs and ensuring their safety and appropriateness. Pharmacists become well acquainted with their regular clients and are required to maintain their medication records on a computer. This means that the pharmacist can check new prescriptions against current drugs and other details such as known adverse effects. Nurses who prescribe should develop good relationships with pharmacists, who often provide advice about over-the-counter drugs, and their knowledge and records may also be of value to the prescriber nurse in preventing possible interactions.

Nurses working in the community, and private nurses, have authority to possess controlled drugs only to administer them in accordance with the directions of a doctor or dentist. Unlike nurses in hospitals, they may not hold a 'stock' of controlled drugs, but may obtain them only on prescription for a specific patient.

Similarly, nurses in community or private practice have no authority to obtain or possess 'prescription only' medicines except on prescription, or to administer them to patients except in accordance with the directions of a doctor or dentist.

## DOSAGE CALCULATIONS

Patients may be prescribed doses of a drug which are not precisely equivalent to a single tablet, ampoule or a 5 ml spoonful. In this case, it is necessary to calculate the quantity of drug preparation which will contain the dose prescribed, and this is a common source of error in drug administration. The ward pharmacist should always be asked to annotate the prescription with the precise quantity of drug preparation which will contain the prescribed dose. If the dose must be given before the ward pharmacist has seen the prescription, then any calculation made must be checked by a second person, and if there remains any doubt, advice must be sought before the drug is administered. Remember that the most common error when calculating drug dosage is a misplaced decimal point, i.e. the patient receives 10 times too much or only one-tenth of the dose.

Dosage calculation is a worry to nurses (and others!) and they may find it helpful to read *Drug calculations for nurses* (1995) by R Lapham and H Agaz, published by Arnold, London.

## SUMMARY OF PHARMACEUTICAL SERVICES AVAILABLE TO NURSES

1. Supply of drugs for use on the ward.
2. Preparation of unusual formulations or doses of drugs.
3. Advice on storage conditions and expiry dates.
4. Advice on legal responsibilities.
5. Ward pharmacy services providing a ready point of contact and enquiry.
6. 24 hour service or on-call service.
7. Advice on preparation and reconstitution of drugs.
8. Advice on addition of drugs to intravenous infusion fluids.
9. Information on physical, chemical and pharmacological properties of drugs.
10. Information on dose, method of administration, effects, side-effects, precautions and contra-indications associated with drugs.
11. Information on drug costs and drug usage in a particular hospital.
12. Seminars and discussions on drugs and their uses.
13. Information to assist with drug projects.
14. Advice about prescribing in the community.
15. Education and training for dosage calculation and administration.

## Further reading

McHale J 2002 Extended prescribing: the legal implications. Nursing Times 98: 36

Humphries J, Green J 2002 Nurse prescribing. Palgrave, Basingstoke

Wright D 2002 Medication administration in nursing homes. Nursing Standard 16: 33

# Chapter 4

# The autonomic nervous system, asthma, 5–hydroxytryptamine and migraine

At the end of this chapter, the reader should be able to:

- give examples of sympathomimetic and parasympathomimetic drugs
- give examples of selective α and β agonists and antagonists
- know the basic anatomy of the autonomic nervous system
- name the neurotransmitters and receptors of the autonomic nervous system
- describe the effects of sympathetic and parasympathetic stimulation on visceral organs
- appreciate that drugs that block the action of acetylcholine have important uses
- describe what the symptoms of migraine are and how they may be prevented and treated

## INTRODUCTION TO THE AUTONOMIC NERVOUS SYSTEM

The autonomic nervous system is that part of the nervous system which supplies the viscera as distinct from the voluntary muscles.

The **viscera** include:

- the gastrointestinal tract
- the respiratory and urogenital systems
- the heart and blood vessels
- the intrinsic muscles of the eyes
- various secretory glands.

The autonomic nervous system consists of two divisions called the sympathetic and parasympathetic systems. Nerves from both these divisions supply most of the viscera. In general they have opposite effects on the various viscera which they supply, and they also differ both in their anatomical arrangement and mechanism of function.

## COMPONENTS OF THE AUTONOMIC NERVOUS SYSTEM

### SYMPATHETIC NERVOUS SYSTEM

The sympathetic nervous system consists of a chain of ganglia lying on either side of the vertebral column and extending from the cervical to the lumbar vertebrae. Sympathetic nerve fibres, after passing out from the spinal cord, leave the anterior nerve root and pass to one of these ganglia. Here they form

a synapse or junction with further nerve cells whose fibres are distributed to the viscera.

Some sympathetic fibres, after leaving the spinal cord, pass through the ganglia and form their synapses in ganglia situated peripherally; the group of ganglia surrounding the coeliac artery is a good example of this arrangement.

### PARASYMPATHETIC NERVOUS SYSTEM

The parasympathetic fibres leave the central nervous system and are distributed with certain cranial nerves (III, VII, IX and X) and with the sacral nerves. The relay ganglia of the parasympathetic system are situated peripherally near the organs supplied (Fig. 4.1).

### SENSORY FIBRES

The autonomic system also carries a large number of sensory nerves, which supply the various organs. These nerves carry information from the organ to the central nervous system (CNS). They enter the spinal cord where they may form a spinal reflex arc with the autonomic nerves leaving the cord or they may ascend to the brain where more complex reflexes

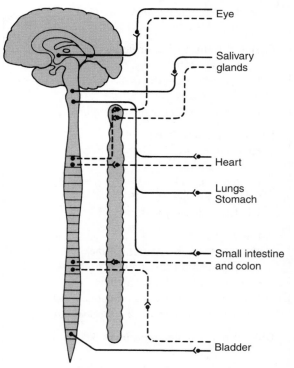

**Figure 4.1**   The anatomy of the autonomic nervous system. Sympathetic, dashed line; parasympathetic, solid line.

are built up which may be influenced by impulses arising from the higher levels of the brain. Some visceral sensation may enter consciousness and events in consciousness may themselves stimulate various visceral effects. The rapid beating of the heart after a fright is a typical example.

## CHEMICAL TRANSMISSION OF NERVE IMPULSES

Stimulation of a nerve liberates a substance called a **neurotransmitter** at the nerve ending which activates a **receptor** in the organ supplied or in another nerve cell. This is known as the chemical transmission of nerve impulses and is an important concept because many drugs act by interfering with this process. In the autonomic nervous system, transmission occurs in this way in both the sympathetic and parasympathetic divisions, but the neurotransmitter released onto the target organ differs, being acetylcholine in the parasympathetic division and norepinephrine (noradrenaline) in the sympathetic division.

### THE PARASYMPATHETIC SYSTEM (Fig. 4.2)

Following stimulation of a parasympathetic nerve, a neurotransmitter called **acetylcholine** (ACh) is librated at the nerve ending; ACh acts on a receptor on the organ supplied by the nerve. To prevent the effect of acetylcholine being too prolonged and powerful there is also present at the nerve ending an enzyme called **acetylcholinesterase**, which rapidly breaks down the acetylcholine and terminates its effect.

### THE SYMPATHETIC SYSTEM (Fig. 4.3)

The sympathetic nerves release the neurotransmitter norepinephrine from stores at the nerve endings in the peripheral tissues. In addition, the sympathetic system releases epinephrine (90%) and norepinephrine (10%) from the medulla of the adrenal gland; these substances enter the bloodstream and produce widespread effects. Norepinephrine and epinephrine produce these effects by combining with specific sympathetic adrenoceptors on the target organs. There are several types of sympathetic receptors:

### ADRENORECEPTORS

Types of adrenoreceptors:

- $\alpha_1$
- $\alpha_2$

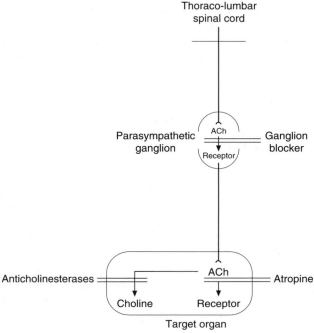

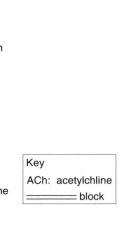

Key
ACh: acetylchline
═══ block

**Figure 4.2** Principal neurotransmitter and its receptors in the parasympathetic division of the autonomic nervous system and sites of receptor blocking drugs.

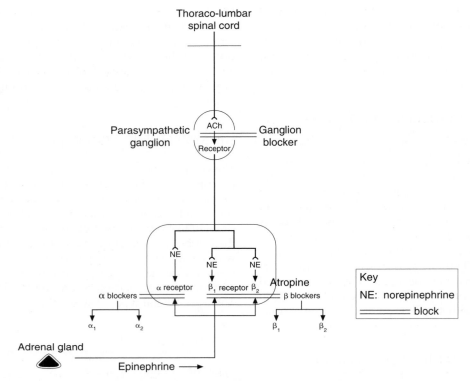

**Figure 4.3**   Neurotransmitters and receptors of the sympathetic division of the autonomic nervous system and sites of receptor blocking drugs.

- $\beta_1$
- $\beta_2$
- $\beta_3$

### $\alpha_1$ Receptors

These receptors occur on target tissues opposite the nerve terminal and are stimulated by norepinephrine released at sympathetic nerve endings and by epinephrine. Stimulation produces: constriction of blood vessels, causing a rise in blood pressure and reflex slowing of the heart, and dilatation of the pupil. Stimulation of $\alpha_1$ receptors is blocked by several drugs (see p. 51).

### $\alpha_2$ Receptors

These receptors occur on the nerve terminal from which norepinephrine is released, and when norepinephrine binds them they limit further release of norepinephrine, thus forming a release control mechanism. $\alpha_2$ Receptors are targets for drugs, such as clonidine, which stimulate them selectively to inhibit further norepinephrine release, and are therefore useful to treat hypertension.

### $\beta_1$ and $\beta_2$ receptors (Figs 4.4 and 4.5)

These receptors are both stimulated by isoprenaline and epinephrine. In addition, the neurotransmitter norepinephrine acts as a $\beta_1$ stimulator on the heart, and the drug salbutamol produces a $\beta_2$ response largely on the bronchi. The effects are:

- $\beta_1$ responses. Increase in rate and excitability of the heart with increased cardiac output.
- $\beta_2$ responses. Dilatation of bronchi and blood vessels.

### $\beta_3$ Receptors

These receptors have only recently been reported in cardiac muscle. They are negatively inotropic, i.e. they depress the rate and force of contraction (Moniotte & Balligand 2002).

Overactivity of the sympathetic nervous system produced by fright or anger causes a mixed picture due to stimulation by norepinephrine and epinephrine of $\alpha_1$, $\beta_1$ and $\beta_2$ receptors (see Table 4.1).

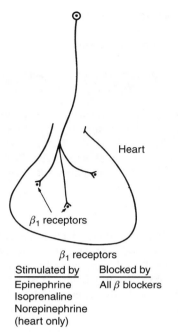

β₁ receptors

| Stimulated by | Blocked by |
|---|---|
| Epinephrine | All β blockers |
| Isoprenaline | |
| Norepinephrine | |
| (heart only) | |

**Figure 4.4** Important β₁ receptors, showing agonists (stimulators) and blocking agents.

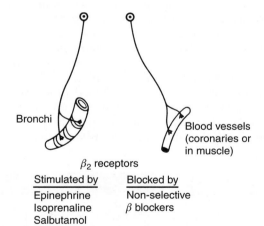

β₂ receptors

| Stimulated by | Blocked by |
|---|---|
| Epinephrine | Non-selective |
| Isoprenaline | β blockers |
| Salbutamol | |

**Figure 4.5** Important β₂ receptors, showing agonists (stimulators) and blocking agents.

## TRANSMISSION AT AUTONOMIC GANGLIA

The nerve that arrives at an autonomic ganglion from the CNS is termed a **preganglionic nerve**. The nerve with which it synapses in the ganglion, and which carries the impulse away to the target organ, is called the **postganglionic nerve**. Acetylcholine is

**Table 4.1** The chief effects of sympathetic and parasympathetic activity

| | Sympathetic activity | Parasympathetic activity |
|---|---|---|
| Heart rate | Increased | Slowed |
| Blood vessels | Constricted | Dilated |
| Stomach and intestine | Decreased activity and secretion | Increased activity and secretion |
| Salivary and bronchial glands | Decreased secretion | Increased secretion |
| Urinary bladder | Body relaxed, sphincter contracted | Body contracted, sphincter relaxed |
| Bronchial muscle | Relaxed | Contracted |
| Blood sugar | Raised | |
| Eye | Pupils dilated | Pupils constricted Accommodates for near vision |

liberated by the preganglionic nerve at the synapses in both sympathetic and parasympathetic ganglia, binds to its receptors on the postganglionic nerve and is thus responsible for the transmission of the nerve impulse.

## SYMPATHOMIMETIC DRUGS

Sympathomimetic drugs have effects similar to those produced by activity of the sympathetic nervous system and comprise:

- epinephrine
- norepinephrine
- isoprenaline
- selective β₂ agonists.

### EPINEPHRINE

Epinephrine (adrenaline) is released from the medulla of the adrenal gland when the sympathetic system is activated. For clinical use, however, it is prepared synthetically. It acts on the sympathetic receptors of the visceral organs. Epinephrine is destroyed by gastric acid and is therefore not effective if taken orally. It is usually given by subcutaneous or intramuscular injection, its effects being produced more rapidly from the latter site.

Following injection, its various actions become apparent within a minute. They are:

- An increase in the force and rate of contraction of the heart ($\beta_1$ effect), so that the patient may report palpitation.
- A rise in systolic blood pressure due to the increased cardiac output ($\beta_1$ effect). The diastolic pressure shows little change as epinephrine produces vasoconstriction only in the skin and in the splanchnic area (mixed $\alpha_1$ and $\beta_2$ effects) and vasodilatation in arteries in muscle ($\beta_2$ effect).
- Epinephrine relaxes smooth muscle, including that of the bronchial tree ($\beta_2$ effect).
- Epinephrine raises blood sugar by mobilizing glucose from tissues.

Following injection, epinephrine is rapidly broken down in the body by the enzymes monoamine oxidase and methyl-O-transferase, and its effects last for only a few minutes.

Epinephrine is used less now than in former times. It is still the best immediate treatment for serious anaphylactic reactions (see p. 409). In anaphylactic reactions, epinephrine causes constriction of blood vessels and thus relieves oedema and swelling and stimulates the heart in cardiac arrest.

### Nursing point

It is important not to inject larger doses of epinephrine into a vein by mistake, as a sudden intravenous injection can precipitate a fatal cardiac arrhythmia. However, epinephrine can be given as an intravenous bolus in smaller doses as a stimulant to the heart in cardiac arrest. Check the *British National Formulary* (*BNF*) for the correct dosages.

## NOREPINEPHRINE

Norepinephrine (noradrenaline) is chemically closely related to epinephrine and is the neurotransmitter released from sympathetic nerves at the target organs and tissues. Its most important action is to produce widespread vasoconstriction and thus a rise in both systolic and diastolic blood pressure ($\alpha_1$ effect). The body rapidly inactivates norepinephrine and to produce a continuous effect on the blood pressure it is given by intravenous infusion.

Norepinephrine has been used in the treatment of various forms of shock, which is usually associated with a very low blood pressure.

### Nursing point

A patient receiving norepinephrine requires careful nursing and observation with frequent estimations of blood pressure, which may fluctuate widely with small changes in the rate of infusion. Care should be taken to avoid extravasation, which can cause necrosis.

Opinion has moved against using norepinephrine to raise blood pressure except in extreme circumstances, for although a satisfying rise in blood pressure can be obtained due to vasoconstriction, this also reduces the blood flow in essential organs, particularly the kidney, with troublesome results.

## ISOPRENALINE

Isoprenaline is a synthetic drug related to epinephrine; but unlike epinephrine, which stimulates all sympathetic receptors, isoprenaline stimulates $\beta_1$ and $\beta_2$ receptors but not $\alpha$ receptors. It is well absorbed from the oral mucosa and following inhalation. It relaxes smooth muscle, including that of the bronchial tree, and also stimulates the heart, but has little or no effect on the blood pressure. It is important to avoid overdosage as it can cause dangerous cardiac arrhythmias. It is rapidly inactivated after absorption and its effects are short-lived.

### Safety point

Isoprenaline was formerly used in the treatment of asthma, both by inhalation and orally. Because it stimulates both $\beta_1$ and $\beta_2$ receptors, its action of cardiac stimulation can precipitate fatal arrhythmias. It has now been replaced for this purpose by safer $\beta_2$ agonists such as **terbutaline** and **salbutamol** (see below).

Isoprenaline can also be given by infusion in severe bradycardia. Adverse effects include palpitation, nausea, headaches and tremors.

## SELECTIVE β₂ AGONISTS

These drugs stimulate predominantly $\beta_2$ receptors, so that although they are effective bronchodilators, they have minimal effects on the heart. This is an important improvement over drugs such as isoprenaline, as the risk of cardiac arrhythmias is removed.

### Salbutamol

Salbutamol is the most widely used $\beta_2$ agonist. It is a powerful bronchodilator. Salbutamol can be given by various routes, but if given orally a considerable proportion is broken down in the liver (first pass effect). Its action lasts about 4 hours. In large doses it may cause tremor and tachycardia and occasionally night cramps.

Salbutamol is used to treat bronchospasm due to asthma or bronchitis. It may be taken to relieve an attack or, on a regular basis, to control the spasm. It can be given via various routes:

- Inhalation is the most commonly used route of administration and given in this way in the treatment of bronchospasm it is possible to get the maximum effect on the bronchi with minimal effects elsewhere. Even so, only 10% of the dose reaches the bronchial tree if the patient inhales directly from the aerosol puffer, the rest being swallowed during self-dosage (Fig. 4.6).
- Orally three or four times daily. Note that a relatively large dose is required because of the large first pass effect (metabolism in the liver; see p. 9), and side-effects are frequent.
- Slowly by the intravenous route to treat a severe asthmatic attack. This is rarely necessary as a nebulizer is usually very effective. Salbutamol through I.V. route requires careful monitoring for cardiac arrhythmias, and the nurse has an important role to play in monitoring the patient for cardiac arrhythmias when salbutamol is administered I.V.

In addition to its use in asthma, salbutamol is used to inhibit premature labour (see p. 224), and for treatment of hyperkalaemia. There are other selective $\beta_2$ agonists, which are very similar to salbutamol, e.g. terbutaline, fenoterol, reproterol and bambuterol.

### Salmeterol and eformoterol

These drugs are long-acting $\beta_2$ agonists. They are effective after about 30 minutes and their action lasts for about 12 hours; therefore they should not

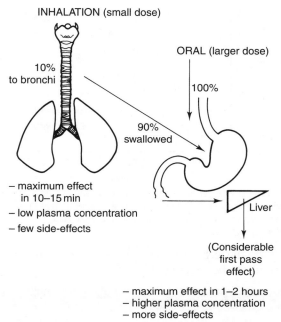

**Figure 4.6**    Comparison of inhalation and oral dosage of salbutamol.

be used for rapid effect in treating an acute attack, but given twice daily, by inhalation, as a preventative. It has been claimed they have some anti-inflammatory action as well as relieving bronchospasm, but this is controversial. They may be combined with an inhaled steroid.

## INHALATION DELIVERY SYSTEMS

Inhalation is a useful and effective way of giving some of the drugs used to treat asthma and other forms of bronchospasm (Fig. 4.7).

There are various delivery systems for inhalation. These delivery systems are:

- pressurized aerosol inhalers
- nebulizers
- delivery systems for children.

### Pressurized aerosol inhalers

These are the most convenient systems for routine use by patients. The drug is dissolved or suspended in a propellant and on pressing the plunger a standard amount is released in the form of fine particles measuring 2–5 µm. It is essential that the patient be

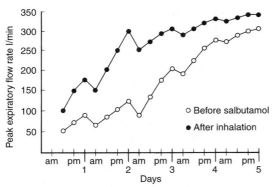

**Figure 4.7** The effect of inhalations of salbutamol on a patient with severe asthma. Note the progressive improvement in respiratory function and the morning dips which are characteristic of asthma.

taught the technique of using the inhaler if the treatment is to be effective (Fig. 4.8).

### Nursing point

Many patients require repeated instruction in the use of aerosols, particularly the young and elderly. Inhalers containing a placebo are available for teaching.

1. Remove the cap from the mouthpiece and shake the inhaler.
2. Breathe out slowly but not fully.
3. Place the mouthpiece in the mouth and close the lips around it.
4. Breathe in slowly and at the same time depress the plunger, thus releasing the drug.
5. Hold the breath for at least 10 seconds and longer if possible.
6. If a second inhalation is required, wait for 1 minute.
7. If steroids and $\beta_2$ agonists are both prescribed give the $\beta_2$ agonist first and wait for 5 minutes.

If inhalations are given on a regular basis they are required 4–6 hourly.

**Spacers.** Some patients lack the coordination required to use a pressurized aerosol. A spacer is a reservoir between the aerosol and the mouthpiece. Pressing the plunger releases the drug into the reservoir from whence it may be inhaled.

## Nebulizers

Nebulizers are used in severe asthma and chronic bronchitis and enable a larger dose to reach the bronchi. Air, or oxygen, is driven through a solution of the drug and the resulting mist is inhaled via a mask. It is important to have the correct particle size, which is best obtained by using an airflow rate of 6–8 litres/minute. Piped air or oxygen may be used; various mechanical compressors are available, which some patients use at home. It is important that these are cleaned regularly to prevent bacterial contamination.

Alternative drugs used in asthma and other types of bronchospasm can be given by inhalation, including corticosteroids (see later), sodium cromoglicate and ipratropium bromide.

### Delivery systems for children

Asthma is a common disease in childhood, affecting about 10% of children. It usually disappears in adolescence. Drug treatment with inhalers may be required but may be difficult to administer.

- Less than 18 months: nebulizers cannot be used
- 18 months to 2 years: nebulizer can be used
- 2–5 years: nebulizer and spacers can be used
- 5–10 years: as above
- Over 10 years: as for adults.

## ASTHMA

### THE CAUSES OF AN ASTHMATIC ATTACK

The cause of the disease is unknown, but asthma is believed to be an autoimmune disease. Patients with asthma have an inherent sensitivity of the bronchi that is probably inherited. The attacks are precipitated by trigger factors such as infection, exercise, various allergies and psychological factors that release substances in the bronchial wall causing spasm and inflammation. It is a common disorder that causes considerable morbidity and some mortality. The attack of asthma, with its characteristic wheeze, is due to narrowing of the bronchi by spasm of the circular muscle in the bronchial wall and inflammation with oedema of the bronchial mucosa.

### THE TREATMENT OF ASTHMA WITH DRUGS

The correct use of drugs, given either regularly to prevent an attack or intermittently to relieve one, plays an important part in the management of

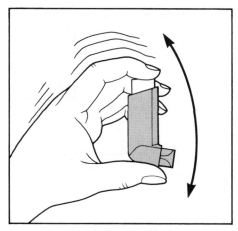

1  Remove the cover from the mouthpiece, and shake the inhaler vigorously.

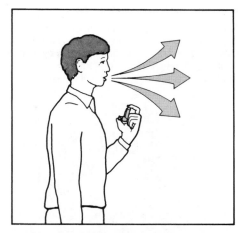

2  Holding the inhaler as shown above, breathe out gently (but not fully) and then immediately...

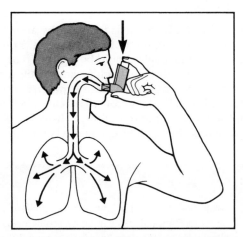

3  Place the mouthpiece in the mouth and close your lips around it. After starting to breathe in slowly and deeply through your mouth, press the inhaler firmly as shown above to release the medication and continue to breathe in.

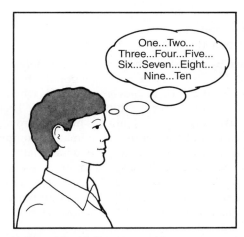

One...Two... Three...Four...Five... Six...Seven...Eight... Nine...Ten

4  Hold your breath for 10 seconds, or as long as is comfortable, before breathing out slowly.

5  If you are to take a second inhalation you should wait at least one minute before repeating steps 2, 3 and 4.

6  After use replace the cover on the mouthpiece.

**Figure 4.8**   How to use an inhaler properly.

asthma (Fig. 4.9). Several classes of drugs are used:

- bronchodilators
- corticosteroids
- sodium cromoglicate
- leukotriene modifiers.

### Bronchodilators

Bronchodilator drugs play an important part in the treatment of asthma. Bronchodilators used:

- inhaled $\beta_2$ agonists
- oral $\beta$ agonists

Attack of asthma with narrowing of the airways

Contraction of the circular muscle of the bronchus. Reversed by $\beta_2$ agonists, methylxanthines and ipratropium

Inflammation and swelling of the mucosa. Prevented and reversed by steroids, cromoglicate and montelukast

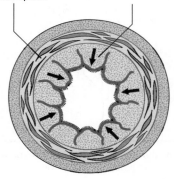

Figure 4.9    The asthma attack and its control by drugs.

High carbohydrate diet (−)
Liver disease (−)
Old age (−)

Drugs
oral contraceptive (−)
cimetidine (−)
erythromycin (−)
barbiturates (+)
alcohol (+)
rifampicin (+)

Smoking (+)

Broken down in liver into

methylxanthine

+ = (low blood levels) increased clearance,
− = (high blood levels) decreased clearance

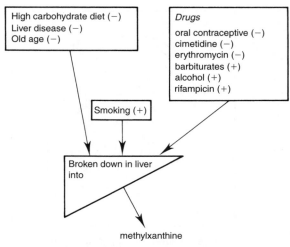

Figure 4.10    Factors affecting the blood level and activity of methylxanthines.

- methylxanthines
- anticholinergic drugs.

**Inhaled $\beta_2$ agonists.**    These drugs are widely prescribed. They are given by inhalation to treat a developing attack or to prevent an attack when it seems likely (e.g. exercise-induced asthma). Their regular use alone as a preventive is more controversial. They do not control the inflammatory component of asthma and there is some evidence that their regular use can lead ultimately to more severe and sometimes fatal attacks. If regular use of a $\beta_2$ agonist is required to control asthma most authorities advise that a corticosteroid (see below) should be added to the regimen.

**Oral $\beta_2$ agonists.**    Salbutamol tablets are not very efficient, but salbutamol controlled-release tablets, at a dose of one at night, have a prolonged action and are useful in preventing nocturnal attacks of asthma.

**Methylxanthines.**    This group of drugs inhibits the enzyme phosphodiesterase in the bronchial muscle, causing it to relax and thus relieve the bronchospasm. **Aminophylline** and **theophylline** belong to this group and, although they are effective, they require careful use, as there is only a small difference between the therapeutic and toxic dose. In addition, their rate of elimination depends on a number of factors, including weight, sex, age, concurrent disease and other medication, and may vary considerably (Fig. 4.10).

**Aminophylline** can be given slowly intravenously to terminate an acute attack. It can also be given as a loading dose followed by an infusion by pump or micropipette. If the infusion is prolonged, then plasma levels should be measured at intervals as a guide to dosage. High plasma levels may result if oral and intravenous administration are combined and this can be dangerous. Therefore, before giving intravenous aminophylline, always ask if the patient is already taking a methylxanthine orally.

**Nursing point**

Taken orally, aminophylline and theophylline may be nauseating but this can be overcome by using slow-release preparations, which require 12-hourly administration. This avoids peaks in plasma levels of these drugs, and is less likely to cause side-effects. Slow-release preparations must be swallowed whole to avoid interfering with the slow delivery system.

Because of inter-individual variation, fixed-dose regimens are not ideal and it is better to control dosage by measuring blood levels to obtain optimal results.

Available preparations include:

- Phyllocontin Continus – contains aminophylline
- Slo-Phyllin – contains granules which can be sprinkled on food for easier administration

*Adverse effects* are dose related and include nausea, anxiety, tachycardia and arrhythmias and convulsions. Interactions are common and effects are increased by cimetidine, erythromycin and oral contraceptives.

**Anticholinergic drugs.** Ipratropium bromide is related to atropine and acts as a bronchodilator by virtue of its anticholinergic action. It is given via an inhaler or a nebulizer. Any of the drug that is swallowed is not absorbed from the intestine. It has a powerful local action on the bronchi but avoids the unwanted side-effects of atropine (see p. 55). It should be used for those patients who have not responded to $\beta_2$ agonists. Its bronchodilator effect begins after about 45 minutes and lasts for 3–4 hours; therefore, it is best taken regularly to prevent an asthmatic attack. It may be combined with a $\beta_2$ agonist or corticosteroids. Adverse effects are an unpleasant taste and a dry mouth due to the blocking of salivation.

## Corticosteroids

Corticosteroids (steroids) reduce the inflammatory and allergic aspects of asthma and decrease bronchospasm in severe and persistent asthma. **Beclometasone** (a steroid that is well absorbed from mucous surfaces) can be given by inhalation. **Fluticasone** has less systemic effects for the same benefit. Occasional candida infection of the mouth may occur, presumably due to the lowering of local resistance by the steroid, and occasionally a hoarse voice develops due to weakening of the vocal cords. This effect usually disappears if the drug is stopped or the dose reduced.

### Nursing point

Patients on inhaled corticosteroids generally do not experience the side-effects associated with those seen after chronic use of tablets or injection (see p. 205), although children on high doses of inhaled corticosteroids may show a reduced growth rate. There is also a report that switching patients from inhaled corticosteroids to inhaled $\beta_2$ agonists such as salbutamol could destabilize their asthma and lead to treatment failure with the latter drug (Editorial 2002b).

In a few resistant cases of asthma oral prednisolone will be required, at the minimal effective dose.

The combined use of $\beta$ agonists and steroids is illustrated in the Case History given below.

## Sodium cromoglicate

Sodium cromoglicate prevents asthmatic attacks by stopping the release from bronchial mast cells of substances such as histamine that are responsible for bronchospasm. It is given regularly by pressurized aerosol or rotahaler. The usual dose is four inhalations daily. It is most effective in young patients with asthma with an allergic history but is of some use in non-allergic asthma.

**Nedocromil** is also a mast cell stabilizer and anti-inflammatory drug, and is very similar to sodium cromoglicate. It is given as a pressurized aerosol and is used to prevent rather than treat attacks.

## Leukotriene modifiers

Leukotrienes are substances that are produced by leucocytes involved in the inflammatory response and which cause spasm of the bronchial muscle. Asthmatic subjects appear to be very sensitive to this action, which plays an important part in the asthmatic attack. Drugs are becoming available which prevent spasm either by blocking the action of leukotrienes or by preventing inflammation. They also diminish hyperactivity of the bronchial mucosa and reduce inflammation. **Montelukast**, for example, can be given orally to adults and children over age 6. At present it is used as a continuous treatment for mild-to-moderate asthma and may reduce the need for other drugs. It is also useful in preventing exercise-induced asthma and that due to aspirin.

## MANAGEMENT OF CHRONIC ASTHMA

The management of asthmatic patients is not easy in spite of the number of remedies available and the various guidelines drawn up to advise on which therapy should be used. It is important that the management involves a partnership between the patient (or for children, including the parents) and the health professional: for example, health visitor and district nurse.

Drug therapy will depend on the age of the patient and the severity and pattern of attacks. The use of drugs in chronic asthma may be approached in stages, with the patient starting at the appropriate level and moving up or down according to the response to treatment. For adults and older children, the following programme is widely used:

*Stage 1:* The patient has occasional episodes of wheezing. These can be treated with an inhaled bronchodilator (usually a $\beta_2$ agonist). Bronchodilators can also be used as a preventative before some known precipitating trigger, e.g. exercise. If several inhalations are required daily, a move is made to the next stage.

*Stage 2:* Regular inhaled low-dose steroid or sodium cromoglicate is given and a $\beta_2$ agonist used as required. If this fails to prevent attacks, treatment should proceed to stage 3.

*Stage 3:* There is some difference of opinion as to the best drug combination at this stage: either high-dose inhaled steroid + a $\beta_2$ agonist as required or low-dose inhaled steroid + a long-acting $\beta_2$ agonist (e.g. **salmeterol**).

*Stage 4:* High-dose inhaled steroid + regular bronchodilator (e.g. $\beta_2$ agonist, methylxanthine or ipratropium used as is most appropriate).

*Stage 5:* Oral steroids are added to the regime.

In young children both the diagnosis of asthma and its management present special problems, which are beyond the scope of this book.

## MANAGEMENT OF STATUS ASTHMATICUS

A prolonged and severe attack of asthma can be very distressing to the patient and may be dangerous (Case History 4.1). The immediate treatment is:

### Case History 4.1

Mr A H was diagnosed as having atopic asthma at the age of 4 years and had several admissions to hospital during acute attacks, which were treated by nebulized $\beta$ agonists such as salbutamol (*Ventolin*), or the atropine-like drug ipratropium (*Atrovent*), all of which dilate the bronchi, and both intravenous and oral steroids which suppress the immune response. As he grew up he was maintained with inhaled steroids such as beclometasone using a space haler and his parents had to use his $\beta$ agonists infrequently, usually when he had a respiratory infection. Unfortunately, as with up to one-half of childhood asthma cases, his problem persisted into his adulthood. He was strongly advised not to smoke and to avoid aspirin and similar drugs such as ibuprofen. Beta blockers as a drug group must also be avoided, since, as explained in the text, they will block the action of the bronchodilators on $\beta$ receptors. As an adult he was maintained on a selective $\beta_2$ agonist

and a corticosteroid given by diskhaler, as he was not very coordinated when using a pressurized inhaler. He was advised to avoid any allergic stimulus known to precipitate his problem and periodic bone scans ordered because of his long-term use of steroids.

---

- Ensure adequate hydration of the patient, if necessary by infusion, as this will prevent the sputum becoming tenacious
- Use bronchodilators such as salbutamol by inhalation or, in very severe attacks, methylxanthines by continuous intravenous (I.V.) infusion
- Hydrocortisone, given I.V., or prednisolone orally, is given to reduce inflammation. Corticosteroids, even if given intravenously, however, take several hours to be effective
- No sedative drugs should be given due to the risk of respiratory depression
- Chest infection frequently complicates the attack and is treated with antibiotics such as amoxicillin
- Oxygen is administered as required
- Occasionally, patients who respond poorly will require artificial ventilation.

---

### Special points for patient education

It is very important that the patients learn to manage their own disease as far as possible and for children the parents should be fully involved. This means that they should be taught:

1. Modify their lifestyle as far as possible to avoid attacks, yet lead a normal life.
2. Understand the use of their drugs, whether they are for an acute attack or used prophylactically.
3. Understand the care and maintenance of their home nebulizer if they use one.
4. Learn to monitor their own disease by means of a peak flow meter and adjust their treatment accordingly. A peak flow of <70% of normal requires step-up treatment. With a peak flow of <50% of normal, the patient's doctor should be called for and corticosteroids started.
5. Recognize (both nurses and patients) the signs of dangerous deterioration in asthma. A rapid pulse (>110 per minute), rapid respiration (>25 per minute), exhaustion and inability to complete a sentence require that the doctor be called urgently and indicate that the patient will probably require hospital admission.

## CHRONIC OBSTRUCTIVE AIRWAYS DISEASE

This common disease differs from asthma in that it is progressive rather than intermittent, affects older people and is clearly related to smoking and air pollution. The small bronchi are obstructed by inflammation and excess mucus production (chronic bronchitis) and, in addition, there is destruction of the walls of the alveoli (emphysema). This reduces the total surface of the respiratory membranes available for gaseous exchange.

Treatment is not very satisfactory and is aimed at minimizing progressive lung destruction and treating acute exacerbations as they arise. It is essential that the patient gives up smoking and avoids air pollution as far as possible.

Bronchodilators are used as for asthma but their efficacy is variable and ipratropium may be better than $\beta_2$ agonists. A newer anticholinergic agent, **tiotropium**, has been reported to give good results in patients with chronic obstructive airways disease (Editorial 2002a).

Inhaled or systemic steroids are worthy of a trial, but if there is little or no improvement over a short course they should be tailed off. Exacerbation occurs, particularly in winter, due to infection of the bronchi and will require antibiotic treatment. Ultimately, a proportion of patients will progress to respiratory failure.

## OTHER SYMPATHOMIMETIC DRUGS

**Amfetamine** and **dexamfetamine** are similar drugs whose main effect is on the central nervous system. They produce some euphoria, abolish fatigue, increase activity and reduce appetite. They are taken orally. They carry a considerable risk of dependence and their therapeutic use is now confined to:

- narcolepsy (recurrent, uncontrollable episodes of sleep)
- some hyperactive children on whom, paradoxically, they have a sedative effect.

They should not be used for appetite control.

## ADRENERGIC BLOCKING AGENTS

It is possible to block α and β adrenergic receptors selectively.

## $\alpha_1$ ADRENERGIC BLOCKERS

Examples of uses:

- hypertension
- bladder neck obstruction.

### Hypertension

$\alpha_1$ Adrenergic blocking drugs are used in the treatment of hypertension. By removing the vasoconstrictor action of norepinephrine these drugs dilate arterioles and thus lower blood pressure. They are considered on p. 75. They are also used in the diagnosis of phaeochromocytoma (a rare epinephrine and norepinephrine-releasing tumour of the adrenal gland) when phentolamine is used.

### Bladder neck obstruction

$\alpha_1$ Adrenergic receptors control the smooth muscle round the neck of the bladder. By blocking these receptors it is possible to relax this muscle and partially relieve bladder neck obstruction due to an enlarged prostate. Several α blockers including doxazosin and terazosin can be used when surgical treatment is contraindicated.

## β ADRENERGIC BLOCKERS

This group of drugs, which block the effects of epinephrine and norepinephrine on β adrenergic receptors, is widely used and is a more important group of drugs than are the α blocking drugs. In general, their therapeutic effects and uses are very similar, but individual members of the group show minor differences:

- Some β blocking drugs block predominantly $\beta_1$ adrenoceptors (i.e. cardiac β receptors) and are called selective β blockers; others block both $\beta_1$ and $\beta_2$ receptors (i.e. cardiac + bronchial + peripheral blood vessel receptors) and are called non-selective β blockers.
- Members of the group differ in their speed and site of elimination and in their duration of action.

Table 4.2    Features of some β blockers in common use

| Drug | Selectivity | Elimination hepatic | Renal | Half-life (hours) |
|------|-------------|---------------------|-------|-------------------|
| Propranolol | $\beta_1 + \beta_2$ | + | − | 3 |
| Oxprenolol | $\beta_1 + \beta_2$ | + | − | 2 |
| Sotalol | $\beta_1 + \beta_2$ | (+) | + | 12 |
| Timolol | $\beta_1 + \beta_2$ | (+) | (+) | 5 |
| Nadolol | $\beta_1 + \beta_2$ | − | + | 16 |
| Metoprolol | $\beta_1 > \beta_2$ | + | − | 4 |
| Pindolol | $\beta_1 > \beta_2$ | (+) | + | 4 |
| Acebutolol | $\beta_1 > \beta_2$ | (+) | (+) | 6 |
| Atenolol | $\beta_1 > \beta_2$ | − | + | 12 |
| Bisoprolol | $\beta_1 > \beta_2$ | (+) | (+) | 10 |
| Betaxolol | $\beta_1 > \beta_2$ | ? | (+) | 16 |
| Esmolol | $\beta_1 > \beta_2$ | ? | ? | Very short |

### Safety point

The first β blocker introduced was **propranolol**, which is still in use, and it revolutionized the treatment of hypertension (see p. 79). It is, however, non-selective, and will block both $\beta_1$ and $\beta_2$ receptors, which makes it dangerous in asthma since it will block bronchodilation.

## General actions of β blockers (Table 4.2)

**Cardiovascular actions.**  When $\beta_1$ receptors in the heart are blocked, the heart rate is slowed, the cardiac output is reduced and the work done by the heart is thus decreased. This is particularly marked when there is increased activity of the sympathetic nervous system such as occurs with excitement or exercise. In addition, the excitability of heart muscle is reduced. β Blockers lower blood pressure.

**Respiratory actions.**  Blocking $\beta_2$ receptors with β blockers cause bronchospasm, particularly in patients with asthma. This is particularly marked with non-selective β blockers such as propranolol. This is usually of little consequence in healthy people, but in patients with asthma it may make bronchospasm worse and increase dyspnoea. Selective $\beta_1$ blockers have less effect on $\beta_2$ receptors.

**Metabolic actions.**  Some β blockers prevent the rise in blood glucose, which normally follows increased sympathetic activity.

**CNS actions.**  It is believed that at least some β adrenergic blockers penetrate the central nervous system. Some sedation is fairly common in patients

receiving β blockers and occasionally this may be severe. In addition, vivid dreams and, more rarely, hallucinations may occur.

Many of the symptoms of anxiety such as palpitations, sweating and tremor are mediated via the sympathetic nervous system. These symptoms can often be relieved by β blockers. Whether this is only a peripheral action or whether in addition there is some other effect on the brain is not known.

### Examples of uses

- Angina of effort (see p. 94), because they reduce the work of the heart, especially on effort or excitement.
- Cardiac arrhythmias, because they reduce the excitability of the heart.
- Hypertension as they lower blood pressure, perhaps by setting the regulation of blood pressure at a lower level.
- Thyrotoxicosis and anxiety, because they reduce the increased sympathetic activity which occurs in these disorders.
- Essential tremor, a rare familial condition characterized by severe intention tremor.
- Prevention of migraine attacks.

### Adverse effects

Adverse effects other than exacerbation of heart failure and of bronchospasm can be troublesome, but are not usually serious. Occasionally they cause vivid dreams and hallucinations, and by decreasing cardiac output they reduce the blood flow to the extremities, causing the patient to feel cold, and are best avoided in peripheral vascular disease. They mask the usual warning symptoms of hypoglycaemia and can be dangerous in patients with diabetes who are taking insulin (see p. 197). Active people may feel less energetic whilst taking these drugs.

**Labetalol** and **carvedilol** are combined $\alpha$ and $\beta$ blockers which are used to treat hypertension (see p. 79). Blocking $\alpha$ receptors dilates the arterioles, thus reducing blood pressure; blocking the $\beta$ receptors prevents the reflex speeding up of the heart ('palpitations') that occurs when cardiac $\beta_1$ receptors are activated in response to the fall in blood pressure.

## PARASYMPATHOMIMETIC DRUGS

Parasympathomimetic drugs have effects similar to those produced by activity of the parasympathetic nervous system. Examples of parasympathomimetic drugs are:

- acetylcholine
- carbachol
- bethanechol
- pilocarpine.

### ACETYLCHOLINE

Acetylcholine is released from the parasympathetic nerve endings throughout the body and also from motor nerve endings in voluntary muscle. Its effects as a result of parasympathetic release are shown in Table 4.1. In addition, acetylcholine activates voluntary muscle when a motor nerve is stimulated and is essential for all voluntary movements. Its action is very short-lived, as it is quickly broken down by cholinesterase to choline and acetate, so it is not used therapeutically. However, a prolonged effect can be produced either by giving an acetylcholine-like drug which is not broken down or by using a drug which inhibits the action of cholinesterase, thus prolonging and intensifying the actions of naturally occurring acetylcholine. This latter type of drug is called an anticholinesterase.

### CARBACHOL

Carbachol is a synthetic substance chemically related to acetylcholine. Its actions resemble those of parasympathetic stimulation. It is not broken down by the body cholinesterases and its actions are therefore much more prolonged than those of acetylcholine. Carbachol may be given by subcutaneous injection or by mouth.

### Uses of carbachol

The most important therapeutic use of carbachol is in the treatment of urinary retention following surgical operation or childbirth when there is no mechanical obstruction. It causes contraction of the bladder muscle, resulting in the passage of urine.

### Administration and effects of carbachol after injection

Carbachol may be given by subcutaneous injection or by mouth. After subcutaneous injection, flushing and sweating appear in about 20 minutes, followed by increased intestinal peristalsis sometimes with colic and contraction of the bladder muscle. These actions last up to an hour.

*Adverse effects* include colic, diarrhoea and a marked fall in blood pressure. These adverse effects are controlled by atropine.

### BETHANECHOL

Bethanechol is another acetylcholine-like drug, which, like carbachol, is not broken down by cholinesterase.

### PILOCARPINE

Pilocarpine is used only as eye drops, where it causes constriction of the pupil.

## THE ANTICHOLINESTERASES

These drugs prevent the breakdown by cholinesterase of acetylcholine produced at nerve endings throughout the body. The actions of acetylcholine are thus intensified at their two sites of action:

- on tissues innervated by the parasympathetic nerve endings
- on voluntary muscle.

It can thus be seen that the final picture produced by these groups of actions is mixed. The actions on tissues innervated by the parasympathetic nerve endings usually predominate, and the action on voluntary muscle is only seen under special circumstances.

## IMPORTANT EFFECTS OF ANTICHOLINESTERASES

- The eye: some anticholinesterases are absorbed through the conjunctiva and following application to the eye cause constriction of the pupil and spasm of accommodation.
- Gastrointestinal tract: anticholinesterases cause increased tone and motility.
- Urinary tract: anticholinesterases cause contraction of the bladder.

## CLINICALLY USED ANTICHOLINESTERASES

Several anticholinesterases are used to treat a variety of disorders depending on where their actions are most pronounced:

- neostigmine
- physostigmine
- pyridostigmine
- edrophonium
- distigmine.

### Neostigmine

Neostigmine is a synthetic anticholinesterase with actions very similar to those of physostigmine, but with an effect on the neuromuscular junction of voluntary muscle and less on the eye and cardiovascular system. It is rapidly effective following subcutaneous or intramuscular injection and is also absorbed after oral administration, although this route requires larger doses. Physostigmine is a naturally occurring anticholinesterase that is relatively short acting.

**Uses of neostigmine.** Neostigmine is used widely in the treatment of disorders in the neuromuscular junction of voluntary muscle (e.g. myasthenia gravis) (see p. 236), and has been used in cases of paralytic ileus and atony of the bladder.

**Pyridostigmine** and **edrophonium** are anticholinesterases used in the treatment of myasthenia gravis. Edrophonium has a very short-lived action.

**Distigmine** has widespread actions and may be used for urinary retention and myasthenia gravis. It can be given orally or by injection.

## ADVERSE EFFECTS OF THE ANTICHOLINESTERASES

All the anticholinesterases produce broadly similar adverse effects due to the prolonged action of acetylcholine. The symptoms include:

- intestinal colic and diarrhoea
- sweating and salivation
- pupils are constricted
- pulse slow
- blood pressure low.

**Treatment.** The immediate treatment is atropine given intravenously.

## NON-CLINICAL USES OF ANTICHOLINESTERASES

There are a number of other anticholinesterase preparations which are not used therapeutically but which are extensively employed as insecticides and are also potential lethal weapons for use in war. As some are absorbed though the intact skin and produce powerful anticholinesterase effects, they have been termed 'nerve gases'. These are the organophosphate anticholinesterases. Examples are malathion and parathion insecticides and the nerve gas sarin. They are dangerous because they combine irreversibly with the cholinesterase enzyme and new enzyme has to be produced. If organophosphate poisoning is suspected, the drug pralidoxime must be administered fast before the poison forms an irreversible bond with the enzyme. With luck, pralidoxime will regenerate some of the enzyme.

## DRUGS INHIBITING THE ACTION OF ACETYLCHOLINE

The drugs that inhibit the action of acetylcholine after it has been released from parasympathetic nerve endings belong mainly to the belladonna group or are synthetic substitutes. **Atropine** was originally extracted from the belladonna plant. Another natural example is **hyoscine**. These drugs produce their effect by blocking the action of acetylcholine on the cholinergic receptors in the organ concerned.

### EFFECTS OF BLOCKADE OF THE PARASYMPATHETIC DIVISION OF THE AUTONOMIC NERVOUS SYSTEM

The blockade of the parasympathetic division of the autonomic nervous system produces the following symptoms:

- Gastrointestinal tract: diminished motility of the stomach and both small and large intestines with relief of spasm.

- Secretions: decrease in salivary secretion and reduction of gastric acid secretion.
- Heart: diminished cardiac vagal tone, leading to an increase in pulse rate.
- Lungs: blockade of vagal (parasympathetic) action, leading to some relaxation of the bronchial muscle; diminished secretion from the bronchial glands.
- Involuntary muscle: relaxation of other voluntary muscles, notably those of the biliary and renal tracts.
- The eye: blockade of the parasympathetic nerve supply to the eye, leading to dilatation of the pupil and paralysis of accommodation with an inability to see near objects clearly.

## ATROPINE

### Uses of atropine

Atropine has several therapeutic uses, the more important of which are:

- *Relief of involuntary muscle spasm*: most forms of smooth muscle spasm are relieved by atropine, given subcutaneously or intravenously. It is useful in the relief of intestinal, biliary or renal colic.
- *Eye conditions*: atropine may be applied locally to the eye as an eye drop to dilate the pupil. Homatropine or tropicamide are often used for this purpose because their effects are not as prolonged as are those of atropine. Ophthalmologists may use a short-acting atropine-like drug such as **tropicamide** to dilate the pupil to facilitate examination of the eye.
- *Preoperative medication (pre-med)*: pre-med is not used as much as previously. Short-acting antimuscarinic agents were given preoperatively by subcutaneous injection to dry up the salivary and bronchial secretions and to protect the heart from undue vagal depression.
- *bronchial spasm*: an atropine derivative (**ipratropium**) is given by inhalation to relieve bronchospasm in asthma (see p. 49).

### Administration, absorption and elimination of atropine

Atropine is well absorbed from the intestine after oral administration; it can also be given subcutaneously, intramuscularly or intravenously. Atropine is largely broken down by the liver. Its effects last 2 hours or longer.

*Adverse effects* are dose related. Dry mouth, constipation, difficulty with micturition (in the elderly) and paralysis of ocular accommodation are common. After toxic doses restlessness, hallucination and delirium can occur. The patient appears flushed and the skin is hot to the touch.

### Safety point

It is important that atropine or similar drugs should not be given to those with a history of glaucoma. In this disorder the drainage of fluid from the eye is reduced and the pressure rises within the eyeball. Atropine further reduces the flow of fluid from the eye and may precipitate an acute attack of glaucoma (see p. 368).

## HYOSCINE

Hyoscine (scopolamine) is the drug traditionally beloved of mystery fiction writers, who call it the 'truth drug'. The peripheral actions of hyoscine are the same as those of atropine. Its action on the central nervous system differs, however, in that hyoscine, even in small doses, is a CNS depressant, leading to drowsiness and sleep. Hyoscine is particularly used for its central as well as peripheral effects. It is used preoperatively by injection and can be taken orally as an anti-emetic. Several proprietary travel sickness preparations contain hyoscine.

## SYNTHETIC ATROPINE-LIKE DRUGS

These drugs were developed to shorten the duration of action of the drug, e.g. tropicamide for use in the eye, or to target certain specific subtypes of the muscarinic receptor. For example, trihexyphenidyl is used clinically to treat Parkinson's disease since it is claimed selectively to target MI muscarinic receptors in the brain.

Among those available are:

- dicycloverine
- mebeverine
- propantheline
- oxybutynin
- flavoxate
- tolteridine.

## 5-HYDROXYTRYPTAMINE

5-Hydroxytryptamine (5-HT, Serotonin) is an important chemical neurotransmitter with actions in the nervous system and elsewhere. 5-Hydroxytryptamine is released by so-called serotonergic nerves and by some tumours, and reacts with several subtypes of 5-HT receptors. Its action depends on the class of receptor which is stimulated and on the organ involved. Drugs that block the actions of 5-HT at its various receptor sites are important in the treatment of various disorders – for example migraine (see below) – and are becomingly increasingly important in the treatment of psychiatric problems.

Abnormalities in the actions of 5-HT are involved in several disorders:

- brain: depression
- brain and gut: vomiting caused by certain cytotoxic drugs
- cranial blood flow: migraine
- carcinoid tumours produce large amounts of 5-HT which causes a variety of symptoms.

## SYMPTOMS OF MIGRAINE

Migraine is characterized by recurrent attacks of moderate-to-severe headache, often unilateral and pulsating, which may be associated with vomiting and preceded by visual disturbances (the aura). Its often-familial attacks may be precipitated by 'trigger' factors such as certain foods, alcohol, stress and hormonal influences, e.g. premenstrual tension, and the taking of the oral contraceptive pill. The aura is caused by a wave of depressed activity passing over the cerebral cortex associated with changes in the cerebral circulation. The headache is due to activation of the trigeminal nerve with release of substances that cause dilation of local blood vessels, leading to pain. Stimulation of 5-HT receptors in this area reverses the vasodilation and thus relieves the headache.

## TREATMENT OF THE ACUTE MIGRAINE ATTACK

Treatment is by non-specific drugs or 5-HT receptor-stimulating drugs.

### Non-specific drugs

- Aspirin
- Paracetamol
- Metoclopramide
- Tolfenamic acid.

The headache often responds to simple analgesics such as aspirin or paracetamol and some NSAIDs (non-steroidal anti-inflammatory drugs). They should be started early in the attack. Metoclopramide (see p. 125) may be given 30 minutes before the analgesic to prevent vomiting and increase the rate of gastric emptying and thus hasten absorption and relief of pain. Tolfenamic acid is an NSAID which, given orally, may be particularly effective.

In addition to the use of these drugs, it may help to lie down in a quiet, darkened room and some patients find a small dose of diazepam useful for promoting sleep. If these measures fail, as they do in about 20% of subjects, a specific remedy should be used.

### 5-HT receptor–stimulating drugs

- Sumatriptan
- Naratriptan
- Zolmitriptan
- Ergotamine.

**Sumatriptan** stimulates 5-HT receptors in the wall of the dilated blood vessels surrounding the brain and on the trigeminal nerve, resulting in vasoconstriction, thus relieving the headache. It is given by subcutaneous injection as soon as possible after the onset of symptoms and relieves the headache within 1 hour in most patients. Its action lasts about 2 hours, after which the headache may return. It can be repeated once after 1 hour if necessary. It is also available for oral use and as a nasal spray. It is effective in about 85% of patients by injection and 60% if given orally. Sumatriptan is undoubtedly effective for treating a migraine attack but it is rather expensive.

*Adverse effects* are rare but a few patients report tightness in the chest. Although clinical evidence of myocardial ischaemia is very rare, it should not be given to patients with coronary artery disease in view of the risk of arterial spasm and it should not be combined with ergotamine. It may also cause dizziness and nausea.

**Naratriptan** and **Zolmitriptan** are similar and are given orally.

### Ergot

Ergot is a fungus that grows on rye. It has a notorious history and was responsible for thousands of deaths due to the consumption of cereals contaminated with the fungus. Ergot contains many pharmacologically active substances, and three of those substances are relevant here. They are:

- ergometrine (see p. 223)
- ergotamine
- methysergide.

**Ergotamine.**    This drug stimulates $\alpha_1$ adrenoceptors of the sympathetic division of the autonomic nervous system and therefore causes vasoconstriction, particularly of small arteries. It may also cause vasoconstriction by reacting with 5-HT receptors. It is not an analgesic but relieves the migraine headache by its vasoconstrictor action.

*Use of ergotamine:*    Ergotamine has been widely used to treat migraine headaches, but its popularity has declined due to its adverse effects and the introduction of newer remedies.

*Administration:*    Ergotamine can be taken orally and has been combined with caffeine as Cafergot. It is also available combined with cyclizine as Migril tablets. Ergotamine is also absorbed rectally and via the respiratory passages and an aerosol inhaler is available.

*Adverse effects:*    These include vomiting, diarrhoea and peripheral vasoconstriction, which can be severe enough to cause vasospasm and consequent gangrene. Tingling and numbness are an indication to stop treatment immediately. The vasospasm can sometimes be treated successfully using infusions of nitroprusside or glyceryl trinitrate. Withdrawal of ergotamine, particularly after heavy dosage, may itself cause headaches. It is contraindicated in coronary disease and pregnancy. Vasoconstriction is increased in patients taking $\beta$ blockers.

## PREVENTION OF MIGRAINE ATTACKS

Frequent attacks of migraine can be very debilitating and can interfere seriously with living a normal life. If, after excluding trigger factors, the attacks occur more than once a week it may be necessary to use continuous drug treatment as a preventative measure. At present there is no clear-cut best drug so the choice is a matter of weighing efficacy against side-effects for a particular patient.

| Special points for patient education in migraine |
| --- |
| 1. Patients must be taught which drugs are used to relieve an acute attack and which are used for prevention. |
| 2. It should be stressed that ergotamine should only be taken to relieve attacks and for a limited number of doses, not taken regularly for prevention as this will lead to serious side-effects and may actually cause headaches. |
| 3. Migraine attacks may be precipitated by a variety of external factors, such as certain foods and the Pill. The patient should learn to recognize these and avoid them if possible. |

Drugs used to prevent migraine attacks:

- $\beta$ blockers
- pizotifen
- sodium valproate
- antidepressants
- methysergide.

### $\beta$ blockers

$\beta$ blockers prevent or reduce attacks in about half of the patients. They probably act by reducing vasodilation and there is no preferred $\beta$ blocker for this purpose. When they are prescribed, their contraindications must be remembered and they should not be combined with ergotamine.

### Pizotifen

This drug is concerned with the action of 5-HT and prevents migraine attacks by reducing the constriction and dilatation of blood vessels. It can cause drowsiness and the initial dose should be given at night. Its main adverse effect is weight gain and it may take up to a month to be effective.

### Sodium valproate

Sodium valproate (see also p. 249) is an antiepileptic agent that can also be used to prevent migraine attacks. It should not be used in pregnancy, owing to the risk of fetal malformation, and, rarely, it can cause liver damage and a reduction of platelets in the blood.

### Antidepressants

**Dosulepin** and **amitriptyline** are effective, even if the patient is not suffering from depression.

### Methysergide

Methysergide blocks the action of 5-HT on receptors in smooth muscle. It is effective but has serious adverse effects and should only be used when safer treatment has failed.

---

### Nursing point

The overuse of simple analgesic drugs, particularly when combined with caffeine or opioids, can itself cause headaches and nurses should enquire about analgesic consumption in those with frequent headaches.

---

### Summary

- Epinephrine is used as an intramuscular (I.M.) injection in the treatment of anaphylactic shock, but be careful not to inject into a vein
- Epinephrine is used I.V. for cardiac arrest, but don't use the same I.V. line used for sodium bicarbonate

---

- Norepinephrine can be used to treat shock associated with large drops in blood pressure, but is not commonly used to raise blood pressure because it reduces blood flow through the kidneys
- Isoprenaline is no longer used to treat asthma because it stimulates both $\beta_1$ (heart) and $\beta_2$ (lung) receptors, and can cause fatal arrhythmias. Selective $\beta_2$ agonists such as salbutamol are used for asthma and to inhibit premature labour
- Inhalation is the preferred route to treat asthma, and pressurized inhalers and nebulizers are the main delivery systems used. Note age restrictions for their use in children
- Note the treatment of status asthmaticus (p. 50)
- $\beta$ Blockers lower blood pressure
- Be careful with the use of ergotamine in migraine. It can cause prolonged vasospasm that may result in gangrene

---

## References

Editorial 2002b Switching from corticosteroids to $\beta_2$ agonists may destabilise asthma. Pharmaceutical Journal 268: 710

Moniotte S, Balligand J L 2002 Potential use of beta(3)-adrenoceptor antagonists in heart failure therapy. Cardiovascular Drug Reviews 20: 19

## Further reading

Barnes P J 1995 Inhaled glucocorticosteroids for asthma. New England Journal of Medicine 332: 868

Chapman K R, Keston S, Szaiai J P 1994 Regular versus as-needed inhaled salbutamol in asthma control. Lancet 343: 1379

Cross S 1997 Revised guidelines for asthma management. Professional Nurse 12: 408

Editorial 1987 Nebulisers in the treatment of asthma. Drug and Therapeutics Bulletin 25: 101

Editorial 1997 Using $\beta_2$ stimulants in asthma. Drug and Therapeutics Bulletin 35: 1

Editorial 1998 Leukotriene modifiers in the treatment of asthma. British Medical Journal 316: 1257

Editorial 1994 Treating mild asthma – when are inhaled steroids indicated? New England Journal of Medicine 331: 737

Editorial 2002a Tiotropium gives good results in patients with chronic obstructive airways disease. Pharmaceutical Journal 268: 278

Fehrenbach C 2002 Chronic obstructive airways disease. Nursing Standard 20: 45

Ferrari M D 1998 Migraine. Lancet 351: 1043

Goadsby P J, Olesen J 1996 Diagnosis and management of migraine. British Medical Journal 312: 1279

Leach A 1994 Making sense of peak-flow recordings of lung function. Nursing Times 90: 34

Lipworth B J 1997 Treatment of acute asthma. Lancet supplement 350: 18

Pearce L 1998 A guide to asthma inhalers. Nursing Times supplement March 1998

Rees J, Price J 1995 Treatment of chronic asthma. British Medical Journal 310: 1459

# Chapter 5

# Drugs acting on the heart

## Learning objectives

At the end of this chapter, the reader should be able to:

- list the factors that determine cardiac output
- describe the causes and consequences of heart failure
- describe the main approaches to the treatment of heart failure and the major types of drugs used
- give an account of the mechanism of action, use and the toxic and adverse effects of digoxin
- describe the overall strategies for care as well as drug treatment of patients with heart failure
- give an account of the normal cardiac cycle of the spread of electrical excitability and muscle contraction
- discuss the nature of arrhythmias due to cardiac overexcitability and conduction defects in the bundle of His
- list the names of drugs used to treat different types of arrhythmias and their basic mechanism of action

Drugs can treat two major disorders of the heart. These disorders are:

- cardiac failure
- cardiac arrhythmias.

## CARDIAC FAILURE

### THE CARDIAC OUTPUT

The heart is a muscular pump receiving blood from the systemic and pulmonary veins and driving it, under pressure, into the pulmonary arteries and the aorta. The volume of blood passing through the

**Figure 5.1** Processes in cardiac failure.

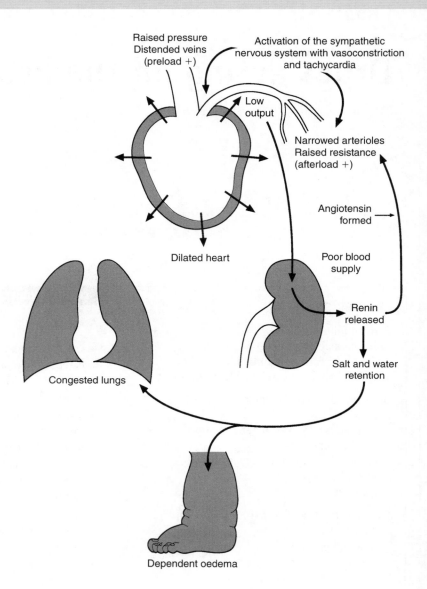

Raised pressure
Distended veins
(preload +)

Activation of the sympathetic
nervous system with vasoconstriction
and tachycardia

Low
output

Narrowed arterioles
Raised resistance
(afterload +)

Angiotensin
formed

Dilated heart

Poor blood
supply

Renin
released

Salt and water
retention

Congested lungs

Dependent oedema

heart each minute is known as the cardiac output. This is largely determined by four factors:

- **The preload** – the pressure in the venous system filling the heart and stretching the cardiac muscle. In health, a rise in venous pressure causes a rise in cardiac output.
- **The afterload** – the arterial pressure that is the resistance against which the heart must pump.
- **The heart rate** – an increase in rate leads to an increased output, except in heart failure when an increased rate decreases cardiac efficiency.
- **The contractile efficiency** of the cardiac muscle.

In good health, the cardiac output varies considerably depending on the needs of the body, being low at rest and rising with exercise. The healthy heart has a great functional reserve and can cope with demands for increased output that occur from time to time.

## CAUSES OF CARDIAC FAILURE

The contractility of the cardiac muscle is reduced through disease:

- the heart muscle may be damaged by previous coronary thrombosis or by cardiomyopathy

• high blood pressure or valve disease may cause an increased workload over a long period, which ultimately causes the heart to fail.

## CONSEQUENCES OF CARDIAC FAILURE

• The ventricles fail to empty properly and the heart becomes enlarged.

• The muscle becomes thicker and stiffer and, in diastole, fails to relax completely; thus, filling of the ventricles is diminished.

• The heart and neck veins become distended with blood and cannot respond to the increased filling pressure (preload) by raising output. At first this is only apparent on exercise but, later, occurs at rest.

• The pump becomes insufficient for the needs of the body and various organs receive an inadequate blood and oxygen supply. This is particularly important in the kidney, where it activates the renin/angiotensin system (see p. 74), causing the kidney to retain salt and water.

• Oedema of dependent parts and lungs develops, the latter being responsible for marked dyspnoea (shortness of breath), which is a common feature of cardiac failure. Angiotensin is also responsible for arterial constriction, which increases the work (afterload) of an already labouring heart. This is further aggravated by an increase in sympathetic activity, causing additional vasoconstriction and tachycardia.

• The low cardiac output carries less oxygen to the tissues. The oxygen supply to the heart and brain is kept up at the expense of other organs, which are starved of oxygen, and this accounts for the fatigue, which may be a prominent symptom (Fig. 5.1).

## DRUGS IN CONGESTIVE CARDIAC FAILURE

Two main approaches are used, either alone or together:

• increase cardiac contractility
• decrease the workload of the heart.

Five main groups of drugs are used:

• Diuretics, which cause the kidney to excrete excess salt and water (see p. 162).
• ACE inhibitors, which act by suppressing the angiotensin/renin mechanism, which is overactive

in cardiac failure. (ACE is the acronym for angiotensin-converting enzyme.)

• Positive inotropic drugs, which are drugs that improve the function of the cardiac muscle so that the heart contracts more powerfully and it empties more completely, thereby raising the cardiac output. This is called a positive inotropic effect.

• Vasodilators, which lower peripheral resistance and thus reduce cardiac work.

• β Blockers, which reduce inappropriate sympathetic activity.

## DIURETICS

Diuretics increase urine flow. They are considered in detail on p. 162. Both thiazide and loop diuretics are used in cardiac failure.

### Mechanism of action

• They help to get rid of oedema and pulmonary congestion by increasing the excretion of salt and water

• They relieve distension of the heart by reducing blood volume.

### Disadvantages

• Renin release by the kidney is activated by reduced blood volume, and this may partially reverse the diuretic's beneficial effects by stimulating the kidney to retain fluid.

• Vasoconstriction will occur in response to reduced blood volume, and this will increase the work of the heart.

• Potassium loss: both thiazide and loop diuretics increase potassium loss via the kidney. If small doses are used this is unlikely to require correction but can occur if large doses of diuretic are used, if dietary potassium is deficient (e.g. in those whose diet is poor, or elderly), or if concurrent digoxin is given.

Nevertheless, the benefits usually outweigh the disadvantages and diuretics are widely used for the relief of chronic cardiac failure. For mild heart failure thiazide diuretics may be adequate but more severe heart failure will require a loop diuretic such as furosemide (frusemide). Non-steroidal anti-inflammatory drugs (NSAIDs) such as aspirin will reduce the efficacy of diuretics.

---

**Nursing point**

Digoxin is associated with potassium loss and potassium deficiency increases digoxin toxicity. Supplementary potassium or a potassium sparing diuretic should be added to the regimen (see p. 166). When patients with heart failure are prescribed thiazides or loop diuretics, the plasma potassium concentration should be monitored and kept above 3.2 mmol/litre.

---

## ANGIOTENSIN-CONVERTING ENZYME (ACE) INHIBITORS (see p. 77)

This group of drugs, which is also used to treat hypertension, has emerged as an important addition to the management of chronic heart failure. ACE inhibitors have considerably improved the treatment of cardiac failure and have prolonged survival.

### Mechanism of action

ACE inhibitors block the overactive renin/angiotensin mechanism (see p. 74). This results in a reduction of salt and water by the kidneys and, in addition, by dilating arterioles ACE inhibitors lower the resistance to blood flow from the heart (afterload), reduce cardiac work and raise cardiac output.

### Disadvantages

The initiation of treatment requires much care. The main danger is a profound fall in blood pressure after the first dose, which is especially liable to occur in patients already taking diuretics, and is due to vasodilatation and a low blood volume resulting from the diuretic treatment.

---

**Nursing point**

The initial dose of ACE inhibitor should be low and the blood pressure should be closely monitored (4 hourly) for 24 hours. ACE inhibitors should not be given to patients with renal failure or in pregnancy. Renal function should be measured at regular intervals for those on long-term treatment.

---

**Nursing point**

When monitoring the blood pressure following the first dose of an ACE inhibitor, it should be remembered that the fall after captopril only lasts a few hours but that after enalapril may be delayed for up to 8 hours and last up to 30 hours.

---

For other adverse effects, see p. 78.

## POSITIVE INOTROPIC DRUGS: DIGOXIN

Digoxin is at present the only important drug for directly strengthening the heartbeat. Doctors have used this drug for hundreds of years. In 1785 William Withering of Birmingham described the use of foxglove in dropsy (oedema) and noted that it appeared to act on the heart. Digoxin was originally extracted from the foxglove plant but is now produced synthetically. (In older textbooks, the term 'digitalis' is used because it refers to the mixture of active principles extracted from the foxglove plant.)

### Mechanism of action

Digoxin has two actions on the heart:

- direct
- indirect.

   **Direct action.** Digoxin acts directly on the heart to strengthen the heartbeat. The strengthening of the heartbeat is called a positive inotropic effect of the drug. Interestingly, these powerful inotropic actions of digoxin are observed only on the *failing* heart.

   **Indirect action.** At lower doses, digoxin slows the heart through activation of the parasympathetic division of the autonomic nervous system, which slows it down. This is known to be the case because this action of digoxin can be blocked by atropine. The indirect action is important, especially in atrial fibrillation (see p. 67), because the slowing of the heart allows for slower and more regular contractions, which increases cardiac output.

### Effects of digoxin on the failing heart

   • Increased force of contraction of the ventricular muscle (Fig. 5.2). This action is due to an increase in calcium ions in cardiac muscle cells (direct action;

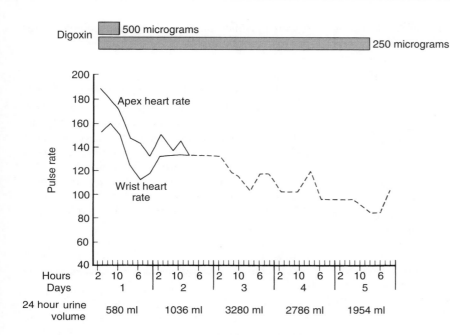

**Figure 5.2** The effect of digoxin in a patient with atrial fibrillation and heart failure. Note the difference between the heart rate at the apex and the rate at the wrist due to weak contractions failing to produce a pulse at the wrist. The difference disappears on treatment with digitalis.

see above). In large doses this may be associated with increased excitability of the ventricle.

- Depression of conduction in the atrioventricular (AV) node and the bundle of His (Fig. 5.3). This action does not affect the heart in sinus rhythm, but in atrial fibrillation it decreases the number of impulses reaching the ventricles from the fibrillating atria, and thus decreases the rate of ventricular contraction.

- Slowing of the heart rate, partially due to increased activity of the vagus nerve (indirect action; see above) and partly to a direct action on the sino-atrial node.

## Diuretic effects of digoxin

Digoxin may cause a powerful diuresis after administration to patients with heart failure. This effect is not seen in patients with healthy hearts. The diuretic effect is due to the inotropic action of digoxin. In patients with heart failure, the increased preload (venous pressure) pushes fluid out of the capillary beds into the tissues and causes oedema. The restored power of the heart reduces the preload, which in turn allows extravascular fluid to re-enter the circulation and be eliminated through normal fluid control via the kidneys.

## Plasma monitoring of digoxin

Plasma levels of digoxin should be monitored, the correct therapeutic range being between 0.9 and 2 micrograms/litre (the sample is taken at least

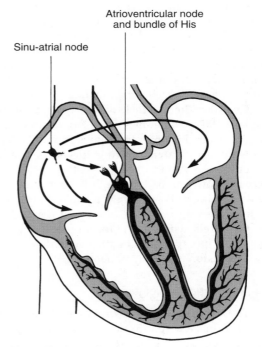

**Figure 5.3** The heart, showing the sinu-atrial node and conducting system (atrioventricular node and bundle of His).

6 hours after dosing). There is, however, considerable interpersonal variation and the estimation of plasma levels is more useful to confirm non-compliance or overdose than in the control of treatment where

clinical observation is usually adequate. It will be noted that the action of these drugs lasts for several days. This is not due only to slow elimination, but because, once bound to cardiac muscle, their action is prolonged.

## Adverse effects and toxicity of digoxin

There is a relatively small difference between the therapeutic dose of digoxin and the toxic dose, i.e. digoxin has a low therapeutic index, so dosage should be carefully regulated. Elderly patients, especially those with renal impairment and with hypothyroidism, are more liable to suffer adverse effects. The nurse should keep a watch for toxicity and should know the common manifestations of overdose:

- **Undue slowing of the heart** due to excessive effect on the conducting system or the sino-atrial node. A pulse rate below 60 indicates that the drug should be omitted for a day or two.
- **Coupled beats**: these are due to ventricular extrasystoles following normal beats. They are felt at the wrist as a double pulsation followed by a pause. The extrasystoles result from increased excitability of the ventricles and are an indication to omit the drug. Continued overdosing may lead to ventricular paroxysmal tachycardia or even ventricular fibrillation, which is rapidly fatal.
- **Complete heart block** with a ventricular rate of about 100 is sometimes seen. An electrocardiogram is required in order to diagnose this disorder.
- **Nausea and later vomiting**: this is due to stimulation of the vomiting centre in the medulla by digoxin. However, as heart failure itself may produce vomiting, it is not a very reliable symptom of an overdose.
- **Coloured vision** in the form of yellow haloes may rarely be experienced with an overdose.
- **Confusion** in elderly patients.

## Drug interactions of digoxin

- The action of digoxin is increased by verapamil (p. 69), diltiazem (p. 75) and amiodarone (p. 70) and the dose should be halved if these drugs are introduced.
- Lowering the level of potassium in the blood increases the toxicity of digoxin. Certain diuretics may cause potassium loss (see p. 165) and their administration may result in the appearance of signs of digoxin overdose in a patient who has been satisfactorily treated for a long time. Any drug that lowers plasma potassium (i.e. diuretics) potentiates the toxicity of digoxin.

## VASODILATORS

Several vasodilators have been used with some success in cardiac failure and include sodium nitroprusside (see p. 78) and nitrates (see p. 94). Vasodilators reduce the work of the heart by lowering peripheral resistance and, by dilating the veins, lower the venous pressure and allow the heart to beat more effectively. However, they are less effective than ACE inhibitors and are usually only used for short-term emergencies.

## β BLOCKERS

The use of β blockers to treat cardiac failure is more controversial. In this condition there is increased activity of the sympathetic nervous system, which may be inappropriate, and β blockers will reduce this activity. Because of their depressing action on cardiac function, however, they can exacerbate cardiac failure. At present, there is probably a place for small and carefully controlled doses of β blockers in certain patients, provided their heart failure is not too severe or of recent onset.

Recently, there have been reports of the discovery of a novel $\beta_3$ adrenoceptor in cardiac muscle, which is negatively inotropic – i.e. reduces the force of contraction of heart muscle – and, if so, it may provide potential $\beta_3$ receptor antagonists to treat cardiac failure (Moniotte & Balligand 2002).

## CARE AND TREATMENT OF PATIENTS WITH CARDIAC FAILURE

The three main objectives in treating cardiac failure are:

- to increase the efficiency and output of the heart, so that there is sufficient blood and oxygen supply to the various organs
- to reduce congestion and oedema
- to try where possible to remove or diminish the factor(s) which caused the heart to fail.

## DIET AND POSTURE

Drugs are only part of the treatment. Patients with cardiac failure are nursed in a sitting position so that the accumulated fluid from oedema drains away from the lungs and abdominal viscera to the legs and does not embarrass respiration. Although the legs may be slightly elevated on a stool when the patient is sitting out of bed, they should not be raised above the horizontal as this may shift fluid to the abdomen and lungs. Constipation may be a problem requiring modification of diet and, sometimes, a purgative or suppository.

These patients usually require easily digested and light foods. Retention of salt is as important as retention of water by the kidneys in producing oedema. Modern diuretics will usually enable the kidneys to excrete salt and a low-salt diet is rarely required. Opinions vary as to the correct fluid intake but it is not usually necessary to restrict it. However, in severe heart failure or when sodium deficiency has developed as a result of prolonged and intensive diuretic treatment, intake should be cut to 1500 ml daily and the regime arranged to minimize the patient's discomfort. Patients in bed with cardiac failure are liable to develop venous thrombosis and it is common practice to give prophylactic treatment with heparin subcutaneously twice daily.

> ### Nursing point
>
> Mistakes with digitalis dosage are not uncommon. Three strengths of digoxin tablet are currently available – 62.5, 125 and 250 micrograms. The paediatric elixir contains 50 micrograms/ml. To avoid confusion, the dose should be written in micrograms.

## TREATMENT OF CARDIAC FAILURE WITH DRUGS

In mild or moderate heart failure treatment is usually started with diuretics, either thiazides for minimal failure or loop diuretics for more severe failure. They are given once daily by mouth. Patients should be weighed regularly at the same time of day and in the same clothes to assess the efficacy of treatment. This may be sufficient treatment and can be carried out at home under the supervision of the patient's primary care team.

There is a tendency to introduce ACE inhibitors into the therapeutic regime early in treatment. They should certainly be used if the response to diuretics is not satisfactory or if cardiac failure is severe, but many doctors think there is a place for their use even in moderate failure, and there is evidence that they not only control symptoms but also prolong life. Digoxin was formerly used extensively in heart failure both to stimulate contraction of the heart and to slow the pulse rate, thus raising the cardiac output. It is now realized that the effect on the contraction is short-lived and less important than it was once considered to be, so its main use in heart failure is to slow the pulse rate, particularly in atrial fibrillation.

Acute failure of the left ventricle, which commonly occurs in patients with high blood pressure or following a cardiac infarct, leads to rapidly developing oedema of the lungs with distress and shortness of breath. It is best treated with a rapidly acting diuretic such as furosemide (frusemide), and with morphine or diamorphine, which sedate the patient. If necessary, these drugs may be combined with prochlorperazine to control vomiting. Vasodilators may also be used. Glyceryl trinitrate dilates the veins and reduces the filling pressure and distension of the heart. Sodium nitroprusside, in addition, relaxes the arterioles, thus reducing cardiac work. Both drugs are usually given by intravenous infusion and dosage requires careful monitoring.

> ### Nursing point
>
> Calcium antagonists may make cardiac failure worse and should be avoided if possible in this disorder; NSAIDs reduce the effect of diuretics and can cause fluid retention with oedema.

## ANCILLARY DRUGS

Various ancillary drugs may be used in the treatment of cardiac failure. A hypnotic drug may be required if the patient cannot sleep. In the very restless and ill patient, morphine is helpful, particularly in acute failure of the left ventricle, but it must be used with care in patients who are cyanosed, as depression of respiration may occur. If cyanosis is a marked feature, oxygen is given at full concentration unless the patient has concurrent chronic respiratory disease, in which case the concentration should be controlled.

It is not easy to remove the cause of the cardiac failure, but some of the precipitating factors can now be treated. Drugs can reduce high blood pressure, and advances in cardiac surgery have enabled many defects of the valves of the heart to be relieved.

## CARDIAC ARRHYTHMIAS

### THE NORMAL CARDIAC CYCLE

In the normal heart the initial stimulus of contraction starts in the sino-atrial node (the pacemaker of the heart) situated at the junction of the superior vena cava and the right atrium (see Fig. 5.3). The rate of discharge from the node is under the control of the vagus and sympathetic nerves. Vagal activity slows the heart rate and sympathetic activity increases it. The wave of contraction spreads over both atria, forcing blood into the ventricles. The stimulus then pauses for a fraction of a second at the atrioventricular (AV) node before passing down the bundle of His and spreading through the muscles of both ventricles, which contract and drive blood into the pulmonary artery and the aorta. The heart then relaxes, refills with venous blood and awaits the next stimulus for contraction.

### SOME USEFUL DEFINITIONS

- **Arrhythmia**: variation from the normal rhythm of the heartbeat, encompassing abnormalities of rate, regularity, site of impulse origin, and sequence of activation.
- **Atrial escape rhythm**: a cardiac dysrhythmia occurring when sustained suppression of sinus impulse formation causes other atrial foci to act as cardiac pacemakers.
- **Atrial fibrillation**: atrial arrhythmia marked by rapid, randomized contraction of small areas of the atrial myocardium, causing an irregular and often rapid ventricular rate.
- **Bradycardia**: slowing of the heart rate; pulse rate falls below 60.
- **Cardioversion**: restoration of the normal rhythm of the heart by cardioversion, which is the application of a controlled direct current shock to the heart of an anaesthetized patient using electrodes placed on the chest wall. The apparatus used is called a cardiovertor.
- **Coupled rhythm**: heartbeats occurring in pairs, the second beat usually being a premature ventricular beat.
- **Ectopic rhythm**: a heart rhythm originating outside the sino-atrial node.

- **Extrasystole**: a premature cardiac contraction independent of the normal rhythm, which arises in response to an impulse outside of the sino-atrial node.
- **Sinus rhythm**: the normal heart rhythm that originates in the sino-atrial node.
- **Supraventricular rhythm**: any cardiac rhythm originating above the ventricles.
- **Tachycardia**: very rapid heart rate.
- **Ventricular fibrillation**: cardiac arrhythmia marked by fibrillary contractions of the ventricular muscle due to rapid, repetitive excitation of myocardial fibres without coordinated ventricular contraction and by absence of atrial activity. It is often fatal.

### DISORDERS OF CARDIAC RHYTHM

Disorders of cardiac rhythm can be divided into:

- those due to **overexcitability of the heart**, which are by far the most common
- those due to **conduction defects** in the bundle of His.

#### Arrhythmias due to overexcitability

These can be divided into:

- extrasystoles (ectopic beats)
- paroxysmal tachycardia
- supraventricular tachycardias
- atrial flutter
- atrial (auricular) fibrillation.

**Extrasystoles (ectopic beats).** Extrasystoles are caused by an excitable focus, either in the atria or ventricles, which stimulates the heart to contract while relaxed and awaiting the next normal stimulus. This normal stimulus then falls on a heart in the unresponsive or refractory phase, which immediately follows a contraction, and there is a pause before normal rhythm is resumed. Extrasystoles are very common in healthy people and although they may be associated with heart disease they are usually of little significance. They may be related to excessive smoking or to the consumption of tea, coffee or alcohol. They rarely require treatment other than reassurance.

**Paroxysmal tachycardias.** These comprise supraventricular and ventricular tachycardias. Paroxysmal tachycardia may arise from the ventricle (ventricular) or from the atria or atrioventricular node

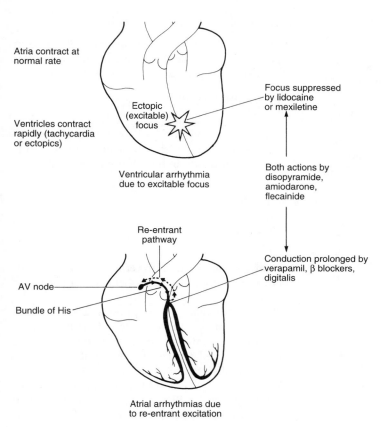

**Figure 5.4**   The mechanisms of paroxysmal tachycardias.

Atria contract at normal rate

Ectopic (excitable) focus

Focus suppressed by lidocaine or mexiletine

Ventricles contract rapidly (tachycardia or ectopics)

Ventricular arrhythmia due to excitable focus

Both actions by disopyramide, amiodarone, flecainide

Re-entrant pathway

Conduction prolonged by verapamil, β blockers, digitalis

AV node

Bundle of His

Atrial arrhythmias due to re-entrant excitation

(supra-ventricular). In ventricular tachycardia an excitable focus in the ventricle stimulates the ventricle to contract regularly at about 160–180 times a minute. It frequently occurs in diseased hearts, for instance after a cardiac infarct (Fig. 5.4).

**Supraventricular tachycardias.** Supraventricular tachycardias are believed to have a rather different mechanism. They are usually due to a rapid circus movement within the AV node which fires off ventricular contractions via the bundle of His at about 160/minute. This is known as a re-entrant phenomenon. If the circus movement is suppressed, the heart returns to normal rhythm. Less commonly, there is an accessory pathway between the atria and the ventricles, which is involved in the re-entrant phenomenon (see Wolff–Parkinson–White syndrome, p. 71).

The terms 'circus' and 're-entrant' (see Fig. 5.4) need explaining. When an area of the ventricular wall is damaged, e.g. through ischaemia (poor perfusion with blood and oxygen starvation), this area is depressed and cannot conduct the impulses that course through the ventricle wall. This can result in a local circular movement of impulses around the damaged area (hence 'circus'). Instead of continuing on their way through the ventricle wall, some of the impulses re-enter the damaged area, thereby setting up a local focus or beat that produces arrhythmias. Interestingly, and usefully, these foci of electricity are more easily suppressed by drugs than are the normal flows of current through the ventricular wall.

Attacks of paroxysmal tachycardia may last for anything from a few seconds to hours or even days. They may occur in quite healthy people or they may complicate heart disease.

**Atrial flutter.** Sometimes the atria may contract at an even higher speed, usually about 240–300/minute. This is called atrial flutter. Under these circumstances the ventricles are unable to 'keep up' with the atria and therefore respond to every other or perhaps every third atrial contraction, a condition known as 2:1 or 3:1 heart block.

**Atrial (auricular) fibrillation.** In atrial fibrillation each individual bundle of muscle fibres in the atria contracts individually at a rate of about 450 contractions/minute. This results in complete disorganization of atrial contraction, and furthermore the ventricles are bombarded, via the bundle of His, with rapid and irregular stimuli and are unable either to fill properly with blood or to contract satisfactorily. Atrial fibrillation, which may be persistent or paroxysmal, is usually associated with heart disease (coronary disease, hypertension, cardiomyopathy and valvular disease). It can complicate thyrotoxicosis, various acute illnesses and alcoholism. Sometimes, there is no apparent cause.

## Arrhythmia due to conduction defects

**Heart block.** Sometimes the bundle of His may fail to transmit the impulse from the atria to the ventricles. This condition is known as heart block. If there is no association between atria and ventricles, the block is said to be complete and, if only a proportion of impulses get down the bundle, the block is said to be partial.

Cardiac arrhythmias are not necessarily associated with cardiac failure, but certain arrhythmias, commonly atrial fibrillation, may, by throwing an extra strain on the heart, either precipitate or augment cardiac failure.

---

### Nursing point

Much of the treatment of cardiac arrhythmias takes place in hospital with continuous monitoring, often in an intensive care unit. Careful observation is required and changes in rhythm must be noted as they may indicate the need to stop a drug or change treatment.

Remember that no mechanical system is perfect and the nurse should check all mechanical aids, particularly infusion pumps administering drugs, at regular intervals.

---

## DRUGS USED TO TREAT ARRHYTHMIAS

Cardiac arrhythmias can be terminated and normal rhythm restored by drugs. If, however, the heart is functioning poorly it is safer to stop the arrhythmia by DC cardioversion or, if it is a conduction defect, to use electrical pacing.

## Arrhythmias due to overexcitability

When the arrhythmia is due to an excitable focus in the heart muscle (usually in the ventricle), drugs that reduce excitability are appropriate and include:

- lidocaine (lignocaine)
- mexiletine.

When the arrhythmia is due to a circus movement, as in supraventricular tachycardias, drugs that slow conduction in the AV node are used. They include:

- adenosine
- verapamil
- β blockers
- digoxin.

Digoxin may also be used in certain cardiac arrhythmias, even if they are unassociated with cardiac failure.

**Atrial fibrillation.** By suppressing conduction between the atria and ventricles, digoxin controls the ventricular rate in atrial fibrillation whether there is associated cardiac failure or not. It does not, however, abolish the fibrillation.

**Atrial flutter.** Digoxin may change the arrhythmia into atrial fibrillation. If the drug is then stopped, normal sinus rhythm may be restored.

See also Wolff–Parkinson–White syndrome (p. 71).

In addition, three drugs that have both actions and can therefore be used in both types of arrhythmia are:

- disopyramide
- amiodarone
- flecainide.

## Lidocaine (lignocaine)

Lidocaine is a local anaesthetic (see p. 237) that suppresses the excitability of the ventricular muscle with only moderate depression of the heart's action; therefore, it is not likely to cause cardiac arrest or a fall in blood pressure except in overdose. Lidocaine is used to treat arrhythmias due to ventricular excitability that are liable to occur in the first few days after a cardiac infarct. It must be given intravenously, because if it is given by mouth it is very rapidly broken down by the liver after absorption from the intestine (first pass effect). Unfortunately, its action lasts only about 20 minutes.

### Nursing point

In patients with cardiac failure or shock the breakdown of lidocaine by the liver is much slower, and dangerous accumulation can occur with continuous infusion. In these circumstances the infusion rate should be slower.

**Contraindications and adverse effects.** Lidocaine should be avoided in shocked patients when it may further depress cardiac function. It should not be given if the conducting system of the heart is damaged, as may happen after cardiac infarction. The most common adverse effects are caused by stimulation of the central nervous system with restlessness, tremor and possibly convulsions. It can also cause a fall in blood pressure and bradycardia, particularly if heart function is already compromised.

**Drug interactions.** A low plasma potassium level reduces the effectiveness of lidocaine and the plasma potassium concentration should be kept above 4 mmol/litre.

## Mexiletine

Mexiletine is similar in its action to lidocaine. It suppresses cardiac arrhythmias and it is particularly valuable because it is effective when given orally. Adverse effects include nausea and dizziness and are frequent.

## Verapamil

Verapamil is a calcium antagonist that acts selectively on the heart (see p. 76). Verapamil blocks the flow of calcium ions into the muscle cells of the heart. This reduces the force of contraction of heart muscle and slows conduction in the AV node, and is thus useful in supraventricular tachycardia as it breaks the circus wave of stimulation.

Because of its depressing effect on cardiac muscle contraction, verapamil should not be used if a β blocker has been given in the preceding 24 hours, as the combination can seriously reduce cardiac efficiency and may cause cardiac arrest. For the same reason verapamil should not be used in cardiac failure. It may also be combined with digoxin to improve the control of atrial fibrillation.

**Drug interactions.** Verapamil reduces the excretion of digoxin, so if the two are combined the dose of digoxin should be reduced.

## β Blockers

**Mechanism of action.** The general pharmacology of this group of drugs is considered on p. 51. By preventing the stimulation of adrenergic receptors by epinephrine, these β blockers decrease the excitability of the heart and thus stop arrhythmias due to an excitable focus or to a supraventricular circus movement as in tachycardia.

β Blockers can be used to prevent ectopic beats or supraventricular tachycardia and to improve the control of atrial fibrillation by digoxin. They are frequently prescribed after myocardial infarction where they improve the prognosis. Sotalol is believed to have an additional action, which is useful in ventricular arrhythmias.

**Drug interactions.** β Blockers may exacerbate the depressing effect on heart muscle of drugs such as verapamil.

### Safety point

It must be remembered that in reducing adrenergic drive to the heart and depressing the heart muscle, these drugs may exacerbate or precipitate heart failure in those patients whose hearts are under stress from some disease. β Blockers should not be used in cardiac failure, except under special circumstances (see p. 64).

## Adenosine

**Mechanism of action and use.** Adenosine suppresses conduction through the AV node and is used to terminate supraventricular arrhythmias. Adenosine is given intravenously. Its action begins very rapidly and only lasts a very short time, but this is usually sufficient to restore sinus rhythm.

**Adverse effects.** Adverse effects are flushing, chest pain and dyspnoea coming on immediately after injection and lasting up to 30 seconds.

## Digoxin

In addition to its use in heart failure, digoxin is sometimes useful in supraventricular arrhythmias, where by slowing conduction it may abolish the arrhythmia or control the ventricular rate.

## Disopyramide

**Mechanism of action.** Disopyramide decreases excitability and slows conduction so it can be used for both supraventricular and ventricular tachycardias. Disopyramide can be given either orally or intravenously. Disopyramide is excreted via the kidneys and reduced dosage is necessary if renal function is impaired.

**Adverse effects.** These include dry mouth, worsening of glaucoma and difficulty with micturition, all due to an anticholinergic action. Disopyramide may also cause nausea, vomiting and diarrhoea.

## Amiodarone

Amiodarone is effective in both ventricular and supraventricular arrhythmias.

**Mechanism of action.** Amiodarone acts by prolonging the refractory period of heart muscle. This is the short period after each contraction of the heart when the muscle will not respond to any stimulus. Its other important property is that, unlike most anti-arrhythmic drugs, it has little depressing effect on cardiac function.

**Adverse effects.** Adverse effects of amiodarone are common and to some extent limit its use. They include:

- Photosensitivity rash and bluish grey pigmentation of exposed areas.
- Amiodarone contains a high concentration of iodine and may cause both hypothyroidism and thyrotoxicosis. Thyroid function tests (TSH, T3 and T4) should be performed every 6 months in those on long-term treatment.
- Pulmonary fibrosis requires chest X-rays every 6 months.
- Deposits in the cornea of the eye occasionally cause visual haloes.
- Rarely, liver damage and neuropathy.
- Rapid I.V. injection causes marked hypotension.

**Drug interactions.** Amiodarone potentiates the actions of warfarin and digoxin.

## Flecainide

**Mechanism of action.** Flecainide reduces excitability and slows conduction in the AV node and bundle of His, so it can be used for both ventricular and supraventricular arrhythmias, including those complicating the Wolff–Parkinson–White syndrome

(see below). Flecainide can be given by slow I.V. injection (over 10 minutes) to terminate arrhythmias. Given orally, it is useful in preventing ventricular arrhythmias.

**Adverse effects.** Dizziness is not uncommon. Flecainide has some depressant effect on heart muscle and should be used with care, if at all, in patients with conduction defects on a pacemaker. Rarely, it actually provokes, rather than diminishes, ventricular arrhythmias. Although flecainide is an effective drug it can induce dangerous arrhythmias in patients who have poorly functioning or damaged ventricular muscle, particularly following myocardial infarction, and should be avoided in this group.

## Propafenone

Propafenone is effective in suppressing both ventricular and supraventricular arrhythmias and those complicating the Wolff–Parkinson–White syndrome. It can be given orally in divided doses and has also been used intravenously. Its efficacy appears similar to that of lidocaine and flecainide. The dose may need to be individualized, as there is considerable interindividual difference in the blood levels for a given dose due to variations in drug metabolism. It has a weak β blocking action and should be avoided in patients who are subject to bronchospasm.

## DIRECT CURRENT CARDIOVERSION

A direct current (DC) shock is applied to the heart via electrodes placed on the chest. This shock obliterates the ectopic focus or circus movement which causes the arrhythmia and allows normal rhythm to be resumed. This form of treatment has been widely and successfully used in treating atrial fibrillation and about 70% of these patients can be converted to sinus rhythm. Unfortunately, in spite of maintenance treatment with anti-arrhythmic drugs many patients relapse within a few months. It is also useful in other arrhythmias.

## ELECTROLYTES AND ARRHYTHMIAS

A low plasma potassium concentration (hypokalaemia) increases the risk of developing an arrhythmia and makes the arrhythmia more difficult to terminate. This is particularly liable to occur after an infarct or in patients taking diuretics.

Magnesium deficiency also predisposes to arrhythmias and in some units magnesium sulphate is infused immediately after a myocardial infarct to reduce cardiac excitability.

## TREATMENT OF INDIVIDUAL ARRHYTHMIAS

In persistent atrial fibrillation an attempt is usually made to restore sinus rhythm, the most effective method being direct current (DC) cardioversion. The patient should be anticoagulated for 4 weeks before and after conversion to reduce the risk of thrombi forming in the atria and becoming emboli. Unfortunately, relapse will occur within a year in about half these patients but maintenance treatment with amiodarone or quinidine reduces the risk. If attempts at DC cardioversion fail or relapse cannot be prevented, the ventricular rate can be controlled with digoxin. Better control may be obtained if digoxin is combined with verapamil or a β blocker. In persistent fibrillation, the ever-present risk of emboli arising in the atria requires that, if possible, patients be anticoagulated with warfarin. Regular aspirin can also be used but is less effective.

In paroxysmal atrial fibrillation, amiodarone or sotalol, taken regularly, may prevent attacks.

### Atrial flutter

Digoxin may restore normal rhythm. It may, however, produce atrial fibrillation, which can then be treated as above.

### Ventricular tachycardia or extrasystoles

Intravenous lidocaine damps down the excitable focus and usually stops this type of tachycardia. DC shock is also very effective and may be preferred if the facilities are available, particularly if the heart is showing signs of strain. Disopyramide or amiodarone or sotalol given orally are used to prevent extrasystoles, although often no treatment is necessary.

### Supraventricular tachycardia

Depressing conduction through the AV node and thus breaking the circuit terminates acute attacks. This may be achieved if the patient performs the Valsalva manoeuvre (expiring against the closed glottis), which causes reflex vagal stimulation and slows AV conduction. A similar effect can be produced by pressure over one carotid sinus.

### Drug treatment

Adenosine, given as a rapid intravenous injection under ECG monitoring, is the treatment of choice. The alternative drug is verapamil but there is some doubt as to its safety. Amiodarone can be tried if other drugs have failed, and is given slowly I.V. β Blockers are used, but due to their negative inotropic effect (depression of the heart muscle) they must not be combined with verapamil.

If drug treatment fails DC shock may be used.

### THE WOLFF–PARKINSON–WHITE (WPW) SYNDROME

The WPW syndrome is an interesting congenital abnormality that occurs in about 0.2% of the population. It is due to an extra (accessory) conducting system between the atria and the ventricles. In itself it causes no trouble but is associated with supraventricular arrhythmias due to re-entry (i.e. down one bundle and up the other) and atrial fibrillation, which are occasionally dangerous.

In treating these arrhythmias it must be remembered that the accessory bundle may not respond to drugs in the same way as the normal conducting system. In particular, digoxin and verapamil enhance rather than depress conduction through the accessory bundle and are therefore contraindicated. Depending on circumstances, amiodarone, disopyramide or flecainide are used.

### ARRHYTHMIAS DUE TO CONDUCTION DEFECTS

Sympathomimetic drugs can sometimes relieve conduction defects. Isoprenaline is most commonly used. In most patients with conduction defects, however, rhythm will have to be maintained by a pacemaker.

Bradycardia, particularly when it occurs following a coronary thrombosis, may be due to failure of the cardiac pacemaker (SA node). Atropine is useful to restore normal function of the pacemaker.

In Chapter 6 we consider the treatment of hypertension, another major disease of the cardiovascular system.

### Special point

Unless the underlying cause can be removed, most patients with chronic heart failure will require some medication for the rest of their lives. It should be explained to them that the main objectives of treatment are to give them a reasonable exercise tolerance and to keep them free of oedema. The importance of taking their drugs regularly should be stressed. Patients should be told of the main adverse effects, particularly those producing symptoms (e.g. nausea in digitalis overdose). All patients with chronic heart failure should be seen regularly, either as outpatients or by their family doctor.

## Reference

Moniotte S, Balligand J L 2002 Potential use of beta(3)-adrenoceptor antagonists in heart failure therapy. Cardiovascular Drug Reviews 20: 19

## Further reading

Coady E 2002 Chromic heart failure. Nursing Times 98: 41
Cobbe S M, Rankin A C 1988 Drug treatment of cardiac arrhythmias. Prescribers Journal 28: 48
Cohn J N 1996 The management of chronic heart failure. New England Journal of Medicine 335: 490
Editorial 1999a The evidence for β blockers in heart failure. British Medical Journal 318: 814
Editorial 1999 β Blockers for mild to moderate heart failure. Lancet 353: 2
Ganz LL, Friedman PL 1995 Supraventricular tachycardias. New England Journal of Medicine 332: 162
Shulman R, Davies R, Landowski R 2002 Drugs used in heart disease. Nursing Times 98: 43

# Chapter 6

# Drugs used for blood pressure

## Learning objectives

At the end of this chapter, the reader should be able to:

- describe how blood pressure is normally controlled
- list the causes of hypertension
- give examples of drugs that:
    lower total peripheral resistance
    lower CO
    decrease blood volume
    act centrally
- describe the treatment of hypertensive emergencies and hypertension in pregnancy
- appreciate the principles and practical aspects of taking blood pressure
- describe the treatment of hypotensive shock and the problems treating peripheral vascular disease.

## THE NORMAL CONTROL OF BLOOD PRESSURE

The blood pressure depends on:

- the peripheral vascular resistance
- the output of blood from the heart
- the volume and viscosity of the blood.

By changing one or more of these factors it is possible to change the blood pressure.

**The peripheral vascular resistance** depends on the cross-section of the smaller arteries (arterioles). The walls of these arteries contain circular muscle fibres, which are controlled by the sympathetic nervous system (see p. 43). Stimulation of this system releases noradrenaline (norepinephrine), which causes these muscles to contract and leads to

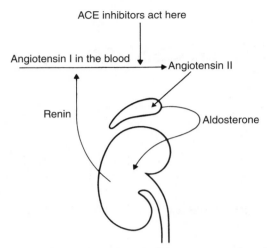

ACE inhibitors act here

Angiotensin I in the blood

Angiotensin II

Renin

Aldosterone

**Figure 6.1**    Renin released from the kidney acts on angiotensin I in the blood to form angiotensin II, which constricts blood vessels and raises the blood pressure. Angiotensin II also releases aldosterone from the adrenal cortex, causing salt and water retention by the kidney. The net result is a rise in blood pressure.

narrowing of the arterioles and a rise in blood pressure. As a counterbalance, the cells lining the blood vessels are continually producing nitric oxide, which acts as a vasodilator and thus tends to lower blood pressure. *Angiotensin* (see below) also causes constriction of blood vessels and a rise in blood pressure.

**The output of blood from the heart** or the cardiac output depends on several factors, but one important control is again the sympathetic nervous system, which, by releasing adrenaline (epinephrine), causes a rise in pulse rate and output of blood.

**The volume and viscosity of the blood** is ultimately controlled by the kidneys. There are receptors which 'sense' changes in the blood volume and if it falls the kidney secretes a substance called renin which, via a complex series of changes, leads to retention of salt and water by the kidneys (Fig. 6.1) and the formation of angiotensin II, which causes vasoconstriction, both of which raise the blood pressure.

In addition to reducing volume, drugs such as the diuretics are used to reduce the body's stores of sodium, which is believed to contribute to hypertension by increasing blood vessel stiffness, possibly through a sodium–calcium exchange that increases intracellular calcium.

## MEASUREMENT OF BLOOD PRESSURE

When blood pressure is measured, two values are noted: namely, the systolic and diastolic pressures.

The **systolic pressure** is the blood pressure at systole, when the ventricles contract and pump blood into the arterial circulation. Here, the pressure of the pumping heart is a major component of the value recorded. The **diastolic pressure** is the pressure recorded at diastole when the heart is filling, and the value obtained reflects predominantly the total peripheral resistance (TPR)[1] in the vascular beds.

A typical 'normal' value obtained might be, for example, 120/75 mmHg (millimetres of mercury), where 120 is the systolic pressure and 75 is the diastolic pressure. Diastolic values of 90 or more are generally accepted to be a red flag, indicating an abnormally high peripheral resistance. Blood pressures measured during periods of stress will often give spuriously high systolic values and the nurse should be aware of the patient's state of mind when taking readings.

## HYPERTENSION

Hypertension is the term used to describe blood pressure that is **chronically** raised above acceptable levels for health. In certain people, the blood pressure is consistently raised above normal limits. This is due to a raised peripheral resistance secondary to vasoconstriction, although the kidneys also play a part. The condition is known as **hypertension**.

### CAUSES OF HYPERTENSION

In the majority of patients the cause is not known, although there are probably inherited and environmental factors, and the condition is then called *essential hypertension*.

Much more rarely, raised blood pressure is secondary to kidney or endocrine disorders. For example:

- phaeochromocytoma, a catecholamine-secreting tumour of the adrenal medulla, that is usually treated surgically by removal of the tumour
- renal artery constriction
- Cushing's disease (see p. 206)
- primary aldosteronism (see p. 204).

The actual elevation of blood pressure, unless severe, rarely produces symptoms, but over a period of time it damages the brain, heart, blood vessels, retina and kidneys, which leads eventually to

---

[1]Note: TPR for nurses is also an acronyom for temperature, pulse and respiration.

coronary thrombosis, heart failure, blindness, strokes and less often to renal failure. It is therefore logical to prevent these complications by lowering the blood pressure and drugs can achieve this.

# HOW DRUGS CAN LOWER BLOOD PRESSURE

Drugs can lower the blood pressure in a number of ways as they can:

- lower the total peripheral resistance
- lower cardiac output
- reduce blood volume and body sodium stores
- act centrally (in the central nervous system).

## DRUGS WHICH LOWER TOTAL PERIPHERAL RESISTANCE

- **Sympathetic blocking drugs**
- **Vasodilators**
- **Angiotensin-converting enzyme (ACE) inhibitors**.

## SYMPATHETIC BLOCKING DRUGS

- **Prazosin**
- **Doxazosin**
- **Terazosin**.

### Mechanism of action and uses

- Prazosin, doxazosin and terazosin block the vasoconstrictor sympathetic nerve supply to the small arteries and arterioles by blocking $\alpha_1$ receptors on the blood vessels, and the resulting vasodilatation causes a fall in blood pressure. With these drugs there is little compensatory rise in pulse rate or cardiac output.
- The fall in blood pressure is inclined to be postural (greater on standing than lying).
- Prazosin is short acting and dosage is required two or three times daily, which makes control of blood pressure difficult. Doxazosin and terazosin have a longer action so once a day dosage is adequate.
- α Blockers improve the flow of urine in patients with bladder neck obstruction and are used in mild cases of prostatic enlargement. These drugs may be combined with other hypotensive agents. Adverse effects are unusual except for postural hypotension. Occasionally, these drugs cause urinary incontinence, particularly in women.

# VASODILATORS

Vasodilators comprise the following groups:

- **calcium channel blockers (calcium antagonists)**
- **diazoxide**
- **hydralazine**
- **minoxidil**
- **sodium nitroprusside**.

## Calcium channel blockers (calcium antagonists)

**Mechanism of action.** The entry of calcium ions into the muscle cell is necessary for muscle fibres to contract. This group of drugs blocks the entry of calcium ions into the muscle cells in the arterial walls, resulting in relaxation of the muscle and dilatation of the arteries.

**Uses**

- Calcium antagonists are used to lower blood pressure in hypertension, to dilate coronary arteries in angina (see p. 94) and one calcium antagonist (verapamil; see below) slows conduction in the AV node and is used to treat cardiac arrhythmias.
- At present there is no clearly preferred drug for hypertension, although the longer-acting preparations are more convenient for patients.
- Calcium channel blockers may be used alone or combined with other hypotensive drugs; for example, nifedipine plus a β blocker is a popular combination.
- Although their actions and uses are similar, calcium channel blockers differ in their duration of action. They are all given orally and are broken down by the liver.

**Short–acting calcium antagonists used for hypertension or angina:**
- **Nifedipine**
- **Nicardipine**
- **Diltiazem**

These need to be administered twice or three times daily.

**Long–acting calcium antagonists used for hypertension or angina:**
- **Amlodipine**
- **Felodipine**

These drugs are usually administered once daily.

**Calcium antagonists used for hypertension only:**
- **Isradipine**
- **Lacidipine**

**Calcium antagonist used for hypertension, angina and cardiac arrhythmias:**

- **Verapamil**

### Adverse effects of calcium antagonists

- Headache, flushing and ankle oedema due to vasodilatation can occur with all these drugs, but are more common with nifedipine and nicardipine. Verapamil has been reported to cause constipation.
- Depression of cardiac function is bound to be a feature of calcium antagonists since they antagonize the entry of calcium ions into the cardiac muscle cell. This effect is particularly marked with verapamil and to a lesser extent with others. For this reason verapamil should not be given intravenously to patients receiving β blockers, since these block the sympathetic cardiac $\beta_1$ receptors.
- Great care is necessary if calcium channel blockers are given to patients with heart failure, as this may be made worse.
- There is some evidence of increased mortality in patients taking large doses of the short-acting preparation of nifedipine, particularly in patients with coronary artery disease. The longer-acting preparations appear safe but ACE inhibitors (see below) are to be preferred in hypertensive patients with diabetes.

The actions of nifedipine and nicardipine are increased by cimetidine, a drug used to treat gastric ulcers (see p. 111).

## Diazoxide

Diazoxide is a drug that is chemically similar to the thiazide diuretics (see p. 163), but it has no diuretic activity. It is, however, a potent dilator of arteries.

### Mechanism of action and pharmacokinetics

- Diazoxide appears to exert its direct vasodilator effect by opening arteriolar potassium channels, and this has the effect of stabilizing the muscle cell membrane at resting levels.
- Diazoxide is extensively bound to plasma proteins, which extends its half-life in the circulation. It is excreted unchanged.

### Uses of diazoxide

- Diazoxide is used to treat hypertensive emergencies.
- It is administered by injection or continuous infusion and is relatively long lasting with a half-life of approximately 24 hours.

- The antihypertensive effect is noticeable after about 5 minutes and lasts for anything from 4 to 12 hours.
- Virtually all patients given diazoxide will respond by the third or fourth dose.
- Diazoxide is extensively protein-bound in the blood, and smaller doses should be administered to patients with renal failure.

### Adverse effects of diazoxide

- Diazoxide is potent and can result in excessive hypotension, and caution should generally err on the side of smaller and perhaps more frequent doses. See the *British National Formulary* (BNF) for dosages.
- The marked hypotensive effect may be accompanied by reflex tachycardia, an increased cardiac output and angina. Patients with ischaemic heart disease may suffer cardiac failure, and the drug should be avoided in these patients.
- Diazoxide inhibits release of insulin from the pancreatic islets, possibly through its action in opening potassium channels. This action of diazoxide renders it generally inadvisable in patients with hyperglycaemia, which is associated with renal failure. This insulin release-inhibiting action makes diazoxide useful in the treatment of hypoglycaemia secondary to an insulinoma.
- Rarely, diazoxide causes salt and water retention.

## Hydralazine

Hydralazine is chemically a hydrazine derivative, which has been clinically available for several years.

### Mechanism of action and pharmacokinetics

- Hydralazine directly dilates arterioles but not veins to produce its antihypertensive effects.
- The hypotensive action of a given dose becomes successively less effective, a phenomenon known as tachyphylaxis. This limits the sole use of hydralazine for hypotension and it is usually prescribed together with other drugs.
- It is administered orally and is well absorbed but rapidly metabolized during first pass metabolism. This reduces its bioavailability considerably.
- The metabolism of hydralazine is partly by acetylation. The general population consists of those who are either fast or slow acetylators of drugs; therefore, fast acetylators will derive less benefit from a single dose than will slow acetylators.
- The half-life of hydralazine is 2–4 hours, although the hypotensive effect may persist after

plasma levels have declined. This is because the drug binds tightly to arteriolar tissue.

### Use of hydralazine

• Hydralazine is generally not used alone but in combination with other drugs – for example, β blockers – to enhance its action and help counteract the reflex tachycardia associated with its use.

• Hydralazine has now been largely replaced by new hypotensive drugs, but is still used in serious hypertension during pregnancy.

### Adverse effects of hydralazine

• Nausea, headaches, palpitations (due to reflex tachycardia) and anorexia are the most common side-effects.

• Hydralazine may precipitate angina or ischaemic arrhythmias in patients with ischaemic heart disease, due to the reflex tachycardia.

• Rarely, hydralazine may cause peripheral neuropathy (functional or pathological changes in the nervous system).

• At high doses, especially in slow acetylators, hydralazine may cause arthralgia (joint pain), myalgia (muscle pain), and fever and skin rashes – a set of symptoms very reminiscent of the disease systemic lupus erythematosus (lupus; SLE). The syndrome is reversible, and symptoms should disappear on ceasing treatment with hydralazine.

## Minoxidil

Minoxidil is a direct vasodilator of arterioles. It is very potent but has some potentially serious adverse effects.

### Mechanism of action and pharmacokinetics

• Minoxidil, like hydralazine, dilates arteriolar but not venous smooth muscle by opening potassium channels.

• Minoxidil is taken orally, and is well absorbed from the gastrointestinal tract.

• After absorption, minoxidil is converted to minoxidil sulphate, the active metabolite.

• The half-life of minoxidil in the circulation is about 4 hours. It is not protein-bound in the blood.

• Despite the relatively short plasma half-life, minoxidil's antihypertensive effects may last up to 24 hours or more, possibly because of a longer half-life of minoxidil sulphate and its binding to arteriolar tissue.

**Use of minoxidil.** The use of minoxidil is confined to patients who are resistant to more usual treatments. It is available only as an oral preparation.

It causes salt and water retention and reflex sympathetic stimulation of the heart, which results in an increased heart rate. Therefore, minoxidil must be prescribed together with a diuretic and a β blocker.

**Adverse effects of minoxidil.** If diuretics and β blockers are not used, or if inadequate doses of these are given, minoxidil causes:

• oedema
• tachycardia
• palpitations
• angina.

Patients may also complain of sweating, headache and hirsutism. This adverse effect has resulted in the use of topical preparations of minoxidil to stimulate scalp hair growth in baldness.

> ### Nursing point
>
> When a patient complains of palpitations, this could be because of a vasodilator drug. When blood pressure falls due to a decrease in the total peripheral resistance, this fall is detected by the CNS, which immediately activates the sympathetic drive to the heart to speed it up (tachycardia). The patient experiences the tachycardia and complains of 'palpitations'. The initial dose of an $\alpha_1$ blocker can sometimes cause a profound fall in blood pressure with fainting, so it is advisable that this dose is given before retiring and that it should be low. Subsequent doses rarely provoke this problem, but the blood pressure should be taken standing and lying down to assess any postural fall. The dose is increased at weekly intervals until satisfactory control is achieved.

## ANGIOTENSIN-CONVERTING ENZYME (ACE) INHIBITORS

## Mechanism of action

ACE inhibitors inhibit the conversion of angiotensin I to angiotensin II in the circulation. This reduces the vasoconstricting effect of angiotensin II and, by inhibiting the release of aldosterone, causes less sodium retention (see Fig. 6.1). The overall effect is a fall in blood pressure. ACE inhibitors are used to treat hypertension and cardiac failure and may actually improve the structure of thickened arteries and failing hearts. They also reduce proteinuria in diabetic patients with kidney disease and slow the decline in renal function.

## Therapeutic use and preparations available

An ACE inhibitor may be used as a single drug to lower blood pressure or combined with other hypotensive drugs such as diuretics. ACE inhibitors are particularly useful if hypertension is complicated by heart failure (see p. 82). Several of these drugs are now available, with similar actions and uses.

## Preparations and uses

**Captopril** was the first to be introduced and is still widely used. It is rapidly absorbed when given orally; its action starts after half an hour and lasts up to 8 hours.

**Enalapril** is a prodrug and is itself inactive, but is converted into an active metabolite in the liver. It therefore takes longer to act (3 hours) but its effects are prolonged (24 hours).

There are a number of other ACE inhibitors, and the reader is referred to the *British National Formulary* (BNF) for these.

> ### Nursing point
>
> Although the BNF is frequently referred to in this book as a source of information, readers should be aware that its companions – the NPF (Nurse Prescribers' Formulary) and the NPEF (Nurse Prescribers' Extended Formulary) – have been introduced.

## Effects of ACE inhibitors after administration

A marked fall in blood pressure occurs occasionally with the first dose of an ACE inhibitor, especially if the patient is already taking a diuretic. For this reason the initial dose should be low and taken before retiring; patients should be warned of the possibility of a sharp fall in blood pressure if they get up during the night. Before starting treatment, electrolytes and renal function should be measured.

## Contraindications for ACE inhibitors

ACE inhibitors are contraindicated in pregnancy, as they may damage the fetus, and the dose should be kept as low as possible in renal impairment.

## Adverse effects and interactions

● A few patients develop renal failure with ACE inhibitors. This is particularly liable to happen in elderly patients and those with stenosis of the renal arteries. Plasma creatinine should therefore be measured in the first few weeks of treatment and thereafter at 6-monthly intervals.

● Dry cough (10%), bronchospasm (5%).
● Fatigue, headaches, diarrhoea.
● Rashes, change in taste (captopril).
● Captopril may produce proteinuria and neutropenia, although this occurs rarely with the lower doses now used.
● Hyperkalaemia in patients with renal disease or who are taking potassium-sparing diuretics or supplementary potassium. Declining renal function if combined with NSAIDs.

## ANGIOTENSIN RECEPTOR BLOCKERS

Angiotensin II is an extremely powerful vasoconstrictor that acts on specific angiotensin II receptors on the blood vessel wall. Antagonist drugs have been developed that bind to the angiotensin II receptor and block the vasoconstrictor action of angiotensin II. These drugs will therefore have similar effects to those of drugs such as the ACE inhibitors. Examples of drugs in use:

● **losartan**
● **valsartan**.

Losartan and valsartan block the action of angiotensin II at the receptor site. Their hypotensive action is thus very similar to that of the ACE inhibitors and trials suggest that they have much the same efficacy. Recent clinical trials of losartan (Editorial 2002) have produced results suggesting that the drug not only reduces blood pressure but also improves left ventricular mass and improves ventricular contractility. The drug is sometimes combined with drugs such as β blockers if it proves ineffective alone (see Case History below).

## Adverse effects

The adverse effects are those of the ACE inhibitors, although angiotensin receptor blockers are much less liable to cause a cough.

## SODIUM NITROPRUSSIDE

Sodium nitroprusside is a very powerful vasodilator used to treat hypertensive emergencies and severe cardiac failure. It dilates both arterial and venous blood vessels, which results in reduced peripheral resistance and venous return.

## Use of sodium nitroprusside

Sodium nitroprusside must be given intravenously and is therefore only suitable for treating a hypertensive crisis and some patients with acute heart failure. It is given by infusion and it is usual to start at the lower end of the dose range and increase it until the blood pressure is satisfactorily controlled. This will require close observation and is usually carried out in an intensive care unit.

---

### Nursing point

There are five important practical points in the use of sodium nitroprusside:

- the contents of the ampoule should be dissolved in 2 ml of 5% dextrose solution and then diluted in dextrose or saline
- the infusion must be protected from the light and discarded after 24 hours
- it should also be discarded if the colour changes from pale orange to dark brown or blue
- infusion should not be continued for more than 72 hours
- if infusion is prolonged, blood cyanide and thiocyanate levels should be measured to guard against the development of cyanide poisoning

---

### Adverse effects of sodium nitroprusside

- Headaches
- Dizziness
- Palpitations
- Chest pain.

## DRUGS WHICH LOWER CARDIAC OUTPUT

### β BLOCKERS

β Blockers will lower the blood pressure to a satisfactory level in about 40% of patients with hypertension, but the hypotensive effect may be delayed for several weeks after starting treatment. It is not known exactly how these drugs produce this effect. By interfering with the sympathetic nervous system they certainly prevent the rise in cardiac output and blood pressure, which occur with excitement or effort. It may be that this damping down of the circulation ultimately causes a permanent fall in blood pressure. β Blockers may decrease renin release by the kidney, which would tend to lower the blood pressure (see p. 74), and some of them (particularly propranolol) have some central sedative action.

The effect of some β blockers is predominantly on the heart by acting on $\beta_1$ receptors and they are called 'selective' β blockers; others also affect the bronchi and possibly the peripheral circulation by acting on $\beta_2$ receptors and are known as 'non-selective' β blockers, although this selectivity is not absolute.

### Therapeutic use of β blockers

There is no evidence that any particular β blocker is more effective in lowering blood pressure, but if the patient is prone to obstructive airways disease a selective β blocker is preferred. Among those used are:

**Selective β blockers**
- Atenolol
- Esmolol
- Metoprolol.

**Non-selective β blockers**
- Propranolol
- Oxprenolol
- Nadolol
- Timolol
- Pindolol.

**Combined α- and β blocker**
- Labetalol

**Combined $\beta_1$ blocker and $\beta_2$ stimulant**
- Celiprolol
- Carvedilol.

**Atenolol**, **pindolol** and **nadolol** can be given once daily. The others are usually given two or three times daily, although such frequent dosage may not be necessary to control blood pressure. There are also slow-release preparations available of propranolol, oxprenolol and metoprolol.

**Esmolol** is a very short-acting selective β blocker used for cardiac arrhythmias and when a controlled reduction of blood pressure is required. It is given by intravenous infusion.

**Labetalol** combines β-blocking activity with some α-blocking effect. The result is that the cardiac output is decreased and at the same time there is some peripheral vasodilatation. This leads to a fall in blood pressure. The initial dose is increased gradually until satisfactory control is achieved. Dosage requirements are variable and this makes treatment difficult. It can also be given I.V. to control a hypertensive crisis.

**Celiprolol** and **carvedilol** combine a selective $\beta_1$-blocking action on the heart with a stimulating $\beta_2$ action on the blood vessels causing vasodilatation. Theoretically, this dual action should be advantageous in lowering blood pressure; however, clinical trials suggest that their efficacy is similar to that of other $\beta$ blockers. They may also play a minor role in treating heart failure (see p. 64).

## Adverse effects of $\beta$ blockers

Serious adverse effects are not common. Some are potentially dangerous or even life-threatening and other effects are more minor.

### Potentially life–threatening adverse effects
- **If used in asthmatics**
- **If used in patients with heart failure**
- **If used in patients with diabetes.**

**Use in asthmatics.** Patients with bronchospasm from asthma or chronic bronchitis may get worse when receiving $\beta$ blockers, which should be avoided in patients with asthma and used with care in patients with bronchitis, for which a selective $\beta_1$ blocker is indicated (see above).

**Use in heart failure.** They may exacerbate heart failure and should be used with care in this disorder (see p. 64).

**Use in diabetics.** Patients with diabetes receiving insulin are at some risk as $\beta$ blockers mask the symptoms of hypoglycaemia and this should be explained to them.

**Less dangerous adverse effects.** Apart from the three dangerous effects mentioned above, $\beta$ blockers have other side-effects, which, although not dangerous, may interfere with the quality of life, an important consideration if treatment is to be continued over long periods.

- Some patients report lacking energy and drive and feel tired and depressed.
- Others may report vivid dreams and, occasionally, hallucinations.
- Owing to the fall in cardiac output, the peripheral circulation decreases and this results in cold hands and feet and can be a serious problem in patients with peripheral vascular disease, in whom $\beta$ blockers should be avoided.
- Occasionally, $\beta$ blockers considerably reduce the resting pulse rate. Provided it does not fall

below 50/minute this is not usually a matter of concern. Lower rates require a change to oxprenolol or pindolol, which allow a rather higher pulse rate at rest.

Labetalol should be used with care in patients with heart failure, as it may exacerbate the condition, and should be avoided in patients with asthma. Other side-effects include stuffy nose, lethargy, vivid dreams and tingling of the scalp.

## Drug interactions

- Myocardial function is reduced if $\beta$ blockers are combined with intravenous verapamil
- $\beta$ Blockers increase the peripheral vaso-constricting action of ergotamine (see p. 57)
- The action of some $\beta$ blockers is increased by cimetidine.

## DRUGS WHICH DECREASE BLOOD VOLUME

### DIURETICS

Diuretics (see also p. 161) are still considered by many to be the drugs of first choice to treat mild-to-moderate hypertension, provided they are not contraindicated by some concurrent disease or pregnancy. The fall in blood pressure is due to a reduction in blood volume and to a vasodilating effect on the walls of the arterioles. They are cheap, relatively easy to use and serious side-effects are rare.

### Therapeutic use of diuretics

Thiazide diuretics are the most suitable and there is no preferred preparation. The dose should be relatively low; raising the dose causes little further fall in blood pressure but increases the incidence of adverse effects.

### Contraindications and adverse effects

- In gout, diuretics cause uric acid retention.
- In diabetes, diuretics decrease glucose tolerance and thus make control of the disease more difficult.
- In pregnancy, diuretics may damage the fetus.
- They cause impotence in about 20% of males.
- High dosage can lead to hypokalaemia, due to increased urinary loss of potassium. This is rare with low dosage but the blood potassium should be checked 1 month after starting treatment.

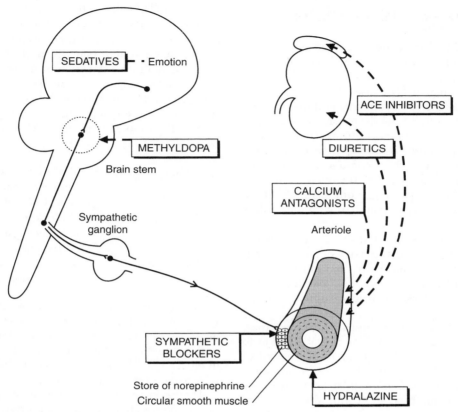

**Figure 6.2**  Site of action of some hypotensive drugs.

## Drug interactions

- NSAIDs reduce the efficacy of diuretics
- Diuretics raise blood levels of lithium and the dose of lithium may require adjustment.

## DRUGS WHICH ACT CENTRALLY

### METHYLDOPA

Methyldopa lowers blood pressure by an action on the brain that results in decreased activity of the sympathetic system.

### Therapeutic use

Methyldopa was formerly used widely in the treatment of hypertension. It is effective and easy to use because the fall in blood pressure is not precipitous. However, it has a number of common adverse effects that patients sometimes find unacceptable and its use has declined considerably. It is still, however, widely used in treating pregnancy-related hypertension.

## Adverse effects

- Drowsiness and depression often occur early in treatment but may pass off after a few weeks
- More rarely, fluid retention producing oedema can be troublesome but is controlled by a diuretic
- Haemolytic anaemia and drug fever have also been reported.

### MOXONIDINE

Moxonidine acts centrally to reduce activity of the sympathetic nervous system. At present, it is indicated if other hypotensive agents are not satisfactory and is given orally, once or twice daily.

### Adverse effects

These include tiredness, headache and nausea.

The sites of action of the various antihypertensive agents are shown in Figure 6.2.

## THE TREATMENT OF HYPERTENSION

When raised blood pressure is detected, it is important to exclude underlying renal or endocrine causes, although essential hypertension is responsible in more than 90% of cases. Hypertension, by itself, rarely causes any symptoms and the object of treatment is to prevent the development of complications, e.g. stroke, coronary thrombosis and cardiac and renal failure. Many hypertensive patients live for years without these complications and this means that the drugs used in treatment should be safe and as free as possible from adverse effects. Unfortunately, no hypotensive drug entirely fulfils these criteria.

It is generally accepted that severe hypertension carries a poor prognosis and adequate treatment considerably reduces morbidity and mortality. It is in patients with milder degrees of hypertension that a decision to embark on drug treatment is more difficult.

In healthy subjects with no evidence of cardiac, vascular or renal complications it is justifiable to observe the patient with regular measurement of blood pressure for 3–6 months because, in some people, it may return to normal levels, particularly when they become used to visiting the doctor. At this stage, non-drug measures may be considered (see *Special points for patient education*, p. 83). If, however, the blood pressure remains persistently above 150/90, and particularly if there are special risk factors (hyperlipidaemias, diabetes, smoking or a family history of cardiovascular disease), it is usual to start treatment with a single drug and, if this fails, a combination should be given. The aim is to maintain the blood pressure around 140/85, though below 160/90 is acceptable.

Ideal blood pressure readings are not easy to achieve and a substantial proportion of treated subjects still have blood pressures well above 140/85.

There have been many trials of hypotensive drugs in this group of patients and the results can be roughly summarized as follows:

- there was some reduction in overall mortality, probably about 20%
- the incidence of stroke was halved, but there was less reduction of coronary thrombosis
- in elderly patients the incidence of stroke was reduced by about 35% and there was some reduction in the occurrence of coronary thrombosis (20%).

It should be realized, however, that most trials to date have used diuretics or β blockers. Although it is logical to believe that other hypotensive drugs would confer similar benefits, trials are still being done and definitive statements cannot yet be made.

A variety of agents are now available and the best drug or combination of drugs for treatment is still being investigated. The usual approach is to start with β blockers in younger or middle-aged patients.

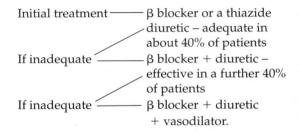

Initial treatment —— β blocker or a thiazide diuretic – adequate in about 40% of patients

If inadequate —— β blocker + diuretic – effective in a further 40% of patients

If inadequate —— β blocker + diuretic + vasodilator.

The combination of β blocker, diuretic and vasodilator are illustrated in the Case history given below. Some authorities prefer to start treatment with a diuretic and this approach is to be preferred in elderly patients and in Afro-Caribbean patients, who respond poorly to β blockers.

There is increasing concern about the quality of life of patients receiving treatment for hypertension, as these regimes may be associated with various adverse effects, which, although usually minor, can be troublesome. ACE inhibitors, though not entirely trouble-free, do not make life a burden and have a place in initial treatment, especially for diabetics in whom they help to preserve renal function. α Blockers and calcium channel blockers may also be used and there are numerous possible combinations where the effects are at least additive. It is usually possible to plan a regime that is therapeutically effective without interfering with the patient's lifestyle.

Elderly patients are a little more prone to side-effects, but usually tolerate treatment well. Low-dose thiazides, ACE inhibitors and calcium channel blockers are all satisfactory.

ACE inhibitors are indicated if there is any evidence of heart failure or diabetes and α blockers may be helpful if there is prostatic obstruction.

A few patients require admission to hospital so that they can be fully investigated and, when treatment is started, frequent observation of blood pressure can be made. In milder hypertension, with no complicating disease, treatment can be started and carried through on an outpatient basis. When adequate control is obtained, further supervision is required by the primary care team or hospital out-patients' department.

Case History 6.1 illustrates the integrated use of different drug approaches to the treatment of hypertension.

### Case History 6.1

Mr WP attended his GP for a routine insurance medical examination as he wished to increase his mortgage. He had not attended the surgery for many years. To the doctor's surprise and the patient's distress he was found to have asymptomatic hypertension, and, following repeated blood pressure readings, the diagnosis was confirmed. Blood and urine tests were normal and so was a kidney ultrasound. A diagnosis of essential (unknown cause) hypertension was made and the GP had to make a decision as to how to treat the condition, remembering that the treatment would be long term and had to do the job and not upset the patient with side-effects. His choices were:

- a thiazide diuretic such as bendrofluazide
- a β blocker such as atenolol or a combined α and β blocker such as carvedilol
- a calcium channel blocker such as amlodipine or nifedipine and
- an ACE inhibitor such as enalapril or captopril
- an angiotensin II antagonist such as losartan or candesartan
- a combination of two or more of the above.

He was started on losartan, and when this only gave partial control, he was changed to a losartan/thiazide diuretic combination and transferred to the GP practice blood pressure clinic for regular checks.

## HYPERTENSIVE EMERGENCIES – RAPID REDUCTION IN BLOOD PRESSURE

Occasionally, it may be necessary to reduce a very high blood pressure rapidly. Sodium nitroprusside (see p. 78) is the drug of choice for initial treatment. Great care must be taken when lowering a very high blood pressure, as a precipitate fall may cause renal failure or cerebral damage due to a sudden reduction of the blood supply to the kidney and brain. The early stages of this treatment should be carried out in an intensive care unit if possible and the blood pressure monitored at frequent intervals. The aim of treatment should be to reduce the diastolic blood pressure slowly to around 100 mmHg. Thereafter, treatment for hypertension should be carried out in the normal way (see above).

If facilities for intensive monitoring are not available and if the clinical situation is less acute, bed rest and a β blocker or slow-release nifedipine are satisfactory and should avoid a precipitous fall in blood pressure.

## HYPERTENSION IN PREGNANCY

Hypertension in pregnancy presents a special problem as occasionally it may progress to pre-eclampsia and eclampsia, with serious risk to both mother and child. Mild transient elevation of blood pressure occurring towards the end of pregnancy rarely needs drug treatment. More severe hypertension, particularly if the patient was hypertensive before the start of her pregnancy, may require drugs to lower the blood pressure. Methyldopa has been found satisfactory for many years. β Blockers are also used, but may retard fetal growth. In severe hypertension, hydralazine orally or intravenously is effective. Diuretics and ACE inhibitors should be avoided.

---

### Nursing point

*Measuring blood pressure*
Nurses frequently measure blood pressure. There are some key points to remember when treating hypertension:

- The blood pressure should usually be recorded with the patient both lying and standing, as some hypotensive drugs cause a much greater fall in blood pressure when the patient is standing than when he or she is lying down. In certain cases it should also be recorded after exercise.
- Some patients are nervous when visiting the doctor and this may cause their blood pressure to rise, the so-called 'white coat' hypertension. Quiet reassurance and a rest period of 5 minutes are necessary before measuring the blood pressure.
- Sometimes it is helpful to teach patients to take their own blood pressure, so a home record can be obtained which will give a better idea of day-to-day fluctuations.
- Because smoking may alter the blood pressure temporarily, patients should be asked to avoid it for 30 minutes before having their blood pressure measured.
- A well-applied cuff and a good stethoscope are necessary for accurate readings.
- Measurements of blood pressure tend to show 'observer bias'. This may happen in trials of new drugs and it is necessary in these circumstances to use a special sphygmomanometer in which the blood pressure is recorded 'blind', so that the recording is not known by the observer.
- It is now possible to record patients' blood pressure as they go about their daily life, with an apparatus they can wear over a long period. This gives a much better assessment of their overall blood pressure and is useful in evaluating 'white coat' hypertension, stress response or the apparent failure of treatment. This approach is becoming more common.

---

### Summary

- Blood pressure can be lowered by lowering (a) total peripheral resistance, (b) cardiac output and (c) blood volume and sodium stores.
- Patients can be fast or slow acetylators of drugs, which will affect the drug's potency and duration of action (e.g. hydralazine).
- Hydralazine can cause arthralgia in high doses, but it is reversible.
- The actions of nifedipine and nicardipine are increased by cimetidine, a drug used to treat gastric ulcers.
- Calcium channel blockers may be used alone or combined with other hypotensive drugs; for example, nifedipine plus a β blocker is a popular combination.
- Palpitations caused by α blockers can be prevented by using a β blocker as well.
- Combining a $\beta_1$ blocker and a $\beta_2$ stimulant is theoretically a good idea since the $\beta_1$ effect is to

lower cardiac output and the $\beta_2$ stimulant lowers total peripheral resistance.

- $\beta$ Blockers must not be used in asthmatics and must be used with caution in patients with cardiac failure or diabetes, as they can mask symptoms of hypoglycaemia.
- In gout, diuretics cause uric acid retention.
- In diabetes, diuretics decrease glucose tolerance and thus make control of the disease more difficult.
- In pregnancy, diuretics may damage the fetus.
- Diuretics also cause impotence in about 20% of males. High dosage can lead to hypokalaemia, due to increased urinary loss of potassium. This is rare with low dosage but the blood potassium should be checked 1 month after starting treatment.
- Diuretics and ACE inhibitors should be avoided in eclampsia of pregnancy.
- The chapter includes details for accurate measurement of blood pressure.

## DRUGS USED TO TREAT PERIPHERAL VASCULAR DISEASE

For many years various drugs, which in normal subjects dilate arteries, were used in vascular disease in the hope that they would increase the blood supply to the ischaemic limb. Unfortunately, vascular disease usually affects the large arteries and these diseased arteries were unresponsive to vasodilators, which are now recognized as being useless in this condition. They are, however, useful in Raynaud's disease, which is due to spasm in the small arteries of the hands and feet brought on by cold.

### TREATMENT

Nifedipine, a calcium antagonist (see p. 75) used as for hypertension, is the most useful drug. Other measures include keeping warm in cold weather. Do not forget that $\beta$ blockers, ergotamine and smoking make peripheral vascular disease worse.

## DRUGS USED FOR PATIENTS IN SHOCK

In a state of shock the output of blood from the heart is acutely reduced, the blood pressure is low

and circulation to the organs of the body is inadequate. Clinically, the patient is pale, sweating and confused, the pulse is rapid, the blood pressure low and the limbs cold; kidney failure may supervene. This state may occur for three main reasons:

- Sudden reduction of blood volume, usually due to bleeding, which is treated by replacing the lost fluid by infusion.
- Reduced pumping action of the heart (pump failure) following damage (e.g. after a myocardial infarct).
- Septic shock, usually due to infection with Gram-negative bacteria (see p. 298). This is commonly found in patients receiving steroids or cytotoxic drugs. Bacterial toxins cause vasodilatation and leaking of fluid from the circulation, which reduces the blood volume, combined with a falling cardiac output. In addition to the usual measures to combat shock, rapid and vigorous treatment with the appropriate antibiotic is necessary, as the condition may prove fatal.

## DRUGS COMMONLY IN USE

Various drugs are being tried to neutralize the bacterial toxin involved but, at present, there is no preferred regime. If the main fault is pump failure, drugs can be given to increase the force of contraction of the heart muscle (positive inotropic effect) and thus improve cardiac output and circulation and raise the blood pressure.

Digoxin is not effective in these circumstances and may precipitate a dangerous cardiac arrhythmia. The most commonly used drugs are dopamine and dobutamine. This type of treatment requires careful monitoring, usually in an intensive care ward.

### Dopamine

Dopamine is a naturally occurring substance, which is changed to norepinephrine in the body. However, it has actions of its own and is used to treat shock, which may follow cardiac infarction or major cardiac surgery.

Dopamine stimulates cardiac $\beta_1$ receptors, and also increases the release of norepinephrine in the heart, thus causing the heart muscle to contract more powerfully. In addition, dopamine stimulates receptors in the renal blood vessels, causing them to dilate and increase both renal blood flow and urinary output. This action is useful since shock often causes a decline in renal function.

Dopamine is given by continuous intravenous infusion (via a central line). It affects mainly the kidneys and is used to improve their function, often combined with a diuretic. Higher doses should not be used as the intense vasoconstriction that develops may cause gangrene of the extremities.

**Drug interactions with dopamine.** Patients receiving monoamine oxidase inhibitors should be given one-tenth of the usual dose of dopamine.

## Dobutamine

Dobutamine is similar to dopamine but has no effect on the kidneys. It is, however, less likely to cause cardiac arrhythmias.

Dopamine and dobutamine may be combined: a low dose of dopamine being used for its effects on the kidneys and dobutamine for its cardiac action.

Both dopamine and dobutamine should be infused via a central vein to minimize peripheral vasoconstriction.

## References

Editorial 2002 Heart function also improved by losartan. Pharmaceutical Journal 268: 864

## Further reading

Bennett N E 1994 Hypertension in the elderly. Lancet 344: 447

Dahlof B, Lindholm L H, Hansson L et al 1991 Morbidity and mortality in the Swedish trial in old patients with hypertension. Lancet 338: 1281

Editorial 1990 Do drugs help intermittent claudication? Drug and Therapeutics Bulletin 28: 1

Editorial 1991 Hypertensive emergencies. Lancet 338: 229

Editorial 1995a Losartan – a new antihypertensive. Drug and Therapeutics Bulletin 33: 73

Editorial 1995b Who needs nine ACE inhibitors? Drug and Therapeutics Bulletin 33: 1

Editorial 1998a Calcium channel blockers. British Medical Journal 316: 1471

Editorial 1998b Treatment of hypertensive patients with diabetes. Lancet 351: 689

Jordan S, Torrance C 1998 Hypertension. Nursing Times 94: 50

Magee L A, Ornstein M P, von Dadelszen P 1999 Management of hypertension in pregnancy. British Medical Journal 318: 1332

O'Brien E, Petrie J C, Littler W A 1997 British Hypertension Society Recommendations on Blood Pressure Measurement, 2nd edn, London

Prasad N, Isles C 1996 Ambulatory blood pressure monitoring. British Medical Journal 313: 1535

Roberts C, Banning M 1998 Managing risk factors for hypertension in primary care. Nursing Standard 12: 39

Simon J R 1996 Treating hypertension: the evidence from clinical trials. British Medical Journal 313: 437

Vallance P, Moncada S 1994 Nitric oxide – from mediator to medicines. Journal of the Royal College of Physicians 28: 209

Chapter **7**

# Atheroma and thrombosis: anticoagulants and thrombolytic agents

## Learning objectives

At the end of this chapter, the reader should be able to:

- list the key stages of the coagulation cascade
- discuss the causes of thrombosis and the prevention and treatment
- give an account of the anticoagulants, and their mechanism, uses and dangers
- describe the causes and treatment of atheroma and arterial thrombosis
- list the drugs used for angina of effort
- understand the treatment and cause of patients with coronary thrombosis
- list the drugs used for fibrinolysis
- appreciate the dangers of platelet clumping and how drugs may prevent this
- discuss how drugs and diet may lower plasma lipids

## COAGULATION AND THROMBOSIS

### COAGULATION

When the wall of a blood vessel is damaged the blood coagulates and this arrests bleeding. Clotting is a complex process, which involves numerous enzymes and other chemicals called clotting factors. Most are present in the blood plasma, some are released by the platelets, and thromboplastin is released from damaged cells. When blood clots, each clotting factor is activated in sequence as part of a cascade of reactions, as shown in Figure 7.1.

The key stages of this series of reactions are:

- The formation of Factor Xa by the clotting cascade which, when activated, converts prothrombin to thrombin.
- Thrombin forms fibrin strands from soluble fibrinogen, which then form a network over the damaged area.

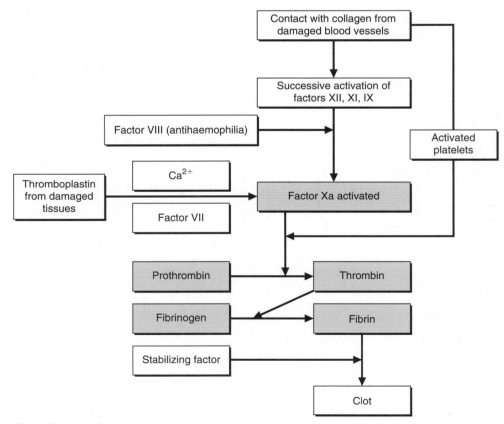

**Figure 7.1** The clotting cascade.

- At the same time, platelets become activated, assisting in the clotting process and aggregate to form clumps which become enmeshed in the fibrin network. The resulting clot plugs the defect in the blood vessel.

## THROMBOSIS

Coagulation or thrombosis may sometimes occur in blood vessels that have not been injured and in these circumstances blockage of the vessel concerned may have serious consequences. There are two types of thrombosis:

- **venous thrombosis (phlebothrombosis)**
- **arterial thrombosis**.

Although both may result in obstruction to a blood vessel, they occur under different circumstances, have different mechanisms and differ in their treatment.

### Venous thrombosis (phlebothrombosis)

This usually occurs in the deep veins of the legs. It is due to stagnation of blood in the veins when a patient is immobile after an operation (particularly if the pelvis or hip is involved), associated with pregnancy or during a severe illness. The risk is increased in obese patients, in patients with malignancy or who have a history of previous thrombosis. Oral contraceptives containing estrogen are also a risk factor and should be stopped 6 weeks before a major operation or any surgery involving the pelvis or hip. It is also apparent that there are genetic factors that predispose to thrombosis. The danger of this type of thrombosis is that part of the clot may break off, forming an embolus which is swept back via the heart to the lungs where it blocks a branch of the pulmonary artery, an event which can be fatal.

In atrial fibrillation a thrombus may develop in the left atrium because of impaired blood flow and fragments can become detached, resulting in emboli to the brain and elsewhere. Anticoagulants, which interfere with the clotting (coagulation) of blood, can be used either to prevent the formation of thrombi or to treat an established venous thrombosis.

## ANTICOAGULANTS

Anticoagulants are drugs that interfere with clotting and are used to prevent and treat venous thrombosis. They include:

- **heparin**
- **hirudin**
- **the coumarins**
  warfarin
  phenindione.

## HEPARIN

Heparin is a complex mixture of acidic substances. It occurs naturally, and is stored in mast cells and basophils. It is a very potent anticoagulant.

### Mechanism of action of heparin

Heparin's actions on the clotting mechanism are multiple and complicated. Briefly, heparin inhibits coagulation by binding to antithrombin III. Antithrombin III is part of the system that regulates clotting. It binds to certain clotting factors (see Fig. 7.1) and renders them inactive. When heparin binds to antithrombin III, this enhances antithrombin's reaction with the clotting factors considerably. The end result is a prolongation of the clotting time. The clotting time is the time taken for blood or plasma to coagulate under controlled laboratory conditions.

### Preparations of heparin

There are two preparations of heparin:

- **unfractionated heparin**
- **low molecular weight heparins**.

Heparin is a large molecule that can be broken down into a number of fragments, not all of which have anticoagulant properties. Those fragments that do have anticoagulant activity are known as low molecular weight heparins. Unfractionated heparin may vary in its potency depending on batches and sources of supply, because of variations in the relative amounts of active and inactive fragments in its structure.

### Emerging advantages of low molecular weight fragments of heparin

- Low molecular weight heparins may be better than ordinary low-dose unfractionated heparin in preventing the venous thrombosis that may complicate surgery, particularly hip and knee replacement.
- Given subcutaneously, they are as effective as intravenous unfractionated heparin in the prevention and treatment of venous thrombosis and pulmonary embolism.

• They have also been used with success in unstable angina.

• As they do not cross the placental barrier, they can be used during pregnancy.

• Since their activity can be more consistently controlled during preparation, patients may not need the same degree of monitoring.

• The mechanism of anticoagulant action of active fragments is very similar to that of unfractionated heparin but the effect is more prolonged than that of unfractionated heparin.

• Lower doses can sometimes be used: for example, for prevention of thrombosis.

## Preparations of low molecular weight fragments of heparin

Preparations available at present include:

• **dalteparin**
• **enoxaparin**
• **tinzaparin**
• **certoparin**.

It seems probable they will replace unfractionated heparin, but they are considerably more expensive than unfractionated heparin.

## Administration

Heparin is not absorbed by mouth and is given by intravenous infusion or subcutaneous injection. The anticoagulant effect of heparin is seen within a minute or two of injection, but passes off within a few hours. Heparin is often used at the beginning of anticoagulant treatment because its effects are so rapid. Low molecular weight heparins are given once or twice daily by subcutaneous injection and the dose can be calculated from the weight of the patient.

**Infusion.** Infusion is given via a syringe pump. If a pump is not available the heparin can be added to 1 litre of saline or 5% dextrose and given as an infusion. Whichever method is used the infusion rate must be carefully controlled. The rate of infusion is monitored by measuring the kaolin cephalin time or activated partial thromboplastin time (APTT) 6 hours after starting infusion and then at least once daily; these should be kept between 1.5 and 2.5 times the control value.

The kaolin cephalin time is a method of measuring the clotting time. Platelet-poor citrated plasma is pre-incubated with kaolin, which is a surface activating agent, and a phospholipid such as cephalin, and calcium. The time taken for clotting is measured.

**Subcutaneous injection.** When used to prevent thrombosis, heparin is given subcutaneously twice daily.

> ### Nursing point
>
> Heparin is injected into the subcutaneous tissue of the abdominal wall via a fine needle (gauge 25, length 16 mm). An inch of skin should be picked up at the site of injection and the needle inserted perpendicularly to its full length. Local pressure is applied for 5 minutes after injection to prevent excessive bruising. Cleansing the skin before injection with isopropyl alcohol (a vasodilator) increases the chance of haematoma formation.

## Adverse effects of heparin

• The only common adverse effect from heparin is bleeding due to overdose. As with all anticoagulants this often first appears as haematuria, but may occur from any site. The treatment is to stop the heparin.

• Prolonged use may lead to osteoporosis.

• Very rarely, severe thrombocytopenia develops and a platelet count should be carried out if the patient receives heparin for more than 5 days.

Osteoporosis and thrombocytopenia are less commonly seen with the use of low molecular weight heparins.

## Protamine sulphate, an antidote to heparin

Protamine sulphate, a basic protein, which reverses the action of heparin, can be given intravenously. This protein neutralizes the acidic heparin.

**Adverse effects of protamine sulphate.** Protamine sulphate may cause a fall in blood pressure.

## HIRUDIN

Hirudin was originally obtained from leeches and has been recognized as an anticoagulant for many years. It can now be made synthetically using recombinant technology. It differs from heparin in its mode of action, being a specific inhibitor of thrombin. It is given by intravenous injection or infusion. Although experience is still limited, it appears to be as effective as low molecular weight heparin, although bleeding may be a problem.

## ORAL ANTICOAGULANTS: THE COUMARINS

There are two substances in this group that are used in anticoagulant treatment, namely **warfarin** and **phenindione**. Historically, this group was discovered when cows developed haemorrhage after eating spoiled sweet clover silage. The active principles were isolated and this led to the synthesis and introduction of warfarin and phenindione. They are often referred to as the oral anticoagulants, since they are active via this route of administration.

### Mechanism of action of warfarin and phenindione

Warfarin and phenindione exert their anticoagulant effects by interfering with the synthesis of vitamin K-dependent clotting factors, namely factors VII, IX, X and XI.

### Administration

Warfarin and phenindione are given orally in tablet form. This makes them very convenient for the patient, who can take anticoagulants at home. Their onset of action is delayed by several hours since they will only be effective after the existing stores of the vitamin K-dependent clotting factors have been depleted. For this reason, anticoagulant therapy is usually initiated with heparin, which acts immediately, followed by oral anticoagulants. Phenindione is shorter acting than warfarin and is now rarely used.

### Monitoring anticoagulant therapy

The initial stages of anticoagulation have been traditionally carried out in hospital, and thereafter controlled on an outpatient basis, but much more is now done in the community. Patients on anticoagulation therapy need to be carefully and regularly monitored for the levels of anticoagulant activity, since excessive activity can result in haemorrhage and insufficient activity can result in clotting.

The prothrombin time should be measured before starting treatment, then daily, and the dose adjusted until the INR (see below) is stabilized. The ratio:

$$\frac{\text{Patient's prothrombin time}}{\text{Normal prothrombin time}}$$

is known as the international normalized ratio (INR) and the dose is adjusted to keep this between 2.0 and 3.5 (depending on the clinical situation),

which gives effective anticoagulation with minimal risk of bleeding.

### Precautions to be taken when prescribing warfarin

- It is very important that strict accuracy is observed in the timing of doses.
- The effectiveness of the drug in interfering with coagulation is measured by prothrombin time estimations.
- The patient's age and state of health. For example, patients with liver disease are more sensitive to oral anticoagulants, because these are inactivated in the liver.
- Poor nutrition, heart failure, previous surgery and concurrent drugs will increase the patient's sensitivity to warfarin and require smaller dosage.

The prothrombin time (PT) is the time taken for clotting to occur in a sample of blood to which thromboplastin and calcium have been added. (Thromboplastin is formed naturally during the early stages of coagulation, and it converts the inactive prothrombin to thrombin.)

### Contraindications

Contraindications to the use of warfarin include active peptic ulcer, severe liver disease and renal failure.

### Adverse effects of warfarin and phenindione

The adverse effects are:

- haemorrhage
- skin rashes, fever and jaundice (phenindione)
- teratogenic effects (fetal abnormalities).

**Haemorrhage** may result from overdosage, and is the most important side-effect of the coumarin group of drugs. An INR of above 5 suggests a risk of bleeding. It is best treated by withdrawal of the drug. If necessary, the effect of the anticoagulant can be reversed rapidly by an infusion of fresh frozen plasma. Alternatively, phytomenadione (vitamin K) intravenously can be given, but takes about 12 hours to become effective. Larger doses of phytomenadione interfere with further anticoagulation for some days. Very rarely, transfusion with fresh blood is required if blood loss has been excessive.

### Use in pregnancy

Warfarin crosses the placenta and may cause fetal abnormalities if given in the first 3 months of pregnancy. If anticoagulation is required during pregnancy, heparin can be used throughout or heparin used up to 16 weeks, warfarin from 16 to 36 weeks and heparin until delivery. Pre-filled syringes of heparin calcium are available for self-injection by pregnant women at home.

## Drug interactions with warfarin

Interactions of oral anticoagulants with other drugs are important because even a small increase or decrease in their effectiveness may render them dangerous or useless.

Warfarin activity is *increased* by:

- antibiotics
- aspirin
- alcohol
- cimetidine
- dipyridamole
- phenytoin.

Warfarin activity is *decreased* by barbiturates. The dangers of taking barbiturates while on anticoagulant therapy are illustrated in Case history 7.1, which highlights the importance of ascertaining the drugs being taken by patients on anticoagulant therapy.

---

### Special points for patient education

1. The dose of anticoagulants is critical – the correct dose must be taken at the correct time.
2. Overdosage is dangerous – any evidence of bruising or bleeding must be reported immediately. In hospital, the urine must be tested daily for blood.
3. As far as possible patients should not alter their lifestyle, but even one night of heavy drinking may alter the efficacy of oral anticoagulants.
4. There are many interactions with other drugs. These (even those obtained over the counter) should not be taken without medical advice.
5. All patients on oral anticoagulants should carry a card and attend regularly for estimations of prothrombin time.

---

This list is by no means complete and, if possible, the use of other drugs with anticoagulants should be avoided. If the drug regimen has to be changed, the prothrombin time must be monitored carefully.

### Case History 7.1

Mrs Y, a 70-year-old widow, was taken into Accident and Emergency after collapsing at home, and after blood tests were taken she was given 4 units of blood. On examination it was found that she was on anticoagulant therapy with warfarin and an overdose was suspected, although the patient was on regular monitoring for clotting time. On further examination it transpired that Mrs Y had borrowed barbiturate sleeping tablets from a friend some months previously and had taken them regularly thereafter. Consequently, the barbiturates had speeded up the rate of elimination of warfarin by inducing the liver enzymes that metabolize warfarin. As a result, her clotting time had changed and the unsuspecting primary care team had increased the dose of warfarin. Soon after that, Mrs Y stopped the barbiturates, which now meant she was getting an overdose of warfarin because the liver metabolizing enzymes were no longer being induced, and she suffered a bleeding episode. It was explained to her that she should not take any medication without first consulting her care team.

## PREVENTION OF VENOUS THROMBOSIS

There is a risk of venous thrombosis under the following conditions:

- immobility
- prosthetic heart valves
- established atrial fibrillation.

Patients **immobilized in bed** as a result of surgery, severe illness or trauma are at risk of venous thrombosis and pulmonary embolism. Overall about 20% of untreated postoperative patients develop a thrombosis and about 1% have a fatal pulmonary embolus. These risks can be considerably reduced by heparin, given subcutaneously twice daily or low molecular weight heparin once daily (see earlier) over the operative and post-operative period. With correct dosage it is possible to achieve thrombus prevention without undue bleeding at operation. The risk of thrombosis for these patients continues for several weeks and although it is usual to stop heparin on discharge from hospital, the possibility of continuing prophylaxis as an outpatient should be considered. The use of full-length anti-embolism stockings further reduces the risk.

Patients with **prosthetic heart valves** require full anticoagulation with warfarin to prevent thrombosis on the valve.

In patients with **established atrial fibrillation** long-term anticoagulation with warfarin is effective in preventing emboli, and aspirin, taken regularly, confers some benefit.

## THE TREATMENT OF VENOUS THROMBOSIS/PULMONARY EMBOLUS

Patients in whom immediate anticoagulant treatment is required should be started on heparin after a baseline APTT and prothrombin time have been obtained. It is usually given by intravenous infusion as detailed earlier.

Some authorities consider twice daily subcutaneous injection to be equally effective. At the same time the patient is started on oral warfarin, the dose being adjusted to produce the required prothrombin time, which, initially, is measured daily. When this is achieved the heparin is stopped. If there is less urgency, treatment should be started with warfarin.

The duration of treatment depends on circumstances, but should be continued (usually on an outpatient basis) for at least 3 months and in some patients (e.g. with recurrent episodes) up to a year or longer.

### Summary

- Heparin is administered first as an anticoagulant because it is active immediately, but must be given by injection as it is inactivated in the gastrointestinal tract.
- Low molecular weight fragments of heparin may be safer than unfractionated heparin but are more expensive at present.
- Overdosing with anticoagulants can cause serious haemorrhage.
- Protamine sulphate is an antidote to heparin but can cause a fall in blood pressure.
- Oral anticoagulants, e.g. warfarin, have a delayed onset of action.
- Patients on anticoagulants have to be monitored closely for clotting time due to risk of underdosing or overdosing.
- Oral anticoagulants have many interactions with other drugs. It is important to discover what other drugs patients are on and know the health (e.g. liver function) of the patient.
- Long-term immobilization of patients in bed puts them at risk of venous thrombosis.

## ATHEROMA AND ARTERIAL THROMBOSIS

An atheroma is a mass or plaque of fatty or scar tissue on the inner lining (intima) of the arterial wall that occurs due to damage and degeneration of the intima.

## CAUSES OF ATHEROMA

Atheroma arises in a rather different way from venous thrombosis. With increasing age the lining (endothelium) of the arterial wall may become damaged by:

- the flow and eddying of blood, stress and strains due to raised blood pressure
- high levels of circulating cholesterol
- possibly other factors, such as irritants from tobacco smoke.

This damage to the endothelial wall leads to the patchy accumulation of cholesterol-containing lipoproteins and macrophage cells under the arterial endothelium, together with the deposition of platelets. Ultimately, the patch may break down, leaving a rough area (atheromatous plaque) on which a thrombus may form and block the artery. Atheroma is widely distributed throughout the vascular system, but it particularly affects:

- the coronary arteries, causing ischaemic heart disease
- the carotid and cerebral arteries, causing strokes
- the legs, causing claudication, which is limping or lameness.

A drug has been recently introduced for the specific treatment of claudication. It is a phosphodiesterase inhibitor called cilostazol (Editorial 2002c). Phosphodiesterase inhibitors keep intracellular levels of cyclic AMP elevated, and this dilates blood vessels and improves circulation in the limbs.

## ISCHAEMIC HEART DISEASE

Advancing age coupled with risk factors such as high blood pressure, smoking and raised plasma cholesterol levels lead to narrowing of the coronary arteries and atheroma, which is the degeneration of arterial walls. If severe, this interferes with the blood supply to the heart muscle. The coronary blood flow is usually adequate when the patient is at rest, but with effort, the increased demands of the heart muscle for oxygen cannot be met by the narrowed coronary arteries. This results in chest pain, which characteristically comes on with effort and is relieved by rest (angina of effort, angina pectoris). In a few patients the coronary artery may also be narrowed by spasm, which can also give rise to chest pain.

If a thrombus forms on a plaque of atheroma (coronary thrombosis) the blood supply to the area of heart muscle supplied by that artery is cut off and the muscle dies (myocardial infarct).

## DRUGS USED IN ANGINA OF EFFORT

Several groups of drugs relieve the symptoms of angina (summarized in Fig. 7.2), but they do not reverse the underlying atheroma:

- the nitrates
    glyceryl trinitrate
    isosorbide dinitrate
    isosorbide mononitrate
- β blockers
- calcium antagonists
- nicorandil.

## THE NITRATES

These drugs act directly on the plain muscle of the body, causing it to relax. This action is particularly marked on the walls of blood vessels. It is due to the release of nitric oxide, which acts as a vasodilator.

Nitrates relieve the pain of angina in two ways:

- by vasodilatation, which is their main action; this reduces the venous return of blood to the heart and thus reduces the heart work and lowers the demand for oxygen
- by dilating the coronary arteries, particularly if in spasm, so that the blood flow through these arteries is increased.

Some drugs in the nitrate group have powerful, but short-lived, actions; others act less powerfully, but over a longer period (Fig. 7.3).

### Glyceryl trinitrate

**Glyceryl trinitrate** is an oily liquid. It is prepared as tablets by mixing with an absorbent base. It is also

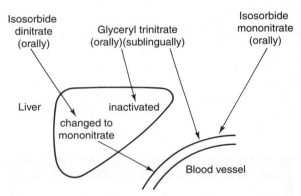

**Figure 7.3** The absorption and metabolism of some commonly used nitrates.

**Figure 7.2** Action of drugs used in angina.

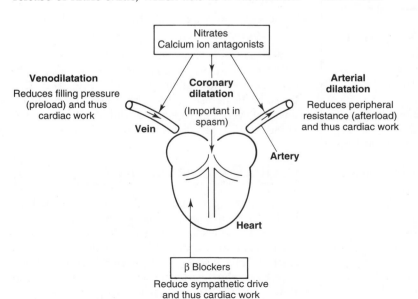

prepared as a metered aerosol, impregnated skin patches or an intravenous infusion.

**Tablets.** These are taken sublingually, the drug being absorbed from the mucous membrane of the mouth. If swallowed whole it is not effective because the drug is rapidly destroyed as it passes through the liver. Its effects start within a minute and last for 15–20 minutes. The tablets lose potency and should not be kept for more than 2 months, and they should be stored in a glass container and not exposed to light or cotton wool.

**Metered aerosol.** A very useful alternative is to give glyceryl trinitrate via a metered aerosol; this acts rapidly. It is sprayed under the tongue and the mouth is then closed.

**Impregnated skin patches.** Glyceryl trinitrate is also absorbed through the skin and impregnated patches are available for application to the skin. They release the drug slowly over 24 hours, thus producing a prolonged effect. They have not proved particularly useful, as it is difficult to control dosage. Headaches can be troublesome and tolerance to the drug's action may develop. If this is suspected, the patches should be removed several times each day.

**Intravenous infusion.** Glyceryl trinitrate can be given by intravenous infusion. This approach is reserved for patients with severe chest pain usually following myocardial infarction, when it may relieve the pain and also improve any complicating heart failure. It is best given in saline or 5% glucose by a syringe pump. PVC containers (*Viaflex* and *Steriflex*) must not be used.

**Effects.** Glyceryl trinitrate causes a marked general vasodilatation with a fall in blood pressure.

## Isosorbide dinitrate and isosorbide mononitrate

**Isosorbide dinitrate** is similar to glyceryl trinitrate. It is broken down in the liver to **isosorbide mononitrate**, which is the active agent, and which is also available for clinical use. Isosorbide mononitrate is given twice daily as its action is quite prolonged. Both the mononitrate and dinitrate are available for intravenous use.

## Clinical uses of nitrates

The main use of nitrates is in the treatment of angina of effort. They can be used in several ways to treat angina. They may be taken intermittently to relieve the pain in an attack or, better, taken before performing some activity, which the patient from experience knows will cause pain. Glyceryl trinitrate is the best drug for this purpose.

One tablet is sucked or placed under the tongue (sublingual) and the dose may be repeated as frequently as is required. In patients who have repeated attacks, a long-acting nitrate such as sustained-release isosorbide dinitrate or isosorbide mononitrate can be given regularly to prevent attacks or diminish their severity. The duration of action of orally administered preparations of nitrates is summarized in Table 7.1.

In patients with severe angina or myocardial infarction, glyceryl trinitrate or isosorbide dinitrate may be given by intravenous infusion.

**Table 7.1**  Duration of action of nitrates

|  | Onset of effect | Duration of effect |
|---|---|---|
| Glyceryl trinitrate | | |
| (sucked or chewed) | 2 minutes | 30 minutes |
| (patch) | 1–2 hours | up to 24 hours |
| Isosorbide mononitrate | | |
| (swallowed) | 20 minutes | 10 hours |
| Isosorbide dinitrate | | |
| (chewed) | 2 minutes | 2 hours |
| (swallowed) | 20 minutes | 5 hours |
| (modified release) | 20 minutes | 12 hours |

## Adverse effects of nitrates

- Flushing
- Headaches
- Palpitations
- A fall in blood pressure which can be particularly troublesome with long-acting preparations when the patient may feel faint
- Rarely, large doses cause methaemoglobinaemias, leading to a cyanotic appearance.

## Tolerance

Tolerance to the action of nitrates occurs with long-acting preparations or frequent dosage, but sensitivity is rapidly restored if the drug is stopped for a few hours. Intravenous infusions should not be given for more than 36 hours without a break. The last dose of sustained-release or long-acting preparations should be taken with the evening meal and the patch removed overnight unless nocturnal angina is a problem. Glyceryl trinitrate is unlikely to produce tolerance, as it is so short acting.

## β BLOCKERS

β Blockers (see p. 79) have proved very useful in treating angina of effort. The rise in heart rate and heart work that occurs on exercise is partially brought about by the activity of the sympathetic nervous system. By blocking this stimulating effect the β blockers protect the heart from overactivity and prevent the development of anginal pain.

### Clinical use

Most β blockers have been used successfully in treating angina of effort and there is no evidence that any one drug is to be preferred. The usual method of giving these drugs is to start with a small dose and increase it until a satisfactory control of symptoms is obtained. The drug is given regularly to prevent pain rather than to treat attacks.

## CALCIUM ANTAGONISTS

The calcium antagonists (see p. 75) are potent dilators of blood vessels. Nifedipine, verapamil and diltiazem are all used to treat angina.

These drugs decrease cardiac work by dilating the peripheral blood vessels and this lowers resistance to blood flow. In addition, they dilate the coronary blood vessels; therefore they are useful in treating angina, particularly if it is believed that coronary spasm is playing a part in producing the symptom. There has been some controversy that the use of the short-acting preparation of nifedipine in patients with coronary artery disease is associated with increased mortality. They are taken regularly to prevent angina. Nifedipine slow release (Adalat retard) is given twice daily, and verapamil and diltiazem are given three times daily.

## NICORANDIL

Nicorandil is a vasodilator that activates potassium channels in the blood vessel membrane; it also acts as a nitric acid donor. It has been in use for angina for many years in Japan and has been relatively recently licensed for use in the UK. At present it is usually reserved for patients who remain symptomatic despite management with other drugs.

### Adverse effects

These include headache, flushing and nausea.

## UNSTABLE ANGINA

Sometimes angina is not clearly related to effort but occurs irregularly and includes attacks at rest. This indicates that a plaque of atheroma on the wall of a coronary artery is becoming detached and may herald a myocardial infarct. Low-dose aspirin is used to try and prevent the formation of a platelet thrombus on the unstable plaque, and is the most important part of treatment. Glyceryl trinitrate relieves pain and β blockers (best given intravenously at first) reduce the risk of a myocardial infarct. Heparin is also used and treatment should not be delayed.

---

### Special points for patient education

Patients with angina can learn to avoid or treat their attacks.

1. If possible, they should avoid situations known to precipitate attacks, e.g. undue exertion, heavy meals.
2. They should differentiate between drugs that are used intermittently to treat an attack or taken immediately before exertion to prevent one, and those which are taken regularly as a prophylactic measure.
3. They should be aware of the main adverse effects they may encounter and it is helpful if the first dose of glyceryl nitrate is taken under supervision so that patients may become familiar with the side-effects.
4. Patients may ask if the drugs will become less effective with continued use. This is unlikely with glyceryl trinitrate, but not for the longer acting nitrates (see text). Tolerance does not occur with β blockers or calcium antagonists.
5. Patients should be told to call their doctor if an attack is prolonged and fails to respond to glyceryl trinitrate.
6. Patients should be encouraged to stop smoking, reduce weight (if obese) and their plasma cholesterol should be lowered (if raised). Provided there are no contraindications, aspirin 75 mg daily should be given to prevent thrombus formation.

---

## DRUGS USED IN THE TREATMENT OF CORONARY THROMBOSIS

When a thrombus forms on an atheromatous plaque, it may block the artery and cut off the blood supply to the relevant area of myocardium, causing an infarct (death) of that segment of muscle. This is one of the most common medical emergencies. Except for a few elderly patients with minimal infarction, patients are nursed in hospital and may spend the first 48 hours in a coronary care unit because this is the period when dangerous complications such as arrhythmias may occur.

## TREATMENTS

• **Relief of pain**, which may be severe. Diamorphine or morphine are the best analgesics, and to prevent opioid-induced vomiting they should be combined with metoclopramide or prochlorperazine.

• **Dissolving the thrombus**: the early use of thrombolytic drugs (see later) reduces the mortality by 25–30 deaths per 1000 patients. It is very important to start this treatment as soon as possible after the onset of symptoms, certainly within 12 hours. Streptokinase is probably as effective as other thrombolytic drugs and a good deal cheaper. If the patient has received streptokinase within the preceding year, alteplase should be used, because, as stated above, patients develop antibodies to streptokinase.

• **Preventing further platelet thrombus formation** (see later) is achieved by giving aspirin, chewed and swallowed, as early as possible after the onset of symptoms, followed by daily oral doses.

• **Preventing arrhythmias**: there is no really satisfactory solution to this problem. Plasma potassium must be kept at about 4.5 mmol/litre; otherwise, arrhythmias are treated in the usual ways (see p. 68) and it is essential to have a defibrillator immediately available.

---

**Nursing point**

Aftercare is important in these patients. Most patients are discharged home within 1 week, so aftercare is important to help them to return to a normal life while minimizing the chances of a further episode. This should include:

• Reassurance and support; many patients are anxious and have lost confidence.
• Patients should be given support to give up smoking.
• Weight should be reduced to the ideal level.
• The plasma cholesterol concentration should be reduced if this is raised above 5.5 mmol/litre.

---

This is achieved most effectively with statins (see p. 101).
• Further studies should be arranged to determine whether a coronary bypass operation would be beneficial.
• Heart failure, if present, can be treated with ACE inhibitors.

## DRUGS TO PREVENT RECURRENCE

Provided there is no contraindication, patients should receive aspirin daily to minimize platelet thrombus formation. Aspirin should be prescribed after a coronary bypass operation, since a recent study found evidence that the treatment reduced postoperative mortality as well as non-fatal ischaemic complications, stroke, renal failure and bowel infarction (Editorial 2002a).

There is some evidence that β blockers improve the long-term prognosis, but they should be avoided in patients with heart failure.

## FIBRINOLYTIC DRUGS

### FIBRINOLYSIS

Normal fibrinolysis is the process that is set in motion when the intrinsic coagulation process is triggered. Essentially, it is the process whereby the blood clot is digested. A plasma globulin protein called plasminogen is deposited on the fibrin strands. Plasminogen activators convert plasminogen into another protein called plasmin, which is able to digest fibrin and fibrinogen amongst other proteins. Enzymes called antiplasmins break down any plasmin that escapes into the circulation. The plasminogen activators have been identified and are now used as fibrinolytic drugs to dissolve thrombi. They therefore complement the use of anticoagulants, which prevent the formation of clots in the first place.

There are several fibrinolytic drugs available:

• **streptokinase**
• **alteplase**
• **anistreplase**.

### STREPTOKINASE

Streptokinase is a non-enzymic protein isolated from β-haemolytic streptococci, which binds to plasminogen, thereby activating it. It has been used for many years to treat venous thrombosis, but is now used mainly to treat coronary thrombosis. Streptokinase is a streptococcal exotoxin. Exotoxins are powerful poisons that are released from bacteria into the surrounding tissues. Endotoxins are poisons that are produced by certain Gram-negative bacteria.

## Therapeutic use

**Administration** is by intravenous perfusion. Patients may be pre-treated with chlorpheniramine and hydrocortisone to reduce allergic reactions. Patients are also given a loading dose of oral aspirin, which should be chewed before swallowing, and this is followed by maintenance doses of aspirin thereafter.

## Adverse effects

- **Bleeding**: This is the main risk with streptokinase, and is particularly liable to occur at sites of recent trauma or invasive vascular procedures, which must be avoided if possible. It is contraindicated in those in whom it might precipitate bleeding (e.g. patients with peptic ulcers, oesophageal varices, severe hypertension or recent head injuries).
- **Allergies** are common and include fever, bronchospasm and rashes.
- **Hypotension** can occur and the blood pressure should be monitored.

## Contraindications

Patients develop antistreptokinase antibodies after about 4 days of treatment, and it should not be used again for at least 12 months to allow these antibody titres to fall, since the antibodies will neutralize the streptokinase and render it useless.

## ALTEPLASE

Alteplase is a tissue plasminogen activator (tPA). It is called this because it is a much more potent plasminogen activator when it is bound to fibrin, and is less active on plasma plasminogen. Circulating streptococcal antibodies do not neutralize alteplase; therefore it can be used in patients who have had streptokinase or a streptococcal infection. It is, however, considerably more expensive than streptokinase. Alteplase may be followed by heparin to prevent re-occlusion.

## ANISTREPLASE

Anistreplase is a plasminogen–streptokinase complex that liberates streptokinase, and after injection is converted to streptokinase. It is therefore a prodrug. It is administered by intravenous infusion over 4–5 minutes, and fibrinolytic activity is sustained for 4–6 hours. It is an expensive drug.

### Summary

On the present evidence streptokinase appears to be at least as effective for patients requiring thrombolytic treatment as the alternative plasminogen activators and is more cost-effective. Alteplase should be used in those with circulating streptococcal antibodies. Anistreplase, which is easy to administer (no infusion required), may have a place for emergency treatment outside hospital where facilities are limited.

### Nursing point

When giving thrombolytic drugs:

1. Avoid intramuscular injections.
2. Avoid subclavian catheters for central venous lines.
3. Use indwelling venous or arterial catheters for access.
4. Look out for bleeding.
5. There are several contraindications to the use of thrombolytic drugs. Check that they have been considered and excluded.

The fibrinolytic drugs are summarized in Figure 7.4.

## STROKES

Strokes are an important cause of death and disability. Most of them (80%) are ischaemic, due to thrombi developing on atheroma, or emboli from atrial fibrillation blocking a branch of the cerebral circulation; the rest are due to haemorrhage.

The use of fibrinolytic agents or anticoagulants immediately after an ischaemic stroke to dissolve the obstruction would seem reasonable but the

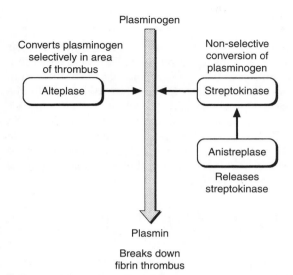

Figure 7.4    The action of thrombolytic drugs.

- after coronary artery bypass grafting
- **atrial fibrillation in patients who cannot take anticoagulants**
- **when there is a high risk of myocardial infarction, e.g. in patients with intermittent claudication, symptoms of atherosclerosis or patients who are recovering from myocardial infarction**.

A new drug is currently being tested for its potential usefulness in reducing mortality in patients undergoing angioplasty following myocardial infarction, and seems promising. The drug is **pexelizumab**, one of the so-called biologic drugs, consisting of an antibody fragment that neutralizes one of the proteins of the complement cascade (Editorial 2002b).

These drugs, as well as certain dietary supplements, are undergoing extensive trials to see whether it is possible to prevent as well as treat thrombotic disease.

results of trials are conflicting, and there is the ever-present danger of causing a bleed.

Preventative measures can considerably reduce their incidence or prevent recurrence and include:

- lowering raised blood pressure, which should not exceed 140/85, if possible
- regularly using antiplatelet agents (e.g. low-dose aspirin), which should be started 6 weeks after either a stroke or a transient ischaemic attack
- lowering raised blood cholesterol with statins (see below)
- using anticoagulants in patients with atrial fibrillation, to prevent emboli
- helping the patient to stop smoking
- taking adequate exercise.

## DRUGS AND PLATELET CLUMPING

Arterial thrombosis such as occurs in coronary thrombosis and strokes is partly due to an aggregation of platelets, which ultimately forms small plugs in blood vessels. Certain drugs have been shown to reduce platelet 'stickiness' so that aggregation is less likely to occur. The main indications for the use of antiplatelet drugs are:

- **acute myocardial infarction**
- **acute thrombotic stroke**
- **after coronary artery angioplasty and stenting**

## ASPIRIN

Aspirin, by inhibiting the production of thromboxane in platelets, prevents them adhering to each other and to atheromatous plaques and so forming or extending a thrombus.

The uses of aspirin in vascular disease so far determined, *provided there is no contraindication*, are:

- in acute coronary thrombosis – combined with streptokinase
- taken regularly following a coronary thrombosis to prevent recurrence
- taken regularly following transient ischaemic attacks or strokes to prevent recurrence
- in angina of effort to prevent vascular episodes
- in unstable angina to prevent progress to myocardial infarction
- in patients with atrial fibrillation, aspirin has some effect in reducing the formation of emboli.

Aspirin may also have a place in preventing eclampsia in pregnancy and in slowing the progress of diabetic retinopathy. A possible disadvantage of aspirin is that it does not block all the pathways to platelet clumping.

There is as yet no conclusive evidence that regular aspirin prevents vascular disease in healthy (low-risk) people. There is a slight chance of gastric bleeding, which is dose-related. There is no increased risk of cerebral haemorrhage.

## DIPYRIDAMOLE

Dipyridamole, like aspirin, prevents platelet clumping. It is not very effective when given alone, but may be combined with aspirin or warfarin.

## GLYCOPROTEIN IIb/IIIa (GPIIb/IIIa) RECEPTOR ANTAGONISTS

The final step in the clumping of platelets is the deposition of fibrin on the platelet surface, leading to the formation of a thrombus, and is due to the activation of a receptor, the glycoprotein IIb/IIIa (GPIIb/IIIa) receptor on the surface of the platelet. Drugs are now available which can block this receptor and thus prevent thrombus formation. An advantage of this approach is that it blocks all pathways to platelet clumping. Several drugs are in development, and some in use include ticlopidine, clopidogrel and abciximab.

### Ticlopidine

Ticlopidine has an efficacy in reducing stroke approximately equal to that of aspirin. It is a pro-drug and works through an active metabolite. Its onset is relatively slow, being about 7–10 days and it is not suitable for long-term use due to adverse effects (diarrhoea and rashes); it is, however, indicated for short-term use under certain circumstances, and it has been used together with aspirin.

### Clopidogrel

Clopidogrel is similar chemically to ticlopidine and has similar adverse effects, but is more potent.

### Abciximab

Abciximab is an interesting drug, whose development reflects a radically new approach to the treatment of disease. It is one of a class of drugs, sometimes referred to as biologic drugs. It is a monoclonal Fab antibody fragment directed against the GPIIb/IIIa receptor. It must be given by intravenous infusion. Evidence suggests that, when combined with aspirin and heparin, it improves the outcome in unstable angina and after coronary angioplasty.

Similar biological drugs are now licensed for use in rheumatoid and psoriatic arthritis, and are proving to be very effective (see p. 156).

## FISH OILS

Inuits have a low incidence of coronary thrombosis and this appears to be related to their large consumption of fish. The fatty acids in fish differ from those of meat and reduce the production in the body of prostaglandins (which promote thrombosis and inflammation) and increase that of prostacyclin (which is anti-inflammatory). The role of fish oil in preventing thrombotic disease and also rheumatoid arthritis and psoriasis is being studied and the results are encouraging.

## THE HYPERLIPIDAEMIAS AND ATHEROMA

The hyperlipidaemias are a group of disorders of metabolism in which there are increased amounts of various lipoproteins in the blood. Lipoproteins are substances that are composed of fats and proteins and are produced by the liver. The concentration of blood lipoproteins is determined partly by the dietary intake of fats and partly by metabolic processes within the body. It is therefore possible to lower the lipoprotein levels either by decreasing the intake or absorption of fats or by changing the metabolism.

The most important lipid in lipoproteins is cholesterol and there is strong evidence that a high level of cholesterol in the blood, especially in the form of low-density lipoproteins (LDL), is associated with an increased risk of atheroma and coronary thrombosis (Table 7.2).

It therefore seems reasonable to lower the blood cholesterol concentration and thereby reduce the risk of coronary artery disease. Reducing raised blood cholesterol levels in patients following myocardial infarction improves their prognosis.

There is also increasing evidence that even in apparently healthy subjects with raised blood cholesterol, lowering the level reduces the risk of coronary

**Table 7.2** Approximate relationship between blood cholesterol levels and coronary thrombosis

| Blood cholesterol level (mmol/litre) | Coronary deaths/1000 |
| --- | --- |
| 4.5 | 5 |
| 6.0 | 8 |
| 7.0 | 12 |

disease. It has been suggested that lowering cholesterol levels, particularly in younger men, by 10% would reduce the incidence of coronary disease by 20–50%. The benefit would be increased if other risk factors (e.g. smoking and hypertension) were also controlled.

Mild hyperlipidaemia (plasma cholesterol 5.2–6.5 mmol/litre) is very common in the adult population of the UK and the problem is largely one of health education and changing people's lifestyle rather than using drugs.

## REDUCING PLASMA CHOLESTEROL LEVELS

There are several ways of lowering plasma cholesterol levels.

## DIET AND WEIGHT REDUCTION

- Reduce total fat intake and decrease intake of saturated (animal) fats relative to unsaturated (fish and vegetable) fats
- Increase consumption of antioxidants by taking, for example, vitamin E (see p. 392), or the preparation called coenzyme $Q_{10}$.

A decrease in the total fat intake and the proportion of saturated (animal) fat to unsaturated (fish and vegetable) fat will reduce plasma cholesterol, but requires adherence to a strict diet. Attempts to lower blood cholesterol using dietary advice alone are disappointing and only achieve a 3–6% reduction with minimal effect on the risks of coronary disease.

## Antioxidants

Until recently, attention had been focused on lowering plasma cholesterol levels by limiting saturated fat intake. It is now realized that other dietary factors are involved, in particular antioxidants. These substances, which are found in green vegetables, carrots and fruit, and include vitamin E, are thought to reduce the ability of LDL to cause atheroma and are also believed to reduce the incidence of some types of cancer. Whether this is true is still debated, but they should form part of a healthy diet. Fruit and vegetables, nuts and alcohol (especially red wine) can all play a part in preventing atheroma.

## DRUGS

### Bile acid–binding resins

Bile acid-binding resins comprise:

- **colestyramine A**
- **colestipol**.

These drugs combine with bile acids and cholesterol in the gut, thus preventing their absorption and increasing faecal excretion. They produce a fall in plasma cholesterol but, being rather gritty powders, are unpleasant to take. They are usually dispersed in fruit juice and given just before meals. They may cause abdominal discomfort and diarrhoea.

### Fibrates

Fibrates alter the metabolism of lipoproteins, and so lower blood cholesterol and triglycerides; they have been shown to reduce the risk of coronary disease. Fibrates are given orally. They can cause headaches, fatigue, rashes and dyspepsia and muscle pain, and should not be given to alcoholics. Fibrates include:

- **bezafibrate**
- **ciprofibrate**
- **clofibrate**
- **fenofibrate**
- **gemfibrozil**.

### HMG–CoA reductase inhibitors (statins)

**Statins**, which block the synthesis of cholesterol in the liver and thus lower the blood level, include:

- **atorvastatin**
- **fluvastatin**
- **pravastatin**
- **simvastatin**.

These drugs are given at night because cholesterol synthesis is greatest at this time. In general, they appear to be most useful drugs for lowering blood cholesterol.

**Adverse effects.** Liver disturbances can occur, and regular liver function tests should be carried out for the first year of treatment. Rarely, severe muscle pain and damage develop.

Cerivastatin, which was mentioned in the last edition of this chapter, has now been withdrawn from use over concerns about muscle toxicity.

## MANAGEMENT OF RAISED PLASMA CHOLESTEROL

Patients with modestly raised plasma cholesterol, found on routine screening and who are symptom-free, will need some encouragement to stick to a strict low-fat diet as it may seem very unexciting; yet, too much pressure may induce anxiety. In these circumstances, the best advice is to avoid animal fats as far as possible, use vegetable oils, develop a taste for oily fish, increase the intake of fruit and vegetables and, if appropriate, enjoy a modest wine consumption.

If however, the patient has blood cholesterol in the higher ranges, has a family history of high cholesterol or already has symptoms of atheromatous disease (usually coronary thrombosis), there is a clear advantage in reducing the blood cholesterol, and this is achieved most effectively by using statins. In addition, other risk factors must be addressed: in particular, smoking, hypertension, obesity and lack of exercise. Other rare and more complex hyperlipidaemias may require different management, usually by a specialized unit.

### Summary

- Routine screening for plasma cholesterol in older patients is important
- Symptom-free patients with moderately raised plasma cholesterol and patients with a family history of thrombosis should be encouraged to stick to a strict low fat diet, take exercise and give up smoking
- Liver function tests should be carried out during the first year of treatment with statins
- Fibrates should not be prescribed for alcoholics
- Bile acid resins may be dispersed in fruit juices to make them more palatable

## References

Editorial 2002a Early aspirin improves survival after coronary bypass operations. Pharmaceutical Journal 269: 705
Editorial 2002b Antibody fragment reduces mortality (Pexelizumab). Pharmaceutical Journal 269: 803
Editorial 2002c Cilostazol introduced for claudication. Pharmaceutical Journal 268: 867

## Further reading

Antiplatelet Trialists' Collaboration 1994 Collaborative overview of randomised trials of antiplatelet therapy. British Medical Journal 308: 81
Editorial 1992 Preventing and treating deep vein thrombosis. Drug and Therapeutics Bulletin 33: 129
Editorial 1992 How to anticoagulate. Drug and Therapeutics Bulletin 30: 77
Editorial 1995a Fish oils and cardiovascular disease. British Medical Journal 310: 819
Editorial 1995b Nicorandil for angina. Drug and Therapeutics Bulletin 33: 12: 89
Editorial 1996a Evidence-based guidelines for the primary care of stable angina. British Medical Journal 312: 827
Editorial 1996b The management of hyperlipidaemias. Drugs and Therapeutics Bulletin 14: 89
Editorial 1997a The emerging role of statins in the prevention of coronary heart disease. British Medical Journal 315: 1554
Editorial 1997b Managing established coronary disease. British Medical Journal 315: 69
Editorial 1997c Antithrombotic agents and thromboembolic disease. New England Journal of Medicine 337: 1383
Editorial 1997d Low molecular weight heparins. New England Journal of Medicine 337: 688
Editorial 1998 Low molecular weight heparins for venous thromboembolism. Drug and Therapeutics Bulletin 36(4): 25
Furberg C D, Psaty B M, Meyer J V 1995 Nifedipine. Dose related increase in mortality in patients with coronary heart disease. Circulation 92: 1326
Gershlick A H, More R S 1998 Treatment of myocardial infarction. British Medical Journal 316: 280
ISIS 3 1992 A comparison of thrombolytic régimes. Lancet 339: 753
Law M R et al 1994 The cholesterol papers. British Medical Journal 308: 363
Lensing A W, Prandoni P, Privis M L et al 1999 Deep-vein thrombosis. Lancet 353: 479
McMurray J, Rankin A 1994 Treatment of myocardial infarction, unstable angina and angina pectoris. British Medical Journal 309: 1343
Manson J E 1992 Primary prevention of myocardial infarction. New England Journal of Medicine 326: 1406
O'Connor P, Feely J, Shepherd J 1990 Lipid lowering drugs. British Medical Journal 300: 667
Opie L H, Messerti F H 1995 Nifedipene and mortality. Circulation 92: 1068
Parker J D, Parker J O 1998 Nitrate therapy for stable angina pectoris. New England Journal of Medicine 338: 520

Tang J L, Armitage J M, Lancaster T et al 1998 Systematic review of dietary intervention to lower blood total cholesterol. British Medical Journal 316: 1213

Turner-Boutle M 1998 Cholesterol and coronary heart disease. Nursing Times 94(15): 46

Weinmann E E, Salzman E W 1994 Deep vein thrombosis. New England Journal of Medicine 331: 1630

Weston C F M, Penny W J, Julian D G 1994 Guidelines for the early management of patients with myocardial infarction. British Medical Journal 308: 767

Wolf P A 1998 Prevention of strokes. Lancet 352 (Supplement III): 15

# Chapter 8

# Drugs affecting the alimentary tract

At the end of this chapter, the reader should be able to:

- appreciate that oral infections are a potential problem for inpatients
- explain how to prevent and treat specific oral infections
- list the treatments for acid reflux
- describe how acid and pepsin are produced
- understand the causes of peptic ulcer
- discuss the antacids and the problems associated with their use
- understand the aims and treatments of peptic ulcer
- give an account of the drugs used to treat chronic inflammatory bowel disease
- list the various classes of purgatives
- appreciate the dangers associated with inappropriate use of purgatives
- describe how to diminish peristaltic activity with drugs
- discuss the significance of the liver in the use of drugs

## THE MOUTH

## SALIVATION

A proper flow of saliva is necessary to keep the mouth fresh and free from infection. Salivary flow will be diminished in fever and dehydration and also by certain drugs, notably those of the phenothiazine group and the tricyclic antidepressants. Antimuscarinic drugs such as atropine will also diminish salivation. Severe oral infection may supervene if salivary flow is markedly decreased. This was a frequent complication in very ill patients in former times when dehydration was not adequately corrected and measures to ensure oral hygiene not practised. Patients receiving cytotoxic drugs are especially at risk as their resistance to infection is lowered and some cytotoxic drugs cause ulceration of the mouth.

## PREVENTION OF ORAL INFECTION

- **Avoid oral infection during surgery**
- **Avoid dehydration**
- **Use mouthwashes**.

**Before major surgery** or any other procedure with a special risk of oral infection, the mouth should be inspected and infected gums or teeth treated. The help of a dentist or dental hygienist may be

needed. **Dehydration** must be avoided and several topical treatments are available.

## Mouthwashes

**Thymol.** Mouthwash solution tablets contain thymol, a mild antiseptic, and are adequate for most patients. One tablet is dissolved in a glass of warm water and used three or four times daily. For patients at special risk various regimens can be used.

**Chlorhexidine gluconate.** A slightly more powerful antiseptic, chlorhexidine gluconate is used in a 0.2% solution (*Corsodyl*). The mouth is rinsed out two to three times daily with 10 ml for about 1 minute. The tongue and teeth may be stained brown, but this can be largely avoided by brushing the teeth before use. Chlorhexidine 1% dental gel is useful for children and handicapped patients. Mouthwash solution can be used every 2 hours in between.

**Artificial salivas.** If dry mouth is a special problem, various artificial salivas are available, instead of or as well as mouthwash solutions. These include *Glandosane* and *Luborant*. In unconscious patients the mouth should be cleaned regularly. Sodium hydrogen carbonate one-quarter teaspoonful in 50 ml is particularly valuable for clearing mucus. (Note that sodium bicarbonate is also called sodium hydrogen carbonate and has the chemical formula $NaHCO_3$.)

**Hydrogen peroxide.** In some hospitals hydrogen peroxide is used to remove debris from ulcers, etc. In seriously ill patients the care of the mouth is a particularly important aspect of nursing care. Hospitals using different regimens and nurses will have to draw their own conclusions as to the most effective treatments.

### Nursing point

In oral infection, prevention is better than cure and recognition that it is a potential problem is important as it can cause considerable discomfort.

## ORAL INFECTIONS AND ULCERATION

In spite of care some patients will develop infections in the mouth; those receiving cytotoxic drugs are at special risk. The main infections are:

- Candida
- oral herpes simplex
- herpes labialis

- non-specific stomatitis with/without ulceration
- aphthous ulceration
- infections of the pharynx and tonsils.

## Candida

This is common and is best treated by **nystatin**, an antifungal antibiotic (see p. 325), which is not absorbed from the intestine. Pastilles of nystatin are dissolved in the mouth four times daily after food; or a suspension can be used. Some patients find the taste unpleasant. Treatment should be continued for 48 hours after symptoms have resolved. An alternative is to use **amphotericin**, another antifungal antibiotic, as lozenges, four to eight times daily. Dentures must be removed during treatment and should be soaked in 1% sodium hypochlorite solution overnight and rinsed before being replaced.

In young children miconazole gel smeared round the mouth is easier, but expensive.

## Oral herpes simplex

For this problem **aciclovir** suspension is used.

## Herpes labialis (cold sores)

This must be treated when symptoms (local burning) just develop. There is no ideal remedy. Aciclovir 5% cream, corticosteroid cream or ice cubes applied locally have all been tried with some success. Aciclovir cream's effectiveness may be enhanced if it is applied as soon as symptoms appear.

## Non-specific stomatitis with/without ulceration

- Dehydration, if present, should be corrected.
- Chlorhexidine mouthwashes should be used as described above.
- Hydrogen peroxide can be used to cleanse ulcers.
- Benzydamine mouthwash (*Difflam*), which acts as a local anaesthetic, is extremely effective in relieving the discomfort of oral ulceration. The mouth should be rinsed out every 2–3 hours with the undiluted solution. If this causes stinging, a 50:50 diluted solution should be used.
- Choline salicylate (*Bonjela*) is a mild local anaesthetic in gel form that may be applied before meals and at night.

## Aphthous ulceration

These small, painful, recurrent oral ulcers are common in healthy people. The cause is unknown, but may be related to stress, and treatment is only partly effective. **Hydrocortisone** pellets dissolved in the mouth four times daily or **tetracycline** mouthwashes are used.

## Infections of the pharynx and tonsils

Infections of the pharynx and tonsils are very common and are usually viral. Most of them require no specific treatment, since recovery is rapid. Many people use gargles, although there is little evidence that they do any good. Compound thymol glycerin, a mild antiseptic, is popular and does no harm. Soluble aspirin is also used as a gargle. It is doubtful whether it has any effective local action but when swallowed will rapidly produce its systemic analgesic and anti-inflammatory effect.

Serious throat infections require the use of the appropriate antibiotic given systemically and there is little indication for the local use of antibiotics in these circumstances.

## THE OESOPHAGUS

## ACID REFLUX AND TREATMENT

The following drugs are used:

- Gaviscon
- Gastrocote
- Mucaine
- $H_2$ histamine receptor blockers
- proton pump inhibitors
- metoclopramide
- domperidone
- cisapride.

Inflammation may occur at the lower end of the oesophagus; it is usually due to reflux of acid from the stomach, and may be associated with a peptic ulcer (see below). Antacids and drugs that block the release of gastric acid can relieve it. Preparations are available which combine an antacid with a local anaesthetic and these are particularly valuable in relieving the pain of swallowing.

**Gaviscon** and **Gastrocote** are combinations of an antacid with alginates which float on the gastric contents. If reflux occurs they protect the mucosa of the lower oesophagus.

**Mucaine** contains the antacids aluminium hydroxide and magnesium hydroxide with oxetacaine, a local anaesthetic, which, it is claimed, relieves the pain arising from the inflamed oesophagus. If reflux is severe and persistent, more active treatment is used. This requires reducing gastric acidity and increasing the motility of the lower oesophagus.

**H$_2$ histamine receptor blockers** (see p. 111) can be combined with antacids, but are less effective than in the treatment of peptic ulcers.

**Proton pump inhibitors** (see p. 111) abolish gastric acid secretion almost entirely and are more effective; they are used in severe cases of reflux oesophagitis.

**Metoclopramide**, which is a drug that stimulates oesophageal motility and thus keeps the oesophagus empty, is also useful. Metoclopramide (see p. 125) is the first choice, but adverse effects may preclude its use. Alternatives are **domperidone** or **cisapride**, which are free from central adverse effects, although cisapride has a number of potentially dangerous interactions with other drugs.

> ### Nursing point
>
> Patients should be advised not to bend after meals and to avoid large meals late at night. Finally, non-drug measures such as weight loss in the obese, elevation of the bedhead and stopping smoking are advised.

## THE STOMACH

The stomach is a hollow organ receiving food from the oesophagus and passing it on to the intestines after a variable interval of between 4 and 6 hours. It is concerned with the mechanical breaking down of the food to render it more easily digested and more easily absorbed. Its muscular walls are capable of powerful waves of peristalsis, which mix and macerate the food. The mucosa lining the stomach secretes hydrochloric acid and pepsin, which together initiate the digestion of proteins.

### DYSPEPSIA AND PEPTIC ULCERS

**Dyspepsia**, which is commonly called indigestion, is discomfort or pain in the abdomen or lower chest after eating. It may be accompanied by nausea and vomiting and is usually ascribed to disordered digestion.

**Peptic ulcers** are lesions of the lining (mucosa) of the stomach (gastric ulcer), the duodenum (duodenal ulcer) or of the oesophagus (oesophageal ulcer). One or a combination of the following may cause them:

● **excessive secretion of hydrochloric acid and pepsin**

● **breakdown of the protective mechanism of the mucosa**
● **a microorganism, *Helicobacter pylori*.**

Hydrochloric acid, which is produced to excess in duodenal but not in gastric ulcers, is responsible for the pain and, for many years, the use of antacids was the mainstay of treatment. The whole approach to the healing of ulcers has changed with the discovery that infection of the stomach lining by the organism *H. pylori* is a major cause of them.

Infection of the lower part of the stomach (the antrum) increases acid production. This acid passes to the duodenum and the combined effect of acidity and damage to the mucosa gives rise to duodenal ulceration and prevents healing. Infection of the body of the stomach is a frequent cause of gastric ulcers and may also lead to gastritis and gastric carcinoma. Eradication of this infection results in healing of the ulcer.

Other factors may be involved, the most important being the resistance of the lining of the stomach to acid and pepsin. Prostaglandin E$_2$, which is formed in the stomach, reduces acidity and helps in the secretion of a layer of mucus which coats and protects the gastric lining. If the production of prostaglandin E$_2$ is inhibited by NSAIDs (see p. 148), the protection is lost and ulcers are liable to develop.

> ### Nursing point
>
> In patients with peptic ulcer, always enquire about the use of NSAIDs.

## THE PRODUCTION OF ACID AND PEPSIN

Acid secretion is a complex process. There are two ways in which it can be provoked (Fig. 8.1):

● Stimulation of the vagus nerve leads to the release of acetylcholine and thus to increased secretion of acid. In healthy people with an intact gastric mucosa this is brought about by the thought, sight or smell of appetizing food. Adequate acid and pepsin are thereby produced to start the digestion of food when it arrives in the stomach. In patients with ulcers, the acid causes the typical pain, particularly if the hoped-for food is delayed.

● Distension of the stomach (for instance by food) causes the production of the hormone gastrin, and this in turn stimulates the stomach to produce acid.

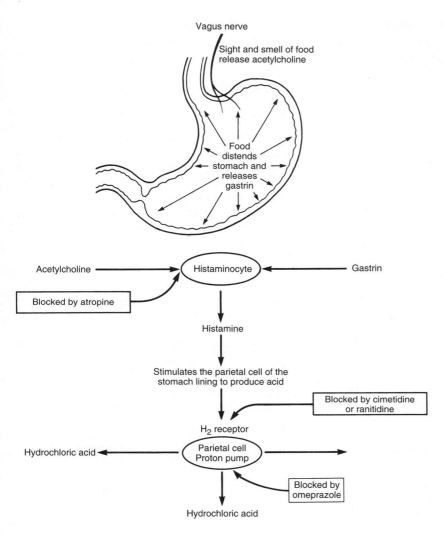

**Figure 8.1**  The mechanisms involved in the secretion of acid into the stomach and the effect and site of action of H₂ blockers.

The common factor in acid production by both these mechanisms is the release in the stomach wall of histamine from cells called histaminocytes. Histamine in turn stimulates the proton pump in the parietal cells, which causes the release of acid in the stomach. The secretory effect of histamine on the stomach is mediated by H₂ receptors.

## TREATMENT OF PEPTIC ULCERS AND DYSPEPSIA

### Approach to the treatment of peptic ulcers

Reducing acidity and protecting the ulcer from acid will relieve the pain of duodenal ulcer and will heal the majority of ulcers, but relapse within a year is very common (75%) unless the associated *H. pylori*

infection is eradicated (see below). It is probably advisable, as demonstrated by Case History 8.1, always to test early for the presence of *H. pylori*. Reducing acidity and eliminating infection is achieved by reducing acid secretion (usually by a proton pump inhibitor) and using a combination of antibacterials (see below). This will cure the majority of patients but a few will require further treatment.

For gastric ulcers the initial treatment may be either with H₂ blockers or the eradication of infection, if present. After the treatment of gastric ulcers, repeat endoscopy is essential to eliminate the possibility that the ulcer may be malignant. Ulcers due to NSAIDs usually respond to an H₂ blocker or omeprazole. For a patient who is at a high risk of developing an ulcer – for example the elderly, those with a previous history of an ulcer, or those taking high-dose NSAID – omeprazole may be co-prescribed. These approaches are summarized in Figure 8.2.

## Aims of treatment

- To reduce acidity, which relieves pain and also helps the healing process
- To protect the ulcer from further damage by acid
- To eradicate *H. pylori* infection
- To discourage the use of NSAIDs.

## DRUGS FOR REDUCING ACIDITY

- Antacids
- Histamine $H_2$ receptor blockers

- Proton pump inhibitors
- Tripotassium dicitratobismuthate (bismuth chelate: *De-Nol*)
- Sucralfate
- Prostaglandins.

## Antacids

Antacids were once widely used in the treatment of peptic ulcers and other forms of dyspepsia. They act by reducing the acidity in the stomach and they also reduce pepsin activity. They are very effective at temporarily relieving the pain from an ulcer, but, unless used intensively, do not accelerate healing. They are also used in various minor gastric upsets; whether they do any good in these circumstances is

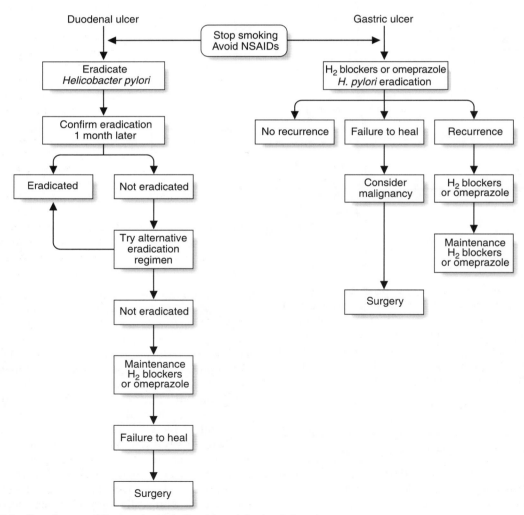

**Figure 8.2** Flow diagram of the management of gastric and duodenal ulcers.

open to doubt, but they are useful placebos. Magnesium or aluminium salts are the most popular. Magnesium is available as magnesium oxide, magnesium hydroxide or magnesium trisilicate.

**Magnesium trisilicate** is a white, gritty powder usually prescribed as a mixture that contains sodium hydrogen carbonate and magnesium carbonate as well. Magnesium salts are very poorly absorbed from the gut and cause diarrhoea.

**Aluminium hydroxide** is a white powder, insoluble in water and usually given as a mixture or a tablet, which is sucked to prolong its effect. In addition to reducing gastric acidity, aluminium salts inactivate gastric pepsin. This antacid is slightly astringent (causes cells to shrink by precipitating proteins from their surface) and can also cause constipation.

The frequency of dosage of antacids is important. They are usually given 1 hour after meals throughout the day and on retiring. This produces a moderate reduction in acidity and keeps symptoms at bay. To accelerate healing, however, larger than usual doses must be given more often.

**Antacid mixtures.** There are many antacid mixtures available. They contain a variety of antacids sometimes combined with substances that protect the mucosa, including anticholinergic drugs or local anaesthetics. Generally, they have little advantage except in special circumstances (see *Gaviscon* and *Mucaine* above) and are usually more expensive.

**Antacids in renal failure and other disorders.** Although the amount of magnesium or aluminium absorbed is very small and harmless in patients with normal renal function, accumulation can occur in patients with renal failure. Some antacids contain fairly large amounts of sodium and cause fluid retention and oedema in patients with cardiac, renal or hepatic failure and also in pregnant women and in infants less than 6 months. Some antacids contain magnesium, and this ion may be dangerous in patients with arrhythmias.

**Drug interactions.** Antacids may interfere with the absorption of digoxin, tetracycline, iron salts, indometacin and isoniazid.

## BLOCKING GASTRIC ACID SECRETION

Gastric acid secretion is reduced in two ways:

- **by blocking the action of histamine at the $H_2$ receptors**
- **by inhibiting the proton pump**.

## Histamine receptor ($H_2$) blockers

The $H_2$ blockers are:

- cimetidine
- famotidine
- nizatidine
- ranitidine.

These drugs block the action of histamine on receptors in the stomach wall and thus reduce the excretion of acid by about 70%. They are given orally, although injections of cimetidine and ranitidine are available.

Ulcer symptoms usually disappear within a week and about 85% of duodenal ulcers heal in a month; gastric ulcers may take rather longer. Unfortunately, about half the patients will develop a recurrence of symptoms after treatment is stopped.

$H_2$ blockers can also be used in reflux oesophagitis (see above) or to prevent the development of ulcers in patients under severe stress.

There is little to choose between these drugs; cimetidine and ranitidine have been in use the longest. Adverse effects are a little more troublesome with cimetidine.

**Adverse effects.** These are rare but with cimetidine include gynaecomastia (enlargement of the breasts in the male) and male impotence due to interfering with the action of testosterone. Cimetidine can cause confusional states in elderly patients.

**Drug reactions.** Cimetidine interacts with various drugs by interfering with their metabolism in the liver. Drugs whose action may be prolonged are phenytoin, morphine, warfarin, methadone, theophylline, labetalol, propranolol, diazepam and metoprolol.

These effects have not been reported with the other $H_2$ blockers.

## Proton pump inhibitors

Proton pump inhibitors are:

- **lansoprazole**
- **omeprazole**
- **pantoprazole**.

These drugs inhibit gastric acid secretion more powerfully than do the $H_2$ blockers. They are used to treat peptic ulcers in patients who have not responded to $H_2$ blockers, and are combined with antibiotics to eliminate *H. pylori*. They are also used in reflux oesophagitis and in the rare Zollinger–Ellison syndrome in which there is gross oversecretion of acid. They are given orally.

**Adverse effects.**    These include headache, nausea, diarrhoea and rashes.

## ULCER PROTECTION

In addition to reducing acid, ulcer healing can be encouraged by drugs that protect the ulcer and increase the resistance of the gastric and duodenal lining to acid. Drugs used:

- tripotassium dicitratobismuthate (bismuth chelate: *De-Nol*)
- sucralfate
- prostaglandins, e.g. misoprostol.

**Tripotassium    dicitratobismuthate    (bismuth chelate:    De-Nol)** is a bismuth-containing compound. It is believed to relieve the symptoms of peptic ulcers by causing coagulation at the base of the ulcer and thus protecting it and promoting healing. It also has some action against *H. pylori*.

This solution has an unpleasant taste and most patients prefer tablets (*De-Noltab*), which are washed down with water. The tongue and stools may appear black and the drug should not be combined with antacids. Treatment is usually continued for 4 weeks and may be repeated after a month.

**Sucralfate** is a compound of aluminium and sucrose that coats the base of an ulcer, protecting it from pepsin and allowing healing to take place.

Prostaglandins (see p. 223) exert some protective effect on the gastric mucosa and this is the reason why drugs that inhibit all prostaglandin production (e.g. NSAIDs) can cause peptic ulcers. **Misoprostol**, which is related to prostaglandins, has been shown to reduce the risk of gastric ulcers in patients at special risk (e.g. the elderly and those with a history of ulcers) who are taking NSAIDs.

## ERADICATION OF *HELICOBACTER PYLORI*

Various triple drug combinations that are effective include:

- Omeprazole + metronidazole + amoxicillin (1 week). This is effective and fairly cheap.
- Omeprazole + clarithromycin + metronidazole (1 week).
- Omeprazole + clarithromycin + amoxicillin (1 week). This is effective but more expensive.

- Ranitidine + amoxicillin + metronidazole (2 weeks). This is cheaper but takes longer.

The use of triple treatment is illustrated in Case History 8.1. Diarrhoea may complicate all these treatments.

### Case History 8.1

Mrs K was in her early thirties when she noticed that she would get indigestion after spicy meals and a little too much alcohol. Initially, this was controllable with over-the-counter antacids when necessary. She then began to notice more pain especially at night and also a couple of hours after eating. As the antacids were no longer sufficient she went to her GP, who prescribed ranitidine (*Zantac*), an $H_2$ blocker. Again, this worked at first, but progressively she had to return to the surgery for more help. Suspecting that his patient's problem might be caused by a *Helicobacter pylori* infection of the stomach, which as well as causing gastric and duodenal ulcers can also cause stomach cancer, the GP referred her to a local gastroenterologist. A biopsy taken at upper gastrointestinal endoscopy confirmed the diagnosis and Mrs K was started on a 1-week course of triple therapy to eradicate the bacteria, which could consist of either of the proton pump inhibitors omeprazole (*Losec*) or lansoprazole (*Zoton*) combined with clarithromycin (*Klaricid*) and either amoxicillin or metronidazole.

### Summary

- Stop NSAIDS in patients with peptic ulcers
- Discourage smoking in patients with peptic ulcers
- Prescribe antacids with care in patients with renal problems
- Do not prescribe antacids for patients taking digoxin, tetracycline, iron salts, indometacin and isoniazid, as antacids interfere with their absorption from the gastrointestinal tract
- Cimetidine is a histamine $H_2$ receptor blocker that can reduce fertility in men
- Proton pump inhibitors can be prescribed for patients that do not respond to $H_2$ blockers
- Misoprostol should be considered for patients who are taking NSAIDs

- H$_2$ blockers and antibacterials may be prescribed together to eradicate *H. pylori* and reduce acid and pepsin secretion
- Patients can also be treated with drugs that coat the ulcer

## NON-ULCER DYSPEPSIA

Non-ulcer dyspepsia may also be associated with *H. pylori* infection but the link is less clear-cut. Patients should be screened for infection and the older age group also endoscoped to exclude cancer. In those with evidence of infection, eradication (as above) can sometimes produce an improvement, although it may be delayed for some months. Those without infection are usually treated with antacids or H$_2$ blockers.

### Special points for patient education for those with peptic ulcer

1. Bed rest helps to heal ulcers but is rarely practical for those who work or who look after young families.
2. Special diets are no longer popular. Patients should be advised to take regular meals (not too widely spaced), avoiding irritating foods and alcohol.
3. Patients should stop smoking.
4. NSAIDs (including aspirin) make ulcer bleeding and perforation more likely, particularly in elderly patients. Steroids in high doses may cause ulcers to develop and make their complications more dangerous. Both drugs should be avoided if possible in patients with a history of peptic ulcers.

## CARMINATIVES

Carminatives are substances which when taken by mouth produce a feeling of warmth in the stomach. They cause relaxation of the cardiac sphincter and allow the 'belching up' of wind and may thus relieve gastric distension. Examples in common use are the oils of ginger and peppermint.

## THE INTESTINES

After food has been partially digested in the stomach, it passes into the small intestine where the digestion of proteins, carbohydrates and fats is completed and absorption occurs.

The passage of food through the small intestine takes about 12–24 hours and the residue then enters the colon where further absorption, largely of water, takes place and the intestinal contents become semi-solid. The filling of the rectum produces the characteristic sensation of the 'call to stool' and the bowels are then emptied by a complicated mechanism, partially voluntary and partially involuntary.

The passage of food through the intestines is brought about by peristalsis, which consists of a wave of contraction preceded by a wave of relaxation. Parasympathetic stimulation increases peristaltic activity and sympathetic stimulation decreases it.

## DRUGS USED IN CHRONIC INFLAMMATORY BOWEL DISEASE

Inflammatory bowel disease is any inflammation of the bowel and includes Crohn's disease and ulcerative colitis. These are chronic autoimmune diseases, in which the immune system attacks the tissues in the absence of any foreign invader. Both Crohn's disease and ulcerative colitis are inclined to run a relapsing course. Crohn's disease is a chronic inflammatory disease of the bowel and may affect any part of the gastrointestinal tract, but commonly affects the small bowel and colorectum. Ulcerative colitis is confined to the colon and rectum. The cause of these diseases is not known.

The usual pattern of treatment is to bring the acute attack under control and then keep the patient in remission. In addition to the use of drugs, other aspects of management include the maintenance of nutrition and electrolyte balance, correcting anaemia (if present) and surgery on occasion to deal with complications or intractable disease.

Drugs used in chronic inflammatory bowel disease:

- corticosteroids
- sulfasalazine
- mesalazine
- immunosuppressants
    azathioprine
    corticosteroids
    infliximab.

## CORTICOSTEROIDS

Corticosteroids are used to induce remission in both disorders. Prednisolone is given orally until the disease remits, then it is reduced stepwise. **Budenoside** (Entocort) is a retarded-release steroid that may have a more marked local action in the terminal small intestine and is preferred by some. In mild ulcerative colitis, if it is confined to the descending colon, prednisolone enemas may be used instead. Corticosteroids are used in Crohn's disease, as illustrated in Case History 8.2. The adverse effects of the corticosteroids are covered on p. 205.

## Case History 8.2

Mr H, aged 22 years, started having lower right abdominal pain associated with diarrhoea and fever. He initially self-treated with antidiarrhoeal agents bought over the counter, but as his symptoms persisted and he started to lose weight and need time off work he visited his GP. Blood tests showed iron deficiency anaemia but no infectious cause for the diarrhoea. A barium examination was made showing narrowing and ulceration of the affected bowel and a diagnosis of Crohn's disease affecting the ileo-caecal junction was made following this. He was started on high-dose oral steroids (prednisolone) 40 mg daily. The symptoms improved rapidly, but on reducing the dose of prednisolone there was a relapse and a 5-aminosalicylic acid-containing drug (*Pentasa* or *Asacol*) more frequently used for ulcerative colitis was added; however, the relapse persisted and to be able to reduce the steroid dose below 10–15 mg daily, the immunosuppressant azathioprine was added. This required regular blood tests since azathioprine affects blood cell production. He was maintained for 2 years in a stable condition, but a further relapse and fistula formation led to a bowel resection of the affected area. The patient was informed of up to a 50% relapse rate after surgery in the first 10 years.

## SULFASALAZINE

Once the patient is in remission after treatment with corticosteroids, sulfasalazine can then be started to keep the patient in remission. Sulfasalazine is a combination of 5-aminosalicylic acid and sulfapyridine and is broken down in the bowel to release 5-aminosalicylic acid, which is the active component. Its action is largely anti-inflammatory. It is effective in maintaining a remission in ulcerative colitis and in colonic Crohn's disease.

**Adverse effects.** These include headache, nausea, rashes and, rarely, blood disorders. Male fertility may be temporarily reduced.

## MESALAZINE

Mesalazine (5-aminosalicylic acid) is also available and has fewer side-effects than sulfasalazine, but is more expensive. Mesalazine enemas can be used to treat distal colitis. Asacol is a delayed-release preparation of mesalazine, useful in distal disease.

## IMMUNOSUPPRESSANTS

Immunosuppressants reduce the activity of the immune system, which is important in causing the inflammation of autoimmune diseases such as Crohn's disease. Immunosuppressants reduce inflammation by inhibiting the production of immune cells and/or by interfering with their production of inflammatory proteins. This approach does weaken the immune system and make the patient prone to infection, but the benefits obtained are often considered sufficiently beneficial to outweigh the risks.

### Azathioprine

Azathioprine, which is also used in rheumatoid arthritis (see p. 156), another autoimmune disease, is sometimes used combined with steroids so that the steroid dose can be reduced to reduce the steroid's side-effects. This approach was used to treat the patient described in the Case History above.

### Methotrexate

This immunosuppressant drug was originally introduced for the treatment of cancer, but is now widely used to treat autoimmune diseases such as rheumatoid arthritis (see also p. 155) and Crohn's disease.

### Infliximab

Infliximab (*Remicade*) is one of a group of newer drugs called biologics (see also p. 156) that block the action of powerful immunoreactive chemicals that are produced by the cells of the immune system. They are now widely used to treat autoimmune diseases and their effects can be dramatic (Kugathasan S et al 2002, Lichtenstein et al 2002).

**Mechanism of action.** Infliximab binds to and inactivates an important inflammatory protein of the immune system called tumour necrosis factor α (TNF-α), which initiates a cascade of production of other chemical inflammatory proteins.

**Administration.** Infliximab is given by intravenous infusion and the patient is usually admitted to a day bed for the procedure. Patients may suffer a relapse within 3 months after the first infusion, but this is generally prevented if the infusion is repeated thereafter at intervals, usually every 8 weeks. After the disease is brought under control, patients can be maintained on other immunosuppressants such as azathioprine.

**Effects.**  The beneficial effects in Crohn's disease can be very rapid and dramatic, especially in patients who do not respond to other treatments. The drug is also effective in healing anal fistulae of Crohn's disease, which are generally unresponsive to other treatments.

**Adverse effects.**  This type of treatment is relatively new, and data about the adverse effects are still being gathered. During the infusion the patient may complain of nausea, shortness of breath or chest pains, and these symptoms usually disappear if infusion is stopped. Since infliximab is a large molecule, it can cause an immune response and patients may develop fever, a worsening of the Crohn's disease and 'flu'-like symptoms. These immune reactions may be severe enough to warrant treatment with other immunosuppressants. Infliximab has been reported to cause tuberculosis (TB) in some patients and is contraindicated in patients who have had TB. Patients should be tested for TB before receiving infliximab. It is also contraindicated in patients with cancer and in patients with existing infections such as abscesses, urinary tract infections or pneumonia.

---

**Nursing point**

In view of the risk of a suppressed blood count with sulfasalazine, mesalazine, methotrexate or infliximab, patients taking any of these should be warned to report sore throat, fever, bruising or bleeding immediately.

---

## Diet

In addition to the drugs detailed above, an elemental diet which contains the essential constituents for nutrition (e.g. carbohydrates, amino acids, fats and vitamins in pure form) given for 2 weeks has a specific therapeutic effect in Crohn's disease, but not in ulcerative colitis.

# PURGES AND THE TREATMENT OF CONSTIPATION

## PURGES

Purges (purgatives) may be defined as drugs that loosen the bowel. They are also called cathartics or laxatives. They are widely used, and a great deal of their use is unnecessary and may even be dangerous. Bowel habits vary considerably, and many people need to open their bowels less frequently than is usually considered 'normal'. For these people, there is nothing to be gained by trying to attain a more frequent bowel action with purges.

Even more dangerous is the indiscriminate use of purges for all types of abdominal pain. In many acute abdominal diseases the use of such drugs aggravates the condition, a classical example being the rupture of an acutely inflamed appendix following a purge. Purges should never be given to patients with undiagnosed abdominal pain.

Bowel evacuation may be achieved using orally administered **purges** or by the use of **enemas** and **suppositories**.

Purges may work in different ways and there are several types:

- bulk purges that are high residue foods, e.g. bran; ispaghula husk (*Isogel*)
- stool softeners, e.g. docusate sodium
- Osmotic purges, e.g. magnesium sulphate, lactulose
- Stimulant purges, e.g. anthracenes; bisacodyl

The **bulk purges** increase the contents of the bowel and thus stimulate peristalsis. The emollient (stool softening) purges aid the passage of faecal material by their lubricating action. The stimulant purges increase peristalsis and thus the intestinal contents pass more rapidly through the bowel and remain more fluid.

## BULK PURGES

High-residue foods contain a high proportion of cellulose, which is not digested or absorbed and thus increases the bulk of the intestinal contents. Common examples are green vegetables, fruit and wholemeal bread.

## Bran

Bran, which is a by-product of milling, contains about 30% fibre made up of celluloses, pectins and lignins, substances which are not absorbed from the intestine and which swell as they take up water and thus increase the bulk of the faeces. The initial dose is one tablespoonful, combined with fluid, daily and this is increased at weekly intervals until a satisfactory result is achieved. The main side-effect is wind.

## Methylcellulose

Methylcellulose is available in a number of preparations either as granules or tablets. It is an effective bulk purge.

## Ispaghula husk

Ispaghula husk is of plant origin and swells on contact with water, thus acting as a bulk purge. It is available as *Isogel* and *Regulan* and other preparations. Combine both with plenty of water.

> ### Safety point
>
> Patients must be warned **not** to take granular preparations that swell in water without first mixing with water. There have been fatalities due to the ingestion of dry granules that swell in the throat and cause asphyxiation.

Bulk purges depend on the ability of the colon to respond to distension and may not be effective in elderly patients.

## STOOL SOFTENERS

## Liquid paraffin

Liquid paraffin has been in use for many years and has been heavily used, especially by elderly patients, who took it chronically and regularly. It is odourless, tasteless and facilitates evacuation in the chronically constipated patient. It is, however, associated with potentially serious adverse effects if taken for long periods. It may cause:

- leaking via the anal sphincter
- lipoid pneumonia in the very young and very old
- interference with the absorption of vitamins A, D and K.

Liquid paraffin should therefore not be used for long periods.

## Docusate sodium

Available as tablets or syrup, docusate sodium acts by softening the stools, which may be sufficient to relieve constipation, particularly if a painful condition such as piles or anal fissure is interfering with bowel evacuation. It may be combined with a stimulant laxative as it takes 2 or 3 days to be effective. It can also be used as a micro-enema in the management of faecal impaction, when docusate in solution is injected into the rectum.

## OSMOTIC PURGES

## Saline purges

The most commonly used saline purge is magnesium sulphate (Epsom Salts). It is poorly absorbed from the intestinal tract. Originally it was thought to make the intestinal contents more fluid, but it is now considered that its purgative effect is a response to magnesium ions reaching the intestine.

A saline purge should be given on an empty stomach (before breakfast is a good time) so that it passes rapidly through the stomach and into the intestine. If it is held up in the stomach, it may not be effective. It is given dissolved in water and the concentration should not exceed 8 g of magnesium sulphate to 120 ml of water as a more concentrated dose may cause closure of the pyloric sphincter and delay the drug leaving the stomach. These drugs are usually effective within 1–2 hours.

Fruit salts usually contain some sodium hydrogen carbonate and tartaric acid. When these are mixed with water, sodium tartrate is formed with the liberation of carbon dioxide. The sodium tartrate acts as a mild purge.

## Lactulose

Lactulose is a sugar that is broken down by bacteria in the large bowel with the production of various acids. These act as osmotic purges, rendering the bowel contents more fluid, and as mild irritants, both of which produce a laxative effect. Lactulose is given in liquid or as a powder, which can be mixed with food or water. It takes several days to act and may cause a certain amount of flatulence and distension. For these reasons it is not a particularly good purge, but is sometimes used in the long-term treatment of constipated elderly patients and for those receiving opioids for intractable pain when constipation may be a problem. It also has a limited use in patients with severe liver disease to reduce the absorption of toxic substances from the bowel.

## STIMULANT PURGES

The anthracene group of purges all contain the anthraquinone, emodin, which is the chief active constituent of the group; the varying properties of the anthracene purges depend on the ease with which this active constituent is released. After liberation in the intestine, emodin is absorbed into the bloodstream and acts on the large intestine, causing increased peristalsis. All members of this group of drugs therefore take about 8–12 hours to act and are best given at bedtime. They may occasionally cause griping (severe abdominal pain) and should be avoided during pregnancy.

### Senna

Senna is usually prescribed as *Senokot*. This is a proprietary preparation that contains the purified principles called sennoside A and sennoside B. It is highly satisfactory and can be used either as granules, tablets or syrup.

### Bisacodyl

Bisacodyl is a preparation that stimulates activity of the colon when it comes in contact with the wall of the bowel. It can be used either orally or as a suppository.

### Co-danthramer

Co-danthramer is a mixture of a stool softener and a stimulant purge (dantron). Unfortunately, it has been shown to produce tumours in rodents with high and prolonged dosage, although there is no evidence that this occurs in humans. Its use is therefore restricted to elderly patients with obstinate constipation or those whose constipation is due to opioid analgesics (e.g. terminally ill patients).

### Sodium picosulfate

Sodium picosulfate is a very powerful bowel stimulant used for preparation before surgery or radiology and not for the long-term treatment of constipation.

## LAXATIVE ABUSE

Some patients become dependent on laxatives because they believe that these drugs wash away poisons from the body. If carried to extremes this can lead to serious electrolyte depletion and damage the bowel with dilation of the colon. In severe electrolyte depletion, intravenous replacement may be required, but for the majority of patients the oral route is satisfactory and preparations containing sodium, potassium, glucose and water in the optimum concentrations are available.

## ADVERSE EFFECTS OF PURGES

- Diarrhoea with loss of fluids and electrolytes
- Dependence on purges with chronic use
- Systemic absorption of purges
- Lipoid pneumonia with liquid paraffin
- Damage to the bowel
- Abdominal pain
- Dangers associated with the use of stimulant purges in pregnancy.

### Summary

- Never give purges to patients with undiagnosed abdominal pain
- Proper diet containing roughage and exercise are important complementary strategies in addition to purgatives
- Bulk purges that swell in water must be mixed with water before oral use
- Powerful stimulant purges should be avoided in pregnancy
- Saline purges such as magnesium sulphate should be taken on an empty stomach
- Liquid paraffin should not be used for long periods
- Purges should be stopped once a regular pattern of evacuation is achieved

## THE TREATMENT OF CONSTIPATION

Before making a diagnosis of constipation it is important to realize that there is considerable natural variation in the frequency with which people open their bowels. The majority vary between twice daily and once every other day.

Constipation has two main causes:

- delayed passage of faeces through the colon
- neglect of the call to stool.

## CAUSES OF DELAYED PASSAGE

Causes of delayed passage are:

- local lesions of the bowel
- disorders that interfere with bowel muscle function such as hypercalcaemia or myxoedema
- pregnancy
- old age
- depression
- weakness of the abdominal muscle
- low bulk diet
- various drugs including opioids, antidepressants and verapamil.

## NEGLECT OF THE CALL TO STOOL

This cause of constipation may occur for social reasons or may be due to illness, surgery or some painful lesion of the anus such as a fissure. As a result the rectum becomes used to distension of its walls by faeces and loses its ability to contract and empty.

In patients who are ill and who have been constipated for a few days, 2–4 *Senokot* tablets at night followed by a glycerin suppository the next day are often sufficient.

In chronic constipation the object of treatment is to re-educate the intestines so that a normal bowel habit is restored. This can be achieved by increasing the bulk of the faeces either by a high fibre content in the diet, i.e. bran or similar substances, or by the use of bulk purgatives such as methylcellulose. A reasonably high fluid intake and exercise are also helpful. This should be combined with regular habits and may require the use of some purgative such as *Senokot* at night until a normal rhythm is regained.

Constipation is a common problem in the elderly, especially those who are institutionalized. It is due to poor diet, inadequate muscle tone and immobility. If faecal impaction occurs it can be relieved by a retention enema of docusate sodium followed by washouts. If this fails or rapid evacuation is required, manual removal may be necessary.

Long-term management needs dietary advice, as much exercise as is practicable, regular habits and the use of a laxative as required. Senna or bisacodyl are cheap and probably as effective as more expensive preparations.

## ENEMAS AND SUPPOSITORIES

The wall of the rectum contains nerve receptors which respond to pressure to produce the normal call to stool, but may also be stimulated by various substances which can be introduced into the rectum as suppositories or micro-enemas to initiate the evacuation of the bowel. Larger-volume enemas distend the rectum and lower bowel, causing contraction, and also have some washout effect.

### Enemas

Enemas may be used to soften the stool and include arachis oil or docusate sodium. To promote evacuation, a phosphate enema, run into the rectum, is useful: for example, before sigmoidoscopy. An alternative is to use a micro-enema such as *Micolette*. This is given rectally and acts as a colon stimulant.

Enemas can also be used to treat conditions of the bowel. In ulcerative colitis, steroids (either prednisolone or hydrocortisone) can be introduced into the rectum and retained if possible for at least 1 hour. A certain amount of steroid is absorbed into the circulation and so both local and general therapeutic effects result.

### Suppositories

Glycerol suppositories, one or two moistened with water and inserted, are quite satisfactory. Other suppositories are available but, in general, offer no advantage.

Purgatives are also used to prepare the bowel before colonic surgery or colonoscopy. Various regimens are used, but essentially a low-residue diet is taken for a few days and one sachet of sodium picosulfate in water is given in the morning and one in the afternoon on the day before the procedure.

## INTESTINAL SEDATIVES

Several drugs may diminish the peristaltic activity of the intestines.

## ANTICHOLINERGIC DRUGS

The anticholinergic drugs decrease gut tone by blocking the action of the parasympathetic nervous system. They are particularly useful in colon spasm.

## OPIOIDS

Opioids actually increase gut tone but reduce peristalsis. They are useful in various forms of diarrhoea. The most widely used is codeine phosphate.

## CO-PHENOTROPE (*LOMOTIL*)

This preparation is a combination of atropine and diphenoxylate hydrochloride. The latter drug is related to the narcotic analgesics. Co-phenotrope is widely used in controlling diarrhoea, but it must be remembered that it is dangerous in overdose, particularly in children, as it can cause depression of respiration due to the action of the opioid.

## LOPERAMIDE

Loperamide decreases large bowel motility. Toxicity is relatively low. It is available for adults and older children without prescription.

## PANCREATIC SUPPLEMENTS

As a result of pancreatic disease (usually cystic fibrosis or chronic pancreatitis) the pancreatic enzymes may be deficient, leading to a failure to digest fat and protein, malabsorption and loose fatty stools (steatorrhoea). The missing enzymes may be given orally, but they are broken down by the acid in the stomach and thus rendered ineffective. This may be circumvented by combining the enzyme with an $H_2$ blocker to reduce gastric acidity or by using preparations that are coated to protect them against acid.
   Available preparations include:

- *Pancrex*, which is supplied as a powder, capsules or tablets and is given before meals (or feeds). The capsules should be broken and mixed with water or milk.
- *Creon* capsules containing coated pellets that may be swallowed whole or opened and the pellets mixed with food. They must not, however, be chewed as they will lose their protective coating. The dose is very variable and is best judged by observing the nature of the stool.

### Nursing point

Maintain a reasonable fluid intake. Some high-strength pancreatic supplements have been associated with bowel strictures. The development of new abdominal symptoms should be reported.

## GALLSTONES

Gallstones are a common finding, although they do not always cause symptoms. They are usually removed surgically either by open operation or by endoscopy. There are, however, drugs that dissolve cholesterol-rich gallstones and they are used to treat selected patients.

## CHENODEOXYCHOLIC ACID AND URSODEOXYCHOLIC ACID

Most gallstones are largely composed of cholesterol. These two drugs, which are bile salts, reduce the concentration of cholesterol in the bile and make it more soluble so that cholesterol-containing stones are slowly dissolved.
   Only small stones are suitable for this treatment. The two drugs are often given together orally as a single dose at bedtime and it may take from 6 to 18 months for the stones to disappear. Relapse is liable to occur when the treatment is stopped. Because of the relatively few patients suitable for this method of treatment and the lengthy supervision required, it has not become popular.

## DRUGS AND THE LIVER

The liver plays an important part in the use of drugs:

- All drugs pass first through the liver via the portal system after absorption from the gastrointestinal tract. Many drugs are activated and inactivated by the liver.
- Liver disease may reduce activation and/or inactivation of drugs, resulting in drug toxicity.
- Some drugs can cause liver damage.
- Drugs are used to treat certain diseases of the liver.

   Drugs pass through the liver either via the portal system after absorption from the intestine or, if the drug has been injected, via the systemic circulation. Many drugs are inactivated by the liver, being either broken down or combined with some substance which renders them inactive.

If the liver cells are damaged by disease or if the portal circulation partially bypasses the liver, as in cirrhosis, the elimination of drugs may be reduced and they will accumulate and produce toxic effects. It is therefore important to consider this possibility whenever drugs are given to patients with liver disease and to adjust the dose as necessary.

A comprehensive list of drugs to avoid or use with care is given in the *British National Formulary*.

Some drugs can cause liver damage. This may be either dose-related or idiosyncratic, although the distinction is not always easy. The drugs involved include:

- paracetamol
- phenothiazines (chlorpromazine)
- methotrexate
- isoniazid
- rifampicin
- pyrazinamide
- halothane.

Recovery usually occurs when the drug is stopped, but in a few cases (e.g. paracetamol overdose) the damage can be severe and fatal.

## CHRONIC VIRAL HEPATITIS

Viral hepatitis B and C present a serious and widespread health hazard that is likely to increase in incidence. Intravenous drug abuse, sexual promiscuity and contaminated blood or blood products transmit hepatitis B virus. The majority of patients clear the virus and make a complete recovery but in about 5% the infection continues and becomes chronic active hepatitis. Hepatitis C infection is also associated with intravenous drug abuse and the injection of blood and blood products. In about 30% of infected subjects the disease progresses as a very slow and indolent hepatitis. Some of these patients will remain as asymptomatic carriers of the virus, but some may develop cirrhosis and, a few, a hepatic carcinoma.

## Interferons

The only specific treatment available at present is with the interferons (see also p. 323). The interferons are peptides that are produced by cells infected with viruses. These drugs stimulate immunity and also have an antiviral action. The interferons are active against a wide variety of viruses, but a particular interferon will be effective only in the species that produced it. There are three types of interferon: namely, interferon alpha from white blood cells, interferon beta from fibroblasts, and interferon gamma from lymphocytes. The course of treatment is prolonged but in about 50% of those with hepatitis B and 25% of those with hepatitis C, the progress of the disease is halted. Interferons may be combined with other antiviral agents.

**Adverse effects.** These include depression, flu-like symptoms and lethargy, and may be very severe.

## Vaccines

For those exposed to the risk of infection with the hepatitis B virus a vaccine is available and there is also a specific hepatitis B immunoglobin ('HBIG') when rapid protection is required. The BNF lists individuals at high risk of infection and nurses are particularly at risk. A combined hepatitis A and B vaccine is also available.

## References

Kugathasan S et al 2002 Infliximab retreatment in adults and children with Crohn's disease: risk factors for the development of delayed severe systemic reaction. American Journal of Gastroenterology 97: 1408

Lichtenstein G R, Bala M, Han C et al 2002 Infliximab improves quality of life in patients with Crohn's disease. Inflammatory Bowel Disease 8: 273

## Further reading

Allbright A 1984 Oral care of cancer chemotherapy patients. Nursing Times 80(21): 40

Amin D 1997 Clinical use of laxatives in general practice. Prescriber, September 1997

Butler M 1998 Laxatives and rectal preparations. Nursing Times 94: 56

Di Bisceglie A M 1998 Hepatitis C. Lancet 351: 351

Editorial 1995 Interferon and hepatitis C. New England Journal of Medicine 332: 1509

Forbes G M, Glaser M E, Cullen D J et al 1994 Duodenal ulcer treated by *Helicobacter pylori* eradication – seven year follow-up. Lancet 343: 258

Forgacs I 1995 Clinical gastro-enterology. British Medical Journal 310: 113

Gorbach S L 1997 Treating diarrhoea. British Medical Journal 314: 1776

Hanauer S B 1996 Inflammatory bowel disease. New England Journal of Medicine 334: 848

Hopkins S 1992 Drugs update: undermining ulcers. Nursing Times 88(16): 62

Langman M J S 1991 Omeprazole. British Medical Journal 303: 481

McCarthy M, Wilkinson M L 1999 Recent advances in hepatology. British Medical Journal 318: 1256

Pope C E 1994 Acid-reflux disorders. New England Journal of Medicine 331: 656

Richmond J 2003 Prevention of constipation through risk management. Nursing Standard 17: 39

Sladen G 1995 The place of laxatives in managing constipation. Prescriber 6(4): 56

Tsai H H 1997 *Helicobacter pylori* for the general physician. Journal of the Royal College of Physicians, London 31: 478

Walsh J H, Peterson W L 1995 The treatment of *Helicobacter pylori* in the management of peptic ulcer disease. New England Journal of Medicine 333: 984

# Chapter 9

# Emetics and anti-emetics, cough remedies, respiratory stimulants

## Learning objectives

At the end of this chapter, the reader should be able to:

- understand what is meant by the vomiting centre and chemoreceptor trigger zone (CTZ)
- describe how they are stimulated
- give an account of the emetics and the classes of anti-emetic drugs
- understand the uses and limitations of cough suppressants
- describe inhalations and mucolytic agents
- explain the term respiratory failure

## EMETICS

## MECHANISM OF VOMITING

Vomiting is a complex series of actions involving the stomach, oesophagus and pharynx with the voluntary muscles of the chest and abdomen, and results in the ejection of the stomach contents. A vomiting centre in the medulla of the brain coordinates these actions. This centre can be stimulated:

- Directly from the labyrinth of the ear in conditions such as seasickness or vertigo.
- By gastric irritation or distension.
- By mental activity (e.g. being sick with fright; imagining something extremely unpleasant).
- Via the chemoreceptor trigger zone (CTZ) which lies close to the vomiting centre in the brainstem and which is stimulated by a number of circulating substances, including certain drugs.

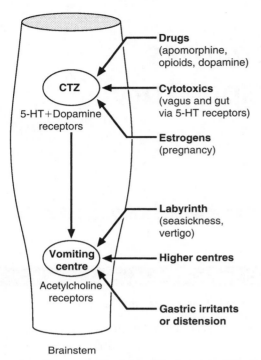

**Figure 9.1** Drugs and other factors stimulating the CTZ and vomitting centre.

• By stimulation of the 5-hydroxytryptamine (5-HT) receptors of the CTZ. Circulating cytotoxic drugs (particularly cisplatin (see p. 344)) release 5-HT from nerve endings, and this activates the CTZ receptors. From the CTZ, impulses travel to the vomiting centre and activate it by acting on muscarinic acetylcholine (ACh) receptors.

The stimulation of vomiting outlined above is summarized in Figure 9.1.

Before the act of vomiting occurs, stimulation of the vomiting centre produces a sensation known as nausea, which is often associated with increased secretion by the salivary and bronchial glands. Drugs that provoke vomiting are called **emetics**.

Emetics are rarely used in medical practice except in cases of poisoning. They may be divided into two types:

• **reflex emetics**, e.g. ipecacuanha
• **central emetics**, e.g. apomorphine.

## REFLEX EMETICS

This group of drugs produces vomiting by irritating the stomach. The only one in common use is ipecacuanha, a plant extract, which is dispensed as ipecacuanha emetic mixture, and vomiting should occur in 15–30 minutes. It may be used as a first-aid treatment for overdose provided that:

• the patient is fully conscious
• overdose is not of corrosive substances or petroleum products when inhalation of vomit could be fatal.

Ipecacuanha can be used up to 1 hour after ingestion of poison and longer for some substances, such as tricyclic antidepressants and salicylates, when gastric emptying is delayed. It is not as effective as a stomach washout, but is particularly useful in children, when the upset caused by the process of lavage should be avoided if possible, and in removing such objects as berries, which cannot be washed out of the stomach. In general, the use of emetics in poisoning is decreasing because there is little evidence, even if used soon after ingestion of poison, that they usefully reduce absorption.

## CENTRAL EMETICS (THOSE ACTING ON THE BRAIN)

**Apomorphine** stimulates dopamine receptors in the CTZ. It is closely related to morphine but has none of its analgesic effects. It has, however, a very powerful emetic action and also produces some cerebral depression. It was formerly used as an emetic but because of its depressing action **it should not be used in treating patients who have taken an overdose**. At present its use is confined to patients with resistant Parkinson's disease (see p. 257).

## ANTI-EMETICS

It is believed that acetylcholine, histamine, dopamine and 5-HT act as intermediate transmitters in the CTZ and vomiting centre. By blocking the action of these substances on their receptors it is possible to prevent or diminish vomiting (Table 9.1).

The classes of anti-emetic agents:

• acetylcholine (ACh) receptor antagonists
• antihistamines
• dopamine receptor antagonists
• 5-HT receptor antagonists
• miscellaneous anti-emetics.

**Table 9.1** The management of vomiting. There are several causes of vomiting and specific drugs are effective for different types

| Types of vomiting | Effective drug | Comment |
| --- | --- | --- |
| Vomiting of pregnancy | Promethazine, sometimes combined with pyridoxine | Dietary management if possible. Keep drugs to a minimum in early pregnancy owing to risk of fetal deformity. Promethazine appears to be safe |
| Motion sickness | Hyoscine | Dry mouth. Blurred vision. Some sedation. Short journey |
| | Cinnarizine | Preferred for longer journey |
| Vertigo | Prochlorperazine Cinnarizine Betahistine | |
| Opioids | Prochlorperazine Metoclopramide Chlorpromazine | |
| | Haloperidol | Less sedating. Long-acting |
| Cytotoxic drugs | Prochlorperazine | Sedative |
| | Domperidone | Not sedative |
| | Metoclopramide | High doses required |
| | Ondansetron Cannabinoids | |
| | Benzodiazepines | Particularly if anxiety is a factor |
| | Dexamethasone | |
| Migraine Postanaesthetic (often opioid) | Metoclopramide Prochlorperazine Haloperidol | |

## MUSCARINIC ACETYLCHOLINE RECEPTOR ANTAGONISTS

**Hyoscine** blocks the action of acetylcholine on the vomiting centre and is useful for the short-term control of motion sickness. It is administered orally or as a transdermal patch. The patch is applied behind the ear for maximum absorption 6 hours before starting a journey. Drowsiness and blurring of vision, due to paralysis of ocular accommodation, can occur.

## ANTIHISTAMINES

Antihistamines commonly used as anti-emetics:

- cyclizine
- promethazine
- cinnarizine.

Antihistamines block the action of histamine on its receptors. Most of the antihistamine group of drugs are not specific and also block ACh receptors. This makes them effective anti-emetics.

Among the most useful are **cyclizine** and **promethazine**, which occasionally has a place in severe vomiting of pregnancy. **Cinnarizine** is an anti-emetic which has found particular favour among yachtsmen and others at risk from seasickness, but it can also be used in other types of vomiting, especially that associated with Ménière's disease. Sedation is not usually a problem.

## DOPAMINE ANTAGONISTS

Several of the phenothiazine drugs (see p. 264) are powerful anti-emetics due to their action in blocking the effects of dopamine on the CTZ. Some do not act only on dopamine receptors – i.e. they are relatively non-specific in action – and therefore have side-effects; for example, they may be sedatives (see Table 9.1). Among those used are:

- prochlorperazine
- chlorpromazine
- haloperidol
- levomepromazine
- domperidone
- metoclopramide.

**Prochlorperazine** suppresses opioid-induced vomiting. It can be given orally or by intramuscular, but not subcutaneous, injection. If given intravenously, it must be well diluted before use. **Chlorpromazine** is similar in action to prochlorperazine. **Haloperidol** is also similar but is longer acting and less sedating. **Levomepromazine** is used, particularly in terminal care, to control vomiting and reduce agitation.

**Domperidon**e is less sedative than chlorpromazine and less liable to produce dystonic reactions (muscle spasms of the face, neck, shoulders, limbs and the trunk) than metoclopramide (see below) because its action on the nervous system is confined to the CTZ. It also enhances gastric emptying. Unfortunately, only about 15% of the oral dose reaches the circulation and a parenteral preparation is not available. It can be used to suppress the vomiting that accompanies long-term treatment with the opioids, levodopa and with the mildly emetic cytotoxic drugs.

**Metoclopramide** increases gastric tone and dilates the duodenum. This causes the stomach to empty more quickly. In addition, it has some central action on the vomiting centre. It is a fairly effective anti-emetic and is administered orally or by intramuscular injection. It is used in postoperative and opioid-induced vomiting and in migraine. In very large doses it also blocks 5-HT receptors and is used to prevent vomiting due to cytotoxic drugs.

Adverse reactions with metoclopramide are rare, but even with normal doses patients may develop dystonia of the facial and neck muscles. This is more common in young people. The spasms pass off within a few hours of stopping the drug and can be controlled by diazepam. Prolonged use of metoclopramide has been reported to cause tardive dyskinesia (involuntary repetitive movements of muscles of the face, mouth and upper trunk brought on by repetitive use of certain drugs, especially antipsychotic drugs; see p. 264).

## 5-HT ANTAGONISTS

**Ondansetron** and **granisetron** probably block the 5-HT receptors associated with the central connections of the vagus nerve in the brainstem in close proximity to the CTZ. They are used to prevent vomiting in patients receiving highly emetic cytotoxic drugs, such as cisplatin, which release 5-HT.

## MISCELLANEOUS ANTI-EMETICS

### Cannabinoids

Cannabinoids are derivatives of *Cannabis sativa* (marijuana); they have an anti-emetic action and have been used with some success in controlling vomiting in patients receiving cytotoxic drugs. They also produce some sedation and occasionally confusion. Cannabis cannot be prescribed at present but **nabilone**, a derivative, is available.

### Betahistine

Betahistine differs from other anti-emetics in that its use is confined to Ménière's disease (see above) in which vertigo and vomiting are due to a disturbance

in the labyrinth of the inner ear. The drug is believed to lower pressure in the inner ear and thus relieve symptoms.

### Dexamethasone

Dexamethasone has proved useful as an anti-emetic during cancer chemotherapy.

### Benzodiazepines

Benzodiazepines (e.g. diazepam – *Valium*) may be used in combination with other anti-emetics. It seems probable that they have no specific anti-emetic effect, but are useful for relieving anxiety (see p. 269).

---

**Summary**

- Do not use an emetic if the patient is not fully conscious
- Do not use any emetic if the ingested material is corrosive or a petroleum product
- It is generally better to pre-treat with an anti-emetic *before* administering an emetic stimulus
- Do not administer a muscarinic antagonist such as hyoscine if that patient is to drive or operate heavy machinery after taking the drug
- Cinnarizine is favoured for seasickness
- Anti-emetics are of major importance in cancer chemotherapy

---

**Nursing point**

As a general rule anti-emetics are best if given at least half an hour before the emetic stimulus. Prevention is easier than cure.

---

## COUGH REMEDIES

### THE COUGHING REFLEX

The cough is a reflex, although one can cough deliberately as well. The stimulus may arise from inflammation or foreign material in the pharynx, larynx, trachea or bronchial tree. It may also be provoked by stimuli arising in the pleura. It is therefore advantageous to aid the removal of foreign material from the respiratory passages and increasing the secretion of the bronchial glands and thus 'loosening' the sputum may achieve this. The cough reflex can also be activated inappropriately by respiratory inflammation or by neoplastic growth in the tract.

The bronchial glands are supplied by the vagus nerve and when nausea or vomiting occurs there is widespread vagal activity and also a considerable increase in bronchial and salivary secretion.

## EXPECTORANTS

Expectorants are drugs that loosen the sputum and thus aid its ejection from the bronchial tree. They are nearly all emetics if given in large enough doses and the theory behind their use is that in smaller doses the emetic action is not provoked but the reflex stimulation of the bronchial glands remains.

There is little if any hard evidence that expectorants in the doses commonly prescribed have any useful action and in general their use should be discouraged. There are many products available over the counter with a powerful and sometimes unpleasant taste that can have a placebo effect and will no doubt continue to be used. Among the ingredients that may be found in such cough mixtures are ammonium chloride, ipecacuanha, guaifenesin and squill, and many can be bought over the counter. In addition, some preparations contain vasoconstrictors such as pseudoephedrine or phenylephrine, which act as nasal decongestants.

There are many mixtures of similar type and efficiency. They are useful in the cold plus cough situation, but it must be remembered that those containing vasoconstrictors must not be used by patients taking monoamine oxidase inhibitors (MAOIs; see p. 280), since this may greatly enhance the activity of sympathomimetic drugs.

As a result of British government action, the antihistamine-decongestant preparations are no longer prescribable under the NHS, but are available on private prescription and many of them can be bought over the counter. The only way to obtain the drugs on the NHS is for the main ingredients to be prescribed separately.

## COUGH SUPPRESSANTS (ANTITUSSIVE DRUGS)

Under certain circumstances it is advantageous to suppress a cough that is tiring the patient and serving no useful purpose. However, undue suppression of a cough can lead to sputum retention and thickening, and antitussives should not be used in patients with chronic bronchitis, bronchiectasis or for cough associated with asthma. It is also debatable whether cough remedies actually work. A recent study published in the *British Medical Journal* found no significant efficacy for cough remedies (Schroeder & Fahey 2002).

## DEMULCENTS

Coughs arising from irritation of the mucous membranes of the mouth and throat may be suppressed through the soothing action of syrup, which forms a protective film over the inflamed tissues. These syrups are called demulcents. **Simple linctus**, which is essentially flavoured syrup, is satisfactory but should be avoided in patients with diabetes as it contains sugar. A sugar-free substitute is available.

## OPIOIDS

For many years the only really effective cough-depressing drugs were those derived from the opioid group, which include morphine, heroin and codeine. These drugs were included in many cough mixtures and, by virtue of this action on the cough centre, were valuable antitussives.

**Codeine**, the most popular of this group, was included in linctus codeine (BPC). This linctus, although widely used, has been found to be not very effective unless given in doses above those usually recommended, in which case it is often constipating.

**Dextromethorphan** is related in structure to levorphanol, which is a synthetic narcotic analgesic. A number of over-the-counter preparations for cough, colds and influenza contain dextromethorphan. It is about as potent as codeine as a cough suppressant and, like codeine, can cause constipation, depending on the dosage and frequency of use.

**Pholcodine** is closely related to codeine and depresses the cough centre. On a weight for weight basis, experimental results suggest it is more active than codeine, although the side-effects are probably similar. Its action lasts 4–6 hours. It is included in various mixtures, including linctus pholcodine (BPC). In terminal care, morphine or diamorphine (heroin) may be required to relieve a distressing cough.

## ANTIHISTAMINES

These drugs have some antitussive effect, partly perhaps by a local antihistamine action, but their antitussive action is more likely to be through a sedative effect on the nervous system.

## INHALATIONS AND MUCOLYTIC AGENTS

Mucolytic agents are those that are used to try and liquefy mucus. In the past, various drugs were inhaled, particularly in the treatment of chronic lung infections, although with the advent of antibiotics this treatment has been largely superseded. **Steam** itself is, however, a very good expectorant as it liquefies the sputum and thus enables it to be coughed up.

### BENZOIN TINCTURE

Benzoin tincture is one of the balsams that contain resins and volatile oils. A tincture, incidentally, is a plant extract in alcohol. When it is added to hot water, the volatile oil is given off and may be inhaled; it exerts a mildly soothing effect on the bronchial mucous membrane and is frequently used in acute bronchitis. Menthol and eucalyptus inhalation can be used in a similar way and produce a considerable outpouring from the bronchial glands and a transient vasoconstriction of the respiratory mucous membrane with clearing of the air passages. It is also often used postoperatively to avoid chest infection.

### Safety point

Great care must be taken when young or elderly patients are inhaling these drugs that they do not spill the hot water over themselves or severe burns may occur.

### Nursing point

Avoiding dehydration, giving hot drinks and physiotherapy are more effective than medicines in 'clearing the chest'.

### PULMONARY SURFACTANTS

Natural surfactants allow the surfaces of the pulmonary alveoli to separate so that the lungs can expand and function immediately after birth. In premature infants this factor may be lacking so the lungs do not function properly and respiratory distress syndrome develops. This is treated by mechanical ventilation and the inhalation via an endotracheal tube of **colfosceril palmitate**, a synthetic surfactant.

## RESPIRATORY FAILURE

Respiratory failure occurs when the lungs are unable to maintain an adequate exchange of oxygen and carbon dioxide. There are two types.

### TYPE I

In type I respiratory failure the balance between circulation and ventilation of the alveoli is disturbed. This results in a reduction of oxygen in the blood, but normal levels of carbon dioxide. It may occur in heart failure, pneumonia and shock lung. Oxygen may be given freely and the underlying disorder should be corrected if possible.

### TYPE II

Type II respiratory failure occurs in obstructive airways disease usually associated with chronic bronchitis and pulmonary emphysema. Pulmonary emphysema results from damage to the alveoli of the lungs. This reduces the surface area for $O_2$ and $CO_2$ exchange and in severe cases the patient becomes breathless. The disease is common among British men and may be due to a combination of advancing age, chronic bronchitis and smoking. The essential abnormality is underventilation of the alveoli, resulting in a low blood oxygen concentration and a raised level of carbon dioxide. Hypoxaemia can be relieved by the inhalation of oxygen, but this may lead to decreased respiration with a further fall in alveolar ventilation and an increased blood concentration of carbon dioxide which causes the patient to become disorientated and, finally, comatose. This situation can be avoided to some extent by giving low concentrations of oxygen, which does not reduce alveolar ventilation. In addition, physiotherapy helps to remove retained bronchial secretions, and antibiotics are used to treat complicating bronchial infections and bronchodilators relieve spasm.

### RESPIRATORY STIMULANT DRUGS

Respiratory stimulant drugs have a limited use in these circumstances. Given intravenously, they increase ventilation for a short period.

**Nursing point**

It is important to avoid sedatives which will further depress respiration and cause a deterioration in the patient's condition.

**Doxapram** is the most effective respiratory stimulant and is given by intravenous infusion. The dose is adjusted depending on response. This treatment requires careful monitoring and every effort should be made to remove retained secretions in the respiratory tract by physiotherapy. In overdose, doxapram can cause convulsions.

**Summary**

- Patients prescribed MAOI drugs must be warned not to take cold preparations containing vasoconstrictors such as pseudoephedrine
- Do not give cough suppressants (which cause sputum retention and thickening) to patients with chronic bronchitis, bronchiectasis or cough associated with asthma
- Cough syrups containing sucrose must not be given to diabetics
- Codeine and pholcodine may constipate the patient
- Oxygen should be used in lower concentrations in patients with type II respiratory failure

## References

Schroeder K, Fahey T 2002 Systematic review of randomised controlled trials of over the counter cough medicines for acute cough in adults. British Medical Journal 324: 329

## Further reading

Editorial 1991 Ondansetron vs dexamethasone for chemotherapy-induced emesis. Lancet 338: 478

Grunberg S M, Hesketh P J 1993 Control of chemotherapy-induced emesis. New England Journal of Medicine 329: 1790

Hawthorn J 1995 Understanding the management of nausea and vomiting. Blackwell, Oxford

Williams C 1994 Causes and management of nausea and vomiting. Nursing Times 90: 38

Chapter **10**

# Narcotic analgesics

## Learning objectives

At the end of this chapter, the reader should be able to:

- understand what is meant by an opioid
- discuss the gating theory of pain
- appreciate the existence of endogenous pain-related opioids and their receptors
- describe what opium is, the important opioid drugs, their therapeutic uses and adverse effects
- list the types of pain control for which morphine is used
- describe the symptoms of morphine and heroin overdosage and emergency treatment
- describe what is meant by an opioid agonist, partial agonist and antagonist and give examples of each
- understand and appreciate the needs and problems of the patient with acute pain
- appreciate the modern, caring attitudes to acute pain treatment
- understand the concept of 'total pain'
- understand the need for individualized pain control programmes
- appreciate the need to determine the cause of pain in patients with terminal disease
- discuss the concept of titration of dose of analgesic against pain
- describe the treatments for opioid non-responsive pain
- be aware of the alternative methods for controlling pain
- be aware of the existence of pain control services and teams

Analgesics are drugs that relieve pain. They are of great importance in patient care, as pain is a common and distressing feature of many conditions. It must be remembered, however, that pain has its uses, both as a warning of the presence of disease and also, by its nature, it may help in localization and diagnosis of the underlying cause. It is debatable whether chronic pain has any physiological role, except as an unwelcome and constant reminder of ongoing tissue damage.

## THE PERCEPTION OF PAIN

The most important principle underlying pain perception is that the brain perceives pain. No matter how bad the damage to the body is, if nerve connections carrying pain signals to the brain, for example through damage to the spinal cord, are interrupted, the patient will feel no pain.

## MECHANISM OF PAIN PERCEPTION

### The gating theory of pain

The mechanism of pain perception is summarized in Figure 10.1. The central nervous system is constantly receiving nerve impulses arising in the body from the skin and internal organs. Under certain circumstances the brain interprets these as pain. There are a number of theories to explain how this occurs and the most popular today is the 'gate' (input control) theory. This states that:

- high-intensity stimulation activates a network of fine nerves at the periphery that terminate centrally in the **posterior horn of the spinal cord**
- from here nerve impulses are relayed via the **spinothalamic tract** to the **thalamus** in the brain where they are felt as pain
- there is then a further relay system to the **cerebral cortex** where discrimination and interpretation occur.

The passage of nerve impulses through the relay 'gate' in the posterior horn is modified by:

- ascending impulses from the periphery to the brain
- descending impulses from the brain to the periphery.

### Ascending impulses from the periphery to the brain

Low-intensity ascending nerve impulses unrelated to pain dampen the transmission of pain impulses. This explains why methods such as transcutaneous stimulation or counter-irritation applied to a painful area can relieve pain by 'closing the gate'. An example is the application of creams containing skin irritants to painful joints or muscles (e.g. *Deep Heat* cream, which contains capsicum extracted from hot chillies). Heat therapy, for example, through the use of lamps and heated pads, is also used to treat pain.

High-intensity impulses from an area of tissue damage (as may occur after surgery) overcome the low-intensity ascending nerve impulses and facilitate transmission through the 'gate' and thus increase painful sensations. This may be reduced by blocking impulses from the area of damage by **local anaesthesia** or by giving an **analgesic** just before an operation.

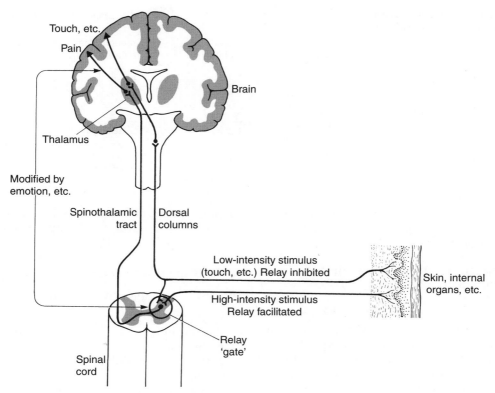

**Figure 10.1**   Pathways involved in perception of pain.

### Descending impulses from the brain to the periphery

Nerve fibres arising in the brain and descending in the spinal cord terminate in the posterior horn and damp down transmission through the gate and thus decrease the sensation of pain.

## DRUGS THAT RELIEVE PAIN

## SITES OF DRUG ACTION

Drugs that relieve pain may act at various sites along the pain pathways:

- They may act on the brain and spinal cord and reduce the appreciation of pain. This is the major site of action of **opioid analgesics**.
- They may suppress conduction in nerves carrying impulses from the painful area. This is where **local anaesthetics** act.
- They may reduce inflammation and other causes of pain in the painful area. This is the site of action, for example, of the **non-steroidal anti-inflammatory drugs** (NSAIDs; see Chapter 11).

**Table 10.1**   Opioid analgesics

| Type | Name |
| --- | --- |
| Natural | Morphine; codeine |
| Synthetic | Diamorphine; methadone; pethidine; phenazocine; dextromoramide; dipipanone; dihydrocodeine, fentanyl |

Analgesics can be broadly classified for practical purposes as:

- opioid analgesics (Table 10.1)
- non-opioid analgesics.

Non-opioid analgesics and local anaesthetics are dealt with in later chapters.

## OPIOID ANALGESICS*

Nearly all the opioids are potentially drugs of dependence and this subject is discussed in more

---

* The term opioid is applied to any substance which has an opium-like action. These drugs are also called *narcotics*.

**Figure 10.2**   Mode of action of opioid agonists, antagonists and partial agonists.

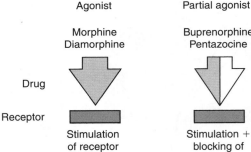

| Agonist | Partial agonist | Antagonist |
|---|---|---|
| Morphine Diamorphine | Buprenorphine Pentazocine | Naxolone |
| Stimulation of receptor | Stimulation + blocking of receptor | Blocking of receptor |

Drug

Receptor

detail on p. 287. The opioids have been called narcotic analgesics because of their well-known soporific effects.

## THE MECHANISM OF ACTION OF OPIOID ANALGESICS AND ANTAGONISTS OF OPIOID ACTION

The body contains chemicals called endorphins and encephalins. These are the body's own type of opioid. Two of these, **β endorphin** and **metencephalin**, act on special opioid receptors in the nervous system, particularly in the midbrain and posterior horn of the spinal cord. When these receptors are stimulated transmission of nerve impulses related to pain are inhibited and the appreciation of pain is suppressed. It seems likely that β endorphin and metencephalin are part of a system in the brain that controls pain appreciation and may be involved in such phenomena as acupuncture. Opioid drugs also react with these receptors and thus relieve pain. There are several types of opioid receptor in the nervous system, but the most important for pain control by opioids are called **μ receptors** and are responsible for the analgesia, euphoria and respiratory depression seen with most opioid analgesics. Although the most important actions of the opioids occur in the central nervous system, there is now some evidence that they may also react with receptors on the peripheral nerves, which augments their analgesic action. Endorphins, incidentally, are released during physical exercise and may be responsible for the feeling of well-being that participation in sports so often engenders.

## OPIOID AGONISTS, PARTIAL AGONISTS AND ANTAGONISTS

Some opioids, for example **morphine** and **diamorphine** (heroin), are full agonists. Some, such as

buprenorphine, are partial agonists. **Naloxone** (see also p. 140) is a drug that is a pure antagonist at opioid receptors (see Fig. 10.2).

### Opioids and related drugs

**Agonists.**   Examples are:

- morphine
- diamorphine
- methadone
- pethidine (meperidine)
- codeine
- dihydrocodeine
- dextropropoxyphene.

**Partial agonists.**   Examples are:

- buprenorphine
- meptazinol
- nalbuphine
- tramadol.

**Antagonists.**   Examples are:

- naloxone
- naltrexone.

## OPIUM – THE SOURCE OF MORPHINE

Opium is obtained from the unripe seed capsule of the poppy *Papaver somniferum*. Opium has been used for thousands of years in the Orient, and was (and possibly still is) smoked in opium dens. The drug produces euphoria and the user slips into a deep sleep, called the 'yen', which is often characterized by vivid dreams. The poppy is now grown in the UK as well (at secret locations) for commercial development of morphine. Crude opium is a brownish gum-like material and contains a number of substances, the most important being **morphine**, codeine and papaverine. Morphine is the most powerful of these alkaloids and the actions of morphine and opium are similar and may be considered together.

## OPIOID AGONISTS

### MORPHINE

Administration of morphine:

- oral
- intramuscular injection
- intravenous injection
- infusion via a syringe pump.

### Oral

Morphine can be given orally as an immediate-release tablet that must be given every 4 hours. For long-term control of pain there are slow-release tablets, which are only needed twice daily, or as an aqueous solution.

When given orally as a single dose, morphine's effect is greatly reduced because the liver breaks down about 75% of the dose through first pass metabolism before the drug reaches the circulation. With repeated oral dosage, however, it is very effective. This may happen because the metabolite morphine-6-glucuronide (see below) is slowly excreted and with repeated doses accumulates sufficiently to help to produce satisfactory analgesia.

### Injection

The modes of injection are:

- subcutaneous
- intravenous
- continuous subcutaneous infusion.

When given by injection, morphine produces analgesia rapidly. The analgesic effect of morphine usually lasts about 4 hours after injection but depends to some extent on the severity of the pain, the sensitivity of the patient to the drug, and on the dose. The dosage in severe pain or in acute left ventricular failure depends on many circumstances, including the age, weight and general health of the patient.

Morphine can also be given slowly intravenously. The analgesic effect starts within 20 minutes of subcutaneous injection and 10 minutes of intravenous injection and peaks after about 1 hour.

Morphine in small doses can also be given by continuous subcutaneous infusion. This allows the dose to be modified as required and can be very useful in severe and fluctuating pain. However, this method needs careful titration of the dose in relation to the therapeutic effect and fixed dose regimens are not very successful.

### Metabolism and excretion

After absorption, morphine is combined in the liver to form several substances, one of which (morphine-6-glucuronide) has powerful analgesic properties of its own. The kidney excretes these substances. Repeated doses of morphine will induce a state of tolerance to the drug so that increasing doses may be required to produce an effect.

### CNS actions

The most important actions of morphine are on the central nervous system: the effects may be divided into **depressant** and **stimulant**. Morphine also causes the development of **tolerance** and **dependence** to its central actions. Drug dependence is discussed more fully in Chapter 22.

### CNS depressant effects

- Morphine depresses the appreciation of pain by the brain and thus acts as a powerful analgesic.
- It relieves all types of pain.
- If the pain is felt at all, it seems to have lost its unpleasant nature.
- Morphine depresses the emotional component of pain, namely anticipation and fear of pain. It is euphoric and allays anxiety.
- It depresses respiration. In large doses; patients are often left in pain through erroneous fears about respiratory depression.
- It depresses the cough centre and thus damps down the cough reflex.
- It is a mild hypnotic and may produce drowsiness and sleep.

### CNS stimulant effects

- Morphine stimulates the chemoreceptor trigger zone (CTZ; see p. 124) in the brainstem causing nausea and vomiting in about 30% of patients, particularly if they are mobile.
- The pupils of the eye are constricted due to an effect on the nucleus of the third nerve.

- Morphine stimulates the vagus nerve. This action is particularly liable to be troublesome when morphine is used for the pain of coronary thrombosis as it may cause undue slowing of the pulse and lowering of the blood pressure.

## Peripheral actions (outside the CNS)

**Constipation.** Morphine decreases the peristaltic activity of the bowel and at the same time increases the tone, leading to constipation.

**Increase in biliary pressure.** Morphine causes spasm of the sphincters, including the sphincter of Oddi at the lower end of the bile duct, and thus produces a rise in pressure in the biliary system.

**Urinary retention.** Morphine interferes with bladder function, which may cause urinary retention, particularly after an operation.

**Histamine release.** Morphine causes some histamine release, occasionally leading to bronchoconstriction.

## Tolerance to morphine

Tolerance may be defined as the phenomenon whereby successively more of a drug is needed to produce the same effect. Tolerance develops only to the CNS actions of morphine, and long-term diamorphine (heroin) addicts take doses (as much as 50 times the therapeutic range) that would normally kill the naïve user. The same addicts still develop chronic constipation (a peripheral effect of morphine) to a much smaller dose that would not satisfy their craving. There are several theories to explain tolerance, but the actual mechanism of tolerance is unknown.

## Common uses of morphine

- **Pain control**
- **Cough**
- **Diarrhoea**.

**Pain control.** Morphine is very useful for pain control in:

- surgical emergencies
- the postoperative period
- following injury
- after a coronary thrombosis
- controlling severe pain in terminal cancer on a regular basis (see p. 142)
- acute failure of the left ventricle with pulmonary oedema.

Morphine is still one of the best analgesics for severe pain of a temporary nature. Not only does it relieve the pain but it also relieves the anxieties and miseries of the patient.

Morphine is useful after a coronary thrombosis. Its mode of action under these circumstances is not clear, though it probably acts by its widespread sedative effect on the central nervous system and by dilating veins and relieving congestion of the lungs.

## Signs of overdosage

A patient who has received an overdose of morphine is drowsy or unconscious. The skin is cyanosed and sweating. Respiration is depressed and the pupils are pinpoint. The treatment for overdosage is immediate endotracheal intubation to aid respiration and administration of an opioid antagonist (see below).

## DIAMORPHINE (HEROIN)

Diamorphine is obtained by chemical modification of morphine. When given by injection it enters the nervous system more rapidly than does morphine so that its action starts a little sooner. Thereafter it is quickly converted to morphine in the body. When given orally diamorphine is all converted to morphine in the liver before it enters the systemic circulation; therefore their actions are similar except that the effects of diamorphine are seen a little earlier after injection. It is more soluble than morphine and this is useful when large doses are required by injection.

Although diamorphine is more popular than morphine among addicts, it is difficult to see a scientific reason for this and it may be for social or mythological reasons.

## Adverse effects of morphine and diamorphine

These adverse effects comprise:

- allergy
- bradycardia
- confusion
- constipation
- dependence
- dry mouth
- hallucinations and nightmares (especially at night)
- hypersensitivity
- nausea
- sedation
- urinary retention.

**Table 10.2**  Adverse effects of morphine, diamorphine and other powerful opioids (Based on the Guys, St Thomas's and Lewisham Formulary)

| Adverse effect | Approximate frequency (%) | Dose related | Tolerance | Comments |
|---|---|---|---|---|
| Constipation | 100 | No | No | Prophylactic laxative (e.g. Senokot) required |
| Nausea | 30 | Yes | Yes (5–7 days) | Prophylactic anti-emetic if needed<br>Give oral or I.M. prochlorperazine or oral haloperidol |
| Sedation | 30 | Yes | Yes (3–4 days) | Usually mild. Wears off in 48 hours |
| Confusion, nightmares hallucinations (particularly at night) | 1 | No | No | Try reducing dose, then consider haloperidol 2–4 mg at night |

Some features of these adverse effects are summarized in Table 10.2.

**Hypersensitivity.**  Certain patients are very sensitive to powerful opioids and a normal dose may produce signs of overdose. The most important of this group are patients whose respiratory centre is under stress, i.e. those with chronic bronchitis and emphysema, and in patients during an asthmatic attack. Patients with liver damage or impaired renal function suffer an exaggerated and prolonged response. Finally, the very old and the very young are especially sensitive and they should only be given a small dose until their sensitivity to the drug is known.

**Dependence.**  This can develop rapidly when narcotics are used in a social context, but they very rarely present a problem when used therapeutically either in an acute painful situation or in terminal disease. However, their use in chronic painful, but non-fatal disorders should be avoided.

**Allergy.**  Morphine is chemically a base, and bases are known to cause allergic reactions.

**Pregnancy.**  Morphine will also cross the placental barrier and affect the fetus, a point of importance in midwifery.

**Drug interactions.**  Opioids increase the effect of other central depressants, as do monoamine oxidase inhibitors (MAOIs), which are particularly dangerous with pethidine (see below).

## METHADONE

Methadone is a synthetic analgesic. Its analgesic action is as powerful as that of morphine, but it has little of morphine's euphoric and tranquillizing effect. Like morphine, it also has a depressing effect on the cough centre, but the effect on the respiratory centre is not so marked. It is a drug of dependence, especially if given by injection. It is rapidly and well absorbed after oral administration or subcutaneous injection and is less liable to produce vomiting than morphine. Its action is longer lasting than that of morphine and this can make repeated dosage difficult. It should not be given more than twice daily to avoid accumulation.

### Therapeutic uses

**Pain.**  Methadone may be used as a substitute for morphine in the treatment of pain.

**Cough.**  In small doses methadone is useful as a cough sedative.

**Heroin withdrawal.**  Methadone is used orally as a substitute for morphine or diamorphine in the treatment of drug dependence. The drug prevents the severe symptoms of withdrawal from heroin. It is rarely required more frequently than every 12 hours in the management of opioid withdrawal.

**Nursing point**

Patients treated with oral tablets of methadone for treatment of heroin dependence have been known to crush the tablets and attempt to inject them intravenously, when the drug produces the euphoric effect. In order to discourage this, opioid antagonists such as naltrexone (see below) have been in some cases added to the formulation of the tablets. This is because the antagonist is ineffective if taken orally, but if injected would immediately precipitate withdrawal symptoms, which all heroin addicts fear (see p. 289). The wisdom of this drastic strategy is, however, debatable. Nurses who work with patients dependent on opioids should be aware of this problem with methadone.

## PAPAVERETUM (*OMNOPON*)

Papaveretum is a mixture of morphine and other opioids. Its actions are essentially those of morphine. It is hardly used anymore.

## PETHIDINE (MEPERIDINE)

Pethidine is a synthetic substance that is related chemically to atropine. It is well absorbed after oral or subcutaneous administration. It is less powerful than morphine, but has less effect in therapeutic doses on the cough or respiratory centre. It causes some spasm of the muscle of the bile ducts. It is not constipating. It does not cause constriction of the pupils and is therefore used in head injuries where observation of the pupil size may be important. Dependence can develop.

### Therapeutic uses

Pethidine is used in the treatment of moderately severe pains, particularly those arising from the viscera. It can be administered orally or by intramuscular injection. For many years it was given to relieve pain in the later stages of labour, as it is short acting, thus avoiding prolonged depression of the infant's respiration immediately after birth. There is now good evidence that, although it produces sedation, it is an ineffective analgesic in these circumstances and is being replaced by epidural analgesia. Its action lasts 2–3 hours.

## FENTANYL

This is one of a group of opioids that are very powerful and are short acting. They are used largely in the intraoperative period to help anaesthetic induction. Their use requires care, as severe respiratory depression is a risk. Fentanyl can also be used as a patch, applied to dry, non-hairy skin, which allows slow absorption for up to 72 hours in the relief of terminal pain. Owing to its complex distribution in the body, the action of fentanyl in these circumstances may continue for 24 hours after removal of the patch.

### Nursing point

Fever can increase absorption from patches and result in symptoms of overdose.

## CODEINE AND DIHYDROCODEINE

Codeine is obtained from opium. It is given orally. It is a mild analgesic, having only about one-seventh of the power of morphine. Its most useful action is its depressing effect on the cough centre and it is about half as powerful as morphine in this respect. Like morphine, it also decreases peristalsis of the intestine.

### Therapeutic uses

These comprise:

- **cough**
- **mild analgesia**
- **diarrhoea**.

**Codeine** is widely used in various cough mixtures for its sedative effect on the cough centre. These cough mixtures usually also contain syrup, whose demulcent action is useful in relieving coughs arising from the pharynx (don't give to diabetics). Codeine will control diarrhoea. It is combined with aspirin or paracetamol as a mild analgesic, although there is some variation in its analgesic efficacy, due to differences among patients in metabolism.

### Nursing point

Increasing the dose of codeine or dihydrocodeine above those given here will not enhance the analgesic effect. Dihydrocodeine and probably codeine given alone are ineffective in postoperative dental pain.

**Dihydrocodeine** is similar to codeine and is used as a mild analgesic. It causes constipation and occasionally dizziness, low blood pressure and nausea. It is administered by intramuscular injection or as tablets.

## DEXTROPROPOXYPHENE

Dextropropoxyphene is similar to methadone but is a much weaker analgesic. It is combined with paracetamol as the compound tablet co-proxamol (*Distalgesic*), which is useful in treating pain that does not respond to aspirin or paracetamol alone. It is slightly addictive and like many drugs in this group it can cause vomiting. Overdose can be dangerous, not only because the paracetamol can cause liver damage (see also p. 428) but also because dextropropoxyphene can cause respiratory depression and collapse.

## PARTIAL AGONISTS

Opioid partial agonists differ from opioid agonists such as morphine in some of their effects. They are powerful analgesics but are less addictive, less likely to depress respiration and are less euphoric.

## BUPRENORPHINE

This analgesic, although only a partial agonist, is as powerful as morphine. It can be given by injection or sublingually, but is not effective orally as it is broken down in the liver in a large first pass action. Its analgesic action lasts longer than that of morphine (6–8 hours) and it is less likely to depress respiration. The risk of dependence is low but it can occur.

Buprenorphine shows a 'ceiling effect' so that increasing the dose above the usual range will not improve its efficacy. Although it competes with powerful opioids such as morphine for receptor sites in the brain, in the therapeutic dose range buprenorphine only slightly reduces the analgesic action of other opioids when they are combined. In higher doses, the antagonistic action of buprenorphine will become apparent if combined with opioid agonists.

### Therapeutic use

Buprenorphine is used to treat moderate and severe pain. It can be given by injection for postoperative pain, but it is slow to take effect. It is also given sublingually every 6–8 hours for various forms of chronic pain.

### Adverse effects

Buprenorphine sometimes causes troublesome vomiting which requires the drug to be stopped. Respiratory depression, although not so marked as with morphine, is only partly reversed by naloxone.

## MEPTAZINOL

This drug is similar in some respects to buprenorphine. When given by injection it has a short action (2–3 hours) and is used in obstetrics where its rapid elimination by both mother and fetus is an advantage. It is also useful for breakthrough pain in the postoperative period. There is a large first pass effect so that only about 10% of the oral dose reaches the circulation and it is only used for moderate pain by this route.

## NALBUPHINE

Nalbuphine has an analgesic action that lasts about 4 hours and it can only be given by injection. Like buprenorphine it also shows a 'ceiling' effect.

## TRAMADOL

Tramadol is a relatively new analgesic. It is a weak opioid and, in addition, reduces pain appreciation by interfering with pain pathways through the spinal 'gate'. It can be given orally or systemically and is about as powerful as pethidine, its action lasting for about 6 hours. Its main use is to treat moderately severe pain – e.g. postoperatively – although it can be used orally for chronic pain. Respiratory depression is not usually marked and its addiction potential is low. Adverse effects include nausea and vomiting, dizziness and a dry mouth.

## MORPHINE ANTAGONISTS

Several substances antagonize the actions of morphine and other opioids. Generally they resemble morphine in their chemical structure and thus compete with it for receptor sites. Having occupied receptor sites, however, they produce little or no stimulation so that the actions of morphine are reversed. They are used to treat overdosage by opioids. The most widely used are naloxone and naltrexone.

## NALOXONE

Naloxone is a pure antagonist, having no stimulating actions. It reverses the effects of both natural and synthetic opioids, but with buprenorphine a larger dose of naloxone may be required. It has no analgesic action. The drug is administered subcutaneously or intravenously and it is very rapidly effective. It can also be used to terminate the action of narcotic drugs in the postoperative period. Its action is relatively short (about 1 hour) and if used to reverse the effects of longer-acting opioids repeated doses might be needed.

## NALTREXONE

Naltrexone is an orally active opioid antagonist used in special clinics in the treatment of opioid withdrawal.

### Summary

- Repeated oral doses of immediate-release morphine tablets are needed to build up effective pain relief
- With continuous subcutaneous infusions of morphine, *fixed dose* regimes are not generally satisfactory to control pain
- Even therapeutic doses of morphine and heroin will cause some respiratory depression
- Emergency treatment for morphine overdosage is endotracheal intubation to aid respiration and an opioid antagonist, e.g. naloxone or naltrexone
- Morphine can cause vomiting
- Morphine slows the pulse and lowers blood pressure, which is potentially a problem in coronary thrombosis
- Opioids constipate the patient
- Morphine can cause an allergic reaction
- There is a danger of causing tolerance and drug dependence with chronic use of opioids
- Opioids suppress cough

## ANALGESICS FOR ACUTE PAIN

Acute pain is frequently generated by surgery, but may occur as a result of trauma or as part of a medical illness such as myocardial infarction or some form of colic.

### ATTITUDES TO ACUTE PAIN RELIEF

Attitudes to acute pain relief on the part of both nurses and doctors have been historically complacent, especially towards pain after surgery. Thankfully, more practical and caring attitudes are emerging. Patients needing opioids for the treatment of acute pain were too easily labelled as addicts and yet dependence and respiratory depression are rarely associated with the treatment of acute pain with opioids. The unimaginative approach of the 'give as necessary' 4-hourly prescription, which is not regularly given, and which does not allow for the opportunity to titrate the dose and frequency against the needs of the patient, can lead to the emergence of extreme pain. The patient then becomes tense, sweaty and exhausted, and needs a large dose of opioid for adequate relief of pain.

### THE PAIN RELIEF PROGRAMME

A programme for pain relief needs to take some important factors into account:

- Patients vary considerably in their sensitivity to pain and response to analgesics, so the programme should be individualized.
- The pain relief programme for an individual patient will depend on the severity, nature and cause of the pain. It may include a wide range of analgesics and, in addition, local anaesthetics and drugs that are specific for certain types of pain (e.g. colchicine for gout; see Chapter 11).

It is impossible to specify regimens for all types of pain, but certain general rules should be followed:

- The programmes must be flexible and aim to keep the patient free of pain.
- Many programmes have a continuous background of analgesia with facilities for a top-up (perhaps with a more powerful analgesic) if the pain breaks through.
- A combination of drugs and treatments should always be considered. This can be very successful.

Thus, paracetamol may be combined with an NSAID (see Chapter 11) and an opioid – and a local anaesthetic technique may be used as well.

● Anxiety markedly exacerbates the perception of pain. Explanation and reassurance are powerful tools with which to reduce anxiety and therefore the perception and distress of pain. Patients undergoing surgery must be given a full description of postoperative pain problems and the steps that will be taken for their relief.

It is recommended that in hospitals there should be specialized teams of doctors and nurses dedicated to the relief of acute pain.

## PATIENT-CONTROLLED ANALGESIA (PCA)

Pain in postoperative and some terminally ill patients can be effectively controlled by the self-administration of analgesia via a syringe pump set up to deliver a pre-set dose of the drug when a delivery button is pressed by the patient (Fig. 10.3). A number of PCA devices are commercially available, all designed so that dose, rate and frequency of administration can be controlled and pre-set. A number of drugs have been used successfully, including morphine and pethidine.

Trials have demonstrated high levels of acceptance of PCA among patients in hospital and the community, where small, portable PCA machines have been used. Part of the success of PCA is related to the feeling of control it gives patients and the confidence that they will not have to wait for the nurse to give an injection to relieve pain. Nursing time is saved as, once the device is set up, it obviates the need to prepare and administer routine injections. However, nurses still have a responsibility for monitoring the adequacy of analgesia and the appearance of side-effects such as nausea or respiratory depression. This is best done by using written protocols that should define the monitoring and actions necessary

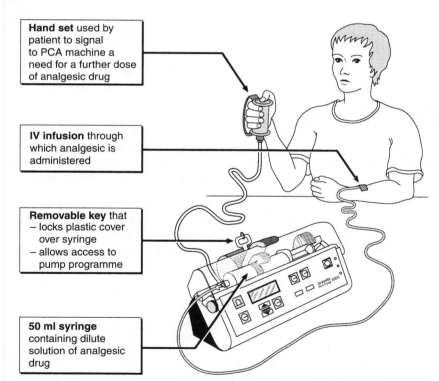

**Hand set** used by patient to signal to PCA machine a need for a further dose of analgesic drug

**IV infusion** through which analgesic is administered

**Removable key** that
– locks plastic cover over syringe
– allows access to pump programme

**50 ml syringe** containing dilute solution of analgesic drug

**Figure 10.3**    An example of a machine/syringe pump used for PCA (patient-controlled analgesia). This machine, a specialized syringe pump, enables small bolus injections of analgesic to be given on demand. The minimum time between injections – the 'lock-out period' – is controlled. If required, a background, low-dose, continuous infusion is possible.

  These machines contain many safety features. The syringe is locked under a plastic cover and cannot, therefore, be interfered with by an unauthorized person. The *pump programme* used to control and alter the bolus size, the lock-out period, the continuous infusion rate and other functions, is only accessible using the same key that locks the plastic cover. The key should, therefore, be kept with ward keys or in some other secure place.

to maintain adequate analgesia and to manage properly the side-effects of the drugs.

Patients must be taught how to use the device before they need it. For surgical patients this should be before their operation as a heavily sedated postoperative patient will not be receptive to lengthy explanations. Patients going home with PCA machines should have the opportunity to become familiar with their use before they are discharged.

## ANALGESICS IN PATIENTS WITH TERMINAL DISEASE

Pain is often a prominent feature of terminal disease, particularly cancer. Although the use of drugs is only part of the management of the dying, the correct use of analgesics can play a very important part in the care of these patients.

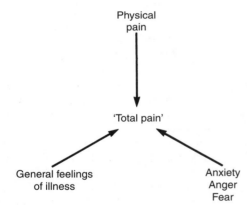

Figure 10.4    Factors which go to make up the concept of 'total pain' or anguish in the terminally ill.

## DETERMINATION OF THE CAUSE OF PAIN

It must be realized that in this type of patient pain can arise in many ways and the cause should be determined as it may have a specific remedy. It may be:

- related directly to the spread of the cancer
- the result of therapeutic measures such as surgery or wound procedures
- due to secondary deposits, particularly in bone
- due to some unrelated cause
- due to a combination of these factors.

## THE CONCEPT OF TOTAL PAIN

Whatever the cause of the pain, unresolved fear or anxiety may make it worse. A vicious cycle of pain and distress is thus engendered, relieved only by resolution of the anxiety as well as the alleviation of physical pain. The concept of 'total pain' introduced by Cicely Saunders to incorporate physical, social and emotional factors is crucial if the patient's problems are to be fully addressed (Fig. 10.4).

## ADJUSTING THE DOSE OF ANALGESIC TO KEEP THE PATIENT PAIN-FREE

The nurse has a fundamental role in the assessment of the patient's pain. Nursing interventions may include regular administration of analgesia and also active listening to the patient's worries and anxieties. Evaluation of the response to such interventions is important in the ongoing care of that individual. Pain cannot be treated in isolation but must be regarded as one facet of the patient's physical and mental state. The nurse is critically important in the titration of the drug against the pain (Fig. 10.5).

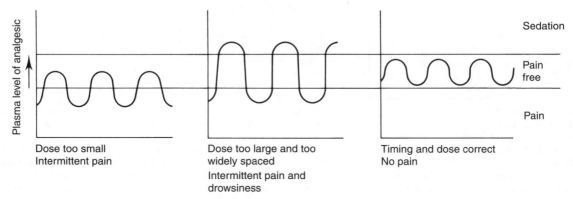

Figure 10.5    Adjusting the dose to keep the patient free from pain.

## MILD PAIN

For mild pain, weak analgesics such as paracetamol may be adequate. Co-proxamol (paracetamol + dextropropoxyphene) or dihydrocodeine are useful and, if given regularly, are a little better than paracetamol. For pain arising from secondary deposits in bone, anti-inflammatory analgesics such as aspirin or naproxen (see Chapter 11) are sometimes very effective alone or combined with opioids.

## MODERATE-TO-SEVERE PAIN

Moderate-to-severe pain should be treated by giving opioid analgesics regularly, titrated against the patient's pain.

The most effective drugs are morphine and diamorphine. As diamorphine is largely converted to morphine in the body, their actions and efficacy are essentially the same. However, diamorphine is more soluble than morphine and is thus better for injection if a small volume is required.

The opioid should be prescribed regularly and given regularly. For the average patient morphine orally as an elixir in chloroform water has been used in the past but is seldom given now. (The shelf life of morphine in chloroform is 3 months unopened, or 1 month if in use.) Immediate-release tablets are usually satisfactory. Lower doses are required in elderly patients, very ill patients and sometimes in those with impaired liver or renal function. Higher doses will be necessary for those patients who are already on, or have recently been on, opioids. The frequency of administration is commonly fixed at every 4 hours, but this, like the dose, needs to be kept under regular review.

At first the patient may need additional doses as required when the pain breaks through. This should be noted and incorporated in the regular 4-hourly schedule. The object is to keep the patient pain-free. It is easier to prevent pain with its attendant fear than to relieve a patient who is already distressed.

Once the correct dose of oral morphine has been established it may be convenient to change to slow-release (SR) morphine tablets which are only required twice daily and may be more effective in controlling the pain at night. If possible the drug should be given orally. This saves repeated injections and also produces a smoother and more prolonged analgesic effect. Dosage schedules should be reviewed every 24 hours and titrated against the patient's pain and well-being.

## SIDE-EFFECTS

Side-effects may develop with the use of narcotic drugs. They should be anticipated and treated as necessary. Constipation may be a particular problem and a stool softener (docusate) combined with a bowel stimulant (*Senokot*) is very effective.

With this regimen, tolerance to the analgesic action of the drug does not usually develop. A need to increase the dose of the drug usually indicates advance of the disease. The risk of dependence is not relevant in the terminally ill patient.

## OTHER ROUTES OF ADMINISTRATION

Sometimes it is necessary to give narcotics by injection intravenously or subcutaneously when the dose should be reduced. In very severe pain or when vomiting makes oral administration impossible opioids can be given by subcutaneous infusion. Diamorphine is used because of its solubility. The procedure is as follows:

- A single 4-hour dose is given subcutaneously before the syringe pump is set up.
- The 24-hour requirement of the analgesic is calculated and dissolved in water.
- The syringe pump is started at a rate adjusted to give the correct dose over 24 hours. It should not be delivered at more than 1.4 ml/hour or absorption may be incomplete.
- Anti-emetics can be included in the syringe. Cyclizine, prochlorperazine or droperidol are effective. Metoclopramide is not particularly effective and haloperidol is now rarely used.
- Careful monitoring of the therapeutic effect and degree of sedation are necessary and adjustment of the dose as required.

Dextromoramide, because of its short and rapid action, can be given orally or sublingually before a painful procedure or for 'breakthrough' pain.

Oxycodone suppositories are useful in relieving pain at night; their action lasts for 8 hours and they are particularly useful for patients cared for at home.

## OPIOID NON-RESPONSIVE PAIN

Certain types of pain respond poorly to opioid analgesics. These include pain due to pressure or infiltration affecting a nerve, or bone pain due to secondary deposits where movement may cause an acute exacerbation of pain that breaks through the opioid control. Nerve pain may respond to steroids, which reduce surrounding oedema or to anticonvulsant drugs that stabilize the nerve and prevent its stimulation. Bone pain can be helped by radiotherapy (if this is possible), NSAIDs and by preventing movements that cause pain.

### Treatments for opioid non-responsive pain

**Entonox** (50% oxygen + 50% nitrous oxide) by inhalation can be used to cover painful procedures. **Chlorpromazine** is not only useful as an anti-emetic, but may increase the effectiveness of analgesics. **Amitriptyline** (see p. 277) is a useful antidepressant to combat the psychotic depression that sometimes develops in these patients.

## OTHER METHODS

The use of analgesics is not the only way to relieve pain in terminal cancer. Radiotherapy is very effective, particularly in treating secondary deposits in bone. In recent years various types of nerve block either at the level of the peripheral nerve or in the spinal cord have been developed which can relieve pain without any systemic effects. These blocks may be temporary or permanent. Finally, much of the comfort and tranquillity of the patient will depend on the character and understanding of the nurse.

## ANALGESICS IN NON-PAINFUL TERMINAL DISEASE

Many patients with malignant disease or dying from other diseases such as renal failure do not have pain, but they may experience considerable malaise and mental anguish. The use of opioids in these circumstances is more controversial. Some people consider that opioids should be used only for pain relief. Others, recognizing their undoubted euphoric action, would give them to reduce the anxieties and discomforts in the terminal stages if necessary. Relatively small doses are usually required in these cases. In these patients, opioids are also useful for controlling cough and relieving the sensation of dyspnoea.

## ANALGESICS AND CHRONIC NON-TERMINAL PAIN

For some types of chronic pain the cause is obvious (e.g. arthritis; see Chapter 11); in others, it is obscure. Psychological factors play some part in most types of pain, but may play a major part in the more obscure varieties. This means that there are many types of treatment, depending on the cause and severity of the pain, and it is only possible here to make some general statements:

- Before starting treatment it is very important to **listen to patients** and to assess their perception of the pain and how it affects their daily life.
- Management with the appropriate drugs will be enhanced by **considerable supportive therapy**, and various techniques for dealing with pain by psychotherapeutic methods are available.
- **Alternative methods** of pain relief, i.e. nerve block and transcutaneous electrical nerve stimulation (TENS), which probably acts by closing the relay gate in the spinal cord, may prove helpful in some patients.
- Do not forget that **depression** often presents as obscure chronic pain. In this case antidepressants are effective.
- It is important to **avoid drugs with a high risk of dependence**. Even so-called 'low-risk' analgesics are not entirely safe, e.g. buprenorphine dependence does occur. In prescribing analgesics the patient should be assessed carefully and prescriptions should not be repeated endlessly. The NSAIDs (see Chapter 11) are free from the risk of dependence, but are not free of adverse effects.

## TERMINAL CARE SERVICES AND THE PAIN CONTROL TEAM

### HOSPICE CARE

The object of hospice care is to help maintain an acceptable quality of life whilst enabling a patient to die peacefully, with special reference to the person's values, preferences and outlook on life. This may be achieved through a team approach in various settings.

The hospice movement has expanded considerably over the last 25 years. There are about 500 units in the UK offering hospice facilities or home palliative care. Referral may be through the general practitioner or district nurse or arranged on hospital discharge (Pickrel et al 2001).

## THE HOSPITAL SUPPORT TEAM

A more recent development is the hospital support team, of which there are now about 370 in the UK. The team is usually multidisciplinary, sometimes working in conjunction with the radiotherapy or oncology departments. The hospital support team provides skills in symptom control and pain relief and can offer emotional support to patients and carers, while fulfilling an educational role within the hospital.

## PAIN CONTROL TEAMS

Pain control teams have been developed to cope with the problem of those in chronic pain. Although many of these patients have terminal cancer, there are other types of chronic pain such as post-herpetic neuralgia, various long-term pains following injury such as amputation, and pain for which there is no obvious cause but where psychological factors may play a part.

The team usually comprises one or two doctors who are interested in the subject (for example anaesthetists), nursing staff (often a sister who is specially trained) and a psychiatrist. They deal with patients who have been referred to them in hospital; they may run an outpatient service and may also undertake home visiting.

Many types of chronic pain are made worse by depression, fear and anxiety and here the psychiatrist can help through explanation, reassurance and the judicious use of drugs such as antidepressants. As in so many areas of treatment, the control of pain is becoming a team activity.

## References

Pickrel L, Duggan C, Dhillon S 2001 From hospital admission to discharge; an exploratory study to evaluate seamless care. Pharmaceutical Journal 267: 650

## Further reading

Addington-Hall J M, McCarthy M 1995 Dying from cancer: results of a national population based investigation. Palliative Medicine 9: 295

Chandler A, Preece J, Lister S 2002 Using heat therapy for pain management. Nursing Standard 13: 40

Editorial 1991 Post-operative relief of pain and non-opioid analgesics. Lancet 337: 524

Editorial 1994 Drug-induced end-stage renal disease. New England Journal of Medicine 331: 1711

Editorial 1994 Pain control, TENS machines. Nursing Times 91: 51

Edwards S 1992 Evaluating syringe drivers. Nursing Times 88(3): 46

Fallon M 2000 Rationale for using alternative drugs to morphine. Palliative Care Today 1: 10

Hodges C 1998 Easing pain in children. Nursing Times 94(10): 55

Jordan S 1992 Drugs update – drugs for severe pain. Nursing Times 88(2): 24

Levy M H 1996 Pharmacological treatment of cancer pain. New England Journal of Medicine 335: 1124

Macleod G A, Davies M T O, Colvin J B 1995 Shaping attitudes to post-operative pain relief – the role of the acute pain team. Journal of Pain and Symptom Management 10: 30

McLintock T T, Aitken H, Downie C F et al 1990 Analgesic requirements in patients previously exposed to positive intra-operative suggestion. British Medical Journal 301: 788

Melzack R, Wall P D 1991 The challenge of pain. Penguin Books, London

O'Neill W M 1993 Pain in malignant disease. Prescribers Journal 33: 250

Reynolds F, Crowhurst J A 1997 Opioids in labour – no analgesic effect. Lancet 349: 4

Richmond C E, Bromley L M, Woolf C J 1993 Pre-operative morphine preempts post-operative pain. Lancet 342: 73

Shady P 1992 Patient-controlled analgesia: can education increase outcomes. Journal of Advanced Nursing 17: 408

Wolfe M M, Lichtenstein D R, Gurkipal Singh 1999 Gastrointestinal toxicity of NSAIDs. New England Journal of Medicine 340: 1888

Wood S 2002 Pain. Nursing Times 98: 41

# Chapter 11

# Anti-inflammatory drugs: treatment of arthritis and gout

## Learning objectives

At the end of this chapter, the reader should be able to:

- describe the basic features of the acute inflammatory and the immune responses
- list the important NSAIDs
- explain the theoretical difference between non-selective and COX 2-selective NSAIDs and give examples of each
- state the main aims in the treatment of rheumatoid arthritis (RA)
- list the main classes of drugs used for RA and examples of each
- explain the meaning of the acronym DMARDs
- describe the newer 'biologic' treatments for RA and psoriatic arthritis and how they are administered
- explain what gout is and the drugs used to treat it

Certain key events of the inflammatory process and of the immune response should be known in order to understand the mechanism of the anti-inflammatory drugs in diseases such as rheumatoid arthritis, lupus and gout.

## THE ACUTE INFLAMMATORY REACTION

The acute inflammatory reaction is the body's defence mechanism against invading pathogens such as bacteria, cells infected with viruses and neoplastic growth. The reaction consists of:

- innate, non-specific and non-immune responses
- acquired specific immune responses.

## INNATE RESPONSE

The innate response consists of the inflammation that is produced at a site of damage. Powerful pain-producing chemicals such as the prostaglandins and bradykinin are released locally from cells to warn of a problem. Non-steroidal anti-inflammatory drugs (NSAIDs) such as aspirin and celecoxib (see below) target the systems that synthesize these prostaglandins. Bradykinin is also a vasodilator and in addition it makes the walls of the capillaries more 'leaky', so that proteins and leucocytes can get out of the blood and into the tissues. Vasodilators such as histamine and nitric oxide are released in order to facilitate the entry of blood cells such as leucocytes and monocytes into the area of damage. These cells will attack and kill any bacteria or neoplastic cells. Cells also release peptides called cytokines that play a major role in the inflammatory response. Knowledge of the cytokines involved in the inflammatory response has led to the introduction of powerful new so-called biologic remedies (see below).

## ACQUIRED RESPONSE

Acquired specific immune responses are the responses of the immune system, which is able to recognize as foreign specific proteins of invading organisms or of neoplastic cells and make antibodies against them. A common example of the clinical use of this mechanism is preventive treatment with vaccines. In autoimmune diseases, such as arthritis, lupus, asthma and diabetes, the immune system turns on certain tissues of the body and attacks them. Several of the disease-modifying antirheumatic drugs (DMARDs; see Case History 11.1) specifically target the immune system.

## THE NON-STEROIDAL ANTI-INFLAMMATORY DRUGS

The NSAIDs comprise:

- **salicylates**
- **paracetamol**
- **non-selective COX inhibitor NSAIDs**
- **selective COX 2 inhibitor NSAIDs**.

This is a large group of drugs. There are at least 50 different drugs available. Their chief use is to treat minor pain, i.e. headaches, etc., and to control the pain and stiffness in rheumatic disorders and osteoarthritis. They are believed to act by suppressing the formation within the peripheral tissues of prostaglandins, which occur naturally and are released by cell damage and during inflammation. One of the actions of prostaglandins is concerned with the production of painful stimuli, and they are also responsible for many of the features of inflammation (i.e. swelling and redness). Most of the NSAIDs have three major therapeutic actions:

- analgesic (pain relief)
- antipyretic (temperature reduction)
- anti-inflammatory (reduce tissue inflammation).

## MECHANISM OF ACTION OF NSAIDs

Two enzymes are concerned with the formation of prostaglandins: cyclooxygenase 1 (COX 1) and cyclooxygenase 2 (COX 2). Prostaglandins produced by COX 2 are responsible for pain and inflammation, whereas those from COX 1 have a protective effect on the stomach lining. Most NSAIDs block both COX 1 and COX 2 and, although they relieve pain and inflammation, may cause peptic ulcers. NSAIDs have been introduced which inhibit COX 2 preferentially (see below), and may possibly be less likely to cause stomach ulceration, although at the time of writing this is a controversial issue.

## THE SALICYLATES

### Aspirin (acetylsalicylic acid)

**Administration and absorption.** Aspirin is usually given by mouth and is rapidly absorbed from both the stomach and the ileum.

**Activation and distribution.** Once in the circulation and tissues, aspirin is converted into the active metabolite salicylate, especially in the liver. Aspirin is therefore a prodrug. In higher therapeutic doses, some of the salicylate becomes bound to plasma proteins. This plasma binding can lead to aspirin allergy. This happens because when aspirin binds to plasma proteins it may combine chemically with the protein by acetylating it. This changes the nature of the protein so that the immune system regards the altered protein as foreign and forms antibodies against it. The next time aspirin is taken, an allergic response may occur. Small molecules such as aspirin that combine with larger molecules such as proteins and turn them 'foreign' are called *haptens*.

**Metabolism and excretion.**  Approximately 25% of aspirin is excreted unchanged. The rest is metabolized, mainly in the liver, and excreted. Urinary excretion of aspirin is enhanced in alkaline urine, since the filtered drug is charged and does not easily get back into the circulation. Thus, in cases of aspirin poisoning, the patient's urine is made alkaline to facilitate aspirin excretion.

**Analgesic and anti–inflammatory action.**  Aspirin's therapeutic effects, as stated above, are due to its inhibition of prostaglandins, which are important in the production of both pain and inflammation. Aspirin is non-selective in that it inhibits both COX 1 and COX 2. The newer, COX 2-selective NSAIDs are described below. Aspirin is effective against pain of low intensity and particularly that of rheumatoid arthritis and acute rheumatic fever, when its anti-inflammatory properties are combined with its analgesic action. It is also useful in other minor pains such as headaches, sore throats and toothache (which can of course can be very severe).

**Antipyretic action (reducing body temperature).**  Aspirin is antipyretic. It will lower a raised body temperature. The control of body temperature is regulated by a centre in the hypothalamus, which balances heat production, resulting from metabolism, against heat loss. This is achieved either by increasing heat production by raising metabolism by such means as shivering, or by increasing heat loss by sweating and by dilating blood vessels in the skin. When a patient develops a fever the heat-regulating mechanism is set at a higher level than normal. Aspirin acts on this centre by inhibiting prostaglandin production in the hypothalamus, and this 'resets' temperature control to normal levels in the hypothalamus as long as the aspirin therapy is maintained. Heat loss is achieved by sweating and by dilatation of blood vessels of the skin. Aspirin is used until the body eliminates the cause of pyrexia (raised body temperature). These effects are only seen in patients with a raised temperature because aspirin does not lower the normal body temperature to any appreciable degree.

**Therapeutic use of aspirin.**  To relieve pain, aspirin is given orally as a tablet, and gastric irritation (see later) may be reduced if it is given with a meal. Aspirin is rapidly metabolized and excreted so that dosage every 4 hours is usually required to keep the patient free of pain. To suppress inflammation, larger doses may be needed. Salicylates in high doses are particularly useful in the treatment of acute rheumatic fever. Within 2 or 3 days of starting the drug the patient's temperature should have dropped to normal levels and the swelling and pain in the joints will have disappeared.

**Adverse effects of therapeutic doses.**  In normal doses aspirin is a gastric irritant and in about 70% of people produces slight bleeding from the stomach. If it is taken continuously over a long period this may lead to anaemia. More rarely, aspirin causes a severe haematemesis (vomiting blood), usually from a superficial erosion of the stomach wall, which results in loss of the protective action of prostaglandins on the gastric mucosa and to local damage. This bleeding may occur with both aspirin and soluble aspirin. Although severe bleeding is rare when considered against the enormous amount of aspirin consumed, it should not be used in:

- those with a history of peptic ulcer
- haemophilia or other bleeding disorders
- liver disease
- patients receiving anticoagulant drugs.

Occasionally aspirin causes bronchospasm and thus an asthma-like attack, due to reduced production of prostaglandins.

**Adverse effects of larger doses.**  In large doses aspirin produces effects on the eighth cranial nerve, i.e. dizziness, tinnitus, deafness and vomiting. This is associated with hyperventilation due to stimulation of the respiratory centre and to acidosis. In very high doses, aspirin can actually *increase* body temperature.

Aspirin should not be given to children under 12 years as it may rarely precipitate Reye's syndrome by causing coma and liver damage that can prove fatal. There is some recent evidence that aspirin should not be given to older children either (Editorial 2002a). The Committee on Safety of Medicines in the UK has recommended that aspirin should not be given to children aged 12–15 who are feverish.

**Treatment of aspirin poisoning.**  In cases of aspirin poisoning, patients suffer acidosis and should receive gastric lavage and forced alkaline diuresis provided renal and circulatory functions are adequate.

## Other preparations of aspirin

**Soluble aspirin** is a mixture of aspirin with calcium carbonate and citric acid. Its actions are similar to those of aspirin. It is more soluble, which aids absorption, and has been claimed to be less irritant to the stomach, but it may still cause bleeding.

**Benorilate** is a combination of paracetamol and aspirin that splits into its component drugs after absorption.

**Drug interactions.** Aspirin increases the effects of anticoagulants and oral hypoglycaemic drugs, partly by displacing them from their plasma-binding sites. Aspirin interferes with the effects of drugs such as probenecid and sulfinpyrazole, which are used to treat gout by increasing urate secretion (see below). In lower doses, aspirin actually inhibits urate secretion, so it should be avoided in gout altogether.

Although aspirin is classically known as a drug for the treatment of pain and inflammation, it is now rapidly becoming a drug that is used more and more for the prevention and treatment of a wider range of problems. Some clinicians regard aspirin as more of a cardiovascular drug, since in lower doses it is used to inhibit platelet aggregation (see p. 99). There is evidence that the regular use of aspirin reduces the risk of colon and rectal cancer, and may also reduce the risk of Alzheimer's disease.

## PARACETAMOL

Paracetamol (called acetaminophen in the USA) is a widely used minor analgesic and antipyretic. Although it has some cyclooxygenase inhibiting properties, this action is very weak in the peripheral tissues and it has practically no anti-inflammatory action. Its analgesic effect may be mediated by some action on the central nervous system, which is not yet understood. Its main advantage is that unlike other drugs in this group it does not cause indigestion or gastric bleeding.

## Therapeutic use

Paracetamol is given orally in tablet form. It is well absorbed and peak plasma concentrations are achieved usually well within 60 minutes. It is partly bound to plasma proteins and inactivated by metabolism in the liver.

Paracetamol is the preferred mild analgesic and antipyretic for children under 12 years old, as it does not cause Reye's syndrome. In this age group it is frequently given as an oral suspension. The child should be over 3 months old, except for post-immunization pyrexia, when 2 months is acceptable.

It is not very effective in rheumatoid arthritis because of its poor anti-inflammatory action.

## Adverse effects

Adverse effects are uncommon at normal dosage but in overdose it causes dangerous liver damage. The margin of safety is relatively low, and doses as low as 2–3 times the maximum therapeutic dose can be harmful to the liver (see p. 428 for treatment of overdosage). There is also some evidence that large doses taken over a long period may damage the kidneys.

**Mefenamic acid** is a mild analgesic but is probably a little more powerful than aspirin. Its action may last longer than that of aspirin, but it may produce diarrhoea. It can also cause acute renal failure in the elderly.

## ANALGESIC MIXTURES WITH ASPIRIN OR PARACETAMOL

There are many analgesic mixtures in which aspirin or paracetamol is combined with a small dose of weak opiate; thus the risk of dependence is minimal. These combinations are a little stronger than aspirin or paracetamol alone and are used for more severe pain. Whether in fact they are more effective than the single drugs is debatable and certainly the risk of adverse effects and of danger in overdose is increased. Nevertheless, they are very popular and some are available over the counter.

Among those in common use are:

- **Co-codaprin** tablets:* codeine phosphate + aspirin. This is also available in a dispersible form.
- **Co-codamol** tablets:* codeine phosphate + paracetamol.
- **Co-dydramol** tablets: dihydrocodeine tartrate + paracetamol.
- **Co-proxamol** tablets: dextropropoxyphene + paracetamol.
- *Tylex*: codeine phosphate + paracetamol.

* Available without prescription.

## NSAIDs AND THE UTERUS

Prostaglandins can cause contraction of the uterus and are important in the initiation of labour. NSAIDs, by preventing prostaglandin formation, are useful in reducing period pains and have also been used to prevent premature labour.

## OLDER NSAIDs

Examples of older NSAIDs are:

- **indometacin (Indocid)**
- **phenylbutazone**.

Indometacin and phenylbutazone have been available for many years. Both are associated with problematic side-effects. Indometacin is an NSAID, which has been used in various forms of arthritis and in acute gout. It is effective but minor adverse effects, particularly on the gastrointestinal tract, are common. Phenylbutazone is a powerful NSAID. Unfortunately it has a number of serious adverse effects, including agranulocytosis, gastric bleeding, salt and water retention and rashes. Its use is therefore restricted to the treatment of ankylosing spondylitis in hospital.

## NON-SELECTIVE COX NSAIDs

These are listed in Table 11.1 with their major adverse effects.

Clearly there are now large numbers of non-selective NSAIDs available for use in rheumatoid arthritis and allied disorders. They are used to reduce the inflammatory element in osteoarthritis, though this use is more controversial as there is a suspicion that although they relieve pain they may hasten the degenerative changes in the joint. They are given to relieve pain in dentistry and that arising from soft-tissue and bony injuries and they can be used for the lesser pains of terminal illness. They provide useful analgesia, particularly after day surgery, when undue sedation has to be avoided. They all act by reducing the production of prostaglandins and thus reduce inflammation.

There are certain general principles that can be applied to this group:

- There is no preferred drug. Patients vary in their preference and if one drug is ineffective after 2 weeks of treatment a change should be made to another. It is useless to give two drugs of this type concurrently.
- If a satisfactory response is obtained, use the lowest dose that is effective.
- All these drugs may cause some gastric irritation and should be given with or after meals.

It is generally accepted that **ibuprofen** in doses usually recommended is rather less likely to produce side-effects than the others of this group, but is perhaps less effective. It is available over the counter. **Azapropazone** has the highest incidence of adverse effects. The rest are all very similar.

Several of these drugs are available as suppositories (e.g. diclofenac, indometacin, ketoprofen) or for injection (diclofenac).

**Table 11.1** Newer NSAIDs

| Drug | Trade name | Side-effects and special features |
|------|-----------|-----------------------------------|
| Azapropazone | Rheumox | High incidence of adverse effects. Use only if other NSAIDs are unsatisfactory |
| Diclofenac | Voltarol | Indigestion, avoid in peptic ulceration. Rashes. Can be given by I.M. injection |
| Etodolac | Lodine | |
| Fenbufen | Lederfen | Indigestion, avoid in peptic ulceration. Produces a therapeutically active metabolite |
| Fenoprofen | Fenopron | Indigestion, avoid in peptic ulceration. Rashes |
| Flurbiprofen | Froben | Indigestion, avoid in peptic ulceration. Rashes |
| Ibuprofen | Brufen Ebufac | Indigestion, avoid in peptic ulceration. Rashes. Low incidence of side-effects but not so active as some of the group. Now available without prescription |
| Ketoprofen | Orudis | Indigestion, avoid in peptic ulceration. Rashes |
| Meloxicam | Mobic | |
| Nabumetone | Reliflex | Converted to active metabolite |
| Naproxen | Naprosyn | Indigestion, avoid in peptic ulceration. Rashes. Twice daily dosage |
| Piroxicam | Feldene | Indigestion, avoid in peptic ulceration. Once daily dosage |
| Sulindac | Clinoral | Rapidly converted to active metabolite in the body. Indigestion, avoid in peptic ulceration. Rashes. Dizziness |

### Nursing point

Some NSAIDs, including ibuprofen, ketoprofen and piroxicam, are available without prescription as gels for topical application. Small amounts penetrate to deeper tissues and they appear to produce some improvement in soft-tissue injuries and arthritis. They should be rubbed in gently over the affected area and the hands washed after application. Occlusive dressings should not be used. Occasionally, excessive application can cause systemic adverse effects.

## Adverse effects

These are similar for all non-selective COX inhibitor drugs:

- Indigestion.
- Gastric bleeding and perforation are particularly common in elderly patients (see Case History 11.1) and are believed to be due to the inhibition of the gastric protective action of prostaglandins. These drugs should not be given to patients with peptic ulcers or bleeding disorders but, if essential, they can be combined with omeprazole or possibly with misoprostol (see p. 112), an oral prostaglandin preparation. These drugs should also be avoided in the elderly, if possible.
- Occasionally, salt and water retention.
- Rarely, bronchospasm. These drugs may make asthma worse.

## Case History 11.1

The patient, an 82-year-old lady, was brought to hospital by her neighbour who had found her on the floor in the kitchen of her house. The patient remembered making a cup of tea and feeling dizzy and light headed. She had sustained bruising to her forehead and left arm. For the preceding 3 weeks she had experienced increasing fatigue and had noticed that whenever she arose from a sitting or lying position she temporarily felt light headed. This sensation would last for 1 to 2 minutes during which she would support herself on any furniture to hand.

She was previously a fit and active lady. Over the last 3 months, she had been treated by her general practitioner for swelling, pain and stiffness of her left knee with Diclofenac Modified Release 75 mg twice daily. The patient reported that these symptoms had been attributed to osteoarthritis. After routine tests, a preliminary diagnosis of gastric ulceration secondary to non-steroidal anti-inflammatory drugs was made. The patient was admitted to the medical assessment unit and tranfused four units of blood. She was placed 'nil by mouth' and given 40 mg of omeprazole intravenously. The following morning she underwent an oesophago-gastro-duodenoscopy (OGD) which confirmed the presence of an ulcer in the gastric antrum. The ulcer was not actively bleeding and biopsies were taken to test for the presence of *Helicobacter pylori* or an underlying malignancy. Both of these were subsequently normal. The patient returned to the ward and was prescribed paracetamol 1 g four times a day and omeprazole 20 mg once a day. Two further haemoglobin concentrations were normal as was her blood pressure over the next 4 days. The patient also noted resolution of her postural symptoms and she was discharged.

## Drug interactions of the non-selective COX inhibitor NSAIDs

These drugs may:

- antagonize the actions of diuretics and hypotensive drugs
- increase the effects of anticoagulants
- decrease the excretion and increase the effect of lithium (see p. 282)

## SELECTIVE COX 2 INHIBITOR NSAIDs

Examples of these drugs are:

- **celecoxib (*Celebrex*)**
- **rofecoxib (*Vioxx*)**.

This is a newer class of drugs that are now prescribed as NSAIDs. These drugs selectively inhibit COX 2 – the isoform of the enzyme that synthesizes prostaglandins, which mediate inflammation – while sparing the COX 1 isoform that protects the stomach from attack by acid. Much publicity surrounded their introduction and claims were made that they were significantly less harmful to the lining of the stomach than the non-selective COX inhibitors. There is little doubt that at relatively low concentrations these drugs act predominantly on COX 2, but at the dose levels prescribed, these drugs may be active enough on COX 1 to cause similar levels of gastric damage as do the other NSAIDs. This controversy is underlined by the fact that the US Food and Drug Administration (FDA) have instructed the manufacturers of celecoxib to remove from their product information the claim that the drug protects arthritis patients from gastric damage (Editorial 2002b).

Therefore the prescriber may have to take the same precautions when prescribing these drugs as is done when prescribing the other NSAIDs. Nevertheless, the principle is sound and several companies are at present feverishly seeking the pure COX 2 inhibitor.

## NSAIDs AND THE KIDNEY

NSAIDs very rarely damage the kidneys in normal subjects. However, in patients with heart failure, cirrhosis of the liver, renal disease or who are taking diuretics they can occasionally precipitate renal failure. This is believed to be due to an alteration of blood flow through the kidneys, which follows inhibition of prostaglandin production. It usually recovers on stopping the drug but rarely NSAIDs cause irreversible renal damage. When this group of patients is given regular treatment with NSAIDs their renal function should be checked after a short period of treatment.

### Summary

- NSAIDs inhibit the COX enzymes that produce prostaglandins
- The aim is to inhibit COX 2 and not COX 1
- Aspirin will reduce fever temperatures
- Aspirin should not be given on an empty stomach
- Aspirin poisoning can be countered by alkalinizing the urine if kidney and circulation are healthy
- Soluble aspirin may still cause gastric bleeding
- Do not use aspirin in gout
- Do not use aspirin in children of 15 years and under
- Paracetamol is the preferred analgesic for children under 12 years old
- Paracetamol is not anti-inflammatory and therefore of little or no use in rheumatoid arthritis
- Paracetamol is toxic to the liver at doses not far above therapeutic
- Analgesic mixtures are not proven to be more effective than either aspirin or paracetamol alone

- Some NSAIDs can be applied topically to the skin
- COX 2 inhibitors are not purely COX 2-selective and may cause gastric irritation by inhibiting COX 1

### Nursing point

Glucosamine and glucosamine sulphate are widely used by sufferers from osteoarthrosis, and several studies support the use of these compounds, which are now sometimes prescribed (Editorial 2002d).

## RHEUMATOID ARTHRITIS

Rheumatoid arthritis (RA) is a common disorder affecting small and medium-sized joints and causing pain. In a proportion of patients it leads to considerable deformity and disability. Although the exact cause is not known, RA is an example of an autoimmune disease in which the immune system, for unknown reasons, attacks soft tissues in the joints and inflames them. The inflammation in the joints is due to prostaglandins and other chemical mediators, which give rise to pain and swelling, and to cytokines, which are responsible for progressive damage to the joints, leading to deformity.

## TREATMENT OF RHEUMATOID ARTHRITIS

Currently, the treatment of patients with rheumatoid arthritis aims to:

- slow the rate of degenerative change and tissue damage and delay or prevent deformity of the hands and feet
- control the symptoms of pain, stiffness and swelling of the joints.

Until recently, therapy was usually started with an NSAID, the choice depending on the doctor's experience and preference. Sometimes it was necessary to add a simple analgesic such as paracetamol to the NSAID, either on a regular basis to improve pain control or when pain became severe. Although this approach has been successful and symptoms are relieved, NSAIDs do not affect cytokines so damage to the joint continues. Anti-inflammatory steroids would be resorted to when flare-ups occur.

Many clinicians would now use a DMARD, either alone or in combination, early in treatment in an attempt to protect the joints from damage and minimize deformity, and Case History 11.2 illustrates the use of this principle of treatment. Opinions differ as to the best DMARD to use initially, but methotrexate and sulfasalazine are preferred at present. Newer drugs (so-called biologic drugs) have become available as DMARDs (see below). The initial results are very encouraging, but the long-term consequences of this approach remain to be discovered.

## Case History 11.2

Shortly after the birth of her second child, Mrs M began to have severe pain in both wrists. She woke up feeling stiff in the mornings and the stiffness might persist all day. She took paracetamol tablets for a while, but the pain and stiffness did not go away. She went to her doctor, who referred her to a rheumatologist, who did blood tests, ordered X-rays and told her she had rheumatoid arthritis. He explained that she had developed an autoimmune disease: the body's immune system begins to regard the soft tissues of the joints as foreign and attacks them, causing inflammation, pain and destruction of the tissues. The doctor told her that we understand very little of why the body decides to do this in some people, and while it was bad luck, there were now treatments available that would not only help alleviate the pain but also slow down the course of the disease. He explained that previously doctors could do little more than treat the pain and give steroids, which over a long period have many adverse effects. Today, arthritis is tackled head-on as soon as it is diagnosed with powerful new treatments that slow the course of the disease. These drugs target the damage-causing mechanisms in the body, and this also alleviates the symptoms. He prescribed a short-course of prednisolone to reduce the inflammation, celecoxib (Celebrex), an NSAID, to help with the stiffness and pain, and methotrexate, a DMARD by once-weekly injection to start the disease-slowing process. The rheumatologist also applied to the local health authority for funds to put the patient onto a course of infliximab. Appointments were made for regular blood tests because of the methotrexate treatment.

Drugs used in treatment of rheumatoid arthritis comprise:

- **NSAIDs**
- **anti-inflammatory steroids**
- **DMARDs**.

NSAIDs are considered above, so discussion is confined to the other two groups.

## ANTI-INFLAMMATORY STEROIDS

The anti-inflammatory steroids have been available for at least 50 years, and are synthetic analogues of the body's own anti-inflammatory steroid cortisol (see p. 204), which is synthesized by the adrenal cortex. These steroids are not only anti-inflammatory but are also immunosuppressants. They therefore have a two-pronged action, since inflammatory diseases such as rheumatoid arthritis and lupus are autoimmune diseases. Hailed as miracle drugs when they were first introduced, they soon proved to be a two-edged sword because of the side-effects associated with the prolonged use of these drugs in comparatively high doses (see p. 205). They are, nevertheless, still used chronically in lower doses, and are used on a short-term basis to deal with flare-ups.

## DISEASE-MODIFYING ANTIRHEUMATIC DRUGS (DMARDs)

This is a mixed group of drugs, some of which inhibit the effects of the immune system on the rheumatic process in various ways: they not only relieve pain but also reduce joint damage. Unlike the NSAIDs, they may take up to 6 months to produce a full response. The main drugs in this class are:

- chloroquine
- gold
- penicillamine
- sulfasalazine
- methotrexate
- biologic drugs.

### Chloroquine

Chloroquine is primarily an antimalarial drug that has been found to be useful in rheumatoid arthritis. About half the patients put onto chloroquine respond to the drug. Chloroquine appears to be of some benefit in treating the morning stiffness and joint pain of rheumatoid arthritis and also in the skin lesions of lupus erythematosus. It is unclear at present whether the drug alters radiographic disease progression. The beneficial effects of chloroquine are not evident until about 1 month after initiation of therapy.

**Mechanism of action.** The mechanism of action of chloroquine is not fully understood. It may exert its effects partly by blocking the production of one or more of the inflammatory mediators, and by interfering with the actions of leucocytes. It also inhibits the proliferation of lymphocytes.

**Adverse effects.** Unfortunately, prolonged treatment may cause corneal opacities and, more seriously, retinal damage. The former may be suggested by the patient reporting haloes round bright lights. Patients should have their eyes examined before starting treatment and be told to report any disturbance of vision. Thereafter, the eyes should be examined if it is considered necessary.

## Gold salts

These comprise:

- **sodium aurothiomalate**
- **auranofin**.

The use of gold salts has largely been supplanted by other DMARDs, especially methotrexate (see below). They are still used, however, and the prescribers and dispensers of these drugs need to know of their existence, uses and adverse effects. The onset of action of gold compounds is slow, and the maximum response is obtained after 3–4 months. Gold reduces swelling and treats the pain and stiffness. Disease progression in terms of joint and bone damage is slowed. Approximately 66% of patients will respond to gold.

**Mechanism of action.** This is largely unknown. Gold is known to inhibit the proliferation of lymphocytes, reduce the migration of leucocytes into the tissues and inhibit the release of chemical mediators of inflammation. Whether these actions mediate its disease-modifying effects is unknown.

**Therapeutic use.** Sodium aurothiomalate is usually given weekly by deep intramuscular injection. Auranofin is given orally. It is less toxic and better tolerated than sodium aurothiomalate, but is less effective. Gold salts concentrate in the joints, and also in the liver, kidney, the cortex of the adrenal glands and in the macrophages. They remain in the body for some time after treatment is stopped.

**Adverse effects.** These are observed in about one-third of patients. They can be serious and may require withdrawal of the treatment:

- Itching followed by rashes, which can progress to exfoliation. This requires treatment to be stopped.
- Renal damage – urine must be tested for protein at each visit.
- Bone marrow suppression requires weekly blood counts and the patient should report bleeding, bruising or sore throat.

- Stomatitis (inflammation of the mucous lining of the mouth).
- Dose-related diarrhoea with auranofin that can be stopped by a high fibre diet.

## Penicillamine

Penicillamine (see also p. 431) has been used with some success in treating rheumatoid arthritis, but other DMARDs such as methotrexate have largely displaced penicillamine. It is a chemically modified form of the amino acid cysteine, which is able to interfere with the action of some enzymes that attack joint proteins and thereby suppress the inflammation. A therapeutic effect may not be noticeable for up to 6 months with penicillamine. Its use is not without risk as it can cause skin rashes, proteinuria, nausea, cytopenia (depression of the blood count) and, rarely, damage to the kidneys. It is therefore necessary to test the urine for protein and to perform a blood count at regular intervals.

## Sulfasalazine

Sulfasalazine (see also p. 114) is interesting in that it was designed specifically to treat rheumatoid arthritis. Chemically, it is a combination of an antibacterial sulphonamide with a salicylate. It has commonly been used as a first choice DMARD for the treatment of arthritis and it suppresses the rheumatoid process. It takes about 3 months to produce its full therapeutic effect, but is less toxic than gold or penicillamine. However, its use necessitates regular blood counts and liver function tests and the patient should be warned to report any sore throat, bleeding or bruising.

## Methotrexate

Methotrexate (see also p. 342) is increasing in popularity as a second-line drug. Chemically, it is an antagonist of folic acid and is cytotoxic (destroys cells by blocking cell division). It was originally introduced for the treatment of cancer, but was found to slow disease progression in RA in terms of joint and bone damage. It acts more rapidly than the drugs discussed earlier and, if given in relatively low doses, toxicity is acceptably low provided renal function is normal. The drug is taken orally or by subcutaneous injection once a week. About 50% of patients on methotrexate stay on it for 5 years or longer.

**Adverse effects.** The main adverse effects are gastrointestinal upsets, liver cirrhosis and pulmonary fibrosis. It may be combined with folic acid to minimize these risks. Regular blood counts and liver function tests are necessary and a chest radiograph if a patient develops a persistent cough or dyspnoea.

> ### Nursing point
>
> Patients usually take these drugs long term and they must be aware of possible adverse effects and the importance of regular checks and of reporting warning symptoms.

## Biologic DMARDs

There comprise:

- **infliximab (Remicade)**
- **etanercept (Enbrel)**.

The term 'biologic' is the US version of 'biological', but since the former is being so widely used in the literature it is being used here as well. Infliximab and etanercept are two relatively new drugs designed to treat inflammatory diseases by neutralizing one of the cytokines – tumour necrosis factor α (TNF-α) – that is a prime activator of the inflammatory response (Simon & Yocum 2000, Emery 2001). Both drugs are proving effective in other previously intractable conditions as well, notably Crohn's disease and psoriatic arthritis. This is a fairly revolutionary approach to the treatment of disease that is proving very potent, and no one yet knows what the long-term effects on the body will be. TNF-α is an important component of the immune system, and interference with its action hinders the work of the immune system, which can result in reduced resistance to infection.

**The nature of infliximab and etanercept**. Both of these drugs are proteins. Infliximab is an antibody raised against TNF-α and when injected it binds to it and renders it inactive. Etanercept is a protein that resembles the cellular receptor to which TNF-α normally binds in order to exert its effects, and when injected, etanercept also mops up any circulating TNF-α, thus preventing it from acting on any cells.

**Administration and therapeutic effects.** Both drugs, being proteins, have to be injected. Infliximab is given by slow intravenous infusion that needs to be done in hospital under supervision by trained nurses. The patient is usually admitted to a day bed and the infusion is administered over a 2-hour period, after which the patient is kept under observation for a further 2 hours before being discharged. Etanercept is administered twice weekly by subcutaneous injection.

Results of controlled studies suggest that in many cases these two drugs work faster and slow degenerative changes better than do other DMARD drugs. Infliximab has been used in at least one study in patients concurrently taking methotrexate and results were better than those on methotrexate alone. A recent follow-up study of patients taking infliximab gave evidence that patients who had stopped taking infliximab after 1 year of treatment still showed a 50% improvement in symptoms several months after treatment was stopped (Editorial 2002c). Infliximab is currently the subject of a nationwide clinical trial in the UK and it will take some years before the results are published.

**Adverse effects.** Adverse effects reported with etanercept include:

- more commonly: fever; chills; sneezing cough; skin rash on scalp, face or stomach
- less commonly: stomach discomfort and/or pain; chest congestion; wheezing; dizziness; fainting; fast heartbeat; headache; joint or muscle pain; joint or muscle stiffness, tightness, or rigidity; lightheadedness; nausea and/or vomiting; frequent or painful urination.

Adverse effects with infliximab include rash; fever; polyarthralgia (pain in several joints); pruritus (itching); oedema; dysphagia (painful swallowing); urticaria; sore throat; headache. Some of these effects may be delayed and be evident some days after the treatment.

It is still too early to know what the long-term effects of these drugs will be. What is fairly certain, however, is that this 'biologic' approach is likely to become far more important in the treatment of autoimmune diseases.

## Other DMARDs

**Azathioprine** and **cyclophosphamide** can also be used when other treatments have failed. Ciclosporin (see p. 347), which suppresses the rheumatoid process by interfering with T-cell function, has also been used. It is particularly liable to cause renal damage.

## CONCURRENT CARE

Concurrent care of patients with rheumatoid arthritis includes various forms of physiotherapy and prevention of deformity, sometimes rest, occasionally surgery, the treatment of complications and advice and counselling. Patients with long-term arthritis have special needs. In advanced cases, they cannot open medicine containers or hold even quite light objects such as bottles and have trouble opening doors. Health professionals who work with these patients need to be acutely aware of these problems. The occupational therapist is particularly important in this respect.

### Summary

- After diagnosis of RA, it is now possible to attack disease progression aggressively with DMARDs
- An important aim is to try and prevent deformity
- Steroids are still used in RA but in lower doses
- Patients should have their eyes examined before starting on chloroquine and should report any disturbance of vision while on the drug
- Methotrexate is given with folic acid and patients must have regular checks of liver function
- Ciclosporin can cause liver damage
- Patients with RA need concurrent care, such as physiotherapy and special equipment at home

### Nursing point

Specialist rheumatology nurse practitioners are playing an increasingly important part in patient management

## GOUT

Gout is a metabolic disorder that tends to run in families. In gout there is an increase in the amount of uric acid in the body, probably due to increased production, and this precipitates around joints (particularly the big toe), producing an acute arthritis. In long-standing cases uric acid may also accumulate in other parts of the body.

## DRUG TREATMENT OF GOUT

The following drugs are used:

- **colchicine**
- **NSAIDs**
- **uricosuric drugs** (increase uric acid excretion in the urine)
- **drugs that block uric acid biosynthesis**.

Treatment has two aims:

- To relieve the acute attack: NSAIDs may be used for this purpose. Indometacin (see above) is very effective. It is used in relatively large doses to produce a rapid effect and then at a reduced dose for 1 week. An older remedy is colchicine.
- To decrease the amount of uric acid in the body and thus prevent further attacks: this can be achieved by increasing its excretion in the urine by **uricosuric drugs** or by preventing the production of uric acid by giving **allopurinol**.

### Colchicine

Colchicine is an alkaloid obtained from the autumn crocus or meadow saffron. An alkaloid is a naturally occurring, nitrogen-containing chemical, which is basic in solution. Other examples of alkaloids are belladonna and ipecacuanha. Colchicine is not an analgesic in the strict sense of the word because it relieves only one type of pain, namely that associated with an acute attack of gout. Its mode of action in gout is complicated, but it probably inhibits some actions of inflammatory cells in gouty tissue.

**Therapeutic use.**   The pure alkaloid colchicine is used in the treatment of gout. It is administered orally in tablet form and is well absorbed.

**Adverse effects.**   These are largely in the gastrointestinal tract. Sometimes toxic effects (vomiting and diarrhoea) may cause premature cessation of treatment. Long-term use may cause blood dyscrasias (abnormalities).

### Uricosuric drugs

Uricosuric drugs increase the excretion of uric acid by the kidney.

**Probenecid** increases the excretion of uric acid by the kidney, probably by an action on the renal tubular cells. It can be given over long periods. Side-effects are rare but gastrointestinal upsets and rashes may occur.

**Sulfinpyrazone** is a very powerful uricosuric agent. Its effects are blocked by simultaneous administration of citrates or salicylates.

### Drugs preventing the production of uric acid: allopurinol

Allopurinol slows the production of uric acid by inhibiting an enzyme (xanthine oxidase), which is concerned with the synthesis of uric acid within the body (Fig. 11.1). It has proved particularly useful in

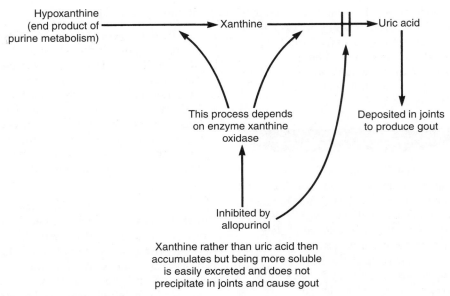

**Figure 11.1** Mode of action of allopurinol.

the long-term management of gout, particularly if the attacks are frequent, and will usually need to be continued for the rest of the patient's life.

**Therapeutic use.** Allopurinol is given orally. It is a prodrug, and is converted into the active metabolite, alloxanthine, which in turn inhibits the enzyme that produced it. It is excreted via the kidneys and care is necessary if it is used in renal failure.

**Adverse effects.** These are relatively few. Skin rashes are particularly common if retention of the drug occurs. It must not be combined with the anticancer agent 6-mercaptopurine, as it prevents the breakdown of this drug and greatly increases its effect.

### Nursing points

1. Uricosuric drugs and allopurinol may cause an acute attack of gout in the first 2 months of treatment, probably because deposits of uric acid are mobilized, and should therefore be combined with an NSAID during this period.
2. If uricosuric drugs are used the patient should be advised to maintain a high fluid intake to prevent the formation of uric acid crystals in the renal tract.
3. Remember that diuretics and pyrazinamide can cause attacks of gout.

### Summary

- Aspirin should not be taken on an empty stomach
- Aspirin should not be given to patients with a history of peptic ulcers, haemophilia, liver disease or those on anticoagulants
- Aspirin should not be given to children under 15. Paracetamol should be used instead
- Aspirin poisoning is commonly treated by gastric lavage and forced alkaline diuresis
- Soluble aspirin may cause gastric bleeding
- Do not use aspirin in patients with gout who are taking probenecid or sulfinpyrazole
- Paracetamol is toxic to the liver in doses not far above those used therapeutically
- NSAIDs are useful for reducing period pains and for preventing premature labour
- Indometacin has a high incidence of adverse gastrointestinal effects
- Wash hands after applying NSAIDs topically to skin
- NSAIDs can precipitate renal failure in patients with heart failure, cirrhosis of the liver, renal disease or who are taking diuretics
- Patients should have their eyes tested before starting on chloroquine and be told to report any visual disturbances

- Patients on DMARDs should have regular blood counts and tests for protein in urine
- Methotrexate is prescribed with folic acid
- Patients given infusions of infliximab must be kept under observation for at least 2 hours before being allowed to go home

- Patients should be advised to report any symptoms after treatment with the biologic DMARDs
- Remember that patients with advanced RA may not be able to open conventional medicine containers

## References

Editorial 2002a Older children should also avoid aspirin. Pharmaceutical Journal 268: 557

Editorial 2002b FDA removes celecoxib's gastric protection claim. Pharmaceutical Journal 268: 861

Editorial 2002c Infliximab exerts prolonged response even after the treatment is stopped. Pharmaceutical Journal 269: 668

Editorial 2002d Glucosamine is allowed on the NHS. Pharmaceutical Journal 269: 705

Emery P 2001 Infliximab: a new treatment for rheumatoid arthritis. Hospital Medicine 62(3): 150

Simon L S, Yocum D 2000 New and future drug therapies for rheumatoid arthritis. Rheumatology (Oxford) 39 (Suppl 1): 36

## Further reading

Akil M, Amos RS 1995 Rheumatoid arthritis – treatment. British Medical Journal 310: 652

Allison M C, Howatson A G, Torrance C J et al 1992 Gastrointestinal damage associated with the use of nonsteroidal antiinflammatory drugs. New England Journal of Medicine 327: 749

Arthur V, Clifford C 1998 Evaluation of information given to rheumatology patients using NSAIDs. Journal of Clinical Nursing 7: 175

Bathon J M, Martin R W, Fleischmann R M et al 2000 A comparison of etanercept and methotrexate in patients with early rheumatoid arthritis. New England Journal of Medicine 343: 1586

Courtney M 1998 Oral analgesics: aspirin and paracetamol. Nursing Times 94(5): 59

Current Problems in Pharmacovigilance 1994 Relative safety of oral non-aspirin NSAIDs 20: 9

Editorial 1995 Methotrexate in rheumatoid arthritis. Drug and Therapeutics Bulletin 33: 17

Editorial 1997 Disease modifying drugs in rheumatoid arthritis. British Medical Journal 314: 766

Editorial 1998 Modifying disease in rheumatoid arthritis. Drug and Therapeutics Bulletin 36(1): 3

# Chapter 12

# Drugs affecting the kidney and renal function

## Learning objectives

At the end of this chapter, the reader should be able to:

- give a definition of diuretics
- list the factors that cause fluid retention
- describe the basic sites of diuretic action in the nephron
- list the main classes of currently used diuretics
- explain the mechanism of action and uses of osmotic drugs
- describe the actions of thiazide diuretics, examples, uses and adverse effects
- describe the actions of loop diuretics, examples, uses and adverse effects
- enumerate the risk factors associated with diuretics and potassium loss
- state the three examples of potassium-sparing diuretics
- provide examples of potassium supplements
- explain the dangers associated with diuretic use in liver cirrhosis and elderly patients
- describe how to alkalinize urine

## INTRODUCTION TO DIURETICS

Diuretics are drugs that cause increased urine production. They are useful in patients who are suffering from retention of water and sodium chloride (salt), which usually accumulates in the tissue spaces and is called oedema. Note that diuretics are not used in

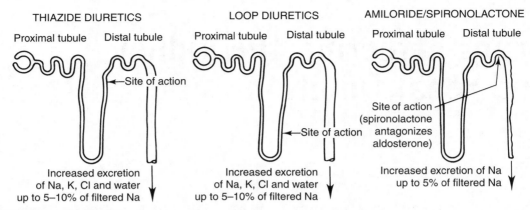

**Figure 12.1** Sites of action of diuretics.

patients who cannot empty their bladders; this is called urinary retention.

## OEDEMA

Oedema occurs most commonly in heart failure, the nephrotic syndrome (severe loss of protein in the urine) and cirrhosis of the liver. Ankle oedema may also develop in individuals sitting with their legs dependent, a common example being elderly people who are confined to their chairs for long periods. It can also complicate the use of calcium channel blockers (see p. 76).

## FACTORS CAUSING FLUID RETENTION

The factors that cause fluid retention are various and depend on the underlying disease. They include:

- **Lowered cardiac output** and underfilling of the vascular system (hypovolaemia), which activates the renin–angiotensin system with increased secretion of aldosterone by the adrenal cortex, leading to salt and water retention by the kidney. This occurs in heart failure, cirrhosis of the liver and the nephrotic syndrome.
- **Raised pressure in the veins and capillaries**. This leads to increased exudation of fluid from the blood to the tissue spaces, and occurs in heart failure, liver cirrhosis and oedema due to prolonged immobility with legs dependent.
- **Low plasma proteins**. This is found in the nephrotic syndrome, where it is due to protein loss in the urine, and cirrhosis of the liver, where there is a failure to make protein.

## RENAL FUNCTION

The role of the kidney is to excrete the waste products of metabolism, drugs, etc., and maintain the correct amounts of water and electrolytes in the body by getting rid of any excesses that may be absorbed or produced by the body. This is effected in two stages (Fig. 12.1):

- glomerular filtration
- tubular reabsorption.

**Glomerular filtration.** At the glomeruli, water along with soluble substances is filtered from the blood. The volume of this filtrate is about 100 litres of water per day and it contains glucose, electrolytes, urea and other substances.

**Tubular reabsorption.** In the renal tubules a selective reabsorption occurs. Glucose is normally completely reabsorbed. Water and electrolytes (including sodium, potassium, chloride and hydrogen carbonate) are partially reabsorbed, whereas urea is almost entirely excreted. The exact amount of each substance finally excreted in the urine is controlled so that the composition of the body fluids remains constant.

## DIURETIC DRUGS

All diuretic drugs produce their effect by decreasing the reabsorption of water and electrolytes by the renal tubules and thus allowing more water and electrolytes to be excreted. The diuretic drugs fall into various classes, depending on their site and mechanism of action:

- osmotic diuretics
- thiazide diuretics

- loop diuretics
- potassium-sparing diuretics.

## WATER

It is common experience that in a normal person, increased ingestion of water results in an increased urine flow. When water is absorbed, it causes the plasma to become more dilute and this in turn decreases the release of antidiuretic hormone (ADH) by the posterior lobe of the pituitary gland (see p. 176). Less ADH reaches the kidney and this causes the tubules to reabsorb less water, so that more is excreted as the urine. In those with fluid retention, for example in heart failure, the normal response to water disappears and so it is of no use as a diuretic under these circumstances.

## OSMOTIC DIURETICS

Any substance that passes through the glomeruli and is not reabsorbed by the renal tubules will increase the concentration of the urine within the tubules. This prevents the reabsorption of sodium chloride and water from the tubule back into the blood and the water is then passed out and produces a diuresis. Osmotic diuretics are now little used to treat oedema. They are more commonly used during cardiovascular surgery to sustain urinary function. A commonly used example is **mannitol**.

### Mechanism of action

The osmotic diuretics are filtered by the glomerulus and increase the osmotic pressure in the tubules. This inhibits the passive reabsorption of water from the tubules. Water is normally able to pass back into the body from the proximal tubule, the descending limb of the loop of Henle and from the collecting ducts, which are therefore the sites of action of the osmotic diuretics. Some sodium is lost as well, but not enough to make the osmotic diuretics useful in conditions associated with salt retention.

The osmotic diuretics must meet certain criteria for use:

- they must be pharmacologically inert
- they must be freely filterable by the glomerulus
- they must not be reabsorbed from the tubules.

## Mannitol

**Administration and therapeutic uses.**  Mannitol and other osmotic diuretics are usually given intravenously. Mannitol is sometimes used:

- during cardiovascular surgical procedures when urine flow through the kidneys needs to be maintained
- to lower raised intracranial pressure after a head injury or in a patient with a cerebral tumour
- to reduce the intraocular pressure in glaucoma.

**Adverse effects.**  These include headache, nausea and vomiting. Osmotic diuretics can cause pulmonary oedema or heart failure in patients who are unable to produce urine.

## THIAZIDE DIURETICS

Thiazide diuretics comprise:

- **bendroflumethiazide (bendrofluazide)**
- **chlorothiazide**
- **cyclopenthiazide**
- **hydrochlorothiazide**
- **indapamide**
- **metolazone**
- **polythiazide**
- **xipamide**

Clearly there are several diuretics in this group. Although there are marginal differences in their actions, the general pattern of their effects is the same and they will be described together. They are all absorbed from the intestinal tract and are therefore effective orally.

## Mechanism of action

The actions of thiazide diuretics on the kidney are:

- They interfere with the reabsorption of salt and water by the early distal tubules by binding to and inhibiting a sodium chloride pump: thus, less sodium chloride is reabsorbed and the salt together with accompanying water passes out of the tubules and causes a diuresis.
- There is an increased excretion of potassium by the kidney (see more on potassium secretion below). This takes place because sodium is normally reabsorbed in the collecting ducts in exchange for potassium; therefore, the more sodium is presented to the collecting ducts, the more will be exchanged for potassium, which is excreted.

## Therapeutic uses

The therapeutic uses of thiazide diuretics are:

- mild cardiac failure
- hypertension
- cirrhosis of the liver with ascites (accumulation of fluid in the peritoneal cavity)
- nephrotic syndrome
- prevention of renal stone formation in idiopathic hypercalciuria.

**Cardiac failure.** The thiazides are used to treat the oedema of cardiac failure. They are not very powerful diuretics and their use is usually confined to mild failure. They are given in the morning as the diuresis lasts throughout the day.

**Hypertension.** The thiazides have some blood pressure lowering action and may be used for this purpose, either alone or with other hypotensive drugs. This is not only due to their diuretic action; they also act as mild vasodilators. For this purpose, small doses of thiazides, e.g. bendroflumethiazide (bendrofluazide) or cyclopenthiazide, may be used. Potassium supplements are not usually required. In the chronic treatment of hypertension with thiazides, blood pressure stays down even after the diuretic action ceases, and this may be due, at least in part, to the vasodilator action of the thiazides.

**Cirrhosis of the liver with ascites.** The thiazides will produce a diuresis in this disorder with reduction in the ascites and oedema. Care is required, however, as their use may be followed by mental changes with disorientation, which it is believed is due to the potassium deficiency produced by these drugs.

**Nephrotic syndrome.** The thiazides can be used to treat the oedema found in this disorder. Frequently, however, a more powerful diuretic will be required: for example a loop diuretic such as furosemide (frusemide) – see below.

**Prevention of renal stone formation in idiopathic hypercalciuria.** The term *idiopathic* refers to a condition whose cause is unknown and which may arise spontaneously. Hypercalciuria is elevated calcium excretion, and calcium salts may be deposited in the kidney as stones and need to be dissolved and flushed out.

**Chlortalidone** is very similar to the thiazides in terms of onset and site of action, but it has a more prolonged action. **Metolazone** is a thiazide which generally has no advantage over others in the group but it will sometimes produce a diuresis when other thiazides have become ineffective. It may be combined with a loop diuretic (see below), particularly in patients with impaired renal function.

## Adverse effects

Generally speaking, the thiazide diuretics are well tolerated, have a high therapeutic index and adverse effects are relatively uncommon. These may include:

- hyperglycaemia
- metabolic alkalosis
- in diabetics, thiazides can actually *reduce* urine flow
- potassium loss; thiazides have in the past been prescribed together with potassium chloride
- increased uric acid secretion and can induce gout
- photosensitivity: patients on thiazides should consider using a sun block in direct sunlight.

## LOOP DIURETICS

The loop diuretics are the most powerful of the diuretics. They are called loop diuretics because they act on the ascending limb of the loop of Henle (see below). The main examples are:

- **furosemide (frusemide)**
- **bumetanide**
- **etacrynic acid**
- **torasemide**.

## Mechanism of action

This group of diuretics is far more powerful than the thiazides. Loop diuretics act on the ascending limb of the loop of Henle (see Fig. 12.1), which is impermeable to water, but where much sodium chloride is usually reabsorbed into the body. Loop diuretics therefore interfere to a greater extent, than do the thiazides, with the reabsorption of salt and water and are the most powerful of all the diuretics. They are sometimes referred to as 'high ceiling' diuretics. Like thiazides these diuretics also increase renal excretion of potassium. This is because much sodium is presented to the collecting ducts, where sodium is normally reabsorbed in exchange for potassium.

## Administration, distribution and metabolism

The loop diuretics are well absorbed from the gastrointestinal tract and are given orally or by injection. They will act within 1 hour after oral administration and their diuretic effect will peak within 30 minutes after intravenous injection. The duration of action of the loop diuretics after oral administration is relatively short (3–6 hours). **Torasemide** is the longest acting and is taken orally once a day.

In the blood, they are strongly bound to plasma proteins. This prolongs their action because only the unbound fraction of the drug can be metabolized in the liver. They are not filtered by the glomerulus. They reach their site of action in the ascending loop by being pumped into the tubular lumen in the proximal tubule, and after exerting the diuretic action are excreted in the urine. The fraction of drug not secreted into the lumen is ultimately metabolized in the liver.

### Clinical use of loop diuretics

Loop diuretics are used in:

- hypertension, especially with renal impairment
- acute treatment of hypercalcaemia
- salt and water overload due to:
    oedema due to chronic heart failure
    nephrotic syndrome
    renal failure
    hepatic cirrhosis complicated by ascites.

### Furosemide (frusemide)

**Furosemide** (frusemide) is probably the most commonly used loop diuretic and is especially useful in:

- Acute left ventricular failure with oedema of the lungs. Given intravenously, furosemide (frusemide) rapidly clears the oedema and pulmonary congestion. In these circumstances it also has a vasodilating action that relieves the load on the heart.
- Patients with congestive heart failure that is no longer responding to other diuretics.
- Oedema associated with the nephrotic syndrome, especially if there is some degree of renal failure. In these cases very large oral doses are sometimes used.
- Large doses may be given when acute renal failure is developing to try and jolt the kidneys into resuming normal function.

### Bumetanide

This powerful diuretic is similar to furosemide (frusemide) in its pharmacological action, although it is distinct chemically. It is given orally and produces a rapid diuresis lasting about 3 hours. For an even more immediate effect it may be given intravenously.

Its therapeutic uses and adverse effects are similar to those of furosemide (frusemide).

### Adverse effects of loop diuretics

Some of these adverse effects are similar to those of the thiazides:

- Hypokalaemia (decreased plasma potassium) due to increased potassium loss by the kidneys; it is more marked with high doses of diuretics (see below).
- Sodium depletion: with large doses of loop diuretics, particularly when given intravenously. The patient's blood volume may be reduced rapidly, causing hypotension and collapse. This can also occur with prolonged oral treatment.
- A large and rapid diuresis can precipitate acute urine retention in those with prostatic enlargement.
- Large doses of furosemide (frusemide) can cause transient deafness.
- Furosemide (frusemide) has been reported to cause photosensitivity.

### Drug interactions: with thiazides and loop diuretics

Drug interactions comprise:

- NSAIDs and steroids reduce the efficacy of these diuretics
- lithium retention (see p. 282)
- renal damage when combined with gentamicin
- increased digoxin toxicity due to hypokalaemia
- hypotension with ACE inhibitors.

> **Nursing point**
>
> When the powerful loop diuretics were first introduced, patients discovered that they were associated with weight reduction, and this led to widespread abuse of the drugs for weight loss purposes. Nurses and other health professionals should be aware of this form of drug abuse, which can be dangerous for the patient.

## DIURETICS AND POTASSIUM DEPLETION

Both the thiazides and loop diuretics cause loss of potassium through the kidneys and if the plasma potassium is lowered excessively (<3.0 mmol/litre) there is a risk of dangerous cardiac arrhythmias. This rarely occurs in patients receiving small doses of diuretics for hypertension or heart failure and it is adequate to check the plasma potassium level 1–2 months after the start of treatment. Note that indapamide does not appreciably affect potassium or uric acid excretion.

## Risk factors

The following risk factors may require more careful monitoring and some form of potassium replacement:

- large doses of diuretics
- poor diet, especially in the elderly
- concurrent use of digitalis – the toxicity of digitalis is increased by potassium deficiency
- immediately following myocardial infarction – low plasma potassium is associated with an increased risk of dangerous arrhythmias
- patients with cirrhosis of the liver are particularly sensitive to potassium depletion
- concurrent use of steroids increases potassium loss.

In all these patients the plasma potassium should be monitored and replacement started if depletion occurs. This may be achieved using:

- potassium supplements
- potassium-sparing diuretics (see below).

**Potassium supplements** should be given in the form of potassium chloride. Unfortunately, this substance is nauseating and can cause ulceration of the gut if given in tablet form. It is therefore formulated as:

- effervescent potassium chloride tablets (*Sando-K*)
- slow-release potassium chloride tablets (*Slow-K*).

Potassium can also be given by intravenous infusion if depletion is severe. This can be a dangerous procedure as hyperkalaemia from too rapid infusion can cause cardiac arrest. Careful monitoring of plasma potassium is mandatory. Certain diuretics are made up as combined diuretic + potassium chloride, e.g. cyclopenthiazide + potassium chloride (*Navidrex K*), but are not recommended as they contain too little potassium to be useful.

## POTASSIUM-SPARING DIURETICS

### Triamterene and amiloride

These drugs increase the excretion of salt and water without producing appreciable potassium loss.

Neither drug is a potent diuretic, and they are usually given with a reduced dose of a more potent diuretic that does cause potassium loss.

**Mechanism of action.** It is thought that this is probably due to a direct action on the renal tubules. Amiloride antagonizes the action of aldosterone on the renal tubule by binding to the sodium channels where aldosterone, the salt-retaining hormone, exerts its actions (see p. 204) and this increases sodium and water excretion with some potassium retention. Triamterene may have the same mechanism of action.

**Administration and absorption.** Both triamterene and amiloride are taken orally or by injection. Triamterene is well absorbed from the gastrointestinal tract, whereas amiloride is poorly absorbed. The effect of triamterene is evident within 2 hours, and lasts up to 15–16 hours, whereas that of amiloride is evident within 6 hours and lasts about 24 hours.

**Clinical use.** A thiazide or a loop diuretic can be combined with a potassium-sparing diuretic in one tablet to prevent potassium loss. Among the preparations available are:

- hydrochlorothiazide + amiloride (*co-amilozide*)
- hydrochlorothiazide + triamterene (*Dyazide*)
- furosemide (frusemide) + amiloride (*co-amilofruse*).

**Adverse effects.** Hyperkalaemia can occur in patients with impaired renal function and those taking ACE inhibitors or supplemental potassium. These preparations are effective and reduce potassium loss but it must be remembered that they have the adverse effects of both constituents. In the case of co-amilozide, both sodium depletion and potassium retention can occur, particularly in elderly patients.

### Spironolactone

Spironolactone is an antagonist of aldosterone at its receptor site inside the tubule cell. Aldosterone is released from the cortex of the adrenal gland in response to a fall in blood volume and in emergency situations such as blood loss through haemorrhage (see also p. 204). It is a sodium-retaining hormone at the expense of potassium, and if sodium is retained, then water is retained with it. Therefore, if aldosterone is blocked, sodium is lost, taking water with it, and less potassium is excreted.

**Administration, absorption and clinical use.** Spironolactone is given orally and is well absorbed from the gastrointestinal tract. It has a very short half-life in the circulation (about 10 minutes), but is converted into an active metabolite called **canrenone**, which has a half-life of about 16 hours. Therefore spironolactone is a prodrug. The diuretic effect has a very slow onset, and may not be observed for some days after administration. **Potassium canrenoate** has been prepared and is administered by injection. Spironolactone, when used, is often combined with other diuretics.

**Adverse effects.**    These are rare but may include:

- *hyper*kalaemia, especially if spironolactone is used on its own
- metabolic acidosis
- risk of carcinogenicity if used in the long term (e.g. in treating hypertension)
- skin rashes
- oestrogenic effects, e.g. gynaecomastia (breast enlargement in the male), testicular atrophy and menstrual disorders.

## Drug interactions

Supplementary potassium or potassium-sparing diuretics should not normally be combined with ACE inhibitors as this causes potassium retention by the kidneys and can be dangerous.

## DIURETICS IN CIRRHOSIS OF THE LIVER

In such cases diuretics carry serious risks of hypokalaemia and hypotension, leading to renal failure. It is best to start with spironolactone and then add a thiazide or loop diuretic cautiously a few days later. All drugs causing fluid retention (e.g. NSAIDs) should be avoided.

## DIURETICS IN ELDERLY PATIENTS

For various reasons, not always sound, one in five people over 65 take diuretics, and they are possibly the commonest cause of adverse reactions in elderly people. These adverse effects are the same as those which occur in younger subjects, but are more severe and may have serious consequences. The most important is sodium depletion, which leads to a marked fall in blood pressure, particularly on standing, causing faints, falls and confusion. As in other age groups, disturbances of potassium and uric acid metabolism occur.

> ### Nursing point
>
> Swollen ankles in the elderly do not necessarily call for a diuretic – they may be due to sitting in a chair all day.
> If an elderly person taking diuretics develops diarrhoea and/or vomiting it is sometimes wise to stop the diuretic temporarily to prevent undue water and salt loss.

> ### Nursing point
>
> The best way to monitor the efficiency of a diuretic is to weigh the patient regularly. Fluid balance charts are not always accurate but can be improved with the cooperation of the patient. Before leaving the hospital the timing of diuretic dosage must be tailored to the patient's daily programme. It is distressing to have a diuresis while stuck in your car in a traffic jam.

## ACETAZOLAMIDE

As a diuretic, acetazolamide is largely of historical interest only. Acetazolamide suppresses the activity of the enzyme carbonic anhydrase, which is present in the renal tubule and the eye. In the kidney this prevents the reabsorption of sodium and water from the tubule and thus causes a diuresis. It is a poor diuretic as its effect is short-lived and it is not now used for this purpose. Acetazolamide increases hydrogen carbonate excretion and thus creates a metabolic acidosis. This limits its action, as the body reacts by limiting hydrogen carbonate loss and the diuretic action of acetazolamide is lost.

### Acetazolamide and the eye

In the eye, acetazolamide reduces the formation of aqueous humour through the inhibition of carbonic anhydrase, and it is useful in lowering the intraocular pressure in glaucoma. It will also help relieve mountain sickness. Hyperventilation, which occurs at high altitude, 'washes out' carbon dioxide from the lungs and causes increased alkalinity of the blood. By increasing the excretion of hydrogen carbonate (alkali) by the kidneys, acetazolamide helps to correct this disorder.

## MAKING URINE ALKALINE

It may be necessary to render the urine alkaline (e.g. to enhance aspirin excretion after overdosage; see also p. 428). Sodium citrate is the substance most commonly used to make the urine alkaline. It is usually given every 2 or 4 hours. Sodium hydrogen carbonate is often combined with sodium citrate and acts in a similar fashion.

### Summary

- Diuretics are not used to treat urinary retention caused by, for example, benign prostatic hyperplasia
- Swollen ankles, especially in the elderly, are not always due to oedema
- Water is useless as a diuretic in patients with oedema
- Osmotic diuretics are of little or no use in conditions associated with salt retention
- Osmotic diuretics can be dangerous in patients who are unable to produce urine
- Thiazides can inhibit urine flow in diabetic patients and may induce hyperglycaemia
- Patients on thiazides and loop diuretics should avoid bright sunlight or wear sunglasses and apply sunblocks
- Diuretics such as thiazides and loop diuretics can cause mental disturbance in patients with liver cirrhosis due to potassium loss
- Potassium loss due to diuretics can increase the toxicity of digoxin
- Check elderly patients carefully for adequate diet when prescribing potassium-losing drugs
- Potassium loss is increased if patients are on anti-inflammatory steroids
- Patients with impaired renal function taking ACE inhibitors or those on supplemental potassium can develop *hyperkalaemia* (raised plasma potassium), which is dangerous, especially in patients with heart conditions
- Spironolactone can cause estrogenic effects, and there is risk of carcinogenicity with prolonged use
- Weight measurement is useful in monitoring patients on diuretics
- It may be prudent to stop diuretics temporarily, especially in elderly patients, if diarrhoea or vomiting occurs, to limit salt and water loss
- Prescribe diuretics so that they are most active when the patient is likely to be at home or somewhere convenient

### Further reading

Allen J E 1993 Drug-induced photosensitivity. Clinical Pharmacology 12 (8): 580

McLean P, Campbell D 2000 Angiotensin converting enzyme inhibitors and congestive heart failure: the pharmacist as facilitator. The Pharmaceutical Journal 265: R23

Brater D C 1998 Diuretic therapy. New England Journal of Medicine 339: 387

Editorial 1988 Diuretics in the elderly, how safe? British Medical Journal 296: 1551

Editorial 1990 Thiazides in the 1990s. British Medical Journal 300: 168

Editorial 1991 Routine use of potassium sparing diuretics. Drug and Therapeutics Bulletin 29: 85

Editorial 1994 Diuretics for heart failure. Drug and Therapeutics Bulletin 32: 83

Loop diuretics 2002 British National Formulary

Chapter **13**

# Endocrine system I. The hypothalamus–pituitary axis

## Learning objectives

- explain the terms endocrine, paracrine and autocrine hormones
- describe the hypothalamus–pituitary axis
- describe the anatomy of the pituitary stalk and the two main pituitary lobes
- give the names, actions and some uses of the hypothalamic releasing and inhibiting hormones
- give the names, actions and some uses of the anterior lobe hormones
- list the posterior lobe hormones and what their main actions are

## HORMONES

The endocrine or ductless glands are organs or small islands of tissue in various parts of the body. Each gland secretes a substance, and in some cases, several substances, called hormones. These are released from the gland and may enter the bloodstream and circulate through the body and act on distant organs or tissues (called an endocrine action); act on neighbouring cells (called a paracrine action); act on the cells that released them (called an autocrine action; see Fig. 13.1).

Some hormones may have two or even all three types of action. Their speed of action is variable; the effects of some hormones are seen immediately after release, whereas others may take hours or even days to show their effects. After release, these hormones act upon a receptor mechanism in the organ or

Figure 13.1 Actions of endocrine organs.

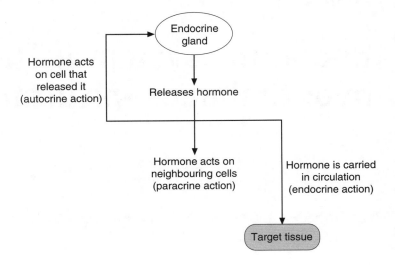

organs they influence, thus producing their specific actions. The actions of the various hormones differ widely: one group is concerned with metabolic processes, another with secondary sexual characteristics and so on. Sometimes a hormone will act on another endocrine gland and stimulate it to produce a further hormone.

Many of these hormones have been isolated and their structure determined. This has made it possible to prepare synthetically either the hormones or analogues which are sometimes more active and more stable than the hormones themselves.

## CLASSIFICATION OF ENDOCRINE GLANDS

For purposes of study, the endocrine glands can be divided roughly into three groups:

- the pituitary gland, which secretes hormones that exercise a controlling influence over much of the rest of the endocrine system, and which, in turn, is largely controlled by the hypothalamus of the brain
- endocrine glands affecting metabolism
- endocrine glands affecting the reproductive system.

The classification is purely for the purpose of facilitating chapter division of this section of the book. It can be argued with much justification that since the pituitary gland controls most other glands, it affects both metabolism and reproduction, which of course it does.

This chapter deals with the hypothalamus–pituitary axis, the hormones of the axis and the drugs derived from them.

## THE HYPOTHALAMUS–PITUITARY AXIS

The pituitary is a small endocrine gland attached to the brain by a stalk and lying, almost surrounded by bone, in the base of the skull. It consists of anterior and posterior lobes. In spite of its small size, it is of great importance. It secretes a number of hormones that not only affect various processes in the body but also the activity of most of the other endocrine glands. It is of interest that the activity of the pituitary itself is influenced by other hormones, both from the brain and from other glands in the body. Those other hormones regulate secretion of pituitary hormones through feedback mechanisms (see below).

The release of the pituitary hormones of the anterior lobe is a complex function and for many of them there is a specific releasing hormone, which is produced in the brain, specifically in the hypothalamus. Some of the hypothalamic hormones do not stimulate but inhibit release of anterior lobe hormones instead (see Table 13.1). The anterior pituitary hormones in turn stimulate the release of hormones from the endocrine glands. Those hormones exert their various effects on the body, and also travel to the brain and to the pituitary gland where they either stimulate or inhibit the release of releasing hormones and/or the pituitary gland hormones. These regulatory actions of the endocrine hormones are called feedback effects, and are of

**Table 13.1**    Anterior lobe hormones and their hypothalamic releasing hormones

| Hypothalamic releasing or inhibitory hormone | Anterior lobe hormone |
| --- | --- |
| Corticotrophin-releasing hormone (CRH) | Adrenocorticotrophic hormone (corticotrophin; ACTH) |
| Gonadotrophin-releasing hormone (GnRH) | Luteinizing hormone (LH) |
| | Follicle-stimulating hormone (FSH) |
| TSH-releasing hormone (TRH) | Thyroid-stimulating hormone (TSH) |
| Growth hormone-releasing hormone (GHRH; somatorelin) | Growth hormone (GH) |
| Growth hormone-inhibitory hormone (GHIH; somatostatin) | Growth hormone (GH) |
| Dopamine (DA) (inhibits release of prolactin) TRH, prolactin-releasing peptide (PRP) (stimulates release of prolactin) | Prolactin |

great importance in the design of several drugs, including the contraceptive pill (see p. 216).

## THE PITUITARY STALK

The pituitary is connected to the hypothalamus of the brain by a stalk. The stalk contains nerves that connect the hypothalamus to the posterior lobe and blood vessels that connect the hypothalamus to the anterior lobe. The blood vessels are called the **portal system** because they carry hormones from the hypothalamus to the pituitary. The nerves to the posterior lobe carry both electrical signals and the hormones **oxytocin** and **vasopressin** (see below), which are stored in the posterior pituitary until released into the general circulation.

## CONTROL OF PITUITARY HORMONE RELEASE

There are two groups of hormones:

- anterior lobe hormones
- posterior lobe hormones.

### CONTROL OF ANTERIOR LOBE HORMONE RELEASE

The release of anterior lobe hormones is governed largely by the hypothalamic releasing hormones. The hypothalamic hormones and the anterior lobe hormones they control are shown in Table 13.1.

The hypothalamic releasing and inhibitory hormones are

- CRH
- GnRH
- TRH
- GHRH (somatorelin)
- GHIH (somatostatin)
- dopamine.

These hormones are all peptides and are important because they or drugs derived from them are used both therapeutically and diagnostically.

### CRH

CRH is corticotrophin-releasing hormone. It is a peptide synthesized in the hypothalamus and it causes the release of ACTH from the anterior pituitary. It is used clinically mainly as a diagnostic tool to test the ability of the pituitary to release ACTH. Cortisol and the synthetic steroids such as prednisolone inhibit its release by a negative feedback mechanism. CRH is now also known to be important in the control of food intake and the problem of obesity, and drugs are being sought to modulate its action in the treatment of obesity, which is a major and growing problem in the UK.

### Safety note

Patients on steroids such as prednisolone must be weaned off them gradually. This is because prolonged use of prednisolone completely suppresses the

CRH–ACTH–cortisol system, which normally protects the patient from stress and is important in glucose metabolism. Gradual reduction in prednisolone allows cortisol levels to rise again (see also below).

## GnRH

GnRH is gonadotrophin-releasing hormone. It is synthesized in the hypothalamus and travels to the anterior pituitary in the portal system of blood vessels (see above). GnRH causes the release of LH and FSH from the anterior lobe. It is therefore the prime hormone of fertility. GnRH is released from the hypothalamus in regular pulses, and this pulsatile release has been used to induce ovulation in certain cases of infertility through the use of synthetic analogues of GnRH (see p. 214). The release of GnRH is subject to the negative feedback effects of the sex hormones (see p. 173), and this negative feedback effect is partly how the combined Pill works (see p. 217).

Paradoxically, if GnRH or its synthetic analogues are used continuously, there is a virtual shutdown of the LH/FSH pituitary system and infertility results. This phenomenon is used to treat certain sex hormone-dependent cancers, particularly prostate cancer (see also p. 346), and other problems where sex hormones need to be suppressed, such as endometriosis, hirsutism and precocious puberty. Continuous suppression of estrogens in women can produce unwanted effects, particularly those normally associated with menopause, such as hot flushes, headache, decreased libido and osteoporosis. GnRH receptor antagonists are also available and are currently being used and tested for various endocrine cancers and for infertility (e.g. see Huirne & Lambalk 2001).

## TRH

TRH is thyrotrophin-releasing hormone. It is synthesized in the hypothalamus and travels to the anterior lobe where it releases thyrotrophin (TSH). A synthetic analogue of TRH, called **protirelin**, is used to test the integrity of the TRH–TSH system and to check for hyperthyroidism. In normal subjects, an injection of protirelin will elicit a release of TSH from the anterior lobe. In hyperthyroid patients, there is elevated thyroxine from the thyroid gland. This has a negative feedback effect on TSH release from the anterior lobe, and so an injection of protirelin will have little or no effect on TSH release. TRH has also been found to cause prolactin release, although the physiological significance of this action of TRH is still unclear.

## GHIH (somatostatin)

Somatostatin inhibits the release of growth hormone (GH) from the anterior lobe. It is thus part of the normal control mechanism for the control of growth hormone release. It is therefore potentially an important tool for the treatment of acromegaly (see below) when there is excess GH release from the pituitary or from a pituitary tumour. A long-acting synthetic analogue of somatostatin called **octreotide** has been introduced for this purpose.

**Uses of octreotide.** By suppressing the release of somatotrophin in acromegaly (see p. 174), octreotide can control the symptoms when surgery is impossible or incomplete. The main problem in its use is that it is expensive. Octreotide also suppresses the release of several hormones in the stomach and intestine and reduces the blood flow to the gut. As a result of these actions it can be given to control certain types of diarrhoea, including that occurring in people with HIV infection, and it is also used to reduce the bleeding from oesophageal varices and in the treatment of certain tumours of the intestine. Adverse effects include gastritis and gallstone formation.

## GHRH (somatorelin)

GHRH is a very powerful hypothalamic hormone that causes the release of GH from the anterior lobe. A synthetic derivative **sermorelin** has been introduced as a diagnostic tool to test the integrity of the GH releasing system.

## Dopamine

Dopamine is an important neurotransmitter, both in the brain and elsewhere in the body, and has also been discovered to be a hypothalamic hormone that is released from nerve endings into the portal blood supply to the anterior lobe where it inhibits prolactin release. It is therefore part of the mechanism that controls lactation (see below). Dopamine is therefore potentially a useful clinical tool for suppression of lactation but cannot be administered as a drug. A dopamine analogue called **bromocriptine** is used instead.

Bromocriptine is an interesting drug that is extracted from ergot. It acts on the pituitary in the

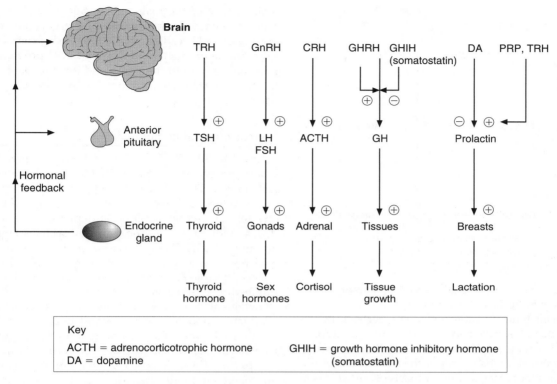

**Figure 13.2**   Hormones of the hypothalamus, anterior pituitary and endocrine glands. For abbreviations see Table 13.1.

same way as the naturally occurring substance dopamine and inhibits the release of various hormones, particularly prolactin and growth hormone (see below). It also stimulates dopamine receptors in the basal ganglia and thus relieves the symptoms of Parkinson's disease (see p. 257). Bromocriptine can be administered orally and is well absorbed. The drug is also used in certain forms of infertility.

**Prolactin-releasing peptide** is a hypothalamic hormone that stimulates prolactin release. Its role in the control of prolactin release is still unclear and is being investigated. No doubt its discovery will generate new drugs for the control of prolactin release.

The relationships between the hypothalamic hormones and those of the anterior pituitary are shown in Figure 13.2.

## HORMONES OF THE ANTERIOR LOBE

These comprise:

- adrenocorticotrophic hormone (corticotrophin; ACTH)

- Luteinizing hormone (LH) } Gonadotrophins
- Follicle-stimulating hormone (FSH)
- thyrotrophin (TSH)
- growth hormone (GH)
- prolactin.

### Adrenocorticotrophic hormone

**Release of ACTH.**   ACTH release from the anterior lobe is under the control of hypothalamic CRH (see above) and of cortisol. CRH causes ACTH release. High levels of cortisol suppress ACTH release from the anterior lobe and they suppress CRH release from the hypothalamus. When cortisol levels fall then more CRH and consequently more ACTH are released. These actions of cortisol both at the level of the brain and the anterior lobe provide a regulatory mechanism for the release of CRH, ACTH and cortisol (Fig. 13.3).

**Stimulation of the synthesis and release of cortisol from the adrenal cortex.**   ACTH rapidly stimulates the synthesis and release of cortisol from the adrenal cortex. It does this by increasing concentrations of

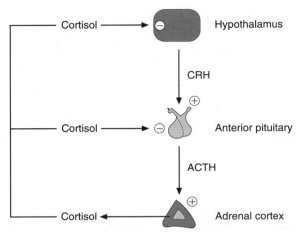

**Figure 13.3** Negative feedback action of cortisol on corticotrophin-releasing hormone (CRH) and adrenocorticotrophic releasing hormone (ACTH) release.

adrenal cholesterol, which is the precursor for all steroid synthesis in the adrenal gland.

**Trophic (growth) action on adrenal cortex cells and regulation of adrenal enzymes that synthesize cortisol.** ACTH actually promotes the growth of the cells that produce cortisol, and of the production of the enzymes that catalyse the synthesis of cortisol. This explains why the adrenal cortex atrophies (shrinks) in patients who receive chronic treatment with glucocorticoids such as prednisolone (see p. 205). In these patients prednisolone shuts down the release of both CRH and ACTH. This is why it is important not to cease steroid treatment suddenly, but to reduce it gradually to stimulate a return to normal adrenal production.

**Uses of ACTH.** ACTH has been used to test the cortisol releasing system and occasionally in some autoimmune diseases such as lupus. ACTH itself is not much used anymore because it is immunogenic, i.e. it stimulates an allergic response. Instead, a synthetic compound, **tetracosactide**, is used, mainly for testing adrenal function.

Tetracosactide is available as a rapidly acting preparation for intramuscular or intravenous use. For testing adrenal function, the drug is injected intramuscularly. Blood levels of cortisol are measured before and 30 minutes after injection. If the adrenals are working properly the injection is followed by a rise in the blood levels of cortisol.

## LH and FSH (gonadotrophins)

LH and FSH are called gonadotrophins because they are concerned with the growth and structural maintenance of the male and female gonads, and with the synthesis and release of the gonadal sex hormones. LH causes ovulation and promotes testosterone production in the male. FSH promotes follicular growth in the ovary and development of the spermatozoa. They are dealt with more fully in Chapter 17, p. 215.

## Thyroid–stimulating hormone

**Release of TSH.** TSH is released from the anterior lobe in response to TRH from the hypothalamus (see above). The release of TSH is regulated by a negative feedback effect of thyroid hormone. If for any reason thyroid function is depressed, e.g. by drugs or disease, then the pituitary secretes large amounts of TSH. The positive effect of TSH on thyroid hormone release, and the negative feedback effect of thyroid hormone on TSH are both used in a number of tests of thyroid function.

**Actions of TSH.** TSH controls every aspect of the production and release of thyroid hormone from the thyroid gland. The thyroid gland releases thyroid hormone, which regulates body metabolism (see p. 181). The actions of TSH on thyroid hormone are covered in more detail on p. 181.

## Growth hormone (somatotrophin; GH)

This hormone stimulates growth both in soft tissue and in bone. Its release from the pituitary is complicated as there are at least two substances from the brain that control its secretion (see above). Unfortunately, most animal somatotrophin is ineffective in humans so human growth hormone must be used. This has now been synthesized using biological technology and the product is called **somatropin**. In patients with dwarfism due to hormone deficiency, treatment must be started before epiphyseal fusion (closure of the ends of the long bones) has occurred and continued until growth is complete. Somatropin is given subcutaneously weekly and the dose adjusted as necessary. It is expensive.

Overproduction of somatotrophin by the pituitary gland will produce gigantism in children and acromegaly in adults.

## Prolactin

**Milk production.** Prolactin, the lactogenic hormone, produces its maximum effect on the breast, which has already been prepared throughout pregnancy

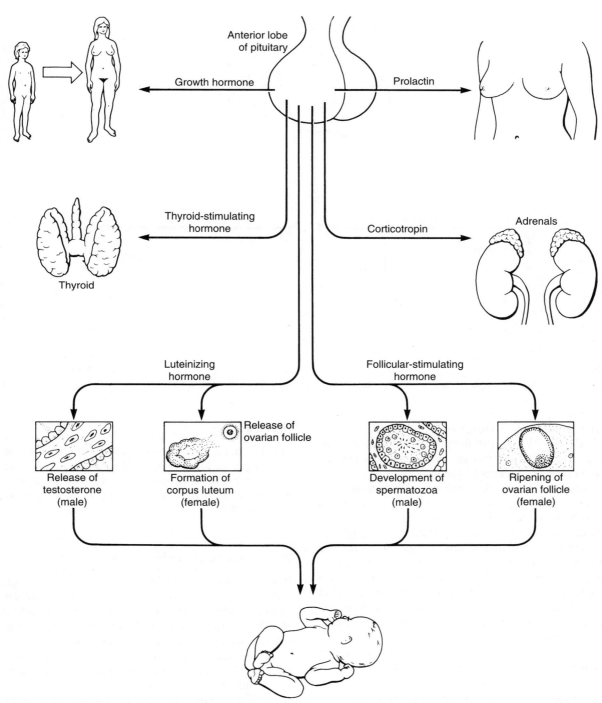

**Figure 13.4**    Hormones released by the anterior lobe of the pituitary gland showing their main sites of action.

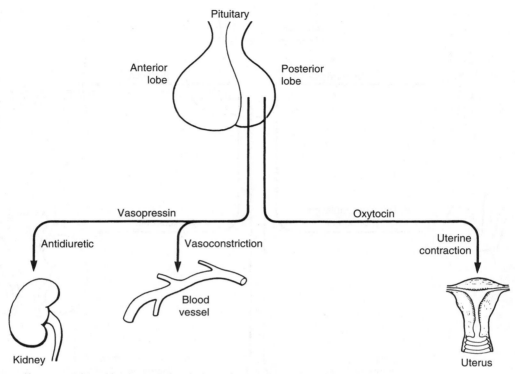

**Figure 13.5** Hormones released by the posterior pituitary gland and their sites of action.

by estrogens and progesterone (see Ch. 17). Its production by the pituitary can be suppressed by bromocriptine (see above), which is used when it is necessary to suppress lactation.

**Inhibition of ovarian function.** Prolactin also has a powerful inhibitory effect on ovarian function, and high blood levels of prolactin during the period of lactation are probably responsible for the delayed return of menstruation after pregnancy. Prolactin levels are also raised in both males and females during stress, and there is evidence from animal studies that this may account to some extent for the reduction in fertility due to stresses caused by, for example, population overcrowding and hierarchical conflicts in communities.

The functions of the various anterior lobe hormones are summarized in Figure 13.4.

## HORMONES OF THE POSTERIOR LOBE

Two important hormones – oxytocin and vasopressin – can be extracted from the posterior lobe of the pituitary. These are both peptides, but they have very different functions (Fig. 13.5).

## Oxytocin

This hormone is released from the posterior lobe as part of the suckling reflex and causes milk ejection from the breast. It causes contraction of the uterus in labour and is considered in more detail in Chapter 17.

## Vasopressin (antidiuretic hormone; ADH)

Vasopressin has two actions. In comparatively large doses it causes vasoconstriction with a concomitant rise in blood pressure, but its more important effect from the therapeutic aspect is concerned with water balance, as it is the antidiuretic hormone.

**Vasopressin release.** If the intake of water is limited, the blood becomes slightly more concentrated, which affects special receptors in the base of the brain. These stimulate the posterior pituitary to secrete more vasopressin. Vasopressin increases the reabsorption of water by the renal tubules and thus decreases the amount of urine and conserves the body water. If the intake of water is increased the production of vasopressin drops and the output of urine by the kidneys is increased, thus balancing the intake and output of water by the body.

**Therapeutic use of vasopressin: diabetes insipidus.** Occasionally damage to the posterior pituitary or closely related structures produces a disease called diabetes insipidus, in which little or no vasopressin is produced. There is thus a continuously high output of urine, which in turn requires the drinking of vast quantities of water if dehydration is to be avoided. Nurses will probably encounter this condition most commonly in patients who have had hypophysectomy (surgical removal of the pituitary gland) and who therefore have no vasopressin.

The disorder can be controlled by the administration of vasopressin, which is given as an injection. It was previously used as a snuff, but has now been replaced by **desmopressin**. Desmopressin is a synthetic drug allied to vasopressin. It can be given orally, nasally or intramuscularly. It has a very long action so that one or two doses daily suffice to control diabetes insipidus and it is now the preferred preparation. Unlike vasopressin it does not cause vasoconstriction. Treatment should aim at reducing the patient's urine output to about 2 litres a day. Desmopressin can also be used to treat nocturnal enuresis, in patients with normal pituitary function, by reducing night-time urine volume. Care must be taken to prevent fluid overload. Desmopressin is administered orally or intranasally at bedtime.

**Therapeutic use of vasopressin: bleeding from oesophageal varices.** The vasoconstrictor properties of vasopressin can be used in the treatment of bleeding from oesophageal varices. The vasoconstriction lowers pressure in the portal vein and allows the bleeding vein to clot. Vasopressin, or somatostatin (see above), can be used and are administered by intravenous infusion.

**Summary**

- Feedback mechanisms are exploited for drug design
- Patients are weaned gradually off corticosteroids
- GnRH shuts down pituitary release of LH if the pituitary is *continuously* exposed to it, and this is used to treat prostatic carcinoma (see also p. 227)
- Feedback mechanisms can be exploited to test the integrity of the feedback system (e.g. using protirelin)
- Somatostatin inhibits growth hormone secretion and is therefore used to treat acromegaly
- Bromocriptine acts like dopamine and can be used to block prolactin release and therefore stop lactation
- Synthetic analogues of ACTH can be used to test the integrity of the cortisol-regulatory system
- Human genetically engineered growth hormone is used to treat dwarfism, but must be started before epiphyseal closure has occurred
- Stress raises prolactin levels and this can cause impotence in men
- Vasopressin or synthetic analogues can be used to treat diabetes insipidus and bleeding from oesophageal varices

## Reference

Huirne J A F, Lambalk C B 2001 Gonadotropin-releasing-hormone-receptor antagonists. Lancet 358: 1793

## Further reading

Editorial 1992 Cyclical breast pain – what works and what doesn't. Drug and Therapeutics Bulletin 30: 1

Editorial 1995 New drugs for hyperprolactinaemia. Drug and Therapeutics Bulletin 33: 65

Lamberts S W, van der Lely A J, de Herder W W et al 1996 Octreotide. New England Journal of Medicine 334: 246

Smail P 1991 The GP, specialist and HGH. Prescriber Issue 38: 28

Chapter **14**

# Endocrine system II. Hormones and metabolism: thyroid, parathyroid glands, calcitonin and osteoporosis

## Learning objectives

At the end of this chapter, the reader should be able to:

- describe the anatomical location of the thyroid gland
- state the role of iodine in thyroid hormone synthesis
- explain how thyroid hormones are stored in the thyroid and how they are released
- give the causes and consequences of hypothyroidism
- state the treatments for hypothyroidism
- describe the symptoms and types of hyperthyroidism
- explain the surgical treatment of thyrotoxicosis
- list the drugs used to treat thyrotoxicosis
- describe the actions of parathyroid hormone (PTH)
- describe the treatment of tetany
- explain how calcium absorption is facilitated and about the role of vitamin D and calcitonin
- explain how osteoporosis is treated and controlled with drugs

## THE THYROID GLAND AND THYROID HORMONES

### INTRODUCTION

The thyroid consists of two lobes connected by an isthmus and is situated in the neck, in front of the trachea (Fig. 14.1). Functionally, the thyroid gland is made up of **follicles** (sometimes called acini), which consist of a single layer of epithelial cells enclosing the follicular lumen. The lumen is packed with a colloidal protein called thyroglobulin, which is the

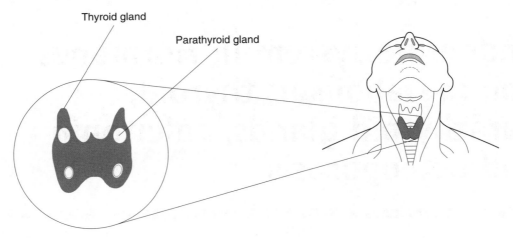

**Figure 14.1** The thyroid and parathyroid glands.

**Figure 14.2** Microscopic view of thyroid gland and follicle.

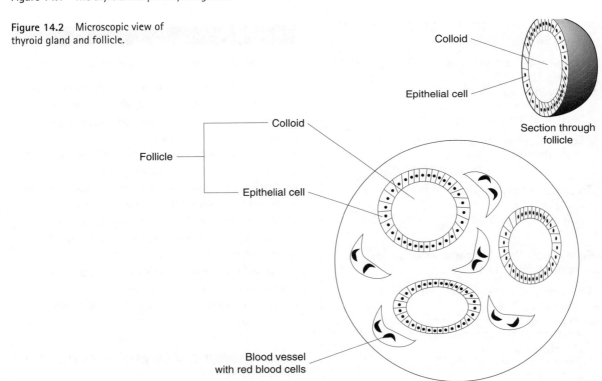

storage vehicle for the thyroid hormones (see below). Circulating iodine is picked up by the epithelial cells of the thyroid gland and incorporated to form two hormones, thyroxine (T4) and triiodothyronine (T3). These are stored in the thyroid as a protein called **thyroglobulin**, which is called colloid (Fig. 14.2). With appropriate stimulation, notably through the action of thyroid-stimulating hormone (TSH), both

thyroxine and triiodothyronine are released into the bloodstream (Fig. 14.3; see also the previous chapter, p. 174).

On reaching the tissues T4 is converted to T3, which is the more active hormone. T3 exerts its effects on the cell by binding both to receptors inside the cell in a manner similar to that of the steroid hormones, resulting in changes in protein synthesis,

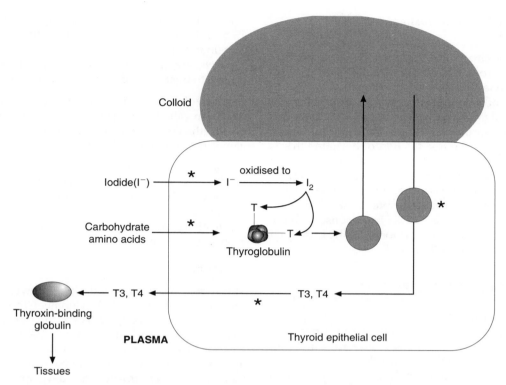

**Figure 14.3**    Production, storage and release of thyroid hormones. Iodide is taken up into the thyroid cell, oxidized to iodine, which is incorporated into tyrosine, on thyroglobulin. The protein is stored as colloid, until thyroid-stimulating hormone (TSH) causes the cell to break down thyroglobulin and release triiodothyronine (T3) and throxine (T4), which are released into the circulation. CHO = carbohydrate, T = tyrosine residue on thyroglobulin, $I_2$ = iodine.

and to receptors on the cell surface (see below). The effect of thyroid hormones is to increase tissue metabolism and thus to raise the basal metabolic rate. They are also important in promoting growth (see below). In healthy people the release of thyroid hormone is nicely adjusted to maintain the metabolic rate at a satisfactory level. When thyroid hormone levels are normal, the patient is described as *euthyroid*. When they are clinically elevated, the patient is *hyperthyroid*. When they are clinically depressed, the patient is *hypothyroid*.

## PRODUCTION AND RELEASE OF THYROID HORMONES

### Uptake of iodide into the thyroid

When iodide ions enter the circulation they are rapidly and powerfully taken up into the thyroid by an energy-dependent mechanism that can pump iodide into the thyroid against a concentration gradient of

anything up to 50:1. In other words, if there is 50 times more iodide in the thyroid than in the plasma, it will still be taken into the thyroid gland.

### Biosynthesis of T3 and T4

Once in the thyroid, iodide is oxidized to iodine and incorporated into tyrosine residues on the protein thyroglobulin such that both T3 and T4 are stored as part of the protein. The hormones are thus stored as part of a protein complex referred to as **colloid**. When circulating TSH from the anterior pituitary gland binds to its receptor on the thyroid cell, this triggers a response whereby droplets of the colloid are broken down in the cell and the hormones are released from colloid and secreted from the cell into the circulation. It is important here to give these processes in some detail, because drugs to treat thyrotoxicosis target some of the steps in the synthesis of thyroid hormones (see below). The process is summarized in Figure 14.3.

## Plasma binding of thyroxin and thyroid function tests

Once in the circulation, a specific thyroxine-binding protein, thyroxine-binding globulin (TBG), takes up the hormones, binds them and they are carried to their sites of action. There is a dynamic equilibrium in the circulation between the bound and free forms of thyroid hormones. This is clinically important since it is only the free fraction of hormone that is available to the tissues, and free levels of thyroid hormones are measured in patients as well as total levels. The levels of TBG are also measured in some tests. As mentioned in the previous chapter, p. 172, the ability of the pituitary to release TSH in response to hypothalamic TSH-releasing hormone (TRH) is also used to diagnose forms of thyroid disease.

## ACTION OF THYROID HORMONES

When T4 reaches its site of action it is converted to T3, which binds to receptors on the cell surface and increases the cell's uptake of amino acids and glucose to increase metabolism. Inside the cell, T3 binds to intracellular receptors in the mitochondria and in the cell nucleus to generate energy and new proteins, respectively.

## ABNORMALITIES OF THYROID FUNCTION

These can be divided into:

- hypothyroidism (thyroid deficiency; myxoedema)
- hyperthyroidism (thyroid excess; thyrotoxicosis).

## HYPOTHYROIDISM

Thyroid deficiency means a reduced availability to the body of thyroid hormone and can result from:

- Impairment of the TRH–TSH system of the brain and pituitary.
- Insufficient iodine in the diet; this is called simple or non-toxic goitre. Insufficient dietary iodine causes an increase in TSH secretion, which in turn causes thyroid growth, causing the goitre in the neck. Non-toxic goitre can also occur through the eating of certain plants, such as cassava root.
- **Hashimoto's disease**, an immunological disorder, when the body reacts against the protein

thyroglobulin, which is the mechanism for storing T3 and T4 in the thyroid gland, or to some other protein in the gland.

- Over-treatment with radioactive iodine, which is used to treat thyroid tumours (see below).

When thyroid deficiency is severe it causes a condition called *myxoedema*. The term myxoedema means thickened skin and gives the disease its name. The symptoms of myxoedema are:

- mental impairment
- slow or slurred speech and deep, low voice
- bradycardia (slowed heart rate)
- lethargy
- sensitivity to cold
- coarse, dry skin.

### Cretinism

The thyroid system is essential in the newborn infant for normal growth and development through the direct actions of T3 on the cells and through the influence of TSH on growth hormone release from the anterior lobe. If severe thyroid deficiency occurs in infants from birth and is left untreated for too long it will give rise to **cretinism**, when development in the baby is stunted, causing dwarfism, mental retardation, and coarsened facial features and skin. It is also called **congenital hypothyroidism**.

### Treatment of hypothyroidism

Hypothyroidism is treated either by increasing iodine in the diet and/or treatment with T3 or T4, both of which are available as oral tablets. Two preparations are effective in the treatment of thyroid deficiency: levothyroxine, which is the pure hormone synthetically prepared and used for long-term treatment, and liothyronine.

### Levothyroxine

Levothyroxine sodium (T4; thyroxine sodium) tablets given orally are absorbed from the intestinal tract, but their full effects are not seen for about 10 days. If they are given to patients with cretinism or myxoedema they will cause them to return to normal metabolic function.

It is important to start treating newborn infants with hypothyroidism as soon as possible because if they are left hypothyroid for too long, the change may be irreversible. In myxoedema it is very important to start with a small dose or the undue stimulating effect on the heart may cause untoward effects, including anginal pain. Early in treatment the patient should be kept warm, hypnotics should be avoided and constipation, which is common, should be relieved.

**Effects of overdosage.**   Large doses will cause an excessive rise in metabolic rate and the symptoms of thyrotoxicosis, with loss of weight, tachycardia, nervousness and tremors. Although the dose can be monitored by the clinical response of the patient, it is preferable to measure the plasma T4 and TSH occasionally to ensure that the correct amount of hormone is being given.

## Liothyronine

Liothyronine is the official name of triiodothyronine (T3). Its actions are similar to those of thyroxine, but are much more rapid in onset, the maximum effect being seen after 3 days. Liothyronine is not as useful as thyroxine in treating myxoedema as the control of the disease is apt to be uneven, but it is useful if a rapid effect is required.

In both cretinism and myxoedema it is usually necessary to continue treatment for the rest of the patient's life.

## HYPERTHYROIDISM (THYROTOXICOSIS)

### Symptoms of hyperthyroidism

The overall effect of hyperthyroidism is a raised metabolic rate, which is manifested by:

- excess T3 and T4 in the bloodstream
- raised temperature and sweating
- excess sensitivity to heat
- nervousness and tremor
- susceptibility to fatigue
- tachycardia (racing heart)
- weight loss with associated increase in appetite
- in some patients, there is protrusion of the eyeballs (see below).

### Types of hyperthyroidism

There are several types of hyperthyroidism, but the two most common types are:

- Graves' disease (diffuse toxic goitre; exophthalmic goitre)
- toxic nodular goitre.

**Graves' disease.**   This is an autoimmune disease, when the patient develops circulating immunoglobulins that stimulate the TSH receptor on the surface of the thyroid gland cell. This results in increased thyroid hormone secretion that is unrelated to the normal demands of the body. In older textbooks, before the identity of the circulating thyroid stimulator was known, it was referred to as LATS (long-acting thyroid stimulator). Aberrant types of the TSH receptor may also be expressed. Patients with this disease have protruding eyeballs (exophthalmos), although the cause of this symptom is not well understood.

**Toxic nodular goitre.**   This is due to a tumour and can develop from simple non-toxic goitres that result from dietary deficiencies of iodine. In a recently published study (Vestergaard et al 2002) smoking was identified as a risk factor for Graves' disease and toxic nodular goitre.

### Thyroid crisis

Thyroid crisis (formerly called thyroid storm) is a term used to describe a severe acute attack of thyrotoxicosis.

## TREATMENT OF THYROTOXICOSIS

### SURGERY

For otherwise healthy patients with thyrotoxicosis either surgery or drug treatment with carbimazole or $^{131}$I (radioactive iodine) produces satisfactory results, and the complications and failure rates are about equal for both methods of treatment. Surgery has the advantage of getting a quick result, but some patients prefer to avoid an operation, and treatment with radioactive iodine is being increasingly used.

Surgery is usually indicated for patients with nodular goitres and when the goitre produces compression of the trachea. It is common practice, prior to surgery, to make the patient euthyroid by treatment with a drug such as carbimazole followed by a short course of aqueous iodine (see below). This pretreatment also makes the thyroid less vascular and easier for the surgeon to handle. The patient may also be treated with β blockers such as propranolol prior to operating. Propranolol is also used in thyroid crisis. The β blocker reduces the severity of cardiac problems such as tachycardia and dysrhythmia. If β blockers are used alone the drug must be continued for 10 days after operation to prevent a thyroid crisis.

The problem faced by a patient and the therapeutic approach used with these drugs are illustrated in Case History 14.1.

## Case History 14.1

Miss K was 22 years old when she noticed that she had a mild tremor of her hands. Within 3 months she noticed a progressive weight loss in spite of a healthy appetite, palpitations, diarrhoea and an alteration in her menstrual cycle. She was upset when a relative complained to her that she was excessively irritable. She went to her GP who suspected an overactive thyroid gland (hyperthyroidism) and sent off blood for thyroid function tests. These showed a decrease in thyroid-stimulating hormone (TSH) and a considerable and abnormal level of thyroid hormone (T4). The GP started her on carbimazole (*Neo-Mercazole*) to control the overactive thyroid and, as the effects take up to a few weeks to be noticed by the patient, propranolol was prescribed to control the symptoms. He referred her to the endocrinology clinic at the local hospital. Antibody tests confirmed an autoimmune thyroiditis and Miss K was warned that it was likely that the overactivity would eventually settle and that her thyroid function might swing to the other extreme and necessitate taking long-term thyroxine (T4). Had she had Graves' disease, which accounts for 75% of the UK's hyperthyroidism, she might have needed surgery for thyroid enlargement or – had she been over 40 years of age – radio-iodine, which is not given to the younger patients to avoid the long-term risk of thyroid cancer.

## USE OF DRUGS TO TREAT THYROTOXICOSIS

The following drugs are used:

- aqueous iodine solution (Lugol's solution)
- radio-iodine (radioactive iodine; $^{131}$I)
- thioureylenes.

### Aqueous iodine solution

Aqueous iodine, also called Lugol's solution, is administered orally and is metabolized in the body to iodide ion, which temporarily inhibits thyroid hormone release. Symptoms of thyrotoxicosis should subside after 1–2 days. In addition, the thyroid gland shrinks and loses some of its vascularity (blood supply). After 10 days or so, the beneficial effect starts wearing off. Aqueous iodine is used mainly as part of the treatment of thyroid crisis and as premedication before thyroid surgery. It does not taste pleasant and is sometimes prescribed with milk to improve the taste.

**Adverse effects.** Patients may develop allergic responses such as skin rashes, sneezing, lacrimation (watering eyes), conjunctivitis and salivary gland pain.

### Radio–iodine

Radio-iodine (radioactive iodine; $^{131}$I) is a radioactive isotope of iodine. As it decays to a more stable form it emits powerful rays that kill cells, particularly cells undergoing cell division. It is a rare example of a 'magic bullet': i.e. a drug that targets one particular organ or group of cells selectively. It does this because of the iodine-concentrating mechanism of the thyroid gland. Also, the thyroid is the only organ that concentrates iodine significantly.

**Administration.**   $^{131}$I is given orally and is rapidly absorbed from the stomach and intestines. The thyroid takes it up in exactly the same way as dietary iodide is taken up and it is incorporated into thyroglobulin. In the treatment of thyrotoxicosis large doses are given to stop production of thyroid hormone.

**Action and use of $^{131}$I.**   The incorporated radio-iodine emits both β-particles and γ-rays. The β-particles have a relatively short path and so their cytotoxic action is confined almost entirely to the thyroid where they have a very powerfully destruction action. Since $^{131}$I is incorporated into T3 and T4, some radioactivity is bound to get into the general circulation; but because the treatment is so powerful, the isotope quickly destroys the tissue that releases it. $^{131}$I has a short half-life of about 8 days, and radioactivity has decayed away completely by about 2 months after the treatment was given.

Because of its powerful destruction of thyroid tissue, $^{131}$I treatment will eventually cause hypothyroidism, especially in patients with Graves' disease, and this is easily treated by administration of thyroxine. In elderly patients or those with some other complicating disease $^{131}$I is very satisfactory.

**Precautions with $^{131}$I.**   Radioactive iodine should not be used to treat thyrotoxicosis during pregnancy or if the mother is breast-feeding. There are doubts about its use in children and young women. Special care is required in the handling of and disposal of urine, etc., from these patients as it will be radioactive. Staff who handle and administer $^{131}$I should wear radioactivity badges and be routinely screened for thyroid radioactivity and patients should be nursed in isolation.

**Other uses of $^{131}$I.**   Radioactive iodine is also used to destroy malignant cells in carcinoma of the thyroid gland.

## The thioureylenes

These comprise:

- **carbimazole**
- **thiamazole (methimazole)**
- **propylthiouracil**.

**Mechanism of action.**   These drugs inhibit thyroid hormone production, possibly by preventing the oxidation of iodide to iodine (see Fig. 14.3). In addition, propylthiouracil blocks the conversion of T4 to T3 in target tissues.

**Therapeutic use.**   The thioureylenes are given orally. After administration carbimazole is rapidly metabolized in the blood to thiamazole (methimazole). Carbimazole is therefore an example of a pro-drug. Thiamazole (methimazole) has a half-life of 5–15 hours. The drugs act quickly to block the oxidation of iodide, but the beneficial effects may not be seen for anything up to 2 months. This is because circulating T3 and T4 have a long half-life, partly because they are strongly bound to plasma proteins and also because the thyroid has large stores of the hormones in the colloid. Propylthiouracil may act faster than the others because of its blocking action on the conversion of T4 to T3 in the target tissue. After thyroid function returns to normal, the thyroid may still be enlarged.

The drug is usually continued but at a reduced dosage for about 18 months, after which treatment may be further reduced and eventually stopped. About 60% of patients will remain well, but 40% will relapse and may require either further drug treatment or surgery.

**Adverse effects.**   These include rashes, joint pains, enlarged lymph nodes and fever. Transient depression of the white cell count develops in around 10% of patients and, rarely, dangerous agranulocytosis; therefore, severe sore throats or other infections should be reported immediately.

Carbimazole should be given with care to pregnant women as excessive dosage may suppress the fetal thyroid, causing goitre and hypothyroidism. It is also excreted in maternal milk and may have similar effects on the newborn.

## Other drugs

β **Blockers** reduce those symptoms of thyrotoxicosis that are due to sympathetic overactivity, including tachycardia, tremor, sweating and anxiety. In addition to their actions on the sympathetic system, they reduce the conversion of T4 to T3 in the tissues. They

are useful for the rapid control of these symptoms, particularly in the preparation for operation and may be continued with digitalis if atrial fibrillation develops. It must be remembered, however, that they do not cure thyrotoxicosis, so that if they are stopped the symptoms will return.

### Nursing point

Patient education in the recognition of the side-effects associated with the use of thyroid drugs is important in monitoring the effectiveness of treatment.

### Summary

- Measurement of the pituitary response to TRH in terms of TSH release, and measurement of circulating T4 and of the free fraction of T4 are important tools in diagnosis
- Treatment of myxoedema should be initiated with small doses of thyroxine to minimize cardiac effects and patient comfort, e.g. adequate warmth attended to
- Cretinism needs to be treated as soon as possible after diagnosis
- Aqueous iodine tastes unpleasant and can be given in milk
- Patients prescribed thioureylenes should be advised to report sore throats or any infections immediately
- Drugs given to pregnant woman to reduce thyroid hormone secretion can also suppress the normal fetal thyroid and make the fetus hypothyroid
- Staff who handle $^{131}$I must be monitored routinely for thyroid radioactive levels
- Patients should be made euthyroid prior to thyroid surgery
- Smoking is a risk factor for Graves' disease and toxic nodular goitre

## BONE METABOLISM, THE PARATHYROID GLANDS AND CALCIUM

Bone metabolism is currently of great medical interest and importance due to increased longevity and the problem of bone loss with ageing. Advances in our understanding of the process of bone remodelling has led to the introduction of powerful drugs that slow the rate of bone loss.

The normal process of bone remodelling is controlled by a balance between osteoblasts that secrete new bone matrix, and osteoclasts, that break down bone matrix. This balance is affected by several chemical factors, notably:

- the turnover of calcium and phosphates
- the action of certain cytokines
- the hormones calcitonin and parathyroid hormone
- the vitamin D family.

## THE PARATHYROID GLANDS AND PARATHYROID HORMONE

The parathyroid glands are situated in the neck in close relationship with the thyroid gland (see Fig. 14.1). They are concerned with the levels of calcium and phosphorus in the blood and their excretion by the kidney. They secrete parathyroid hormone (parathormone; PTH), which is a polypeptide. A fall in the level of blood calcium concentration stimulates the parathyroids to produce more PTH, which mobilizes calcium from bone and decreases its loss through the kidney, thus returning the blood calcium level to normal. This in turn reduces the release of PTH (Fig. 14.4).

### ACTIONS OF PARATHYROID HORMONE

The overall effect of PTH is to increase plasma concentrations of calcium. It does this by:

- mobilizing calcium from bone
- increasing production of calcitriol, a member of the vitamin D3 family (see also p. 187), which in turn increases calcium absorption from the gastrointestinal tract
- enhancing calcium reabsorption from the kidney tubule
- increasing phosphate excretion.

### PARATHYROID HORMONE AND CALCIUM DEFICIENCY

Parathyroid hormone deficiency results in an increase in blood phosphorus and a decrease in

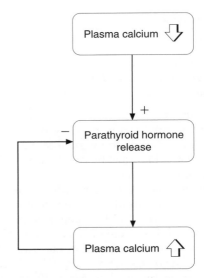

**Figure 14.4** Control of parathyroid hormone (PTH) release.

blood calcium levels. Lowering of the blood calcium causes a disorder known as **tetany**, which is characterized by increased irritability of muscles with spasm of the hands and feet (carpo-pedal spasm) and of the larynx. A decrease in blood calcium may result from:

- parathyroid hormone deficiency
- lack of calcium in the diet, particularly if the patient is also deficient in vitamin D
- alkalosis.

Alkalosis, although not necessarily associated with low blood calcium, causes a decrease of ionized calcium in the blood and it is the ionized fraction that is important in preventing tetany.

### TREATMENT OF TETANY

In cases of tetany due to parathyroid deficiency, several treatments are available:

- calcium
- parathyroid hormone (PTH)
- vitamin D.

### Calcium

Giving calcium salts may quickly relieve acute attacks of tetany due to low blood calcium. They are usually administered as the **calcium gluconate** or **calcium chloride**. Calcium gluconate if given slowly I.V. produces rapid but short-lived relief. Calcium salts can also be given orally, not only to relieve tetany, but also to prevent chronic calcium deficiency developing, particularly in those who absorb calcium poorly and after menopause.

**Calcium absorption.** Poor calcium absorption can occur under the following conditions:

- rickets (vitamin D deficiency)
- following gastrectomy
- in steatorrhoea (abnormally fatty faeces)
- in elderly subjects.

Prolonged calcium deficiency may lead to decalcification of bones, which may become bent or may fracture.

> **Nursing point**
>
> Calcium salts should never be mixed with sodium bicarbonate in a syringe or infusion as the calcium will precipitate. Note that they both may be used intravenously in cardiac arrest.

## Parathyroid hormone (PTH)

PTH is destroyed in the intestinal tract and should be given by injection. Its maximum effect appears about 6 hours after injection. It causes a rise in the blood calcium and a decrease in blood phosphorus levels. It is not satisfactory for long-term treatment, as increasing doses are required to produce the desired effect and it may cause allergic reactions.

## Vitamin D (see also p. 186)

Plasma calcium levels can also be raised by vitamin D, which increases the absorption of calcium from the intestine. Vitamin D may be required:

- if the diet is deficient in the vitamin
- in various disorders in which resistance to the action of vitamin D occurs
- in parathyroid hormone deficiency.

Vitamin D (calciferol) itself can be used, or substances that have a similar action such as dihydrotachysterol or alfacalcidol. These drugs are considered in more detail on p. 391.

## CALCITONIN

Calcitonin is a hormone produced in the so-called C cells of the thyroid gland, but which is concerned with calcium balance. It inhibits the action of bone osteoclasts, which are concerned with bone resorption. Therefore calcitonin lowers the concentration of calcium in the blood and increases its deposition in bone. It is used therapeutically in disorders where there is a rapid breakdown of bone, such as Paget's disease, or to control malignant deposits in bone where they release excessive amounts of calcium into the blood causing hypercalcaemia. It is prepared from either pig or salmon and is given by injection.

Paget's disease is named after the British surgeon James Paget (1814–1899). Three diseases are named after him: Paget's disease of bone, which is marked by abnormally high bone turnover; Paget's disease of the nipple, which is a form of cancer of the nipple; and Paget's disease of the vulva, which resembles in some ways the disease of the nipple.

A form of calcitonin from salmon, called salcatonin, is given by subcutaneous or intramuscular injection. The dose and frequency of administration depend on the disorder being treated. Adverse effects include nausea, vomiting and flushing after the injection and pain at the site of injection.

## OSTEOPOROSIS AND ITS TREATMENT

In this condition the rate of bone resorption exceeds that of bone replacement so there is a loss of bone mass resulting in a tendency to fractures, particularly of the vertebrae, the upper end of the femur and the lower end of the radius. It is responsible for a great deal of morbidity and some mortality among elderly people. With increasing age, bone mass diminishes and there is a markedly rapid loss of bone in women after the menopause (Fig. 14.5).

Members of this group are especially prone to fractures. Osteoporosis can also result from various endocrine disorders, malabsorption of calcium, rheumatoid arthritis and the prolonged use of steroids such as prednisolone.

Prevention and control of osteoporosis are achieved using:

- hormone replacement therapy (HRT)
- the bisphosphonates
- calcium and vitamin D.

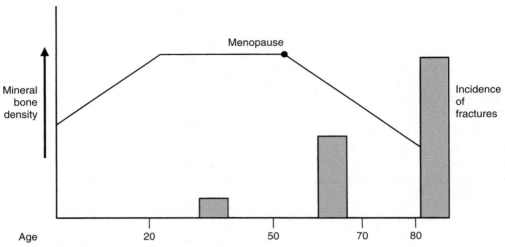

**Figure 14.5** Bone density and the incidence of fractures related to age for women. (Based on a figure first published in Peel N & Eastell R 1995 ABC of rheumatology: osteoporosis. British Medical Journal 310: 989.).

## HORMONE REPLACEMENT THERAPY

This is the regular taking by women of small doses of estrogen alone or with synthetic progestagens, and is covered also on p. 221. HRT is very effective in preventing bone loss. There are, however, concerns about the possible effects of HRT therapy on the incidence of cancer in some women.

## THE BISPHOSPHONATES

These comprise:

- **disodium alendronate**
- **disodium clodronate**
- **disodium etidronate**
- **disodium pamidronate**
- **disodium risedronate**.

This group of drugs is now increasingly used to treat osteoporosis in those with Paget's disease of the bone, in the elderly and in women after menopause.

### Mechanism of action

The bisphosphonates mimic the action of a body chemical called pyrophosphate, but they are more stable. They are absorbed onto the calcium-containing crystals in bone and slow both their rate of formation and dissolution. It should be appreciated that bone is not an inert structure, but is always being broken down and reformed. In Paget's disease and in malignant disease involving bone, this process accelerates, resulting in pain and in the release of calcium into the blood with consequent hypercalcaemia. Bisphosphonates, by slowing bone 'turnover', relieve pain and control hypercalcaemia. They inhibit osteoclast activity and promote osteoblast activity in bone. They have been found in several clinical trials to be very effective in reducing the incidence of fractures in the elderly. It will be remembered that osteoclasts are cells that resorb bone and osteoblasts form new bone.

### Clinical use

Etidronate was the first of these drugs to be tested. The doses needed were high and many patients on etidronate developed osteomalacia (softening of the bones). Eventually alendronate (*Fosamax*) was tested and found to be 1000 times more potent than etidronate in slowing bone resorption. The drug has a very long half-life – more than 5 years – because it binds so strongly to bone. Many trials of the drug found that alendronate significantly improved bone density in the hip and the spine after 2–4 years, and most of the improvement occurs within the first year of treatment.

**Disodium etidronate** has been given orally in the treatment of Paget's disease, although it may cause osteomalacia in these patients (see below). Food should not be taken for 2 hours before and after treatment. **Disodium pamidronate** is given by intravenous infusion to treat bone pain or hypercalcaemia due to secondary malignant deposits in bone. Sodium clodronate is similar but can be given orally.

Many of the clinical trials of bisphosphonates have been conducted in women over the age of 75, although they are prescribed for younger women, and it has not yet been resolved as to whether they are more effective in preventing bone loss than is HRT.

## Oral administration of alendronate

Some precautions must be taken. Alendronate is taken orally as a single tablet with a large glass of at least 150 ml of water. It must be taken standing up and the patient should not lie down for at least 30 minutes after taking it. This is because alendronate is damaging to the oesophagus and must be washed down well. Lying down (or doing early morning exercises, e.g. touching the toes) within 30 minutes of taking alendronate may allow some of the drug to re-enter the oesophagus.

The patient should not eat for at least 30 minutes before taking alendronate because the drug binds to minerals in the food and drug absorption may be reduced. If the patient is on calcium supplements, these are best taken in the afternoon, well after taking alendronate.

## Adverse effects

The adverse effects of the bisphosphonates vary to some extent due to the chemical differences between them. Etidronate has been reported to cause osteomalacia in patients with osteoporosis and Paget's disease. Alendronate may cause ulceration of the oesophagus (see above), and both alendronate and pamidronate have precipitated an acute phase reaction when administered intravenously. Minor adverse effects reported include nausea and diarrhoea.

## OTHER STRATEGIES IN OSTEOPOROSIS

Other preventative measures include regular weight-bearing exercise, an adequate intake of calcium and vitamin D, and giving up smoking.

**Summary**

- Patients must be well informed on the precautions when taking alendronate
- Patients with osteoporosis should be prescribed calcium with vitamin D and should be encouraged to take exercise and give up smoking
- Patients should be informed about the importance of regular bone density scans after menopause and about the importance of taking calcium supplements

## Reference

Vestergaard P, Rejnmark L, Weeke J et al 2002 Smoking as a risk factor for Graves' disease, toxic nodular goitre, and autoimmune hypothyroidism. Thyroid 12: 69

## Further reading

Boyle I, Ralston S 1990 The treatment of hypercalcaemia. Prescribers Journal 30: 180

Brent GA 1994 The molecular basis of thyroid hormone action. New England Journal of Medicine 331: 847

Brownlow I 1992 Transformed by thyroxine. Nursing Times 88(8): 40

Compston J E 1994 The therapeutic use of biphosphonates. British Medical Journal 309: 711

Eastell R, Peel N 1998 Osteoporosis. Journal of the Royal College of Physicians, London 32: 14

Franklyn J A 1994 The management of hyperthyroidism. New England Journal of Medicine 330: 1731

White J, Jordan S 1998 The endocrine system. Hyperthyroidism. Nursing Times 94: 50

Toft A D 1994 Thyroxine therapy. New England Journal of Medicine 331: 174

Chapter **15**

# Endocrine system III. Hormones and metabolism: insulin, diabetes mellitus and obesity

## Learning objectives

At the end of this chapter, the reader should be able to:

- explain the basics of the actions, release and mechanisms of action of insulin
- state the two types of diabetes mellitus
- list the types of insulin available for treating IDDM
- explain the basic principles underlying the choice of insulin
- describe how insulin is given by injection
- give the standard strength of insulin injections
- recognize the existence of other ways of giving insulin
- explain the basics of monitoring treatment with insulin
- recognize the signs of hypoglycaemia
- describe the use of insulin in special circumstances such as pregnancy and diabetic coma
- describe the principles of dietary management in NIDDM
- list the different types of oral hypoglycaemic agents
- describe the actions of glucagon
- explain the management of patients with obesity

## THE PANCREAS

The pancreas is a relatively large gland lying across the upper part of the posterior abdominal wall (Fig. 15.1). It produces a number of digestive enzymes that drain into the duodenum and help digestion. Scattered throughout the gland are small collections of tissue known as the islets of Langerhans. These

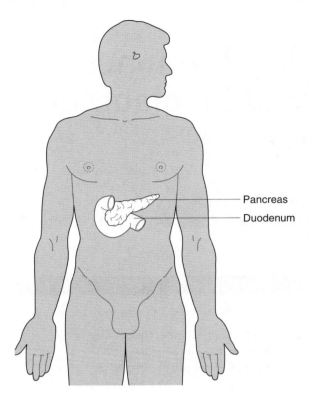

Figure 15.1  Anatomical location of pancreas.

islets contain two important types of cell called alpha and beta cells. The alpha cells secrete glucagon and the beta cells secrete insulin. Insulin and glucagon are important components of the body's mechanism for controlling glucose metabolism. D cells produce somatostatin.

## THE NORMAL CONTROL OF GLUCOSE METABOLISM

Circulating concentrations of glucose are monitored and controlled by the endocrine system. When circulating glucose concentrations rise – for example after a meal – insulin is released from the beta cells of the pancreas into the bloodstream and causes glucose to be taken up into the tissues, where it is converted into energy stores such as liver glycogen and fat or used to generate metabolic energy.

When circulating concentrations of glucose fall, then insulin release is suppressed and other hormones, namely glucagon, epinephrine, the adrenal glucocorticoids and thyroxine stimulate the breakdown of fats and glycogen to glucose, which enters the circulation.

Insulin is therefore the only endocrine hormone that is *hypoglycaemic*: i.e. lowers plasma glucose. Glucagon, epinephrine, the adrenal glucocorticoids and thyroxine are *hyperglycaemic*. A hormone such as insulin that promotes the conservation of energy and tissue growth is termed *anabolic*. Hormones that promote the breakdown of tissues to provide energy are termed *catabolic*.

## INSULIN

Insulin is a protein hormone whose release from the pancreatic beta cells is stimulated by glucose. It was the first hormone to be discovered and crystallized, and its discovery meant that many thousands of children who would otherwise have died from diabetes could be treated.

## ACTIONS OF INSULIN

Insulin lowers the concentration of glucose in the blood by:

- stimulating the uptake of glucose by the tissues
- converting glucose to glycogen in the liver, where it is stored
- increasing the production of fat and protein.

These actions are summarized in Figure 15.2.

### Release of insulin

Insulin is released from the beta cells when the concentrations of glucose in the blood rise, for example after a meal. A number of other chemical agents – for example amino acids, carbohydrates and fatty acids – will stimulate insulin release, but the most important insulin releaser for proper maintenance of circulating glucose is glucose itself.

### Mechanism of action of insulin

Insulin binds to a specific insulin receptor on cell membranes and this triggers the cell's response. An important response is the transport of glucose and other sugars away from the blood and into the cell. Glucose is transported into the cell across the cell membrane by so-called glucose transporters, and insulin increases the activity of the glucose transporters.

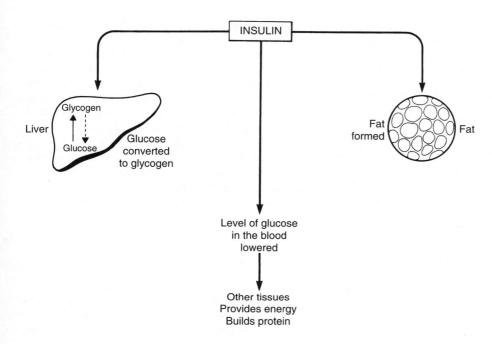

Figure 15.2  The metabolic effects of insulin.

## DIABETES MELLITUS

The term 'mellitus' is derived from the Latin word *mel*, meaning honey. There is a popular tale that in bygone days doctors diagnosed the disease by tasting the patient's urine, which tasted sweet because of the glucose in it.

## TYPES OF DIABETES MELLITUS

Diabetes mellitus is a disease caused by insulin deficiency. There are two types:

- insulin-dependent diabetes mellitus (IDDM; type I)
- non-insulin-dependent diabetes mellitus (NIDDM; type II).

### Insulin-dependent diabetes mellitus

Insulin-dependent diabetes is an autoimmune disease in which the immune system attacks and destroys the beta cells. There is now evidence that a virus, the Coxsackie B4 virus, may cause this form of diabetes in children by infecting the pancreatic islet cells. The disease occurs predominantly in young people. This deficiency leads to a rapid rise in the blood glucose concentration with subsequent loss of large amounts of glucose accompanied by water and salt in the urine. In addition, fats in the body are broken down, releasing ketoacids, which cause acidosis. Protein is also lost and weight loss may be marked. If not treated, the patient will lapse into a coma (hyperglycaemic ketoacidosis). The only treatment is with insulin (see below).

### Non-insulin-dependent diabetes mellitus

Non-insulin-dependent diabetes mellitus has traditionally occurred in middle-aged or elderly people who are frequently overweight. An alarming modern development in Western societies, including the UK, is the appearance of obesity and NIDDM in young people, even in some teenagers. This may possibly be due to the large increase in food intake, particularly the eating of fast foods. In some societies, notably among the Native Americans, the situation has become so bad that upwards of 60% of an entire community may suffer from obesity and NIDDM through the ingestion of vast amounts of carbohydrates and fats that are not part of a traditional diet. These people have the added disadvantage of a genetic predisposition to diabetes.

In this type of diabetes there appears to be resistance to the action of insulin coupled with a deficiency of the hormone due to an exhausted pancreas. The blood glucose concentration is raised with glycosuria, but ketoacidosis is less common and the symptoms are often those of the late complications of diabetes, such as infection. The treatment of NIDDM is given below.

## LATER COMPLICATIONS OF BOTH TYPE I AND TYPE II DIABETES MELLITUS

● Disease of the small arteries leads to damage to the retina of the eye, declining renal function and serious interference with the circulation to the legs, sometimes requiring amputation, and various peripheral nerves may be damaged (peripheral neuropathy).

● Patients with diabetes are particularly prone to infection and these infections may, in turn, exacerbate the diabetes, sometimes leading to ketoacidosis and coma. Good control of the diabetes reduces the severity of the complications but does not entirely prevent them.

## TREATMENT OF INSULIN-DEPENDENT DIABETES MELLITUS

### DIETARY MANAGEMENT

Patients with IDDM require insulin replacement to replace the deficiency and a diet suited to their lifestyle and work to maintain them in good health as judged by their subjective feelings, their weight (which should be kept at the correct level for their age and height) and to keep their blood glucose levels near normal (Fig. 15.3).

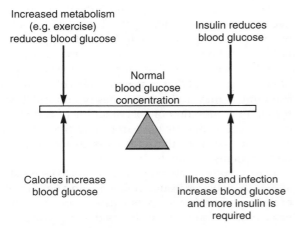

**Figure 15.3** Balancing patients with diabetes.

There are many dietary schemes and with changing fashions it is too lengthy a subject to discuss here in detail. Briefly, about 50% of the calories in the normal, healthy diet should be from carbohydrate in forms that are slowly absorbed such as wholemeal bread, potatoes and other starchy vegetables, but not rapidly digestible sugars such as sweets and cakes. About 35% of the calories may come from fat and the rest from protein.

Because they are at special risk from atheroma, patients with diabetes should avoid foods that have a deleterious effect on plasma lipids. Hypertension, if present, should be treated, exercise encouraged and smoking avoided.

## INSULIN

### Source of insulin

Insulin is available in many preparations that vary in their duration of action. Previously, insulin was extracted from the pancreas of cows (bovine) or pigs (porcine) and needed extensive purification. It is now possible to produce human insulin, either by modifying porcine insulin or, more usually, by a recombinant method involving bacteria. The code for synthesizing human insulin can be inserted into bacteria (*Escherichia coli*), which then multiply and produce human insulin. Virtually all insulin now used is human insulin.

### Short-acting insulins (soluble insulins)

These are used for the treatment of diabetic coma (ketoacidosis), to cover operations and illnesses in patients with diabetes and sometimes in the long-term control of diabetes, combined with longer-acting insulin. They are the only insulins suitable for intravenous injection. Following subcutaneous injection their action starts after about 30 minutes and continues for 8 hours. After intravenous injection their onset is more rapid, but only lasts for about half an hour: they include *Humulin* and *Human Actrapid*.

**Insulin lispro** and **insulin aspart** are modified forms of human insulin, which are very rapidly mobilized from the subcutaneous injection site. They act even more quickly than soluble insulin (15 minutes against 30 minutes) and their duration of action is only 4 hours. Their place in the management of diabetes is not settled but may be useful, if given immediately before a meal for controlling the rise in blood sugar and thus mimicking more closely the response of the normal pancreas.

## Intermediate–acting insulins

These insulins act for varying periods, depending on the mix of rapid and slow-acting components. The blood glucose starts to fall in 1–2 hours after injection and this effect continues for 16–24 hours. They are usually given once or twice daily and may be combined with soluble insulin.

**Insulin zinc suspension (IZS).** It was found that if insulin was buffered with acetate its action was prolonged, and a further two types of insulin could be prepared: **amorphous**, in which the particles were small, and a **crystalline** form with larger particles. The action of amorphous insulin is rapid and short-lived, but that of crystalline insulin is more prolonged. By using a mixture of these insulins a smooth and prolonged effect can be achieved. Among those available are *Human Monotard* (30% amorphous, 70% crystalline) and *Human Ultratard* (crystalline).

**Biphasic isophane insulins.** Biphasic isophane insulins consist of insulin complexed with protamine. This can then be mixed with varying amounts of soluble insulin to produce an immediate and a longer effect. These include *Human Mixtard 30/70* and *Humulin M1, M2, M3, M4* (varying proportions of soluble and isophane insulin).

**Insulin glargine.** Insulin glargine (*Lantus*) is a new product. It is a preparation of insulin as an acidic solution that is given subcutaneously once daily at bedtime and forms micro crystals under the skin. The micro crystals dissolve slowly and release insulin into the bloodstream. The onset of action is 1 hour after injection, and full activity is reached within 4–5 hours. This activity is maintained at a constant level for 24 hours. In contrast to insulin zinc suspension (*Lente*) and isophane insulin (NPH), insulin glargine produces no significant insulin peaks in the bloodstream. *Adverse effects* of insulin glargine are similar to those of NPH insulin and include hypoglycaemia, reactions at the injection site, rashes, pruritus and allergic reactions. The incidence of hypoglycaemias is similar to that produced by NPH insulin. Insulin glargine has been claimed to produce less nocturnal hypoglycaemia than does once daily NPH insulin.

Readers are referred to the company's literature for more information about the use of this insulin preparation.

## Long–acting insulins

**Protamine zinc insulin (PZI).** This is produced by adding protamine and zinc to insulin. Its action is prolonged, starting after 6 hours and lasting for 24–30 hours. It is bovine insulin and may give rise to skin rashes and painful lumps at the site of injection. If soluble and PZI insulin are mixed in the syringe before injection, some of the soluble insulin becomes PZI insulin. To minimize this, the soluble insulin should be drawn up first and the mixture of insulins injected immediately.

**Human Ultratard.** Alternatively, the crystalline form of human insulin zinc suspension (*Human Ultratard*) also has a prolonged action and is not immunogenic.

## Choice of insulin

If a patient is satisfactorily controlled on a certain type of insulin, that preparation should usually be continued. Human insulin is the least immunogenic and it should be used in the following circumstances:

- for patients starting treatment
- if the patient develops generalized allergies to unpurified insulin
- if injection causes severe local reactions
- if very large doses are required, a situation which suggests that antibodies have been produced by the impure insulin and are interfering with its action
- if the patient is pregnant (impurities in the older types of insulin can cross the placenta and affect the islet tissue of the fetus).

If a change is made from animal to human insulin it should be remembered that human insulin acts a little more rapidly and its effect lasts a shorter time, so that some readjustment of dosage may be necessary. Also, only 80–90% of the previous dose may be needed.

## Giving insulin

Because insulin is broken down in the stomach it has to be given by injection. One regime is to give short-acting insulin 15–30 minutes before the three main meals and intermediate-acting insulin at night; alternatively, both short- and intermediate-acting insulin can be given before breakfast and the evening meal. In some patients, provided the dose is small, a single injection of intermediate-acting insulin is adequate. The type of insulin, dosage and frequency of administration are modified in the light of the patient's response until optimum control is obtained.

## Strength of insulin preparations

The introduction of U100 insulin has greatly simplified insulin dosage. All insulins are now of standard strength – 100 units in 1 ml. The U100 syringes are marked in units of insulin and so it is only necessary to draw up the required number of units (Fig. 15.4).

**Storage.** Insulin should be stored in the refrigerator (not the freezing compartment), but the bottle in current use can safely be kept at room temperature.

## Injection of insulin

If at all possible, patients receiving insulin are instructed how to inject themselves and this instruction is usually given by the nurse.

The best sites for injection are the front of the thighs, the abdomen and the outer side of the upper arm and the insulin is given subcutaneously. A different site should be used each time, but it must be remembered that the rate of absorption of insulin into

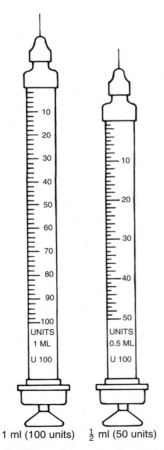

1 ml (100 units)    ½ ml (50 units)

**Figure 15.4**  The U100 syringe marked in units of insulin.

the circulation varies with different parts of the body. Therefore, it is better to use the same area, but not exactly the same site, at the same time of day. For example, the morning dose can be given into the thigh and the evening dose into the arm.

Other points of note about injecting insulin are:

- A microfine I.V. needle and syringe or a 25 G × ⅝ inch should be used. The skin should be pinched up and the needle introduced at an angle of 90°.
- No spirit should be used for skin cleaning as it hardens the skin and the injection site should not be massaged after injection.
- Special syringes are available for those with poor eyesight or other disabilities.

## Other injection apparatus

**Insulin pens** are devices that contain a cartridge of insulin which is automatically injected. A wide range of insulins are available in cartridges and they may be more convenient for the patient.

**Syringe pumps** give a continuous subcutaneous infusion of insulin. The patient wears the pump and the rate of infusion is modified to the patient's needs, thus producing a very fine control of the diabetes. This is used more often in hospitals to cover surgical and other stressful procedures.

## MONITORING TREATMENT

Patients should be taught to monitor their response to treatment by measuring glucose levels in the blood.

## Glucose concentrations

In normal subjects the blood glucose concentration varies from 3 to 7 mmol/litre. The object of treatment is to keep the blood glucose as near as possible to these levels. In patients receiving insulin this is best achieved by measuring the blood glucose using the drop of blood from a finger prick. The blood is applied to a special indicator and the resulting colour change can be read against a colour chart or by a meter. This enables patients to measure their own blood glucose levels and is usually carried out once daily at different times of day. The blood glucose concentration should be kept between 4 and 9 mmol/litre.

The proportion of haemoglobin in the red cells that is glycosylated (i.e. combined with glucose) (**HbA1**) provides an index of the blood glucose concentration over a period of time. Ideally, the HbA1 should be kept below 8.8% and this can be used to monitor treatment.

In patients not on insulin or for whom strict control is not considered practical, the urine is tested for glucose before breakfast, before the midday meal, before retiring, using some dipstick method or using Clinitest tablets. This gives a less precise picture of how the blood glucose level is being controlled since glucose does not appear in the urine until the blood level is about 10 mmol/litre, which is higher than normal. Also it gives no indication if the blood glucose is too low. Nevertheless, it is easy to perform and adequate for some patients, particularly those with NIDDM. It is, however, preferable to measure glucose concentrations in blood.

If the diabetes is seriously out of control, the urine will show the presence of ketones as well as glucose. This means a dangerous situation is developing and immediate treatment is required (see later).

## HYPOGLYCAEMIA

Overdosage with insulin causes an undue decrease in the blood sugar. This leads to faintness, dizziness, tremor, sweating and abnormal behaviour, which may be mistaken for drunkenness. If no treatment is given convulsions, coma and death may occur. It can quickly be relieved by giving sugar or glucose: 4 teaspoonfuls or lumps of sugar in half a glass of fruit juice followed by two biscuits is effective. Glucose solution can also be given by slow intravenous infusion into a large vein using a large gauge needle, but care must be taken as glucose is irritant in higher concentrations if extravasation occurs.

**Glucagon** (see below) by injection is also effective and is useful if the patient is too drowsy to swallow. Glucagon may be administered through most routes by injection, e.g. I.M. or S.C., and can also be given by I.V. injection or infusion. It is often prescribed on an 'if necessary' basis for inpatients being treated with insulin, so that the nurse can rapidly use it if there is a hypotensive emergency.

About a quarter of patients with long-term diabetes may not be aware that they are becoming hypoglycaemic. Alcohol and β blockers may aggravate this condition; it has been suggested that it is more likely to occur when human insulin is used, but proof is lacking.

**Driving a car.** A patient may lose control of a vehicle as a result of hypoglycaemia through excess insulin. Special care is therefore necessary, and patients who are being treated with insulin should check their blood sugar before setting out and at 2-hourly intervals during a long journey. Sugar should always be available in the car.

## INSULIN IN SPECIAL CIRCUMSTANCES

Details of the methods used under the following circumstances vary, but the general principles are the same.

### Pregnancy

During pregnancy, the metabolic rate rises, and this increases the demand for insulin. In fact, the condition may first manifest itself during pregnancy. Human insulin is preferable. It is necessary to control the diabetes as well as possible, usually giving insulin two or three times daily. Poor control increases the incidence of fetal abnormality and perinatal problems. After delivery of the placenta, insulin requirements fall and dosage adjustment will be necessary.

### Serious intercurrent illness

The patient's insulin requirement will rise because of an increased metabolic rate through stress, and this situation is a potent cause of diabetic coma; therefore, it is important not to reduce insulin dosage. It may be necessary to change the regime to 1–6 units/hour of soluble insulin given by intravenous infusion, together with fluid and glucose as determined by blood glucose estimations.

### Major surgery

It is easiest if the patient is first on the morning operating list. The morning dose of insulin is not given, but at least an hour before surgery an infusion of glucose with a suitable dose of potassium is started. Human Actrapid is commenced at the same time. The precise dose will depend on factors such as the patient's weight. Check the *BNF* and a specialist physician for all doses and concentrations of solutes. The rate of insulin infusion is subsequently adjusted depending on the blood glucose levels.

## Diabetic coma (hyperglycaemic ketoacidosis)

Patients with diabetes who are not treated, or who develop some infection during treatment, may rapidly pass into a diabetic coma. These patients not only have a very high blood and urinary glucose level but also are producing large quantities of ketone bodies, which can be detected in the urine and, being acids, lead to an acidosis. The excessive diuresis produced by the glucose in the urine leads to severe depletion of sodium, potassium and water.

Soluble human insulin (*Humulin S* or *Human Actrapid*) is given intravenously by an infusion pump. The rate is adjusted to produce a fall in the blood glucose concentration of about 5 mmol/hour. The aim is to reduce the level to about 11 mmol/litre and maintain it until oral feeding and subcutaneous injection of insulin can be introduced. At the same time water and electrolyte imbalance are corrected by giving an infusion of normal saline containing a suitable level of potassium chloride. Restoration of electrolyte and water balance is usually sufficient and the kidneys will correct the acidosis by excreting acid urine. Occasionally, however, the acidosis is so severe that it is necessary to infuse sodium hydrogen carbonate until the degree of acidosis is improved. Frequent examination of the urine for sugar and ketones, of the blood sugar hourly and of the electrolytes is important in controlling treatment. Subsequent doses of insulin are determined by the blood glucose concentration.

The possibility of infection as a cause of diabetic coma should not be forgotten, and if this is found it is treated by the appropriate antibiotic. Deep vein thrombosis is a common complication and prophylactic subcutaneous heparin may be prescribed.

## MANAGEMENT OF PATIENTS WITH NON-INSULIN-DEPENDENT DIABETES

## AIMS OF TREATMENT

The main objective in treating NIDDM is to prevent the development of the late complications of the NIDDM. These are myocardial infarction, vascular disease, renal failure, retinopathy and neuropathy. This is best achieved by controlling plasma glucose, lipids and blood pressure (if raised) and by avoiding risk factors such as smoking and obesity. Seventy-five per cent of these patients will be overweight and initially the treatment of choice is diet, which aims to reduce the patient's weight to the ideal level. Sucrose and glucose should be largely avoided and most carbohydrate taken in the form of polysaccharides (vegetables, cereals, pasta, etc.). The intake of saturated animal fat should be low. When the appropriate weight has been reached the diet may be increased to maintain it at that level. Regular exercise, tailored to the abilities of the patient, is beneficial by increasing insulin sensitivity.

This regime is intended to keep the fasting blood sugar below 9 mmol/litre and the plasma cholesterol below 6.5 mmol/litre. Blood pressure control is important and, if the blood pressure is raised, it should be reduced to 145/85, if possible. ACE inhibitors (see p. 77) are the preferred hypotensive drugs as they decrease renal damage. In elderly patients the requirements may be relaxed a little.

If, after 6 months, these objectives are not achieved, treatment with oral agents will be necessary. Most patients are given one of the sulphonylureas, although if obesity is a problem metformin (see below) may be preferred. Adherence to the diet remains important as the sulphonylureas may cause some weight gain. A number of patients may still fail to attain the desired objectives, in which case the two types of drug may be combined. There are now also newer types of drugs available (see below). Finally, if this fails, injections of insulin will be needed. There is a group of NIDDM patients for whom insulin is the only way to control the disease.

## ORAL HYPOGLYCAEMIC AGENTS

Oral hypoglycaemic agents include:

- the sulphonylureas
- metformin
- thiazolidinediones
- prandial glucose regulators
- acarbose.

### The sulphonylureas

These drugs are:

- chlorpropamide
- glibenclamide
- gliclazide
- glipizide
- gliquidone
- tolbutamide.

**Mechanism of action.** This group of drugs is related to the sulphonamides. They lower blood glucose levels by increasing insulin production by the pancreas. They may also increase the sensitivity of the tissues to insulin.

**Clinical use.** Sulphonylureas are all given orally and differ largely in their duration of action. They are used in patients with NIDDM who are usually middle-aged or elderly and obese. They supplement, but do not replace, treatment by diet. They have no place in the treatment of the young patient with diabetes who requires insulin or in the treatment of diabetic coma.

**Gliclazide, glipizide** and **glibenclamide** are now the most commonly prescribed, of which gliclazide is the one most used. Its effects last up to 24 hours and it rarely causes hypoglycaemic episodes. Also, it can be taken once or twice daily. The drug takes about 5 hours to achieve a peak response. This means that it can be taken before breakfast and gives good cover for lunch and supper.

**Tolbutamide** and **chlorpropamide** are not used now as much as before. Tolbutamide is very safe and satisfactory if used correctly. Its duration of action is about 6 hours and for this reason it is particularly recommended in elderly patients as the risk of hypoglycaemia is reduced and it is given orally two or three times daily. Chlorpropamide is similar to tolbutamide, but its action lasts a full 24 hours, so once daily dosage is appropriate. Because of adverse effects it should only be used for patients who have been successfully treated with it for some time.

**Adverse effects.** These include:

- gastrointestinal upsets
- blood dyscrasias (abnormalities)
- fluid retention
- hypoglycaemia
- skin rashes.

**Drug interactions.** NSAIDs, including aspirin, enhance the effect and thiazide diuretics reduce the effect of sulphonylureas.

## Metformin

Metformin belongs to a group of chemicals called biguanides. It is at present the only biguanide in use in the UK to treat NIDDM.

**Mechanism of action.** This is not completely understood but metformin may:

- reduce glucose absorption from the gastrointestinal tract
- stimulate uptake of glucose into muscle

- inhibit gluconeogenesis (biosynthesis of glucose from non-carbohydrate sources, e.g. amino acids)
- reduce glucose release from the liver.

### Other effects

- Metformin inhibits plasma low-density lipoproteins (LDL). It may, therefore, reduce the danger of atheroma in some patients.
- Metformin does not reduce the production of ketone bodies
- Metformin does not cause hypoglycaemia
- Metformin does not cause weight gain, possibly because it does not stimulate appetite.

**Clinical use.** Its main use is combined with one of the sulphonylureas when the patient is not responding satisfactorily to diet or to these drugs alone. Metformin is also occasionally used combined with insulin in patients with IDDM whose disease is proving difficult to control.

### Adverse effects and contraindications

- Transient gastrointestinal disturbances (the most common).
- Long-term use may interfere with vitamin $B_{12}$ absorption.
- Rarely, metformin may cause lactic acidosis, which is potentially fatal. Therefore it should not be prescribed for patients with pulmonary or cardiac disease, or renal disease.

## Thiazolidinediones

Examples of thiazolidinediones:

- **pioglitazone**
- **rosiglitazone**.

The thiazolidinedione drugs belong to a group of chemicals called glitazones. The first such drug to be marketed in the UK was troglitazone, which had to be withdrawn due to liver toxicity.

**Mechanism of action.** They seem to reduce tissue resistance to insulin.

**Clinical use.** They have been very satisfactory in controlling NIDDM when combined with other agents, and are, at the time of writing, licensed for use in the UK only in combination with either metformin or sulphonylureas. They are not licensed for use with insulin.

The onset of action is slow, and patients may need encouragement to persist with treatment. About 25% of patients do not respond, and these tend to be the more obese patients with long-standing insulin resistance and lower pancreatic reserves.

**Adverse reactions.**    There are not many reports of liver toxicity. Nevertheless, liver toxicity tests should be carried out before starting patients on these drugs. Weight gain has been reported as well as an increase in plasma LDL levels with rosiglitazone, although the manufacturers claim that this happens with a nonatherogenic fraction of LDL.

**Contraindications.**    These comprise:

- **pregnancy**
- **breast-feeding**
- **liver disease**
- **history of heart failure**
- **do not give with insulin**.

**Drug interactions.**    Pioglitazone induces an enzyme that is partly responsible for its metabolism. The same enzyme metabolizes a number of other drugs, including calcium channel blockers, erythromycin, ciclosporin, statins and glucocorticoids such as prednisolone. Therefore, concurrent use of these drugs must be carefully considered.

## Prandial glucose regulators

**Nateglinide** and **repaglinide** are relative newcomers and although their names sound similar they are not members of the same chemical family and they also have different mechanisms of action. They are unique in that they act postprandially, i.e. they deal with the rise in circulating glucose that occurs immediately after a meal.

**Actions.**    Repaglinide stimulates insulin release from the pancreas in the same way the oral sulphonylureas do, but in contrast to the latter it does not promote insulin release in the absence of glucose. Nateglinide works by restoring early-phase insulin release. Both drugs are quickly absorbed from the gastrointestinal tract and both are very short acting. Nateglinide synergizes with metformin, i.e. the drug increases the effects of a given dose of metformin.

**Clinical use.**    Both drugs are taken before a meal, and both are omitted if the meal is missed.

**Adverse effects.**    Anorexia and nausea are troublesome and may lead to the abandonment of this form of treatment. More serious but rare is lactic acidosis with drowsiness, abdominal pain, vomiting and shock. The mechanism of this side-effect is not understood, but it is more liable to occur in alcoholics and those with liver, renal and cardiac failure.

## Acarbose

**Mechanism of action.**    Acarbose is an inhibitor of the enzyme intestinal α-glucosidase. This enzyme is part of the gastrointestinal mechanism for converting carbohydrate to glucose.

**Clinical use.**    Taken orally before meals, this agent inhibits the digestion of complex carbohydrates such as sucrose and starches, thus preventing their absorption, but it does not interfere with glucose absorption. The postprandial rise in the blood sugar is reduced. However, the unabsorbed carbohydrates in the bowel may cause flatulence and diarrhoea. The role of this drug in diabetes is not yet determined, but it may be a useful adjunct to treatment in NIDDM.

## INSULIN

Insulin may be used in combination with other agents if the patient's own pancreatic reserve is exhausted.

The practical problems associated with the management of NIDDM are illustrated in Case History 15.1. The reader is referred to Dixon (2002) for further information about antidiabetic preparations.

### Case History 15.1

Mr T had a strong family history of non-insulin dependent diabetes, but this unfortunately did not stop him becoming obese and having a high carbohydrate and fat diet. He himself had noticed progressive tiredness, nocturia and an increasing thirst, unfortunately quenched mainly by high-sugar fizzy drinks. His diabetes went undiagnosed for 2 years until a routine urine test at his GP clinic showed a high level of glucose and the diagnosis was confirmed with a fasting blood glucose and glycosylated haemoglobin (HbA1c), which measures whether the average blood glucose has been satisfactory or not over a 3–4 month period. He was referred to a dietician and a specialist district nurse saw to it that his diabetes remained stable and controlled. With adequate motivation, he managed to lose weight and maintain a satisfactory diabetic control. Unfortunately his resolve weakened and his sugar control became poor; he was started on a sulphonylurea drug orally. A choice was available between gliclazide (*Diamicron*) or glibenclamide (*Daonil* or *Euglucon*). This was only partially successful and the biguanide drug metformin (*Glucophage*) was added: this drug is not usually helpful in non-obese diabetics. A promising new type of drug in the group thiazolidinediones (rosiglitazone or pioglitazone) which increase the sensitivity to the body's naturally produced insulin may be added to his oral medication.

## GLUCAGON

Glucagon, a polypeptide, is a hormone secreted by the alpha cells of the pancreatic islets of Langerhans.

### RELEASE OF GLUCAGON

Glucagon is released in response to high plasma levels of amino acids, especially arginine, e.g. after a high protein meal. It is also released in response to circulating epinephrine and increased sympathetic or parasympathetic activity. Release is inhibited by another hormone, somatostatin, which is released from other cells in the pancreatic islets called D cells. In contrast to insulin, however, plasma concentrations of glucagon do not fluctuate but remain fairly steady throughout the day.

### ACTIONS OF GLUCAGON

Glucagon:

- stimulates glycogen breakdown to glucose in the liver
- stimulates gluconeogenesis
- inhibits glycogen synthesis
- inhibits glucose oxidation
- causes lipolysis in fat
- increases breakdown of muscle
- increases release of insulin.

The overall result is to increase blood glucose. Glucagon's actions oppose those of insulin. It also limits its own actions by stimulating insulin release.

### CLINICAL USE

Glucagon is used to raise blood sugar in patients who are hypoglycaemic, e.g. after an overdose of insulin. It can be administered intramuscularly, subcutaneously or intravenously.

## THE NURSE AND THE PATIENT WITH DIABETES AT HOME

The management of patients with diabetes is a team activity involving the patient, the doctor, the nurse, the dietician and often laboratory staff. Increasingly, people with diabetes are stabilized and controlled in the community. District nurse specialists supervise treatment in the home with the back-up of the primary care team or the hospital. This has the advantage that treatment can be geared to the patient's lifestyle and, most importantly, the family can be involved particularly in planning meals, etc.

Education is very important for the patients, who must realize as far as possible the implications of their illness and its treatment.

## APPETITE SUPPRESSION AND OBESITY

Obesity is a serious health hazard and is increasingly common throughout the Western world. Fifteen per cent of the population of the UK are obese (i.e. they have a body mass index (BMI) of over 30). It is strongly associated with heart disease, hypertension, NIDDM and arthritis of weight-bearing joints.

The essential cause is an imbalance between calorie (food) intake and energy expenditure (exercise). Normally, various mechanisms within the body keep these in balance, but even a small disturbance in this balance can lead to increasing deposition of fat. This is particularly liable to occur with a sedentary occupation and the consumption of energy-rich foods, which are, unfortunately, features of a modern lifestyle. Genetic factors play a part in maintaining the balance between calorie intake and energy expenditure, and obesity often runs in families.

### MANAGEMENT

The definitive treatment is to decrease calorie intake and increase energy expenditure. In spite of extensive literature on all types of diet, it remains essential to eat less. The actual composition is less important than its calorie content, and a normal, mixed diet, low in fat and sugar, is adequate. The diet should be combined with a programme of exercise related to the age and health of the patient to increase energy expenditure.

For the average adult, not doing heavy work, a daily intake of 750 kcal will result in the loss of

1.0 kg/week, which is ideal. The aim should be to reduce the weight to the correct BMI, given as:

$$BMI = \frac{\text{Weight in kilograms}}{(\text{Height in metres})^2}$$

which should be between 20 and 25.

**Orlistat** has been introduced to treat obesity. It inhibits the action of lipase in the intestine, thus reducing fat absorption. It has been shown, in trials, to reduce weight but it causes steatorrhoea. Orlistat will not enable those who wish to lose weight to eat what they like but, combined with a low-fat diet, it seems to be a useful adjunct to treatment.

## Summary

- Children should be encouraged to limit the intake of fast foods that are rich in carbohydrates and fats
- Good dietary management is critical in diabetes
- Slowly absorbed carbohydrates such as potatoes and wholemeal bread are preferable to sweets and cakes
- In IDDM insulin lispro or aspart may be useful if given immediately before a meal for controlling the rise in blood sugar
- Intermediate–acting insulin may be combined with soluble insulin
- Try to avoid overmixing soluble insulin and protamine zinc insulin in the same syringe
- Human insulin is the least immunogenic and is preferable in certain cases (see p. 195)
- Human insulin is preferable in pregnancy
- Human insulin acts faster and has a shorter duration of action than does animal-derived insulin
- The sites of injection with insulin should be varied and the site should be massaged after injection
- Spirits for cleaning injection sites cause skin hardening
- Special syringes are available for patients who are disabled or who have poor eyesight
- Some patients find insulin pens more convenient
- Patients need to know how to monitor their own glucose levels and how to restore glucose after overdosage with insulin
- Patients new to insulin must be warned to check glucose levels before driving and at regular intervals during a long car journey if driving
- ACE diuretics are preferred in patients with NIDDM
- Patients may need encouragement to persist with thiazolidenediones
- Liver toxicity tests should be done before starting treatment with thiazolidenediones
- Prandial glucose regulators such as nateglinide and repaglinide are effective only before a meal
- Patient education in diabetes is a critically important responsibility of the health team
- Obesity is a growing problem in the UK and health workers should play a large part in educating patients about balancing calorie intake and exercise

## References

Burden M 2003 Diabetes: new treatments and guidance. Nursing Times 99: 30

Dixon N 2002 Antidiabetic agents. Pharmaceutical Journal 268: 538

## Further reading

Editorial 1990 Insulin injection technique. British Medical Journal 301: 3

Editorial 1991 Hypoglycaemia and diabetic control. Lancet 338: 853

Editorial 1991 Treating obesity. British Medical Journal 302: 803

Editorial 1997 Humalog – a new insulin analogue. Drug and Therapeutics Bulletin 35(8): 57

Editorial 1998 Combined blood pressure and glucose in Type 2 diabetes. British Medical Journal 317: 693

Editorial 1998 Appetite suppression and valvular heart disease. New England Journal of Medicine 339: 765

Fernez R E, Alberti K G 1989 Sulphonylurea treatment of non-insulin dependent diabetes. Quarterly Journal of Medicine 73: 987

Horwitz M S, Bradley L M, Harbertson J et al 1998 Diabetes induced by Coxsackie virus: initiation by bystander damage and not molecular mimicry. Nature Medicine 4: 781

Lebovitz H E 1995 Diabetic ketoacidosis. Lancet 345: 767

Thomas B 1994 Manual of diabetic practice, 2nd edn. Blackwell, Oxford

Wang P H 1993 Tight glucose control and diabetic complications. Lancet 342: 129

Wilding J 1997 Obesity treatment. British Medical Journal 315: 997

Williams G 1994 Management of non-insulin-dependent diabetes mellitus. Lancet 343: 95

# Chapter 16

# Endocrine system IV. Hormones and metabolism: the adrenal glands

## CHAPTER CONTENTS

## Learning objectives

At the end of this chapter, the reader should be able to:

- list the different classes of adrenocortical hormones
- explain the consequences of aldosterone excess
- recognize that the common term 'steroids' often refers to the glucocorticoids
- recognize that cortisol and cortisone are the natural glucocorticoids
- recognize that hydrocortisone is a preparation of cortisol for clinical use
- give examples of synthetic glucocorticoids
- describe the physiological actions of cortisol
- explain how cortisol and progesterone are carried in the blood by the plasma protein corticosteroid-binding globulin (CBG) and the implications of this
- describe the phases of the survival response to stress and the role played by cortisol
- understand that the *physiological* actions of cortisol are not the same as the *pharmacological* actions of clinically used glucocorticoids
- explain the consequences and dangers associated with prolonged use of glucocorticoids
- recognize and explain the dangers associated with the sudden cessation of long-term glucocorticoid therapy
- list some important uses of the glucocorticoids, including replacement therapy in Addison's disease

The two adrenal glands are situated at the upper pole of the kidneys. They consist of an outer layer or cortex and a central portion or medulla (Fig. 16.1).

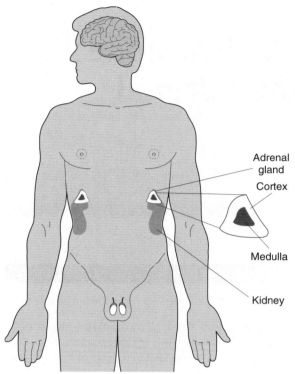

**Figure 16.1**    Anatomical location and structure of the adrenal gland.

These two parts of the adrenal gland produce hormones of very different composition and function and they will therefore be considered separately.

## THE CORTEX

A number of hormones are produced by the adrenal cortex. They also belong to the class of chemical substances known as steroids. Three main groups may be identified:

- mineralocorticoid hormones
- adrenal sex hormones
- glucocorticoid hormones (also called corticosteroids or simply 'steroids').

**Mineralocorticoid hormones** are concerned with salt (sodium) and water control; the most important is **aldosterone**. Aldosterone increases reabsorption of sodium by the kidney, thus raising the amount of sodium in the body, which in turn causes water retention. The main trigger to the release of aldosterone is the renin mechanism (see p. 74) and its main function is to ensure that the volume of fluid in the circulation and tissue spaces is kept constant.

Excess of aldosterone gives rise to hypertension and sometimes oedema. Very rarely, aldosterone-producing tumours arise in the adrenal gland causing Conn's syndrome, which is characterized by hypertension and low plasma potassium with muscle weakness. Many of the synthetic steroids, such as prednisolone and dexamethasone, which are widely used to treat inflammatory conditions, will in higher doses cross-react with the aldosterone receptor and cause oedema. Aldosterone is not available for clinical use as a drug.

Loss of the adrenals is potentially lethal because of the lack of the salt-retaining hormone. The adrenals may need to be removed in patients with breast cancer to remove any source of sex hormones and these patients need to be given salt replacement therapy.

**Adrenal sex hormones** are only secreted in small amounts and are of comparatively little importance as sex hormones when compared with the role of the gonadal sex hormones in sexual reproduction. Both male and female sex hormones are secreted. Excessive secretion of male sex hormones such as androstenedione and testosterone, for example from adrenal tumours in women, leads to virilism (see also p. 221).

**Glucocorticoid hormones (corticosteroids, steroids)** are concerned with metabolism of carbohydrate, fat and protein and will also modify the response of the body to injury. The chief glucocorticoid released from the adrenal is **cortisol**. Another, minor corticosteroid, namely cortisone, is released as well.

## GLUCOCORTICOID HORMONES

### CONTROL OF CORTISOL RELEASE

Cortisol release is controlled by corticotrophin (adrenocorticotrophic hormone; ACTH), which is produced by the anterior pituitary (see p. 173). The release of ACTH is in turn stimulated by corticotrophin-releasing hormone (CRH), a hypothalamic releasing hormone. The mechanism is such that when the amount of cortisol in the blood increases it 'switches off' the release of corticotrophin by the pituitary and the release of CRH in the hypothalamus. This is a negative feedback action that prevents large changes in the blood cortisol concentration (see Fig. 13.3).

### CLASSIFICATION

In addition to cortisol and cortisone, there are a number of synthetic compounds with similar actions to those of cortisol. The members of the whole group are commonly called the corticosteroids, glucocorticoids or simply the 'steroids'.

Naturally occurring corticosteroids (glucocorticoids):

- **cortisol**
- **cortisone**.

Synthetic glucocorticoids:

- **betamethasone**
- **dexamethasone**
- **fludrocortisone**
- **methylprednisolone**
- **prednisolone**
- **prednisone**
- **triamcinolone**.

## ACTIONS OF CORTISOL AND OTHER CORTICOSTEROIDS

These can be considered as:

- physiological actions
- pharmacological actions.

### Physiological actions of cortisol

Cortisol is the major naturally occurring glucocorticoid hormone in humans. In the blood, cortisol is carried mostly bound to a specific protein, corticosteroid-binding globulin (CBG). CBG also binds progesterone (see p. 12). Only the free, unbound fraction of cortisol is available to the tissues; CBG thus acts as a buffer, preventing excess amounts of cortisol from gaining access to the cells.

It is important to distinguish between the physiological and pharmacological actions of the corticosteroids. These are often confused. The physiological actions are those of the hormone cortisol after it is released from the gland in order to perform its normal role in the body. Cortisol:

- raises blood glucose
- promotes survival responses to stress
- controls ACTH and CRH release.

**Effects on blood glucose.** Cortisol has both anabolic and catabolic actions. In the liver it stimulates the production of several key enzymes involved in gluconeogenesis, i.e. production of newly synthesized glucose. This is an anabolic action. In fat and muscle, however, cortisol stimulates the breakdown

of these tissues to mobilize energy. This is a catabolic action that also results in an increase in glucose synthesis.

**Survival response to stress.** Cortisol plays a critical role in the body's response to stress, and if one understands the stress response it makes the actions of cortisol much easier to understand. The body's response to stress is called the general adaptation syndrome (GAS) and has three components: (1) an alarm reaction, followed by (2) resistance to the stress, which is followed by (3) exhaustion. The alarm reaction involves the release of epinephrine and norepinephrine from the adrenal medulla (see below) and the release of norepinephrine from sympathetic nerve terminals. At the same time the corticosteroids are released from the adrenal cortex and these permit the released catecholamines to exert their full effects. The resistance phase involves the prolonged effects of cortisol in stimulating gluconeogenesis in the liver and the breakdown of energy stores from fat and muscle. If the stress is prolonged, this will induce the signs of the third phase of exhaustion (which is also seen after prolonged use of corticosteroids in therapy); i.e.

- muscle wasting
- suppression of the immune system and atrophy of its tissues
- hyperglycaemia
- gastric ulceration
- vascular damage
- reduced sensitivity to insulin.

**Control of ACTH and CRH release.** This has already been covered in more detail on p. 173.

Notice that the normal physiological actions of cortisol do *not* involve the notorious effects of glucocorticoids when used at high doses for prolonged periods. For example, cortisol will not normally cause clinically important oedema and will not cause significant muscle wasting and suppression of the immune system.

### Pharmacological actions of cortisol and the synthetic glucocorticoids

Prolonged use of high doses of the glucocorticoids will result in:

- atrophy of the adrenal cortex
- effects on carbohydrate metabolism
- bone thinning and osteoporosis
- muscle weakness and wasting

- effects on electrolytes – oedema
- suppression of inflammatory responses
- suppression of immunity
- gastric ulceration
- suppression of stress responses
- growth retardation in children
- skin thinning, acne and striae (stretch marks)

- psychological effects (euphoria)
- reduced response to stress
- 'moon face'
- diabetes
- hirsutism
- raised blood pressure
- masked infection.

**Adrenal cortical atrophy.** Prolonged treatment with steroid hormones causes atrophy of the adrenal cortex. If this treatment is stopped suddenly or if the requirement is increased by stress or infection the adrenal cortex cannot produce adequate amounts of cortisol and a shock-like state develops (see also below). It may take the adrenal cortex up to 2 years to recover after prolonged steroid treatment.

**Effects on carbohydrate metabolism.** Glucocorticoids stimulate the production of glucose from protein and decrease sensitivity to insulin. Prolonged treatment may rarely give rise to diabetes mellitus.

**Effects on electrolytes.** Glucocorticoids cause retention of sodium and water and loss of potassium via the kidneys, although they are not as powerful as aldosterone. They do this in part by cross-reacting with the aldosterone receptor in the kidney. The retention of sodium and water may lead to oedema and hypertension in some patients. Potassium loss may be replaced by potassium supplements (see p. 166) in patients who are receiving large doses over long periods.

**Effects on inflammation.** Glucocorticoids suppress all inflammatory processes and also the generalized reactions of inflammation such as pyrexia (raised temperature) and malaise. This action may be very dangerous, for inflammation is the body's method of dealing with infections. If no inflammatory reaction occurs the bacteria can spread widely without the seriousness of the position being apparent to the practitioner or the patient. Such patients require urgent treatment with antibiotics and an increase in steroid dosage (see also Masked infection below).

**Effects on the stomach.** Glucocorticoids may increase gastric acidity and at times appear to exacerbate ulcers already present. Antacids may be prescribed. It is doubtful if enteric-coated glucocorticoid tablets have any advantage. If perforation of the ulcer occurs, the damping effects of glucocorticoids on inflammation may mask the symptoms of the perforation, with disastrous results.

**Effects on immunity.** The immune reaction is suppressed and patients become more vulnerable to infections. This is partly due to damping down the antigen–antibody response and possibly also to the reduced production of antibodies. For the same reasons allergic reactions of various types are inhibited. Glucocorticoids cause atrophy of tissues of the immune system. They inhibit mitosis and therefore suppress production of cells of the immune system.

**Effects on bone.** Glucocorticoids reduce bone production and prolonged treatment can cause osteoporosis. Avascular necrosis of bone, producing severe pain and usually affecting the hips, is a very troublesome complication.

**Psychological effects.** Glucocorticoids usually produce a feeling of well-being (euphoria). Occasionally, however, serious mental disease may follow their administration. This usually occurs in those with a background of mental ill health.

**Responses to stress.** Stress causes an increased secretion of cortisol. In patients on high doses of glucocorticoids this stress response is suppressed. Failure of this response can lead to a shock-like state if the patient is stressed, particularly if glucocorticoids are stopped suddenly (see below).

**Masked infection.** Any infective disease may spread rapidly and yet produce minimal signs in patients on chronic glucocorticoid treatment. Such an infection requires prompt treatment with antibiotics, together with an increase in the dose of steroid. Chickenpox, which is usually a mild disease, may become life threatening in patients taking steroids if they have no immunity from a previous attack. Such patients should avoid contact with chickenpox or herpes zoster. A similar risk applies to measles.

**Miscellaneous effects.** In large doses glucocorticoids will produce a picture similar to that of Cushing's disease. The patient will develop a round 'moon-like' face, hair on the face and body, a tendency to acne and purple striae on the trunk (Fig. 16.2). Occasionally, muscle weakness and wasting occur and the skin becomes thin and very susceptible to bruising. There is redistribution of body fat that can result in the so-called 'buffalo hump'. Patients may develop raised blood pressure and diabetes. Urine should be checked regularly for the presence of glucose. The presence of infections may be masked. Patients may develop cataracts or glaucoma.

Figure 16.2    Side-effects of the steroids.

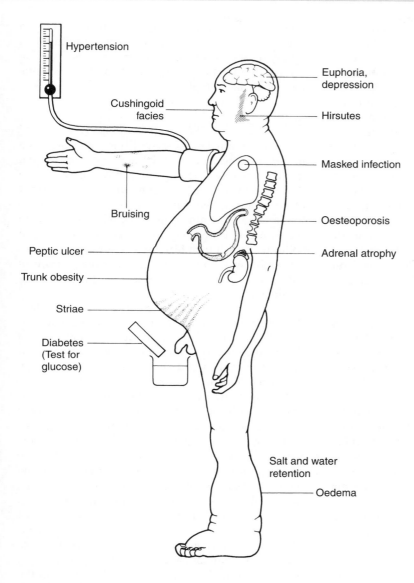

Hypertension

Euphoria, depression

Cushingoid facies

Hirsutes

Bruising

Masked infection

Peptic ulcer

Oesteoporosis

Trunk obesity

Adrenal atrophy

Striae

Diabetes (Test for glucose)

Salt and water retention

Oedema

The various adverse effects are summarized in Figure 16.2. It must be stressed that many of these effects are only seen if glucocorticoids are given in large doses and not at the physiological levels normally found in the blood.

## THE CLINICAL USE OF THE CORTICOSTEROIDS

The therapeutic uses of corticosteroids may be considered under two headings:

- suppression of some disease process
- replacement of steroid hormones which, for some reason, are deficient.

### Suppression of disease processes

These comprise:

- anti-inflammatory action
- anti-allergic action and suppression of immunity
- antitumour action
- idiopathic thrombocytopenic purpura
- certain acute haemolytic anaemias
- certain types of the nephrotic syndrome.

**Anti-inflammatory action.**    This effect is used in treating certain patients with systemic lupus erythematosus, polyarteritis nodosa, temporal arteritis and, rarely, rheumatoid arthritis. In these disorders, pharmacological doses are used that are much higher concentrations than those of naturally released cortisol. It must be stressed that these drugs are only useful in certain types of inflammation. In inflammation due to bacterial infection they may actually favour spread of infections and are thus dangerous. The best drugs to use when anti-inflammatory effects are required are those with little sodium-retaining action such as **prednisolone**.

When the inflammatory steroids were first introduced they were used in high doses for rheumatoid arthritis (RA) and caused their distressing side-effects. Nowadays their use in RA is restricted mainly to short-term treatments to give patients a 'holiday' from pain, or, more usually, in much lower daily doses (1–4 mg daily) for long-term anti-inflammatory effects with much reduced incidence of side-effects.

**Anti–allergic action.** By suppressing allergic reactions these drugs are useful in such disorders as asthma, hay fever and eczema. In asthma, they are reserved for those patients who do not respond to more usual measures. In status asthmaticus, cortisol (hydrocortisone) intravenously and repeated every 6 hours may be life-saving. In the long-term treatment of asthma, steroids such as **beclometasone** can be given by inhalation to produce a maximum local action with minimum systemic effect. In hay fever and eczema, cortisol (hydrocortisone) may be applied locally and it is also used as eye drops. Hydrocortisone is the name given to a pharmaceutical preparation of cortisol.

**Suppression of immunity.** Glucocorticoids have been used to suppress immunity and thus prevent rejection after organ transplant.

**Antitumour actions.** Steroids have some anti-lymphocyte action and are used in combination with cytotoxic drugs to treat lymphomas and some leukaemias. Large doses of prednisolone, for example, are given over 1 or 2 weeks. Dexamethasone is given in the palliative treatment of either primary or secondary cerebral tumours. It probably acts by reducing oedema.

**Miscellaneous uses.** Steroids produce an improvement in idiopathic thrombocytopenic purpura, in certain acute haemolytic anaemias and in certain types of the nephrotic syndrome. In these disorders large doses are usually required.

Ideally, steroids should be given with food at breakfast. At this time natural steroid production is at a maximum so causes least suppression of adrenal function. In children, long-term treatment with steroids retards growth, which may be minimized by giving the hormone on alternate days. Evening dosage should be avoided, as this may keep the patient awake at night.

### Replacement therapy

In these circumstances steroid hormones are used to replace the normal secretions of the adrenal glands because the adrenals have either been destroyed by disease (**Addison's disease**) or removed at operation. When this occurs, the kidneys are no longer able to retain sodium, which is excreted in the urine, and the body thus becomes depleted of sodium. This in turn leads to collapse, with vomiting and low blood pressure. A curious feature of Addison's disease is widespread pigmentation, particularly in the mouth.

The aim of treatment in this disorder is to replace the missing hormones. In an acute Addisonian crisis with a collapsed and severely ill patient, cortisol (hydrocortisone) is given intravenously and repeated as required. Saline and glucose are infused and any concurrent infection is treated vigorously.

For maintenance treatment it is important to use a steroid with sodium-retaining properties. Cortisol (hydrocortisone) morning and night is satisfactory and may be combined with fludrocortisone to further reduce salt loss. A rough check of adequate replacement can be achieved by measuring the blood pressure supine and erect. If inadequate, there will be a large postural fall in blood pressure. Other indications are the weight and well-being of the patient.

Any stress such as an acute infection will increase the requirements of steroids by these patients and the dose should be increased over the period of the acute episode.

### TOPICAL STEROIDS (see also p. 377)

Steroids may be applied to the skin in the treatment of various dermatological conditions. The best vehicle for the drug is soft white paraffin and between 5 and 10% of the applied dose is absorbed through the skin. The most active steroids for this purpose include betamethasone and triamcinolone. Prolonged application can produce atrophy of the skin and a tendency to bacterial or fungal infection.

## Nursing point

Nurses should wear gloves to apply steroids and wash hands afterwards, as these drugs are easily absorbed through the skin.

## THE ADRENAL MEDULLA

The adrenal medulla produces both epinephrine and norepinephrine, which are released into the circulation. The properties of these substances are discussed in more detail on p. 43. Tumours of the medulla occur rarely and may produce both these substances in excessive amounts.

## Nursing points

1. Patients receiving long-term steroids will require double their usual dose if they develop a moderate illness and treble their usual dose for a severe illness. They must be taught to recognize stress situations
2. Before the operation, the surgeon and anaesthetist must be informed if the patient is receiving steroids. Patients must also inform their doctor and dentist if they are receiving steroids.
3. If treatment with steroids lasts more than 10 days, withdrawal must be gradual as adrenal suppression will have occurred. Patients must be taught not to stop taking steroids suddenly.
4. All patients receiving long-term steroids should carry a card detailing their treatment.
5. Careful monitoring of adverse effects (see Fig. 16.2) is important.

## Summary

- The adrenal glands are situated at the upper pole of the kidneys
- High doses of glucocorticoids have aldosterone-like effects
- Prolonged use of glucocorticoids will reduce the body's ability to respond to stress
- Do not allow patients to stop taking glucocorticoids suddenly. This will leave them defenceless against stress. The dosage should be gradually reduced
- Low daily doses of glucocorticoids are now widely used to treat rheumatoid arthritis
- The patient's urine should be checked for glucose regularly if they are on long-term steroids
- Prescribing steroids for patients with ulcers is dangerous
- Patients on long-term steroid treatment should have bone scans periodically
- Patients on long-term steroid treatment should avoid contact with herpes zoster, measles and chicken pox
- Prednisolone is often the steroid of choice because it has relatively little salt-retaining activity
- Low-dose steroids can be used for prolonged steroid treatment of RA with reduced incidence of adverse effects (van Everdingen et al, 2002)
- Steroids are best taken in the morning with breakfast. Evening doses may cause insomnia
- Do not encourage long-term topical use of steroids

## Reference

van Everdingen AA, Jacobs J W, Siewertsz Van Reesema D R et al (2002) Low-dose prednisone therapy for patients with early active rheumatoid arthritis: clinical efficacy, disease-modifying properties, and side effects: a randomized, double-blind, placebo-controlled clinical trial. Annals of Internal Medicine 136: 1

## Further reading

Editorial 1990 Corticosteroids – getting replacement right. Prescribers Journal 28: 71

Griffiths H, Jordan S 2002 Corticosteroids: implications for nursing practice. Nursing Standard 17: 43

# Chapter 17

# Endocrine system V. Hormones and reproduction

## Learning objectives

At the end of this chapter the reader should be able to:

- describe the main phases of the menstrual cycle and the roles of the various hormones
- explain the usefulness of the negative feedback actions of the sex hormones regarding the design of the oral contraceptive pill
- list the clinical uses of GnRH, its synthetic analogues and the gonadotrophins
- describe the uses of inhibitors of gonadotrophin release such as danazol and of estrogen receptor antagonists such as clomifene
- list the three main estrogens and the names of some synthetic estrogens
- list the therapeutic uses of the estrogens
- list the different types of oral contraceptive Pill and a few examples of each
- explain the mechanisms of action and administration of the different types of oral contraceptives
- describe the beneficial and reported adverse effects and the controversies surrounding the use of oral contraceptives
- describe the symptoms of menopause, the types of preparations used for HRT and how they are used
- understand the obstetric use and risks associated with the use of prostaglandins, ergometrine and oxytocin
- list the drugs now used for pregnancy termination
- explain what tocolytic agents are
- describe the treatments for menorrhagia and dysmenorrhoea
- describe the premenstrual syndrome (PMS) and its symptoms
- explain how the nurse can help the patient cope with severe PMS
- describe the use of testosterone and synthetic analogues in the treatment of carcinoma of the breast
- give an account of the treatment of male erectile dysfunction (impotence)

## THE FEMALE SEX HORMONES

It is important to understand the hormonal background of the normal menstrual cycle and of pregnancy before considering the individual hormones.

## THE MENSTRUAL CYCLE

The primary purpose of the menstrual cycle is to grow an ovarian follicle and its enclosed ovum to a point when the ovum is released from the follicle and is ready to be fertilized, while at the same time preparing the female reproductive tract for the entry of the male sperm and for the implantation of the fertilized egg into the inner wall or endometrium. The critical event is the explosive rupture of the follicle at mid-cycle and the release of the ovum into the fallopian tubes where the egg will be fertilized by one of the spermatozoa if these are present. The fertilized egg will travel down to the uterus, dividing as it goes, where it will implant itself in the endometrium of the uterus. If the ovum is not fertilized and implantation does not occur, progesterone secretion stops and this may be one of the triggers for menstruation. The entire process is superbly orchestrated by the combined and synchronized actions of hormones from the brain, the anterior pituitary and from the ovary itself.

### Hormonal control of the menstrual cycle

This is facilitated by:

- a hypothalamic hormone: gonadotrophin-releasing hormone (GnRH)
- anterior pituitary gonadotrophins: follicle-stimulating hormone (FSH) and luteinizing hormone (LH)
- ovarian sex hormones: estradiol-17β and progesterone.

The menstrual cycle and ovulation are made possible through the operation of feedback systems involving the hypothalamus, anterior pituitary and the sex hormones estradiol-17β and progesterone, which are released by the ovarian follicle and corpus luteum, respectively. The feedback systems are similar in principle to those that govern the secretion of thyroid hormone and cortisol in that hormones act on the pituitary and the hypothalamus to suppress the release of hormones that cause sex hormone release from the gonads. They differ from systems that control, for example, thyroxine release, in that there are also positive feedback effects at the level of the pituitary and the hypothalamus in operation to cause more release of sex hormones at critical times of the menstrual cycle. The menstrual cycle has three main components: the **proliferative** phase, the **luteal** phase and **menstruation**.

## Proliferative phase of the cycle

In primates, including humans, the hypothalamus synthesizes and once every 60–90 minutes releases into the pituitary portal system a peptide called gonadotrophin-releasing hormone or GnRH (see also p. 172). This intermittent release of GnRH is called a 'pulsatile' release. GnRH acts on anterior pituitary cells called gonadotrophs, causing them to release FSH into the general circulation. In the ovary, FSH promotes the growth of the follicles. Each follicle contains an ovum, and for some reason, one follicle (and sometimes two follicles) develops faster than the other and it becomes the Graafian follicle, and the other follicles degenerate. The Graafian follicle synthesizes the powerful estrogenic hormone estradiol, which is released into the general circulation. Another two estrogenic hormones released into the circulation are estrone and estriol.

As the Graafian follicle matures, it releases more and more estradiol-17β into the circulation. Estradiol travels throughout the body where it works busily to prepare the reproductive tract for the coming ovulation:

- In the uterus it causes the regeneration of the endometrium or inner lining of the uterus.
- In the anterior pituitary, though a negative feedback effect, it prevents GnRH from causing a release of LH from gonadotroph cells, thus preventing LH from reaching the follicle before the follicle is ready to be ruptured.
- Estradiol works to prepare the gonadotrophs of the anterior pituitary so that they become more sensitive to hypothalamic GnRH.
- Another important job of estradiol is to cause a large increase in the concentration of progesterone receptors in the endometrium, anterior pituitary and hypothalamus. This is done to prepare these tissues for the rise in progesterone secretion that will occur after ovulation. This period before ovulation is called the follicular or proliferative phase of the cycle.

## Ovulation

Ovulation occurs about halfway through the normal 28-day menstrual cycle due to a mid-cycle explosive discharge of luteinizing hormone (LH) from the anterior pituitary. This occurs because estradiol has made the anterior pituitary gonadotrophs exquisitely sensitive to hypothalamic GnRH. In addition, for some unknown reason, the powerful negative feedback effect of estradiol on LH release is overcome. This LH surge causes the rapid swelling and rupture of the follicle and the egg is released. The ruptured follicle now becomes the corpus luteum (Latin for yellow body). Knowledge of these events during the menstrual cycle has made it possible to advise on how to optimize the chances of falling pregnant.

## The luteal phase

The part of the cycle following ovulation is called the luteal phase. The corpus luteum produces the hormone progesterone, which has a number of critical actions:

- progesterone causes further thickening of the endometrium through the build-up of glands and laying down of glycogen; this is called a secretory endometrium
- progesterone exerts a negative feedback effect on the anterior pituitary, suppressing the release of LH
- the hormone, perhaps by an action on the hypothalamus, causes an increase in body temperature of about 0.5°C, its so-called thermogenic effect
- progesterone is responsible for some water and salt retention and is mildly anabolic
- progesterone ensures that any incoming sperm will find a hostile environment by making the cervical mucus more viscid and less alkaline.

The endometrium now passes into what is called its secretory phase. If implantation of the fertilized ovum does not occur, the corpus luteum regresses and the superficial part of the endometrium breaks down and is discharged as the menstrual flow (Fig. 17.1).

## Conception

It is not always easy for couples to conceive, and the information available about the menstrual cycle enables the nurse to give advice. It is most important to ascertain when ovulation occurs. This can be done by taking the temperature throughout the cycle. As stated above, the temperature rises after ovulation by about 0.5° due to the thermogenic action of progesterone. Couples should have intercourse anywhere from 4–5 days before ovulation to 24 hours afterwards, with the best chances of conception if intercourse is within the time window of 24 hours before or after ovulation. The figures arrived at above are based mainly on the fact that spermatozoa live

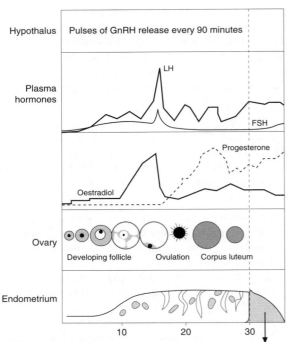

**Hypothalus** — Pulses of GnRH release every 90 minutes

**Plasma hormones** — LH, FSH

Progesterone

Oestradiol

**Ovary** — Developing follicle, Ovulation, Corpus luteum

**Endometrium**

10  20  30

**Figure 17.1** Events of the 'average' menstrual cycle.

up to 72 hours after entry into the female reproductive tract. The most fertile days for a woman with the 28-day cycle are days 12–18, with ovulation occurring on day 14.

## Pregnancy

If a fertilized ovum is implanted in the uterus the corpus luteum does not immediately regress, but continues to produce its hormones. This function is eventually taken over by the placenta. Throughout pregnancy large quantities of progesterone and estrogens are produced by the placenta, and can be recovered from the urine. The human placenta produces a gonadotrophic hormone called chorionic gonadotrophin during the early months of pregnancy and its presence in the urine forms the basis of various tests for pregnancy. The placenta also produces large amounts of the estrogenic hormone estriol, and levels of estriol are used to monitor the growth of the fetus. The most important clinical monitoring aid for fetal development, however, is through the use of ultrasound.

Just before parturition the production of progesterone ceases and this may be concerned with the start of labour.

The reader will appreciate that knowledge of the various negative feedback mechanisms governing LH

and FSH release can and has provided the rationale for the design of the oral contraceptives (see below).

## THE MALE SEX HORMONES

The hypothalamus of the postpubertal male puts out its regular pulsatile dose of GnRH and in response the anterior pituitary puts out FSH and LH. FSH promotes the development of the spermatozoa and LH promotes the production of testosterone by the interstitial Leydig cells of the testis. Testosterone exerts androgenic and anabolic effects (see below) and also has a negative feedback effect on LH secretion from the anterior pituitary, thus regulating its own production in the testis.

## CLINICAL USE OF GnRH ANALOGUES

GnRH is a strange hormone. It is a peptide, and if it is administered to the pituitary in pulsatile fashion it ensures normal anterior pituitary function and continued fertility. If GnRH for some reason is not produced infertility results. If, on the other hand, the pituitary receives a *continuous* exposure to GnRH it actually shuts down gonadotrophin production by the anterior pituitary cells. These phenomena have been exploited either to restore fertility or to prevent sex hormone production by the gonads. GnRH has been prepared synthetically and more stable and powerful analogues introduced.

### Synthetic GnRH and GnRH analogues

These comprise:

- **gonadorelin**, which is synthetic GnRH
- **buserelin**
- **goserelin**
- **leuprorelin**
- **nafarelin**, which is about 200 times more powerful than GnRH.

The last four drugs are synthetic analogues of gonadorelin. An analogue of a hormone is a synthetic compound with a (usually) slightly modified chemical structure but the same biological actions. The analogues mentioned above all act on the GnRH receptors on anterior pituitary cells and are therefore also called *agonists*.

### Therapeutic uses

Gonadorelin is used to induce ovulation in some cases of infertility. It is given as a pulsed injection every 90 minutes using a miniaturized pump.

## GnRH analogues

GnRH analogues are usually given as subcutaneous, long-acting implants. They initially increase the release of gonadotrophins, followed by a falling off of gonadotrophin secretion due to pituitary desensitization. This results in decreased activity of the male and female gonads and reduced secretion of the sex hormones. GnRH analogues are used for the treatment of severe cases of endometriosis and carcinoma of the prostate. The aim is to shut down the production of the sex hormones, which aggravate both conditions. They are also used together with iron supplements to treat anaemia due to uterine fibroids.

---

### Safety note

When these GnRH analogues were first introduced and implanted into men with carcinoma of the prostate, the initial stimulus to gonadotrophin release caused a sometimes-fatal acceleration of the carcinoma due to increased testosterone production. To counteract this, patients are also treated with a drug such as **cyproterone acetate** (see below), which blocks the action of androgens on their receptors.

---

## CLINICAL USE OF GONADOTROPHINS AND ANTAGONISTS

These comprise:

- FSH
- human chorionic gonadotrophin (HCG)
- human menopausal gonadotrophin (HMG: FSH + HCG)
- clomifene
- danazol
- gestrinone

These hormones and synthetic compounds are used therapeutically and will be considered in detail (Fig. 17.2).

### FSH and LH

FSH is available as **urofollitropin** and as **follitropin alpha** and **beta**. It is extracted from the urine of postmenopausal women. In the female it causes ripening of the ovarian follicles and the production of estrogen, and in the male it is necessary for the production of spermatozoa. It is given by injection. Pituitary LH is not used, but its actions are available as HCG. It is extracted from the urine of pregnant women. In the female it produces the corpus luteum and in the male it stimulates the interstitial cells of the testis to produce androgens. It is given by injection.

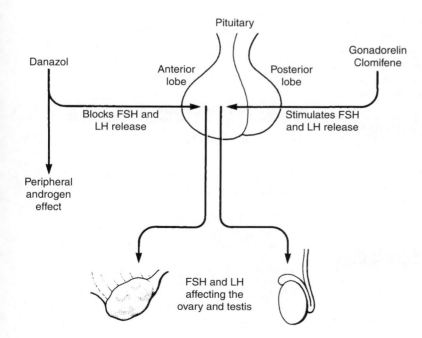

**Figure 17.2**    Drugs modifying the release of follicle-stimulating hormone (FSH) and luteinizing hormone (LH) and thus modifying gonadal activity.

In **female infertility**, FSH and HCG are given by injection to induce normal ovarian function. FSH is given first to produce an ovarian follicle, followed by HCG to induce ovulation, or they may be given together as HMG. They will only be successful if infertility is due to lack of normally secreted gonadotrophins and not if there is primary ovarian failure.

## Clomifene and cyclofenil

Clomifene is a synthetic compound that blocks the action of estradiol on its receptors (see more below). This releases the anterior pituitary from estradiol's negative feedback effects, and large amounts of LH and FSH are released. Clomifene stimulates increased secretion of gonadotrophins and is used in the treatment of **infertility due to failure of ovulation**. It is given daily for 5 days early in the menstrual cycle. It may be so successful that it results in twins, but multiple pregnancies can be avoided by careful dosing. Adverse effects include flushing, headaches, nausea, weight gain and visual disturbances.

## Danazol and gestrinone

Danazol and gestrinone inhibit both GnRH and gonadotrophin release and are used to treat endometriosis and various benign breast disorders: for example, **cyclical breast pain**. This is due to swelling and tenderness of the breasts, which occurs during the second half of the menstrual cycle and is associated with the corpus luteum. If the symptoms are severe, danazol is effective in prevention, but its adverse effects are troublesome. The adverse effects reflect the fact that these compounds are androgen derivatives and cause abnormal hair growth, greasy skin, acne, fluid retention, weight gain and nausea.

### Nursing point

Patients may ask about gamolenic acid, which is extracted from evening primrose oil; this may decrease the sensitivity of the breasts to hormones and may thus also be effective, but relief is delayed for about 3 months.

### Summary

- GnRH analogues are used to treat endometriosis and prostatic carcinoma

- When GnRH is started in patients with prostate carcinoma, they should take an androgen receptor blocker as well
- FSH and HCG (or HMG) will be successful in treating infertility only if infertility is caused by a lack of normally secreted gonadotrophins
- Clomifene is used to treat infertility due to failure of ovulation and can cause multiple births
- Danazol and gestrinone are used to treat cyclical breast pain, although danazol has unpleasant side-effects

## THE ESTROGENS

As mentioned above, **estradiol** is the main female sex hormone and the most potent. **Estrone** is also a female sex hormone but is shorter acting. **Estriol** is produced in large amounts during pregnancy, but its function is obscure.

### THERAPEUTIC USE OF ESTROGENS

The estrogens comprise **natural estrogens** and **synthetic estrogens** (Table 17.1). Estradiol-17β is the principal estrogen secreted by the ovary, but there are a number of estrogens that are used therapeutically. Estrogens are used for:

- oral contraception
- hormone replacement therapy
- (rarely) controlling cancer of the prostate and breast
- atrophic vaginitis (as a cream).

## ORAL CONTRACEPTION

There are two main types of oral contraceptive pill (the Pill):

- the combined oral contraceptive pill
- the progestogen-only pill.

**Table 17.1** Estrogens

| Natural estrogens | Synthetic estrogens |
|---|---|
| Estradiol-17β | Ethinylestradiol |
| Estrone | Mestranol |
| Estriol | Dienestrol[a] |

[a] Used topically in the vagina.

# COMBINED ORAL CONTRACEPTIVE PILL

The combined oral contraceptive pill is very widely used and is the most effective method of preventing conception. It is a combination of an estrogen and a progestogen and acts in several ways. The estrogens used are ethinylestradiol or mestranol (a few). The progestogens used are desogestrel, gestodene, ethynodiol, levonorgestrel, or norethisterone.

## Mechanism of action

- The estrogen inhibits the release of FSH by a negative feedback effect, thus inhibiting follicular development.
- The progestogen inhibits the release of LH, so that ovulation cannot occur. Together, the two chemicals render the endometrium hostile to implantation.
- Both chemicals may upset the coordinated contractions of the fallopian tubes, uterus and cervix.

Usually the composition of the pill is unaltered throughout the full monthly course, but there are a few preparations in which pills of varying composition are given sequentially: namely, the biphasic and triphasic preparations. Of the many preparations now available the most effective and widely used are those in which both an estrogen and a progestogen are given throughout the course, with a failure rate of less than 0.5 per 100 women years. Table 17.2 shows the estrogen and progestogen content of some of the preparations in use.

## Using the combined pill

- It is usual to start with the lowest-dose formulation because the risk of thrombosis (see later) is related to the estrogen content. Preparations containing 20–35 micrograms of ethinylestradiol are usually prescribed.
- The Pill is started on the first day of the menstrual cycle (first day of bleeding) and continued for 21 days, then stopped for 7 days during which bleeding occurs. The regime is then repeated.
- The Pill must be taken regularly. If the dose is taken 12 hours late, other contraceptive precautions should be used for the next 7 days.
- If a low-dose combination Pill fails to control the cycle after 3 months, alternatives such as triphasic preparations should be tried.

- After childbirth, the Pill should be started 3 weeks postpartum if the woman is not breast-feeding. If she is breast-feeding a progestogen-only Pill or a different method of contraception is advised.

Table 17.2    Oral contraceptives

| Progestogen only | | | |
|---|---|---|---|
| Norethisterone | Micronor | 350 micrograms | oral |
| Levonorgestrel | Microval | 30 micrograms | |
| Medroxyprogesterone | | 150 mg | depot |
| Norethisterone | | 200 mg | |

| Combined preparations | | |
|---|---|---|
| | Estrogen micrograms | Progestogen micrograms |
| *Ethinylestradiol + norethisterone* | | |
| Loestrin 20 | 20 | 1000 |
| Ovysmen | 35 | 500 |
| Brevinor | 35 | 500 |
| Norimin | 35 | 1000 |
| *Ethinylestradiol + levonorgestrel* | | |
| Microgynon 30 | 30 | 150 |
| Ovranette | 30 | 150 |
| Eugynon 30 | 30 | 250 |
| Ovran 30 | 30 | 250 |
| Ovran | 50 | 250 |
| *Ethinylestradiol + desogestrel* | | |
| Mercilon | 20 | 150 |
| Marvelon | 30 | 150 |
| *Ethinylestradiol + gestodene* | | |
| Femodene | 30 | 75 |
| Minulet | 30 | 75 |
| *Ethinylestradiol + norgestimate* | | |
| Cilest | 35 | 250 |

| Triphasic preparations | | | |
|---|---|---|---|
| *Ethinylestradiol + norethisterone* | | | |
| Trinovum | (7 days) | 35 | 500 |
| | (7 days) | 35 | 750 |
| | (7 days) | 35 | 1000 |
| *Ethinylestradiol + levonorgestrel* | | | |
| Trinordiol | (6 days) | 30 | 50 |
| | (5 days) | 40 | 75 |
| | (10 days) | 30 | 125 |
| Logynon | (6 days) | 30 | 50 |
| | (5 days) | 40 | 75 |
| | (10 days) | 30 | 125 |
| *Ethinylestradiol + gestodene* | | | |
| Triadene | (6 days) | 30 | 50 |
| Tri-minulet | (5 days) | 40 | 70 |
| | (10 days) | 30 | 100 |

Nurses working in family planning clinics and health centres have an important role in teaching women about taking oral contraceptives and allaying anxieties. If concerned, women should be advised to seek advice from specially trained nurses or their doctor. Stopping the Pill may result in an unplanned pregnancy. Women should be encouraged to express any dissatisfaction they may have so that they do not stop the Pill suddenly with unfortunate consequences.

## Beneficial effects of the combined contraceptive pill

There is a reduced risk or incidence of:

- intermenstrual bleeding
- amenorrhoea
- iron deficiency
- irregular periods
- anaemia
- premenstrual tension
- benign breast disease
- uterine fibroids
- functional ovarian cysts
- thyroid disease
- unwanted pregnancy.

Some authorities (see Baird & Glasier 1993) regard the combined oral contraceptive pill as safe for most women during their reproductive years. Women who smoke or suffer from obesity or hypertension do have a slightly higher risk of adverse effects (see more below).

## Reported adverse effects and unanswered questions about the combined Pill

- Weight gain due to anabolic effects and fluid retention
- Temporary amenorrhoea after stopping the Pill
- Dizziness, flushing, nausea, irritability and depression
- Gastrointestinal upsets
- Acne and skin pigmentation (rare)
- Gallstones
- Cardiovascular problems
- Thrombosis
- Delayed conception in older women
- Cancer?

**Nausea.**   It is probably related to the estrogen dosage and can usually be relieved by changing to a preparation with less estrogen.

**Weight gain.**   Although weight gain doesn't often happen, if it does, it usually settles after a few cycles.

**Thrombosis.**   There is now clear evidence that taking oral contraceptives carries a slightly increased risk of venous and cerebral thrombosis. In addition, there is a slightly increased risk of cerebral arterial disease. The overall mortality is about 2 per 100 000. Older women who smoke heavily are especially at risk from thromboembolic complications. Heavy smokers in the 40–44 age group have an excess mortality of 54 per 100 000 women, and they should therefore use some other form of contraception. Thrombosis is believed to be due to the estrogen in the Pill. For this reason the estrogen content of these preparations is kept as low as possible.

The associated arterial disease is due to the progestogen fraction of the Pill, which alters the blood lipids. The new progestogens desogestrel and gestodene are less likely to cause changes in plasma lipids and, therefore, might be expected to reduce the risk of vascular disease (e.g. coronary thrombosis and strokes). However, evidence has emerged that they may actually increase the incidence of venous thrombosis in the legs and, thus, the risk of pulmonary embolism.

The incidence of venous thrombosis is approximately:

- 5 per 100 000 women per year – no contraceptive
- 15 per 100 000 women per year – with older progestogens
- 25 per 100 000 women per year – with desogestrel or gestodene (third-generation Pill)
- 60 per 100 000 women per year – in pregnancy.

In view of this very small risk of thrombosis with the third-generation Pill, which is considerably less than that of pregnancy, they can be prescribed after a discussion with the patient. However, there is a case for avoiding contraceptives containing desogestrel or gestodene in those who are overweight, immobile or have a history of thrombosis.

Occasionally patients taking oral contraceptives develop hypertension. This is common in older women, but usually improves on stopping the Pill.

**Breast cancer.**   Many studies have been undertaken to determine whether oral contraceptives could cause cancer and there are conflicting reports. There have been reports that in those who are taking the Pill there may be a slightly increased risk of breast cancer. This appeared to be related to the age at which it is stopped rather than to the duration of exposure. At the time of writing, a study of over 9000 woman in the United States gives results suggesting that current or former use of oral contraceptives is not associated with an increased risk of breast cancer (Editorial 2002a).

**Cancer of the cervix.**   There is some evidence that cancer of the cervix is more common in those taking oral contraceptives. There are many complicating factors and the case is not proven. However, women who have taken oral contraceptives for more than 5 years should have an annual cervical smear.

> **Safety note**
>
> In the UK women are advised to have cervical smears every 3 years.

**Cancer of the ovary and uterus.**   The use of oral contraceptives reduces the risk of endometrial and ovarian cancer.

Other side-effects, real or imaginary, of oral contraception must be set against the fact that many women feel better while taking these preparations, and also the potential reduction in therapeutic termination and unwanted and uncared-for children.

Ten years after discontinuation of the Pill there appear to be no long-term ill effects.

> **Nursing point**
>
> It is important to point out that many different Pills are available, and it is usually possible to find one that suits a potential user.

## Drugs that interfere with oral contraceptives

Certain drugs when taken with oral contraceptives will increase the rate of breakdown of the estrogen they contain and thus decrease their efficiency and lead to unwanted pregnancy. The most troublesome drugs in this respect are the antibiotics, because they are so widely prescribed, and the prescriber should check whether the patient is taking any other drugs when prescribing the Pill. Other drugs such as phenobarbital, carbamazepine, phenytoin, isoniazid and griseofulvin have also been implicated. In addition, broad-spectrum antibiotics may interfere with estrogen absorption. The occurrence of breakthrough bleeding may give a warning that the contraceptive is ineffective. If this occurs, a preparation containing 50 micrograms of estrogen can be tried or an alternative contraceptive method used. The Pill reduces the efficacy of antihypertensive treatment.

## PROGESTOGEN-ONLY PILL

It is also possible to give preparations which only contain a progestogen, but although they impair fertility, they only prevent ovulation in about half the menstrual cycles so are less efficient as contraceptives. If used correctly, the combined pill provides the most effective contraceptive available and failure rarely occurs.

This method, which inhibits ovulation and changes the character of the cervical mucus, is less 'safe' than the combined pill, but has virtually no risk of thrombotic disease (see above) and may be preferred in older women or those at special risk from thrombosis. The Pill is started on day 1 and taken at the same time each day throughout the cycle with no break.

Progestogens can also be given as depot injections lasting 2–3 months or as capsules containing a progestogen, which is slowly released (Norplant). These capsules are inserted into the upper arm under a local anaesthetic and are effective for about 5 years. If side-effects occur, the implants can easily be removed.

The main adverse effects of the progestogen-only Pill are

- Amenorrhoea, which is common in women taking this form of the Pill. It is essential to teach them the early signs and symptoms of pregnancy to avoid anxiety.
- Spotting – slight blood loss – may occur through much of the cycle.

### Intra–uterine progestogen coil

This releases a progestogen, levonorgestrel, directly into the uterine cavity, and is used as a contraceptive and to treat primary menorrhagia (abnormally heavy bleeding at menstruation). The effects are essentially local in the uterus to prevent endometrial proliferation and to thicken the cervical mucus. The device itself may contribute to the contraceptive effect.

### Contraindications to the use of oral contraceptives

Contraindications include:

- thromboembolic disease, past or present
- carcinoma of the breast or uterus
- severe liver disease or recent viral hepatitis, previous cholestatic jaundice of pregnancy

- pregnancy
- hypertension (diastolic pressure >100 mmHg)
- porphyria
- herpes gestationis
- focal migraine.

The reader is referred to the *British National Formulary* (*BNF*) for a full list of contraindications. In addition to these contraindications, the following may be made worse:

- migraine
- epilepsy
- depression.

## Postcoital contraception (Yuzpe method)

The risk of pregnancy after unprotected sexual intercourse is about 1:20. It is possible to reduce the risk of pregnancy by using the oral contraceptive as a 'morning after' pill. Two tablets of *Schering PC 4*, a high-estrogen preparation, are taken immediately and repeated after 12 hours. These measures must be instituted within 72 hours of intercourse. Nausea may be a problem. Postcoital contraception can be obtained in family planning clinics and from pharmacies without the need for a prescription.

The patient should be told that a barrier method of contraception will be required until the next period. An alternative is to give levonorgestrel (a progestogen). It is usually effective if given up to 48 hours after exposure. Readers are referred to the *BNF* for dosage and use.

## Summary

- The combined Pill is the most effective oral contraceptive if taken correctly.
- Always start with the lowest-dose formulation of the combined Pill.
- If a dose of the Pill is 12 taken hours late, other precautions should be taken for 7 days.
- If a low combination pill fails to control the cycle by 3 months, try, for example, a triphasic Pill.
- After childbirth, start the Pill 3 weeks postpartum if not breast-feeding; if breast-feeding, use a progestogen-only Pill or use alternative contraceptive methods.
- Patients about to start on the Pill should first be fully briefed on possible adverse effects, such as weight gain and about the risks and unanswered questions, especially about thrombosis.

- There may be a case for avoiding oral contraceptives that contain desogestrel or gestodene in patients who are overweight, immobile or who have a history of thrombosis.
- Women who have taken oral contraceptives for more than 5 years should have annual cervical smears.
- There is evidence that taking oral contraceptives reduces the risk of endometrial and ovarian cancer.
- Oral contraceptives reduce the efficacy of antihypertensive treatment, and their potency may be reduced by drugs such as some broad-spectrum antibiotics that reduce the absorption of estrogens. Drugs such as phenobarbital, carbamazepine, isoniazid, griseofulvin, phenytoin and rifampicin (the most troublesome in this respect) enhance the breakdown of estrogens by the liver.
- The occurrence of breakthrough bleeding may give a warning that an oral contraceptive is ineffective and it may be necessary to use a Pill that contains more estrogen.
- The progestogen-only Pill is not as efficient as the combined Pill, but carries virtually no risk of thrombotic disease.
- Progestogen-only contraceptives can be given as depot injections that are effective for about 5 years.
- Amenorrhoea (the absence or stopping of menstrual periods) is common with the progestogen-only Pill and women should be taught the early signs and symptoms of pregnancy to avoid anxiety.
- Migraine, epilepsy and depression may be worsened if oral contraceptives are used.

## HORMONE REPLACEMENT THERAPY (HRT)

The menopause commences with a woman's last menstrual period: she is considered to be post-menopausal 1 year after her last menstrual period. Nevertheless, women are advised to take contraceptive precautions for at least 1 year after menstruation ceases.

The menopause may be associated with a number of disorders.

## MENOPAUSAL SYMPTOMS

Menopausal symptoms fall into two groups:

- symptoms definitely due to estrogen deficiency
- symptoms, often emotional, whose aetiology is unknown but may be caused by estrogen loss.

Symptoms due to estrogen deficiency respond to HRT with an estrogen, but in the other symptoms the response is variable.

### Symptoms due to estrogen deficiency

These symptoms comprise:

- atrophy of the uterus
- dryness of the vagina, which may cause dyspareunia (difficult or painful sexual intercourse for a woman)
- osteoporosis
- hot flushes.

**Osteoporosis.**    Loss of protein from bone, with subsequent risk of fracture, is a serious problem in postmenopausal women. Estrogen treatment is possibly the most effective way of preventing this. In addition, HRT appears to give some protection against coronary artery disease, stroke and, possibly, Alzheimer's disease. The treatment of osteoporosis is dealt with more fully in Chapter 14, p. 187.

**Hot flushes.**    Their cause is unknown, but may be due to the rise in circulating LH. They respond to treatment with estrogen, which brings LH levels back down again.

## AIM OF HORMONE REPLACEMENT THERAPY

The aim of HRT is to replace the sex hormones lost due to cessation of ovarian function at menopause, and the approach favoured is to restore, approximately, the chemical pattern of hormone presence in blood during the menstrual cycle of younger years.

## PREPARATIONS

HRT preparations comprise:

- estrogen–progestogen combinations
- estrogen patches
- conjugated estrogens
- raloxifene
- tibolone.

Most patients receiving HRT will have an intact uterus. The unopposed action of estrogens stimulates the endometrium and may ultimately cause a carcinoma of the uterus. To prevent this happening, the **estrogen is combined with a progestogen** to mimic the normal menstrual cycle, with regular shedding of the endometrium. A monthly course consists of an estrogen given daily and a progestogen for the last 10–14 days of the cycle. Withdrawal bleeding may occur. A convenient preparation is *Prempak C* in which an estrogen is given throughout the cycle and a progestogen (norgestrel) for the last 12 days. It is presented in a specially designed pack to avoid confusion. Other similar preparations are available.

Estrogens can also be given as a **patch** applied to the skin. The patch available in the UK contains estradiol, which diffuses through the skin and is effective for 3–4 days when the patch is replaced. Cyclical progestogen treatment causing monthly bleeding is still required. If the patient has had a hysterectomy the progestogen is not needed and replacement can be with an estrogen alone, e.g. **conjugated estrogens** (Premarin).

**Tibolone** is a synthetic androgenic hormone that will control postmenopausal symptoms and limit osteoporosis without stimulating the endometrium, and thus eliminate the risk of causing uterine cancer. There is therefore no need for a progestogen and no monthly bleeding. Tibolone may, however, have the androgenic side-effects such as hirsutism that one might expect from such a preparation.

**Raloxifene** has effects similar to estrogens on blood and lipids, but blocks estrogen action on the breast and uterus. It reduces osteoporosis and its use is not associated with menstrual bleeding. Its effect on breast cancer and heart disease is not known. It may cause hot flushes, and there is an increased risk of thrombosis.

## FACTORS TO CONSIDER WHEN PRESCRIBING HORMONE REPLACEMENT THERAPY

### Symptoms to be treated

On balance, HRT is indicated in postmenopausal women if they have symptoms (vaginitis, flushing) or are at special risk of osteoporosis or cardiovascular disease. Before starting treatment a full examination is necessary to exclude cancer, gynaecological abnormalities and thrombotic disease, which may be made worse by HRT, and the patient should be given a full explanation of the implications of the treatment. Nurses play an important role here.

## Duration of treatment

Duration of treatment depends on the therapeutic objectives. To relieve menopausal symptoms, 5 years is usually adequate. To prevent arterial disease, stroke and osteoporosis, lifelong treatment might be desirable, but 10 years is perhaps more practical because of the slight risk of breast cancer which is related to the duration of treatment. For preventing osteoporosis, HRT may be delayed, as it is still effective late in life. There are now serious concerns over use for longer than 5 years.

## Risks

Many practitioners consider that most women should use HRT, provided there are no contraindications. However, possible problems, which must be weighed against the benefits are:

- there may be a slightly increased risk of carcinoma of the breast, particularly in older women and those taking hormones for more than 5 years
- there is a slight risk of venous thrombosis
- HRT appears not to offer protection against heart attacks, although it appears to be safe in heart disease (Editorial 2002b).

## ADVERSE EFFECTS OF HORMONE REPLACEMENT THERAPY

Adverse effects include nausea, weight gain, headache and fluid retention. Breast swelling may occur early in treatment but usually subsides within 3 months.

### Summary

- If a woman has had a hysterectomy, a progestogen is not needed for HRT, and a preparation such as *Premarin* that contains only estrogens may be used
- There is evidence for an increased risk of thrombosis with raloxifene
- HRT is indicated in postmenopausal women who have an increased risk of osteoporosis

- Before starting HRT treatment, there must be a full examination to exclude cancer, gynaecological abnormalities or thrombotic disease and patients must be given a full explanation of the implications of the treatment
- HRT treatment is usually adequate to relieve menopausal symptoms
- Lifelong treatment may be desirable to prevent stroke, arterial disease and osteoporosis, although 10 years may be more practical because of the slight risk of breast cancer
- HRT treatment may be delayed for prevention of osteoporosis as it is still effective late in life
- Recent evidence suggests that HRT appears not to offer protection against heart attacks

## USES OF ESTROGENS IN CANCER

Estrogens are more usually associated with a worsening of breast cancer, but they have been used with some success for the treatment of two types of neoplasm: advanced breast cancer and prostate cancer.

A proportion of patients with **advanced carcinoma of the breast** obtain temporary, but sometimes striking remission of their disease with estrogens, which are most successful in postmenopausal patients.

In **carcinoma of the prostate** estrogens act by suppressing the production of male hormone, which stimulates the neoplasm. Large doses are required. Diethylstilbestrol, a synthetic estrogen, is given by mouth or pellets of the hormone may be implanted subcutaneously. Some patients report nausea and hypertrophy of the breasts with pigmentation of the nipple. Fluid retention may be troublesome and there is an increased risk of venous thrombosis. An alternative is cyproterone, which directly blocks the action of androgens on the prostate or gonadorelin analogues (see also p. 214), which reduce androgen secretion.

## TOPICAL USE OF ESTROGENS

Estrogens can also be applied locally. They are used in atrophic vaginitis, which occurs in postmenopausal women due to estrogen deficiency. Dienestrol cream is applied daily for 1 week and then reduced.

## DRUGS THAT AFFECT UTERINE SMOOTH MUSCLE

These comprise:

- the prostaglandins
- ergometrine
- oxytocin
- syntometrine.

## THE PROSTAGLANDINS

These interesting substances are formed by most cells of the body and are released as a result of a number of stimuli. They usually produce their effects locally rather than at distant sites in the body, and many of them are removed from the circulation when they pass through the lung.

### Prostaglandins and pathology

Prostaglandins have been implicated in a number of pathological processes.

**Inflammation.** Prostaglandins of the E series are the mediators of some of the changes (swelling, redness and pain) seen in inflammation. This is important, since drugs such as aspirin and other NSAIDs, which block the production of prostaglandins, reduce the symptoms and signs of inflammation.

**Thrombosis.** Two types of prostaglandins or chemically related compounds appear to be involved in thrombosis. Thromboxanes stimulate clumping of platelets and constriction of blood vessels and thus encourage thrombosis, whereas prostacyclin has the reverse effect. It seems possible therefore that increasing the availability of prostacyclin and decreasing that of thromboxanes would guard against thrombosis, and a great deal of research is being done in an attempt to achieve this effect.

**Effects on uterine muscle.** Prostaglandins cause contraction of the uterine muscle and are concerned with both menstruation and childbirth. Prostaglandins are responsible for much of the pain associated with dysmenorrhoea. Prostaglandin $E_2$ can be used to induce labour or terminate pregnancy by causing the uterus to contract (see later).

**Effects on the stomach.** Prostaglandins increase mucous secretion by the cells lining the stomach and thus protect the mucosa against ulcer formation.

### Therapeutic uses of prostaglandins

**Dinoprostone** (prostaglandin $E_2$) is used to terminate pregnancy and to induce labour. It can be given by extra-amniotic injection to terminate pregnancy or by vaginal tablets or gel to induce labour.

> **Safety note**
>
> Dinoprostone increases the effects of oxytocin and these drugs should never be given together. The bladder should be emptied before insertion and the patient should lie down for 15 minutes after insertion.

**Gemeprost** (prostaglandin $E_1$ analogue) pessaries are inserted into the vagina to soften the cervix and thus facilitate abortion during the first 2 months of pregnancy. Adverse effects include nausea, vomiting, diarrhoea, headache and fever.

**Carboprost** is given by intramuscular injection. It is used to treat postpartum haemorrhage when ergometrine and oxytocin have failed to control bleeding.

### ERGOMETRINE (see also the ergot alkaloids, Chapter 4, p. 57)

Ergometrine is rapidly absorbed either from the intestinal tract or from the site of injection. This is the chemical that was responsible for the spontaneous abortions suffered by those who ate contaminated rye. Its chief action is to cause contractions of the uterus. With small doses these contractions are rhythmic, but with larger doses they become very powerful and more or less continuous. They are brought about by a direct action of ergometrine on the uterine muscle. The uterus is especially sensitive to ergometrine at the time of childbirth. It has little effect on other smooth muscle throughout the body.

### Therapeutic use of ergometrine

Ergometrine is given after childbirth to cause the uterus to contract and thus prevent bleeding. It should not be given before delivery, even if the uterus is sluggish, as it may produce such powerful contractions that the uterus is ruptured, or the fetus asphyxiated. Increased contractions of the uterus are seen within 5 minutes of intramuscular injection.

### OXYTOCIN

Oxytocin (see also p. 176) is a hormone released from the posterior pituitary gland. It causes contraction of the muscle of the uterus. This effect is not marked until the later stages of pregnancy and at parturition, when extremely small amounts will cause powerful uterine contractions.

### Therapeutic use of oxytocin

Oxytocin is used to induce labour. For this purpose it is usual to use synthetic oxytocin (**Syntocinon**), for the naturally prepared oxytocin contains a small amount of vasopressin. The oxytocin is given by intravenous infusion in saline and the rate of infusion is regulated according to the response of the patient. There is a risk of rupture of the uterus with oxytocin and it should only be used to induce labour under expert supervision. Oxytocin is also used after delivery of the placenta to cause uterine contraction, but its effects are not as prolonged as those of ergometrine. For this reason it is sometimes combined with ergometrine as **Syntometrine** (see later). Whole posterior pituitary extract should not be used, because of its vasopressor effects.

### Adverse effects of oxytocin

In addition to producing powerful uterine contractions, oxytocin can cause a rise in blood pressure and water retention. It should not usually be combined with prostaglandins to induce labour.

## SYNTOMETRINE

Syntometrine is a mixture of ergometrine and oxytocin. It is given intramuscularly and combines the rapid action of oxytocin on the uterus with the prolonged contraction caused by ergometrine. It is commonly used after the expulsion of the placenta to prevent bleeding.

## TERMINATION OF PREGNANCY

The termination of pregnancy has possibly generated more medical interest and preoccupation than any other reproductive issue apart from fertility itself and has undoubtedly been responsible for many fatalities among pregnant girls and women. Today, however, thanks to modern drugs and other products, the procedure can be carried out safely under professional supervision.

Drugs used to terminate pregnancy in the first trimester are

- **mifepristone**
- **prostaglandins**.

Mifepristone blocks the action of progesterone at its receptors in the uterus. Most terminations of pregnancy are carried out in the first trimester.

- first 9 weeks: mifepristone, as above, or vacuum aspiration – both are equally effective.
- 9–13 weeks: vacuum aspiration; this may be preceded by the insertion of a gemeprost pessary to soften the cervix.

There is a risk of infection after termination. Prophylactic antibiotics can reduce this.

## TOCOLYTIC AGENTS (DRUGS INHIBITING UTERINE CONTRACTIONS)

Stimulation of $\beta_2$ receptors in uterine muscles will diminish uterine activity. The $\beta_2$ agonists **salbutamol**, **terbutaline** and **ritodrine** are sometimes used in the management of premature labour between 24 and 33 weeks of pregnancy and are usually given by intravenous infusion for this purpose. There is a real risk of fluid overload.

## MENORRHAGIA

Heavy bleeding during a period is very common and may sometimes be serious enough to require a hysterectomy. The majority of patients have no underlying pelvic disease but a significant proportion have a mild inherited bleeding disorder. It is believed to be due to a functional defect in the mechanism that normally controls uterine bleeding. **Mefenamic acid**, a weak NSAID, is widely used, with some success, to control pain and reduce bleeding.

**Tranexamic acid**, which inhibits the breakdown of fibrin, is more effective. It is given orally when bleeding has started and continued for 3–4 days. Like the progestogen coil it is useful in the treatment of menorrhagia. Adverse effects include nausea, vomiting and blurred vision. It is contraindicated in thromboembolic disease.

## DYSMENORRHOEA

Dysmenorrhoea can be primary or secondary.

Most women experience dysmenorrhoea at some time, but occasionally periods become so painful and heavy that they disrupt everyday life. Most women manage with a hot water bottle and mild analgesics. However, a nurse may be approached for

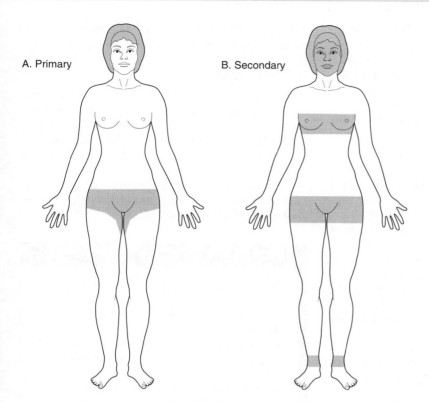

A. Primary

B. Secondary

**Figure 17.3** (A) Primary and (B) secondary sites of discomfort in primary and secondary dysmenorrhoea.

advice so the type of dysmenorrhoea must be established (Fig. 17.3).

## Primary dysmenorrhoea

Primary dysmenorrhoea is common in young women whose usual symptoms are low backache and colicky pain in the pelvic area. This is due to the cyclical release of prostaglandins in the uterus, leading to contraction of the uterine muscle and constriction of the arteries supplying the muscle, with consequent ischaemia. Other symptoms include nausea, vomiting, diarrhoea and faintness. NSAIDs e.g. **ibuprofen** or **mefenamic acid**, should give relief by inhibiting prostaglandin synthesis. Ideally, they should be taken after menstrual bleeding has commenced to avoid the ingestion of drugs by a possibly pregnant subject. If this fails, oral contraceptives (estrogen + progestogen) are frequently effective.

## Secondary dysmenorrhoea

Secondary dysmenorrhoea affects women in their late 20s and 30s, causing a dragging pain often preceded by headaches. As its name implies, this occurs in response to some pathological condition

**Table 17.3** Symptoms of premenstrual tension (PMS)

| Emotional symptoms | Physical symptoms |
|---|---|
| Depression | Headache |
| Tension | Breast swelling and discomfort |
| Crying | Bloating |
| Aggression | Backache |
| Failure to concentrate | |

(fibroids, endometriosis) and treatment is by removal of the cause.

## PREMENSTRUAL SYNDROME (PMS)

The cyclical appearance of a cluster of symptoms in the second half of the menstrual cycle which terminate abruptly with the onset of menstruation is known as the premenstrual tension syndrome (PMS). Although PMS is very common, only about 5% of women experience symptoms severe enough to disrupt their lives. The symptoms are legion and are both emotional and physical (Table 17.3).

The range of these symptoms suggests that there is more than one cause and, in keeping with this theory, women respond differently to prescribed treatments, but its relationship with the menstrual cycle indicates that it is probably related to the hormonal and metabolic changes which occur.

A selection of possible aetiological factors and treatments is given below:

- *Changes in water and salt balance*. Although feelings of bloating and swelling are frequent symptoms, there is some controversy over whether fluid retention actually occurs. Diuretics are often prescribed, but are rarely beneficial.
- *Elevated prolactin levels*. Prolactin is released from the anterior pituitary and stimulates lactation. When a woman is not lactating a hormone inhibitor suppresses prolactin secretion. Some women with PMS have raised prolactin levels. Bromocriptine, which inhibits prolactin release, has been found useful for some symptoms, especially breast discomfort, but adverse effects may be troublesome.
- *Diminished progesterone levels*. These have been suggested as an aetiological agent, but injection of progesterone or of a synthetic substitute has not been shown to be beneficial.
- *Changes in prostaglandin E₁ levels*. This appears important in hormone balance and it has been suggested that PMS is a manifestation of deficiency. Gamolenic acid (evening primrose oil) is converted into prostaglandin $E_1$ and, given as *Efamast*, it has been shown to be effective sometimes. Conversely, prostaglandin synthesis inhibition by mefenamic acid can improve headaches and aches and pains.
- *Brain neurotransmitters*. Attention is now directed to the relationship between ovarian hormones and neurotransmitters in the brain. It is thought that progesterone or, more probably one of its metabolites, interacts with the GABA or serotonin (5-HT) systems and a disorder of these interactions is responsible for PMS.
- *Diet*. Various dietary modifications have been tried. Fluctuation in blood glucose levels can be avoided by giving a high starch diet every 3 hours, which may relieve symptoms, but weight gain can be a problem. Pyridoxine has been used, but with high doses there is a danger of neuropathy.

In summary, there is no overall regime to control PMS. In patients with mild symptoms it is probably best to employ self-help measures combining symptomatic treatment and dietary modifications, or gamolenic acid can be tried. With more severe symptoms, fluoxetine, alprazolam, an oral contraceptive or goserelin may be used.

## Self-help measures

The nurse can do much to help the individual to gain insight into her problem. Keeping a diary of the menstrual cycle with daily accounts of the main symptoms and when they occur is useful. It can be used to predict the appearance of PMS in subsequent months, confirm a physical basis for the symptoms and exclude suggestions of neuroticism. It can also allow the patient to plan her life so that PMS does not clash with events such as holidays.

### Summary

- Dinoprostone and oxytocin should never be given together.
- Ergometrine should never be given before delivery.
- Oxytocin is not effective until the later stages of pregnancy, and is extremely potent at onset of labour.
- There is a risk of rupture of the uterus with oxytocin and it should be used with care.
- Oxytocin can cause a rise in blood pressure and water retention, particularly if it is used in the form of a pituitary extract, which could well contain vasopressin.
- Oxytocin should not usually be combined with prostaglandins to induce labour.
- Syntometrine is commonly used after expulsion of the fetus to prevent bleeding.
- The risk of infection increases as pregnancy progresses. The wide availability of 'home' pregnancy testing kits and the awareness of the importance of 'catching' the situation early enough for medical or surgical procedures means that septic abortion has become uncommon. If there is confusion over dates, then ultrasound should resolve this and appropriate action should be taken.

## MALE SEX HORMONES

### TESTOSTERONE

The interstitial cells of the testis produce the male hormone testosterone. It is responsible for the secondary male sex characteristics, including distribution of hair, deepening of the voice and enlargement of the penis and seminal vesicle. It can be isolated from the testis, but is usually prepared synthetically. Its synthesis and release from the testis is controlled by luteinizing hormone (LH; see p. 215). The actions of testosterone that virilize are called androgenic actions.

## Therapeutic use

Testosterone or synthetic analogues are used in the treatment of testicular hormone deficiency and carcinoma of the breast.

**Testicular hormone deficiency. Testosterone** is used in the treatment of testicular hormone deficiency. This may be of an unknown origin or due to injury or disease of the testis, or it may be secondary to lack of gonadotrophic hormone following pituitary gland disease. **Mesterolone**, which is similar to testosterone, is given orally. Unlike testosterone it does not cause jaundice or depress spermatogenesis. Esters of testosterone (*Sustanon*) can be given intramuscularly every 3 weeks and are released slowly from the injection site.

**Carcinoma of the breast.**    Testosterone is effective in about 30% of premenopausal patients with advanced carcinoma of the breast for relieving symptoms and causing temporary regression of secondary deposits. It does, however, have virilizing effects. When given to women, testosterone causes the growth of facial hair, deepening of the voice and acne.

## ANDROGEN ANTAGONISTS

**Cyproterone acetate** and **flutamide** block the action of testosterone at its receptor. They are used in various endocrine disorders where there is overproduction of male hormone, causing hirsutism in the female (when it may be combined with an estrogen) and hypersexuality in the male. They are also used in treating carcinoma of the prostate.

**Finasteride** blocks the enzyme 5α-reductase that converts testosterone into a powerful androgenic metabolite called 5α-reductase in the prostate gland, thus causing the prostate to decrease in size. It is used to treat benign enlargement of the prostate.

## Carcinoma of the prostate

The structural and functional integrity of the prostate depends on continued stimulation by testosterone and this also applies to carcinomatous tissue in the prostate. When widespread deposits have developed, strategies that interfere with hormone stimulation of these secondaries can control the disease. This can be achieved by giving an estrogen (usually diethylstilbestrol), but adverse effects (feminization and fluid retention) can be troublesome. Alternatively, a gonadorelin analogue may be used. This initially causes increased testosterone activity, which can be controlled by cyproterone (see also p. 214), but after about 2 weeks, LH release is inhibited, resulting in a fall in testosterone levels and a regression of the tumour.

## ANABOLIC HORMONES

The structure of these male sex hormones has been modified so that they have little masculinizing effect but have considerable anabolic action and are capable of building up protein in bone and other tissues. They are used occasionally to hasten convalescence and in senile osteoporosis, which is due to lack of protein in bone. Their effectiveness in these conditions is not proven. They also produce an increase in muscle bulk and have been used by athletes to improve their performance. This is undesirable: it is not only dishonest, but also carries the possibility of adverse effects.

## MALE ERECTILE DYSFUNCTION (IMPOTENCE)

Impotence is a common disorder. Its incidence increases with age and it may have a considerable effect on the well-being of the individual. The cause can be psychological, physical or a combination of both.

Erection depends on the relaxation of the penile smooth muscle, with subsequent engorgement with blood following psychological or tactile stimulation. The autonomic nervous system is involved and it is believed that nitric oxide is an important mediator in the vascular relaxation.

There are two aspects involving drugs:

- drugs may interfere with sexual performance
- drugs can also improve performance.

### Drugs that interfere with male sexual performance

Among those implicated are various centrally acting drugs (alcohol, tricyclic antidepressants, neuroleptics), antihypertensives (particularly thiazides) and cimetidine (due to its estrogen-like action).

## Drugs to provide an erection

An effective method is the intracavernosal injection of **papaverine** or **prostaglandin E$_1$**, which relaxes smooth muscle and produces a very satisfactory erection. After preliminary training the drug can be self-administered. The erection should not be allowed to continue for more than 4 hours. Alternatively, a small pellet of prostaglandin E$_1$ can be inserted into the urethra and enough is absorbed to achieve an erection in a proportion of subjects.

**Sildenafil** (*Viagra*) is an oral preparation that is a specific inhibitor of phosphodiesterase 5 in the blood vessels of the penis, leading to vasodilatation and enhanced erection when taken an hour or two before intercourse. It is effective in the majority of subjects with impotence, whatever the cause, and will probably largely replace other methods.

Adverse effects are rarely serious and include headache, flushing and occasional disturbances of colour vision. It should not, however, be combined with nitrate-containing preparations such as glyceryl trinitrate, which are known to be used recreationally.

In addition to drugs, various mechanical treatments are available.

## References

Baird D T, Glasier A F 1993 Editorial: hormonal contraception. New England Journal of Medicine 328: 1543

Editorial 2002a Oral contraceptives not associated with increased risk of breast cancer. Pharmaceutical Journal 269: 6

Editorial 2002b HRT offers no protection against heart attacks but appears safe in heart disease. Pharmaceutical Journal 269: 6

## Further reading

Beral V, Banks E, Reeves G et al 1997 Hormone replacement therapy and high incidence of breast cancer between mammographic screens. Lancet 349: 1103

Beral V, Hermon C, Kay C et al 1999 Mortality associated with oral contraceptive use: 25 year follow up of cohort of 46 000 women from Royal College of General Practitioners' oral contraceptive study. British Medical Journal 318: 96.

Berga S L 1998 Understanding premenstrual syndrome. Lancet 351: 465

Catalona W J 1994 Management of cancer of the prostate. New England Journal of Medicine 331: 996

Dunn N, Thorogood M, Faragher B et al 1999 Oral contraception and myocardial infarction: results of the MICA case–control study. British Medical Journal 318: 1579

Editorial 1990 Medical termination of pregnancy. British Medical Journal 301: 352

Editorial 1992 New gonadotropins for old? Lancet 340: 1442

Editorial 1993 Gonadotrophin releasing hormone analogues for endometriosis. Drug and Therapeutics Bulletin 31: 21

Editorial 1994 Oral contraceptives and cancer. Lancet 344: 1378

Editorial 1995 Advising women on which pill to take. British Medical Journal 311: 1111

Editorial 1996 Hormone replacement therapy. Drug and Therapeutics Bulletin 34(11): 81

Editorial 1998 Termination of first trimester pregnancy. Drug and Therapeutics Bulletin 36(2): 13

Editorial 1999 Replacing testosterone in men. Drug and Therapeutics Bulletin 37(1): 3

Glasier A 1997 Emergency postcoital contraception. New England Journal of Medicine 337: 1058

Goldstein I, Lue T F, Padma-Nathan H et al 1998 Oral sildenafil in the treatment of erectile dysfunction. Sildenafil Study Group. New England Journal of Medicine 338: 1397

Greendale G A, Lee N P, Arriola E R 1999 The menopause. Lancet 353: 571

Hillard A 1998 Managing the menopause. Nursing Standard 12(27): 49

Kirby R S 1994 Impotence. Management of male erectile dysfunction. British Medical Journal 308: 957

Knowledon H A 1990 The Pill and cancer. Journal of Advanced Nursing 15: 1016

Mills A M, Wilkinson C L, Bromham D R et al 1996 Guidelines for prescribing combined oral contraceptives. British Medical Journal 312: 121

O'Brian P M S 1993 Helping women with premenstrual syndrome. British Medical Journal 307: 1471

Rittmaster R S 1994 Finasteride. New England Journal of Medicine 330: 120

Spitzer W O 1997 Balanced view of the risks of oral contraceptives. Lancet 350: 1566

Wagner G, de Tejeda I S 1998 Update on male erectile dysfunction. British Medical Journal 316: 678

# Chapter **18**

# CNS 1. General anaesthesia, local anaesthetics and resuscitation

## Learning objectives

At the end of this chapter, the reader should be able to:

- give an account of the role that drugs have in the preoperative preparation of the patient for general anaesthesia and surgery
- describe the main elements of general anaesthesia and have an understanding of the groups of drugs involved
- explain how muscle relaxants work and how their effects may be reversed using drugs
- describe the ways in which local anaesthetics may be used and of some of the differences between the different drugs available
- describe which drugs may be used in cardiorespiratory resuscitation and what value they have in this role

## HISTORY

Three important drugs, capable of producing general anaesthesia when inhaled in sufficient quantity, were introduced to medicine within a time span of 5 years in the mid 19th century. These inhalational anaesthetic agents are:

- ether
- nitrous oxide
- chloroform.

In 1842 William E. Clark of Rochester, New York, used ether to provide general anaesthesia for the extraction of a tooth. It is a drug that is still in use in parts of the world where more recent and expensive agents are unavailable. Nitrous oxide was first used as a general anaesthetic in 1844 by Horace Wells, a dentist from Hartford, Connecticut. He had first persuaded a travelling lecturer in chemistry to give him nitrous oxide while a fellow dentist took out one of his teeth before he then used it successfully on his own patients. James Y. Simpson of Edinburgh introduced the use of chloroform in 1847 for general surgery and obstetrics and he administered it to Queen Victoria in 1853 at the birth of Prince Leopold. Chloroform remained popular for over 100 years but is no longer used as a general anaesthetic.

## PREMEDICATION

Premedication is the administration of drugs to patients an hour or two before anaesthesia and surgery. Nowadays it is used much less than previously. The objectives of premedication are:

- to relieve anxiety
- to reduce the production of saliva
- to reduce the volume and increase the pH of the gastric contents.

Premedication is rarely essential nowadays, and it is common practice not to administer any drugs to patients for the above purposes before anaesthesia and surgery. If drugs are used then they are generally given orally and rarely by intramuscular or intravenous injection. Intramuscular premedication, in particular, is not tolerated well by children. Some drugs may still sometimes be necessary before surgery, for example steroids and antibiotics.

## RELIEF FROM ANXIETY

Most patients are anxious before anaesthesia and surgery. Many feel a general sense of nervousness or apprehension. Others have more specific fears which may be of:

- injections
- pain after surgery
- waking up in the middle of the operation
- dying and not waking up at all
- the embarrassment of nakedness
- talking aloud while asleep (and perhaps giving away personal secrets)
- the loss of control over themselves and their environment

- having the wrong operation
- what the surgeon may find wrong with them.

The best treatment for anxiety is to listen to patients carefully; to give clear, simple and accurate explanations in response to their concerns and questions; and to give reassurance whenever possible.

Drugs used for premedication include:

- anxiolytic drugs
- antimuscarinic drugs to reduce secretions
- drugs to raise gastric pH.

### Anxiolytic drugs

Several of the benzodiazepine group of drugs may be used to help reduce anxiety before anaesthesia and surgery. **Temazepam** is the most commonly used. It is well absorbed and effective given orally (there is no injectable preparation). **Midazolam** is only available as an injection solution, but this can be used orally. It is, however, more effective if given intranasally or sublingually, and is sometimes given by these unusual routes in children. The injection solution is extremely bitter and needs to be diluted with something like neat blackcurrant squash immediately before use by all of these routes. It has a shorter duration of action than temazepam. Other drugs in this group that can be used are **diazepam**, which has a slightly longer action than temazepam, and **lorazepam**, which has an even longer action than temazepam. Alimemazine (trimeprazine) may still sometimes be used for oral premedication in children. It can cause marked pallor and a tachycardia. It is a phenothiazine.

**Opioids.** **Morphine** and other opioid analgesics, although good anxiolytics, are only used for premedication for patients who are in pain before surgery.

### REDUCTION OF THE PRODUCTION OF SALIVA

Excessive salivation can present problems in safe airway management, particularly during the induction of anaesthesia. It is a more common problem in children than in adults. Premedication with drugs that reduce these oral secretions is occasionally used, especially in preparation for an awake fibreoptic intubation, before certain complex examinations of the upper airway in children and before the use of ketamine. Antimuscarinic anticholinergic drugs are used for this purpose.

> **Nursing point**
>
> After ketamine has been used, let the child wake up peacefully, preferably in a quiet room with subdued lighting. This will reduce the likelihood of the child experiencing unpleasant nightmares and hallucinations while he is waking up.

## Atropine

Atropine markedly reduces salivary secretions. It is usually given by intramuscular injection but it can also be effective when given orally and this is the preferred route for administration in children. The oral dose is about twice the intramuscular dose. The intravenous route is not used for premedication. It crosses the blood–brain barrier and causes central nervous system (CNS) stimulation, although this is only a mild effect.

**Glycopyrronium (glycopyrrolate)** may be given intravenously minutes before the induction of anaesthesia to reduce secretions immediately. It is not absorbed if given orally. **Hyoscine**, although effective in reducing secretions, is no longer used for premedication because of its marked sedative action. It may also cause confusion and restlessness, particularly in the elderly.

## REDUCTION OF THE VOLUME, AND INCREASE IN THE pH, OF GASTRIC CONTENTS

A reduction in the volume of and an increase in the pH of gastric contents reduces some of the risks of vomiting, regurgitation and of subsequent inhalation of gastric contents during general anaesthesia. Drugs are commonly used to achieve these effects during labour when women face the possibility of elective or emergency surgery under general anaesthesia. They may also be used in other patients known to have significant gastro-oesophageal reflux.

**Metoclopramide** hastens gastric emptying. It is given on the morning of, or a few hours before, delivery in obstetric patients, or general anaesthesia. It may be given orally or intravenously. **Sodium citrate** raises the pH of gastric contents by neutralizing acid in the stomach. It is given orally about 30 minutes before general anaesthesia.

**Ranitidine** also raises the pH of gastric secretions. It is an $H_2$-receptor antagonist that reduces gastric acid production and so increases the pH of gastric contents. It is usually given on the night before, and the morning of, delivery in obstetric patients or general anaesthesia. It can be given orally or intravenously.

> **Nursing point**
>
> Always give patients the opportunity and time to ask all the questions they wish to ask, and to express as fully as possible any anxieties they may have before they undergo anaesthesia and surgery.

## INTRAVENOUS INDUCTION AGENTS

### Thiopental

Thiopental was first used in 1934 and is still in widespread use. It is a barbiturate.

**Onset and duration of action.** Unconsciousness occurs about 20 seconds after injection and continues for several (5–10) minutes. The termination of its action occurs as the drug is redistributed away from the brain into other tissues, particularly muscle and fat. It is metabolized very slowly (several hours) and so cannot be used as a continuous intravenous infusion as it would then accumulate and lead to prolonged sleepiness or unconsciousness when discontinued (compare with propofol).

**Effects on muscle, respiration and blood pressure.** Loss of muscle tone and therefore of normal airway control occurs immediately after injection, as does a short period of hypoventilation (respiratory depression) and sometimes apnoea. It is therefore essential to have facilities for pulmonary ventilation and the delivery of oxygen immediately at hand whenever it is used. Thiopental causes a small drop in blood pressure mainly due to a reduction in peripheral resistance. A marked fall in blood pressure may occur if the injection is given too rapidly, the dose is too large or the patient is elderly, has significant cardiac disease or is hypovolaemic.

**Accidental intra–arterial injection.** This results in immediate and severe pain in the arm distal to the site of injection and, if concentrations of greater than 2.5% are used, this may be followed by arterial spasm, loss of peripheral pulses and permanent ischaemic damage to parts of the arm. Injecting the drug into a vein on the dorsum of the hand reduces the risk of this occurrence. Extravascular injection can also result in tissue damage.

## Etomidate

Etomidate was first used in 1973. It is not a barbiturate. It is metabolized more quickly than either of the two barbiturates and recovery is probably faster than from either barbiturate. It has little effect on blood pressure and for this reason is sometimes chosen for use in patients with cardiac problems. It is otherwise not commonly used.

## Propofol

Propofol is a widely used agent. It was first used in 1977, although it was not released for general use until 1986. It is dissolved in the oil phase of an emulsion of soybean oil and purified egg phosphatide and is an opaque white fluid that looks like milk (like *Diazemuls*; see p. 274). Recovery from its effect is more rapid and complete than from any other intravenous induction agent. It is therefore particularly suited to use in day surgery units and for short procedures. It is very rapidly metabolized (in a few minutes) and can be used as a continuous low-dose intravenous infusion to provide prolonged periods of anaesthesia or to sedate patients for hours or days in intensive care units. Injection of propofol is followed by a short period of apnoea and a small drop in blood pressure. Like etomidate, propofol causes pain on injection, which can be markedly reduced by mixing it with lidocaine (lignocaine).

## Ketamine

Ketamine is unique among the induction agents. Some of the differences between ketamine and the other induction agents are:

- It can be given intramuscularly as well as intravenously.
- It has potent analgesic activity and produces a state known as dissociative analgesia in which the patient looks dreamily awake and may move around but is, in fact, unaware of his surroundings and is free of any pain.
- Muscle tone is maintained and therefore the patient retains the ability to maintain his own airway despite being unconscious. Respiration is generally not depressed. It is thus of particular value when access to the head and neck is not possible as occurs in children receiving radiotherapy, some civilian transport disasters and in casualties in the field of battle.
- It causes a rise in blood pressure and is therefore popular for use in children with cardiac disease.

- During recovery nightmares and hallucinations, referred to as emergence phenomena, are common, except, apparently, in children. These effects are so unpleasant in adults that the drug is rarely used in adults except in the unusual circumstances referred to above.

> **Nursing point**
>
> After ketamine has been used let the patient wake up peacefully, preferably in a quiet room with subdued lighting, and don't prod or shout at the patient to wake him up more quickly. This will reduce the incidence and severity of emergence phenomena – nightmares and unpleasant hallucinations.

## MAINTENANCE OF ANAESTHESIA

### INHALATIONAL ANAESTHETICS

**Nitrous oxide** is the original 'gas' or 'laughing gas', so called because it causes some patients to laugh during the induction of anaesthesia if it is used on its own. It is a faintly smelling gas that is compressed and stored as a liquid in cylinders (coloured blue in the UK). Even in concentrations of 80% it is only a weak anaesthetic and it needs to be combined with other inhalational agents or intravenous drugs. Unlike the other inhalational anaesthetics, it has a strong analgesic effect in concentrations less than those required to produce unconsciousness.

**Entonox** takes advantage of the analgesic properties of nitrous oxide. It is a 50:50 mixture of nitrous oxide and oxygen, stored as a compressed gas in cylinders (coloured blue and white in the UK). It is used for pain relief in labour, and by ambulance crews and others who treat pain outside hospital. It is also useful for rapid but potentially painful procedures, such as when very painful dressings are applied.

**Halothane, enflurane, isoflurane** and **sevoflurane** are potent halogenated hydrocarbons and have similar structures and effects. Some of the differences between them are listed in Table 18.1. They are also referred to as volatile anaesthetic agents as they are liquids at room temperature and it is the vapour from the liquid that is inhaled as the anaesthetic. They require a carrier gas, usually oxygen and nitrous oxide, to deliver them, and vaporizers capable of delivering accurate concentrations in the

Table 18.1   Volatile anaesthetic agents

| Parameter | Halothane | Enflurane | Isoflurane | Sevoflurane | Desflurane |
|---|---|---|---|---|---|
| First use in humans | 1956 | 1966 | 1970 | 1981 | 1988 |
| Boiling point | 50°C | 56°C | 49°C | 58.9°C | 23.5°C |
| Equipotent | 0.8% | 1.7% | 1.2% | 2.0% | 7.3% |
| Cardiac output | Falls | Falls | Falls a little | Falls a little | Little |
| Recovery | Slow | Moderate | Fast | Fast | Very fast |
| Metabolism | 20% | 2.5% | 0.2% | 0.02% | 4% |
| Relative cost | Low | Moderate | High | Very high | Very high |

range of 0.25–8.0%. Unlike nitrous oxide they have no analgesic properties in sub-anaesthetic concentrations. Halothane is the oldest, but is now little used as it causes cardiac arrhythmias and, very rarely, severe hepatitis. Isoflurane is the most commonly used. It has little effect on cardiac output and is associated with a rapid recovery from anaesthesia. Sevoflurane is the most expensive. It is particularly suitable for inducing anaesthesia in children as it has a weak and not unpleasant smell and, in a high concentration of 8%, induces anaesthesia within a few respirations.

### Nursing point

Nurses should make a point of knowing when an inflammable inhalational anaesthetic is going to be used, as may happen in less-developed countries where ether and other inflammable gases may still be used, and ensure that qualified electricians have checked for properly earthed equipment. This is much less of a problem in the UK where inflammable anaesthetics are avoided where possible. It is also important to know that some anaesthetics accumulate in rubber tubing and accidental overdose can occur. In the UK these problems are more of historical interest (or should be).

**Desflurane**, another recently introduced halogenated hydrocarbon, is not widely used. Its place in general anaesthetic practice has yet to be established.

**Ether** is an historically important drug but is no longer used except in a few parts of the world where resources and skills are limited. It is cheap, potent and fairly safe and can be used with simple and portable equipment using room air instead of cylinder oxygen. Induction of, and recovery from, anaesthesia are, however, very slow and it has a pungent and unpleasant smell. It is explosive.

## SHORT-ACTING OPIOID ANALGESICS

Long-acting opioids such as morphine are described elsewhere (p. 135). In patients whose lungs are ventilated during anaesthesia, potent and short-acting opioids are commonly used and safe. They have three valuable actions that contribute to anaesthesia:

- profound analgesia
- sedation, and in large doses, anaesthesia
- intense respiratory depression (in this situation a useful effect).

They have little effect on blood pressure and cardiac output and in large doses they reduce the need for inhalational anaesthetic agents to a minimum. **Fentanyl** is the most commonly used. Others include **alfentanil** and the only significant differences between all of them are their doses and duration of action (Table 18.2).

As with the longer-acting opioids, their action may be reversed at the end of anaesthesia using **naloxone** (see p. 140). This may be necessary to correct any respiratory depression but, of course, it will also reverse any analgesia and may leave the patient in pain.

**Remifentanil** is a new and different class of opioid with μ-opioid activity. Unlike any other opioid it is rapidly metabolized by non-specific esterases and thus its elimination is unaffected by renal or hepatic function. The action of remifentanil is so short that it can only be administered as a continuous

Table 18.2   Short-acting opioids

| Opioid | Approximate duration |
|---|---|
| Alfentanil | 10 minutes |
| Fentanyl | 30 minutes |
| Remifentanil | A few minutes |

infusion. Once an infusion is discontinued the effects of remifentanil are gone within 3–6 minutes. If post-operative analgesia is required it should be given as, or before, the infusion is stopped using other longer-acting opioids such as morphine. Because of its potency, short action and lack of cardiovascular side-effects it has a useful place in the management of general anaesthesia for major operations on patients with heart disease whom it is planned to wake up quickly at the end of surgery. It does not have a place in the management of postoperative pain.

## MUSCLE RELAXANTS

The introduction of muscle relaxants into anaes-thetic practice in the 1940s has been claimed as the greatest single advance in anaesthesia made in the 20th century.

**Curare** was the first such drug to be used and is an alkaloid extracted from the bark, leaves and vines of the tropical plant *Chondrodendron tomentosum*, found around the upper reaches of the Amazon River. Crude preparations of this plant have long been used by South American Indians to poison the tips of their arrows and blow darts. Since the 1940s many new relaxants have been produced and those in current use, and some of the differences between them, are listed in Table 18.3.

Most anaesthetics involve the use of muscle relax-ants. There are three main indications for their use:

● To facilitate intubation of the trachea with an endotracheal tube at the beginning of anaesthesia.

● To relax muscles sufficiently to make surgery possible. This applies particularly to abdominal surgery for which relaxed muscles are necessary for easy access to, and closure of, the abdomen.

● To permit artificial ventilation. There are many situations in anaesthesia in which it is better to ventilate lungs mechanically rather than let patients breath spontaneously and these include chest sur-gery, anaesthesia in patients with severe cardiorespi-ratory disease and lengthy surgery of any nature.

## THE NEUROMUSCULAR JUNCTION

Muscle relaxants act at the neuromuscular junction (or motor end plate) by blocking the transmission of nerve impulses from the nerve to the muscle (Fig. 18.1). When a nerve supplying a voluntary muscle is stimulated, acetylcholine is liberated from vesicles in the nerve ending and acts on special receptor sites on the muscle to produce changes that are known as depolarization. This is followed by contraction of the muscle fibre. The acetylcholine is then rapidly broken down by the enzyme cholinesterase and

**Table 18.3**  Muscle relaxants

| Drug | Type of blocker | Duration of action | Reversal of action | Other points |
|---|---|---|---|---|
| Atracurium Vecuronium | Competitive | 20–30 minutes | Neostigmine (with atropine or glycopyrronium) | The most commonly used |
| Cisatracurium | Competitive | 20–30 minutes | Neostigmine (with atropine or glycopyrronium) | Causes less histamine release than atracurium |
| Rocuronium | Competitive | 20–30 minutes | Neostigmine (with atropine or glycopyrronium) | Fastest onset of action of all competitive blockers |
| Mivacurium | Competitive | 10–15 minutes | Neostigmine (with atropine or glycopyrronium) | Often causes marked histamine release leading to cutaneous flushing and tachycardia |
| Gallamine Pancuronium | Competitive | 45–60 minutes | Neostigmine (with atropine or glycopyrronium) | Older, rarely used drugs. Should not be used in renal failure as renal secretion is significant |
| Suxamethonium | Depolarizing | 2–5 minutes | Cannot be reversed with drugs | Causes postoperative muscle pains and tenderness. Prolonged action in 1 in 2800 patients |

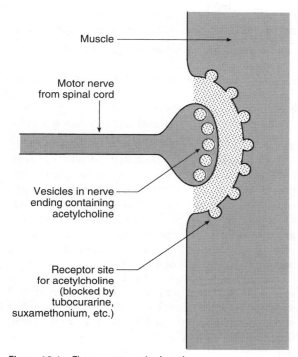

Muscle

Motor nerve
from spinal cord

Vesicles in nerve
ending containing
acetylcholine

Receptor site
for acetylcholine
(blocked by
tubocurarine,
suxamethonium, etc.)

**Figure 18.1** The neuromuscular junction.

repolarization of the muscle occurs. The muscle is now ready to be stimulated again. Should depolarization persist (see depolarizing muscle relaxants), then the muscle remains unresponsive to further stimulation.

## COMPETITIVE MUSCLE RELAXANTS

Two types of block of the neuromuscular junction are produced by muscle relaxants. Most muscle relaxants are competitive or non-depolarizing blockers. These drugs occupy the receptor site for acetylcholine and so render ineffective the acetylcholine released following nerve stimulation. There are two groups of competitive muscle relaxants: the aminosteroid group, which includes pancuronium, rocuronium and vecuronium; the benzylisoquinolinium group, which includes atracurium, cisatracurium, gallamine and mivacurium.

**Atracurium,** with vecuronium, is one of the most commonly used of these drugs. Atracurium has a medium duration of action of 30–60 minutes. It is associated with some histamine release, which can cause skin flushing and a slight tachycardia and drop in blood pressure. It breaks down under the

influence of body temperature and pH and thus its elimination is independent of renal or hepatic function.

**Cisatracurium** is a single isomer of atracurium and causes less histamine release than atracurium (atracurium is a mixture of 10 isomers) but it is otherwise very similar to atracurium.

**Vecuronium** also has a medium duration of action of 30–60 minutes. It is not associated with histamine release and has no effect on cardiac function or blood pressure. A small amount is excreted renally but, nevertheless, it can safely be used in patients with renal failure.

**Rocuronium** has the fastest onset of action of all non-depolarizing relaxants, particularly if given in a high dose, and is therefore sometimes used as an alternative to suxamethonium when rapid intubation of the trachea is indicated at induction of anaesthesia. It is excreted unchanged in the urine and is therefore not suitable for use in patients with poor or no renal function.

**Mivacurium** has a short duration of action of 15–30 minutes. It causes considerable histamine release, with consequent marked skin flushing, tachycardia and hypotension.

**Pancuronium** and **gallamine** are older drugs with a longer duration of action of 60–90 minutes. They are excreted predominately by the kidney and should therefore not be used in patients with renal failure. Pancuronium is sometimes used for long procedures and in the management of patients on ventilators in the intensive care unit. Gallamine has a vagolytic effect that leads to a significant tachycardia.

## DEPOLARIZING MUSCLE RELAXANTS

**Suxamethonium** is the only representative of this group in current use. It also occupies the receptor sites for acetylcholine and initially stimulates the muscle into contracting, visible as the 'twitching' or fasciculation that occurs almost immediately after it is injected. It then produces a state of persistent depolarization of the muscle cell membrane during which no further stimulation of the muscle fibre is possible. There are several special points to note about suxamethonium:

● It has a quick onset of action of about 60 seconds; therefore, it is used in patients who may have full stomachs in whom rapid tracheal intubation is indicated.
● It has a short duration of action of 5–10 minutes.

● It is normally rapidly broken down by the enzyme plasma cholinesterase. About 1 in 3000 of the population have a familial and genetically determined variant of this enzyme which breaks down suxamethonium more slowly and leads to a prolonged period of paralysis of up to 2–3 hours. This is referred to as **suxamethonium apnoea**.

● A common side-effect of the drug is muscle pain and tenderness, particularly in the chest and abdomen. It can be severe and occurs about 24 hours after it has been given. It is likened to the pain and tenderness experienced after severe, unaccustomed exercise and is usually seen in young fit adults. It is rare in children.

● A marked bradycardia is sometimes seen following a second injection of suxamethonium in adults and following the first injection in children. It is easily treated with atropine or glycopyrronium.

● In certain situations, such as following major burns or trauma or in acute peripheral neuropathies, it can cause a dangerous rise in serum potassium with consequent life-threatening cardiac arrhythmias.

● There are no drugs that can be used to reverse its actions.

---

### Nursing point

'Suxamethonium pains': look out for patients, usually young adults, who complain of pain and tenderness in their muscles, particularly of their chest and abdomen, about 24 hours after surgery. These symptoms may be due to the use of suxamethonium but are often attributed to other factors. They can be very severe.

---

## REVERSAL OF MUSCLE RELAXANTS

The effects of the competitive, non-depolarizing muscle relaxants may be allowed to wear off spontaneously. However, the effects can be reversed more quickly by using an **anticholinesterase**. Anticholinesterases act at the neuromuscular junction where they temporarily inhibit the enzyme cholinesterase, which normally breaks down acetylcholine, and allow the concentration of acetylcholine to rise and so help the return of normal neuromuscular transmission and muscle strength.

Unfortunately, anticholinesterases also have effects at sites other than the neuromuscular junction, namely at peripheral parasympathetic nerve endings. The most important effects of this are:

● a bradycardia, which can be severe and therefore dangerous
● an increase in salivation and in tracheobronchial secretions
● an increase in peristaltic activity in the gut that causes colic and diarrhoea and possibly disrupts bowel anastomoses following surgery.

Fortunately these unwanted effects of anticholinesterases can be prevented by the administration of one of the anticholinergic group of drugs (see below) that must be given at the same time as, or before, the anticholinesterase. Thus a common mixture used to reverse the effects of competitive muscle relaxants at the end of anaesthesia is that of neostigmine and glycopyrronium.

**Neostigmine** has a maximal effect after 5–7 minutes, although an initial effect may be seen after 2 minutes. Its action lasts about 30 minutes. As noted above, it must be preceded by, or given at the same time, as an anticholinergic drug, usually glycopyrronium.

**Edrophonium** is also effective in reversing muscle relaxants, although it is not commonly used for this purpose. It possibly has a quicker onset of action and a slightly shorter duration of action than neostigmine. It may also be used in the assessment and management of patients with myasthenia gravis.

## ANTICHOLINERGIC DRUGS

These drugs temporarily block the effects of acetylcholine, particularly at postganglionic parasympathetic nerve endings, and have three uses during anaesthesia:

● to increase the pulse rate
● to reduce tracheobronchial and salivary secretions
● to prevent the increase in peristaltic activity that occurs after the administration of neostigmine or edrophonium.

**Atropine** is the best established of these drugs, although it is not so widely used as glycopyrronium during anaesthesia. It can be given orally as part of premedication. It has a slight central stimulant effect.

**Glycopyrronium (glycopyrrolate)** is widely used during general anaesthesia. Its onset of action is slower, and its duration of action is longer, than atropine. Its effect on reducing secretions is more potent than that of atropine. In the doses generally used it causes less tachycardia than atropine. It is not used for premedication before anaesthesia, as it is not absorbed from the gastrointestinal tract. It does not cross the blood–brain barrier and so does not cause any CNS stimulation.

## MALIGNANT HYPERPYREXIA

Susceptibility to this extremely rare disorder is familial and genetically determined. Malignant hyperpyrexia may be triggered by exposure to suxamethonium (but not to any of the non-depolarizing muscle relaxants) and to any of the halogenated hydrocarbon inhalational anaesthetics – halothane, enflurane, isoflurane, sevoflurane or desflurane – but not to nitrous oxide or, curiously, almost any other drug.

Malignant hyperpyrexia starts with excessive metabolic activity in muscle cells, which leads to muscle rigidity, a high temperature and widespread severe metabolic disturbances. It used to have a high mortality.

**Dantrolene**, if given promptly and combined with aggressive treatment of the metabolic problems, markedly reduces mortality from this disorder. It is a skeletal muscle relaxant that acts at an intracellular level (but not by blocking the neuromuscular junction) and reduces the excessive metabolic activity seen in muscle cells during malignant hyperpyrexia. Every operating department should stock sufficient stocks of the drug to treat at least one patient. It may take 20 minutes to prepare for use and is expensive.

## LOCAL ANAESTHETICS

Local anaesthesia for surgery was first used in 1884 when Carl Koller, in Vienna, used cocaine for ophthalmic surgery. The use of cocaine for nerve blocks was first described by William S. Halstead in 1885; unfortunately, Halstead later became addicted to cocaine after he had experimented on himself with too many nerve blocks.

Local anaesthetics produce a reversible inhibition of conduction along nerves and, in sufficient concentration, produce a complete sensory and motor blockade. However, the fine, unmyelinated, nerve fibres that conduct pain sensation are more easily blocked by local anaesthetics than the thicker, heavily myelinated, motor fibres that supply muscle, and so it is possible to provide good analgesia without loss of too much motor function. This is best illustrated by observing the effects of an epidural during labour in which there is good pain relief and yet the patient is still able to move her legs.

There are several routes by which local anaesthetics can be given:

- direct application to mucous membranes
- direct application to the skin
- intradermal injection
- local infiltration of subcutaneous tissues, muscles, other soft tissues or periosteum
- infiltration around local nerves
- extradural injection (an 'extradural', 'epidural' or 'caudal')
- subarachnoid injection (a 'spinal')
- intravenous injection – intravenous regional anaesthesia (Bier's block).

Intravenous regional analgesia, otherwise known as a Bier's block, in an arm is established as follows. The arm is elevated for a few minutes to encourage the drainage of as much blood as possible. Further exsanguination may be achieved by applying a bandage around the arm. A previously applied orthopaedic tourniquet is inflated to well above arterial blood pressure and maintained at that pressure for the duration of the block. Then, 40 ml of 0.5% prilocaine is injected into a previously inserted cannula in a vein in the dorsum of the hand. The prilocaine now spreads throughout all the vessels in the arm below the tourniquet and after a few minutes this will produce complete analgesia of the arm below the cuff. The tourniquet is not released for at least 20 minutes to prevent toxic doses of prilocaine reaching the heart or brain.

**Lidocaine (lignocaine)** is the most commonly used local anaesthetic. It has a rapid onset of action and duration of action of 1–2 hours. By mixing it with epinephrine its duration of action can be usefully prolonged. It is available in various concentrations and preparations, including an aerosol spray for use on mucous membranes such as in the mouth, pharynx or trachea.

Lidocaine also depresses myocardial excitability and is used to suppress ventricular arrhythmias such as may follow myocardial infarction or cardiac arrest. For this purpose it is given as a bolus intravenous injection or as a continuous, low-dose infusion. It will, though, like all local anaesthetics, cause myocardial depression in overdose.

**Prilocaine** is similar to lidocaine but has a slightly longer action than lidocaine. It is less toxic than lidocaine and is therefore the preferred drug for intravenous regional anaesthesia. It is commonly used, mixed with felypressin, for dental blocks. In doses twice the recommended maximum it causes cyanosis due to the formation of methaemoglobin.

*Emla* **cream** (**eutectic mixture of local anaesthetics**) is a unique preparation. If powders of lidocaine and prilocaine are mixed together, then a *eutectic* mixture is created – that is the mixture changes consistency from a powder to a paste. Substances are then added to this paste to make a cream containing 2.5% lidocaine and 2.5% prilocaine suitable for application to the skin. Absorption through the skin is slow, but application for at least 45 minutes produces adequate analgesia and *Emla* cream is now used extensively to allow pain-free venepuncture, particularly in children, and for other minor procedures.

**Bupivacaine** has a slow onset of action, sometimes taking up to 30 minutes to have its maximum effect. It has about twice the duration of action of lidocaine and its effects may last 2–4 hours. It is particularly popular and suitable for continuous epidural analgesia in labour and for postoperative pain relief. It is more toxic on the heart than other local anaesthetics and must therefore never be used for intravenous regional anaesthesia. It should never be used for Bier's block.

**Ropivacaine** is similar to bupivacaine in structure and effect. It has a marginally shorter duration of action, and is less cardiotoxic, than bupivacaine. More interestingly, it is associated with less motor blockade for the same degree of sensory blockade. Thus an epidural or spinal anaesthesia produced using ropivacaine leaves the patients with greater power in – and more use of – their legs than they would have had if bupivacaine had been used to provide the analgesia.

**Levobupivacaine** has been recently introduced. It is an isomer of bupivacaine that is probably less cardiotoxic than but otherwise has similar properties to bupivacaine.

**Tetracaine (amethocaine)** has a slow onset and long duration of action. It is too toxic to be used by injection or to be used on highly vascular mucous membranes where its rapid absorption may quickly lead to toxic effects. It is mostly used for conjunctival anaesthesia in the eye. It may also be used to provide skin anaesthesia for venepuncture (see below). It is a good vasodilator.

**Tetracaine gel (Ametop)** is a preparation, like *Emla* cream, that is designed to enable pain-free venepuncture. It contains tetracaine (amethocaine) only. It may have a quicker onset of action than *Emla* cream and it may cause more vasodilatation

and so make venepuncture easier. It should be removed after 60 minutes as it can cause marked skin irritation if left on too long.

**Oxybuprocaine** is only used as a local anaesthetic in the eye. It causes less initial stinging sensation and has a shorter duration of action than amethocaine.

**Cocaine,** the first of the local anaesthetics, is a very different drug from all other local anaesthetics. It is an alkaloid obtained from the leaves of a tree, *Erythroxylon coca*, found in Bolivia, Brazil, Peru and other South American countries. For centuries it has been chewed by the peoples of these countries to produce euphoria and to increase their capacity for physical work.

Cocaine is absorbed well by mucous membranes and is used to provide surface analgesia for eye surgery and throat and nose surgery where its intense vasoconstrictor effect is also a useful feature. It is available as a paste, and as a solution of various concentrations, for these purposes. It is too toxic to be used by injection.

Cocaine has widespread sympathomimetic actions, causing mydriasis (dilatation of the pupil), marked vasoconstriction, hypertension, tachycardia and ventricular arrhythmias. In overdose, sudden death due to ventricular fibrillation occurs. Headache, nausea, vomiting and abdominal pain are common. It causes excitement, restlessness, euphoria and confusion, and with increasing dosage, CNS depression, coma and convulsions. It is a drug of addiction and, not surprisingly, a controlled drug.

There are many other local anaesthetics, both old and new. **Procaine** is an old drug that is now rarely used. **Mepivacaine** and **articaine (carticaine)** are used in dentistry. **Benzocaine** is used as a constituent of proprietary drug mixtures, particularly those used for sore throats, mouth ulcers and musculoskeletal conditions.

## VASOCONSTRICTORS AND LOCAL ANAESTHETICS

Most local anaesthetics are also vasodilators, which, by increasing local blood flow, hasten the removal of the drug from the site of action. If epinephrine is mixed with the drug, then the vasoconstriction it produces will delay the removal of the drug and so prolong its duration of action.

Epinephrine must never be used with prilocaine when used for intravenous regional anaesthesia because of the obvious danger that, if the cuff were to deflate unexpectedly, then large doses of epinephrine could reach the heart. Neither should vasoconstrictors be used with local anaesthetics for blocks around the base of the penis or for 'ring' blocks of the fingers or toes; they may severely interrupt the blood supply and cause permanent ischaemic damage to the penis or digit. And particular care should always be taken when injecting local anaesthetics mixed with epinephrine not to inject the drug intravenously by accident.

**Felypressin (octapressin)** is a safer alternative to epinephrine. It is an analogue of vasopressin and is a powerful vasoconstrictor but has none of the potentially serious effects that epinephrine has on the heart. It is generally only used, mixed with local anaesthetics, for dental blocks.

> **Nursing point**
>
> Do not forget that the patient will be conscious during procedures carried out under local anaesthesia. Conversation between staff should be at a minimum, but the patient should be reassured throughout.

## TOXICITY OF LOCAL ANAESTHETICS

All local anaesthetics have dangerous side-effects at doses only a little above those that may be used for some of the more extensive regional blocks. Care must therefore be taken in calculating the total dose used when establishing any block. The development of toxicity is not only dependent on the total dose of local anaesthetic given but also on such factors as:

- the concentration used
- the route by which it is given
- the vascularity of the tissues being injected
- the age and weight of the patient
- the time period over which the local anaesthetic is administered.

The most common cause of life-threatening systemic toxicity is the accidental injection of a local anaesthetic into a vein.

> **Nursing point**
>
> A 1% solution equals 1 g in 100 ml or 10 mg in 1 ml. Only by knowing this can the amount of drug given be calculated.

## Signs of toxicity

Early signs of toxicity are tingling of the tongue and lips, tinnitus, tremor, light-headedness and drowsiness; they progress to unconsciousness and convulsions and then cardiac and respiratory depression. Convulsions may also be the presenting feature of toxicity and cardiac arrest may be the first sign of toxicity due to bupivacaine.

## DRUGS USED DURING CARDIORESPIRATORY RESUSCITATION

### BASIC LIFE SUPPORT

No drugs are used in basic life support. Basic life support is the term used to describe the initial attempts at resuscitation following cardiac or respiratory arrest. Nurses are taught these skills very early during training.

Basic life support starts once it is has been established that a patient is unconscious and unresponsive. The situation is recognized through specific procedures such as the taking of pulse, inspection of the pupils for dilation, lack of respiration.

Action takes three parts and consists of:

- *Airway*: the patient's airway must be cleared and kept open.
- *Circulation*: if there is no pulse, then cardiac massage is started.
- *Breathing*: if the patient is not breathing, then his lungs should be ventilated using mouth to mouth, or other, techniques as appropriate.

> **Nursing point**
>
> This brief account of basic life support is not intended to supplement or replace the training that is given, but is presented to show that drugs are of secondary importance.

### ADVANCED LIFE SUPPORT

Once equipment and drugs appropriate for resuscitation become available, as would happen in any hospital, then advanced life support is started. The initial actions may be divided up into three main parts:

- *Oxygen*, rather than the resuscitator's expired air, is used to ventilate the lungs. A self-inflating bag or other bag system is used to deliver this oxygen.

*Tracheal intubation* may also be undertaken to further improve the efficiency of lung ventilation.

- *ECG monitoring* is established in order to determine the cardiac rhythm. If the rhythm is that of ventricular fibrillation, or of a ventricular tachycardia in a patient with no palpable pulse, then defibrillation is undertaken.
- *Intravenous access* is created so that drugs and fluids can be given as part of the continuing attempts at resuscitation.

Note that the use of drugs comes third in the list above. Although drugs may play a significant part in cardiorespiratory resuscitation (CPR), ventilation of the lungs with oxygen and the appropriate use of defibrillation are far more important in achieving successful resuscitation. The drugs used are epinephrine, amiodarone, lidocaine, adenosine and atropine.

**Epinephrine** is widely used during CPR. It has several useful effects in this situation: it elevates the blood pressure generated during chest compressions and so increases coronary artery perfusion; it improves myocardial contractility and heart rate; it increases the vigour of ventricular fibrillation and makes it easier to terminate by defibrillation; and it helps to redirect blood flow to the brain. It is given in a large dose immediately a diagnosis of asystole is made or if the first three attempts at defibrillation fail to terminate ventricular fibrillation or ventricular tachycardia. Thereafter, it is given every 3 minutes during CPR, whatever the cardiac rhythm, until resuscitation is successful.

---

**A warning note**

EPINEPHRINE is also known as adrenaline.

Do not confuse EPINEPHRINE with EPHEDRINE, which is another sympathomimetic drug used to raise blood pressure, particularly for the treatment of hypotension associated with general anaesthesia and with the use of epidural and spinal anaesthesia.

---

**Nursing point**

*A drug concentration oddity*:

1 mg of epinephrine = 1 ml of '1 in 1000' epinephrine
or 10 ml of '1 in 10 000' epinephrine

---

This information is important to know during cardiopulmonary resuscitation. It is unfortunate that the concentration of epinephrine is still given in such a curious manner. '1 in 1000' means one gram in a 1000 millilitres (1 g in 1000 ml). The concentration of no other drug is indicated in this way.

---

**Amiodarone** is an effective and relatively safe anti-arrhythmic drug that is given to patients with ventricular fibrillation if the first three attempts to terminate this rhythm by defibrillation fail. It is given as a single quick bolus during CPR, which contrasts with the slow infusion over 20 minutes to 2 hours that is the normal method of giving the drug in patients not requiring CPR. Amiodarone is also used in the treatment of several peri-arrest arrhythmias such as ventricular tachycardia, supraventricular tachycardia and atrial fibrillation.

**Lidocaine** is an alternative anti-arrhythmic drug that may be used in the management of ventricular fibrillation and ventricular tachycardia. Unlike amiodarone it may be used as continuous, low-dose infusion after a bolus injection in the peri-arrest scenario.

**Adenosine** is used in the treatment of acute supraventricular tachycardias. It has a very short half-life (less than 10 seconds) and duration of effect of less than 2 minutes. To be effective it must be given as a rapid intravenous injection. After its injection supraventricular tachycardia is usually terminated rapidly and is followed by a transient profound sinus bradycardia. Hopefully, normal sinus rhythm then resumes.

**Sodium hydrogen carbonate** may be used to correct the metabolic acidosis that occurs as a consequence of cardiorespiratory arrest, particularly prolonged arrest. It is not used during the early stages of CPR but may be considered as an option following a prolonged period of CPR or in response to a measurement of arterial pH that indicates a severe metabolic acidosis. It can increase arterial carbon dioxide concentration and intracellular pH, both of which may depress cardiac function. Sodium hydrogen carbonate administration has not been shown to improve survival from CPR, and is not much used for this purpose in the UK.

**Atropine** increases the heart rate by blocking the vagus nerve. It may be used in the treatment of asystole if initial attempts at CPR, including the use of epinephrine, have failed. It is also used if the heart rate during CPR remains inappropriately slow despite all other treatment.

> ### Nursing point
>
> Remember that a 1% solution contains 1 gram in a 100 millilitres. This is the same as 10 milligrams in 1 millilitre. So:
>
> - 5% glucose contains 5 g of glucose in each 100 ml
> - a 1% preparation of lidocaine contains 10 mg of lidocaine in each ml

## ROUTE OF ADMINISTRATION OF DRUGS DURING CPR

The drugs can be administered by the following notes:

- intravenous
- endotracheal tube
- intraosseous
- intracardiac.

The most common route of administration of drugs during cardiopulmonary resuscitation is through a **peripheral vein** since this is usually the most easily and safely established form of intravenous access. The circulation will be slow during cardiac resuscitation and it is therefore essential that each injection of a drug is followed by a generous flush of 20 ml of normal saline or 5% glucose so that there is a good chance the drug will reach the heart where its action is required.

The ideal route is through a cannula placed in a **'central' vein**, i.e. a vein in the neck or groin, from where drugs can more easily reach the heart than from a peripheral vein. However, it is more dangerous and more difficult to place cannulae into these veins in an emergency so that it is not recommended that this route is tried except by experienced practitioners.

Lidocaine and atropine are also absorbed fairly reliably via the respiratory route (by inhalation) if given in twice the usual dose via an **endotracheal tube**. This route may therefore be worth using if intravenous access cannot be established. However it is doubtful if sufficient epinephrine is absorbed by this route, although it is sometimes used during resuscitation. Amiodarone and sodium hydrogen carbonate cannot be administered through the lungs.

The **intraosseous route** is just as effective as the intravenous route. It involves a specialized but not difficult technique that inserts a stout needle into bone marrow, usually in the tibia. It is generally only used in children in whom the bone is soft enough for the technique. There are no exceptions to the drugs that can be given by this route (there used to be a few exceptions quoted but it is now accepted that there are none) and it can also be used for administration of fluid and the transfusion of blood.

Finally, the *intracardiac route*, using a long needle inserted through the chest wall directly into the heart, is no longer used. It is far too unreliable and dangerous.

The procedures for adult advanced life support are shown in Figure 18.2.

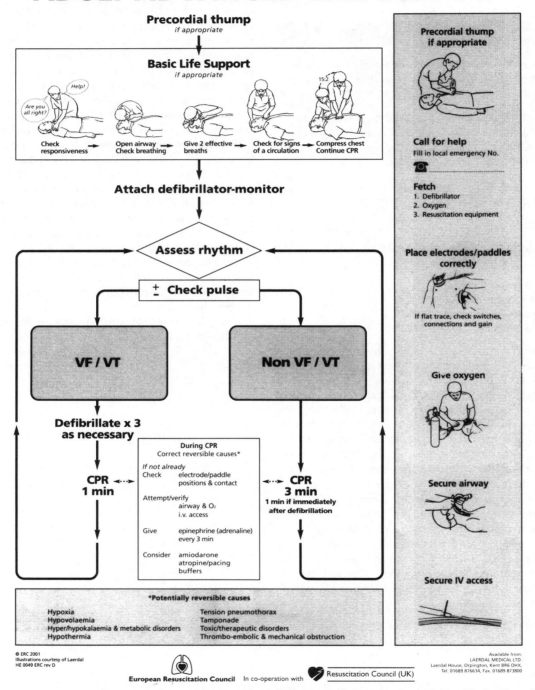

Figure 18.2   Adult advanced life support (from the European Resuscitation Council in co-operation with Resuscitation Council (UK)).

## Summary

- Premedication is not as much used as before, but certain drugs such as steroids and antibiotics may still be required
- Patients may have many diverse fears before surgery and should be listened to carefully and be reassured
- Opioids should only be used as premedication before surgery for patients who are in pain and not as anxiolytics
- Children who have had ketamine should be allowed to wake up peacefully in a quiet, darkened room as this will reduce the possibility of nightmares
- In children, oral administration is the preferred route
- Hyoscine is not commonly used for premedication because of its sedative properties
- Increasing the pH of gastric contents with an $H_2$ antagonist before surgery will reduce the chances of regurgitation and subsequent inhalation of vomit: for example during labour under general anaesthesia
- Thiopental should not be administered by continuous infusion
- It is essential to have oxygen and facilities for pulmonary ventilation to hand when thiopental is administered
- Injection of thiopental or other I.V. induction agents into a vein on the dorsum of the hand minimizes the danger of accidental intra-arterial injection
- Propofol is particularly suited to use in day surgery units
- Entonox is useful in labour
- Nurses who work under more primitive conditions should be aware of the dangers associated with the use of inflammable general anaesthetic gases
- Short-acting opioid anaesthetics are useful in anaesthesia of ventilated patients

- Muscle relaxants are a very important part of general anaesthesia
- Some muscle relaxants such as mivacurium will cause histamine release
- No drugs will reverse the actions of suxamethonium
- Anticholinesterases have very many effects, since they act at every site where acetylcholine is released as a neurotransmitter
- Atropine is a long-acting drug and may not be suitable for short procedures
- Suxamethonium may trigger malignant hyperpyrexia in some patients
- Bupivacaine should never be used for intravenous regional anaesthesia
- Tetracaine is too toxic to be used by injection or on highly vascular mucous membranes
- Epinephrine if injected with a local anaesthetic will cause local vasoconstriction; this will delay removal of the drug from its site of action and thus prolong its duration of action
- Felypressin is a safer alternative to epinephrine
- It is very dangerous to inject a local anaesthetic accidentally into a vein, and care should be taken to check that the needle is not in a vein by withdrawing the plunger briefly before injecting; if blood is drawn up into the syringe, remove the needle immediately
- Epinephrine should not be confused with ephedrine; the two names are very similar
- The most common route of administration of drugs during cardiopulmonary resuscitation is via a peripheral vein, but circulation will be abnormally slow, and the drug must be flushed in with at least 20 ml of sterile saline; the ideal route is via a 'central' vein, e.g. in the groin or neck, but this procedure is more dangerous and should be used only by specially trained practitioners

# Chapter 19

# CNS 2. Epilepsy and Parkinson's disease

## Learning objectives

At the end of this chapter the reader should be able to:

- give an account of the different age-related causes of epilepsy
- explain the terms used to describe epilepsy and the seizures
- list the three main approaches to the treatment of epilepsy with drugs
- provide examples of well-established and newer drugs and their adverse effects and contraindications
- appreciate the importance of phenytoin monitoring
- describe the treatment of absence seizures with drugs
- describe the use of drugs to treat status epilepticus
- explain how to treat febrile convulsions and about reassuring parents
- give an account of antiepileptic drugs, pregnancy and eclampsia
- appreciate the epileptic patient's special needs and problems, e.g. driving
- describe the chief symptoms and other visible clinical features
- describe the various causes of symptoms, including about brain degenerative changes
- give the two main approaches to the treatment of Parkinson's disease with drugs and be able to give examples
- give an account of the problems associated with the use of levodopa and other drugs

- understand the latest surgical interventions in Parkinson's disease
- appreciate the problems and the special needs of the patient and of the patient's family carers

## EPILEPSY

### INTRODUCTION

The word **epilepsy** is derived from Late Latin *epilepsia*, from the Greek *epilambanein*, which means to seize or attack. Hippocrates wrote about epilepsy in about 400 BC, calling it the 'sacred disease', since people experiencing seizures were assumed to be possessed by or communicating with the gods. These days, although much more is known about epilepsy, it is still not fully understood and it is still incurable.

Epilepsy affects at least 350 000 people in the UK. About 30 000 people develop epilepsy every year and epilepsy affects about 1 in 20 people at some time during their lives. Many studies have found a slightly higher incidence among men.

### CAUSES OF SEIZURES

Some causes (see also Michael 1999a) of epileptic seizures are summarized below.

#### Neonatal onset

- Congenital brain malformation
- Asphyxia or hypoxia or intracranial trauma during delivery
- Infection
- Intracranial haemorrhage
- Electrolyte or metabolic disturbances.

#### Childhood and adolescence

- Brain tumours or trauma
- Cerebral degenerative disease or cerebral palsy
- Congenital brain malformation
- Febrile convulsions (see below)
- Chemical toxicity, e.g. lead, drugs
- Hereditary, e.g. tuberous sclerosis
- Hydrocephalus
- Idiopathic
- Infection
- Lennox–Gastaut syndrome (see below)
- Other diseases, e.g. renal disease.

#### Adult

- Birth trauma
- Brain trauma or tumours
- Cerebral degenerative disease
- Cerebral vascular disease, e.g. infarction
- Congenital disease
- Drug toxicity, drug abuse and withdrawal, including alcohol
- Idiopathic
- Metabolic disturbances.

Clearly, there is overlap among the various age groups.

### DRUGS THAT MAY CAUSE SEIZURES

- **Anaesthetics**, e.g. enflurane, halothane, ketamine
- **Antibiotics**, e.g. amphotericin, cephalosporins, chloroquine, cycloserine, fluconazole, isoniazid, penicillins
- **Antidepressants and antipsychotic drugs**, e.g. baclofen, cocaine, lithium, tricyclics
- **Cardiovascular drugs**, e.g. intravenous lidocaine (lignocaine), procaine
- **Endocrine drugs** e.g. desmopressin, insulin, oxytocin, prednisolone
- **Radiographic contrast media**, e.g. certain meglumine derivatives, metrizamide
- **Stimulant drugs**, e.g. aminophylline, caffeine, theophylline.

This list is far from comprehensive, but alerts the reader to the fact that many drugs are capable of producing seizures in some patients.

### TERMS USED TO DESCRIBE SEIZURES

The following terms are used:

- focal
- petit mal (absence seizures)
- grand mal (tonic–clonic)
- psychomotor epilepsy
- partial seizures
- generalized seizures.

### TYPES OF EPILEPSY

There are several varieties of epilepsy and they vary in their response to drugs. In **focal epilepsy** the attack arises from a focal electrical discharge in the brain. This may produce a brief aura, which is a feeling or movement. If the discharge becomes generalized the patient falls unconscious and passes through the typical tonic and clonic phases, regaining consciousness after a varying interval. This is known as a **tonic–clonic (grand mal) seizure.** Sometimes the spread of the discharge is limited (**partial seizure**), producing psychological disturbances (**psychomotor seizure**) or various involuntary movements, but without loss of consciousness. When a seizure starts as a partial seizure and then spreads to become generalized, this is often referred to in the literature as 'secondary generalizations'. In some patients, mainly children, the electrical discharge is widespread from the start, and causes absence (**petit mal** or **absence**) seizure, which is a brief interference with consciousness. The object in treating epilepsy is to abolish the attacks completely by means of drugs.

Readers will encounter the terms **myoclonus** and **myoclonic jerks** when reading about epilepsy. These terms refer to the sudden jerking of the limbs that occurs in patients with epilepsy and in those with degenerative neurological disease. Some healthy people experience nocturnal myoclonic jerks when falling asleep.

Although there are now a number of drugs that are useful in controlling epilepsy, it is usually best to start treatment with one drug (called 'monotherapy') and use multiple drug regimens only in resistant cases. The initial dose should be low and it should be increased until control of the seizures is achieved or adverse effects develop.

> ### Nursing point
>
> Patients with epilepsy should be warned against driving vehicles, swimming and working under conditions where a seizure could produce disaster.

## GENERAL MECHANISTIC APPROACH TO THE TREATMENT OF EPILEPSY

Currently used drugs aim to control epilepsy through one of three main mechanisms:

- enhancement of the activity of the inhibitory brain neurotransmitter gamma-aminobutyric acid (GABA)
- inhibition of the activity of the excitatory brain neurotransmitter glutamate
- directly blocking sodium and/or calcium channels in the nerve cell membrane.

Some drugs, such as gabapentin (see below) are effective but the mechanism is still not well understood.

## WELL-ESTABLISHED DRUGS USED IN TONIC–CLONIC AND PARTIAL SEIZURES

For more information see also Michael 1999b.

### Phenytoin

Phenytoin is a member of the hydantoin group of compounds, which are structurally related to barbiturates such as phenobarbital (see below).

**Mechanism of action.** Phenytoin sodium appears to act by blocking sodium channels in nerve membranes. This reduces the excitability of nerve cells and prevents the abnormal discharge from spreading in the brain.

**Therapeutic use.** Phenytoin is well absorbed by mouth and does not produce drowsiness or sleep. Its effectiveness as an anticonvulsant and the incidence of side-effects depend largely on the plasma level of the drug. Finding the correct dose may be difficult for several reasons:

- Patients vary considerably in the rate at which they break down phenytoin, so there is a wide variation of dose requirements between patients.
- The relationship between dose and plasma level is not linear; this means that a small increase in the dose may cause a considerable rise in the plasma level (Fig. 19.1).
- Because phenytoin is slowly broken down, once daily dosage is adequate, it takes about a week for the plasma level to become steady. Therefore, the dose should not be altered at less than fortnightly intervals.

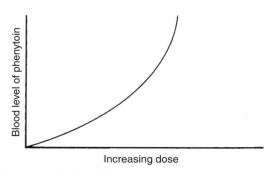

**Figure 19.1**    Relationship between dosage and blood level of phenytoin.

**Adverse effects of phenytoin.** These are fairly common with phenytoin and include:

- if dosage is too high the patient is sedated, ataxic and may show nystagmus (rapid, involuntary eye movements)
- greasy skin and hirsutism may cause problems in women
- macrocytic anaemia due to folic acid deficiency
- gum hypertrophy; dental care is important
- lymph node enlargement
- a variety of rashes.

**Drug interactions with phenytoin.** These are common and underline the need for regular measurement of plasma levels of phenytoin:

- Phenytoin is largely bound to plasma proteins in the blood, and can be displaced from these proteins by other drugs such as sodium valproate, which is another antiepileptic drug (see below) and by aspirin. This will increase the concentration of free phenytoin in the blood and therefore effectively increase the dose. Increasing the unbound fraction of phenytoin in the blood also increases the amount of phenytoin that can be metabolized in the liver, and all this results in highly unpredictable levels of phenytoin in the circulation.
- Phenytoin induces liver enzymes that metabolize drugs such as hydrocortisone, oral contraceptives, theophylline, tricyclic antidepressants and thyroxine among others. This will decrease the efficacy of those drugs.

**Patient compliance and phenytoin monitoring.** As already mentioned above, it is necessary to measure plasma levels of phenytoin regularly. This is necessary not only because of phenytoin's interactions with other drugs and because of the non-linear relationship between dose and plasma levels but also because patients, especially elderly patients, may not be taking the drug as prescribed.

**Fosphenytoin,** which is a prodrug that is converted into phenytoin in the body after injection, has been introduced, and is also mentioned below in the following (newer drugs) section.

## Carbamazepine

Carbamazepine is a drug that is chemically related to the tricyclic antidepressants. It is believed to act by blocking sodium channels in the nerve membrane and keeping the conducting nerve in an inactive state.

**Therapeutic uses.** Carbamazepine is widely used in the control of tonic–clonic and partial seizures.

It is also used to relieve the pain of trigeminal neuralgia and in the treatment of bipolar depression (see p. 282). Carbamazepine is given orally and is fairly slowly absorbed from the intestine. Its rate of breakdown in the body increases with prolonged use because, like phenytoin, it induces the liver enzymes that break it down. Estimation of plasma levels may help to determine the correct dose, although the correct dose is more usually decided on by the patient's response than the plasma levels of the drug. Children may break down the drug rapidly so they may require three or four doses daily. The drug is introduced at a lower dose and this is gradually increased over a month. There is a slow-release or 'retard' formulation of carbamazepine that may be used at higher dosages, and also a suppository for when the oral route is not feasible.

**Adverse effects.** Up to one-third of patients who take carbamazepine experience adverse effects, but only about 5% of patients have to discontinue treatment. The most common adverse effects include rashes, dizziness and drowsiness, blurring of vision, depression of the leucocytes of the blood and occasionally jaundice and excessive salivary secretion. At higher doses, carbamazepine can have an antidiuretic effect and cause dyskinesia, photosensitivity and arrhythmias. It should be used with caution in cases of renal failure and the dose should be reduced in patients with liver disease.

**Interactions.** These occur with warfarin and erythromycin.

## Phenobarbital

Phenobarbital, the oldest drug in use for epilepsy, is a barbiturate. Phenobarbital reduces the spread of electrical excitation in the brain in several ways, but its principal action is by enhancing the action of the inhibitory neurotransmitter GABA by binding to sites on the GABA receptor. It also inhibits the action of the excitatory neurotransmitter glutamate.

**Therapeutic use.** Phenobarbital is not the drug of choice in epilepsy, because of its potential neurotoxicity. It is generally prescribed only when patients cannot tolerate other drugs. It is, however, still widely used in developing countries, because of its low cost.

Phenobarbital is slowly absorbed. The major portion is broken down in the body and the rest slowly excreted by the kidneys. Its action is therefore prolonged over about 12 hours. Phenobarbital is particularly effective in the treatment of tonic–clonic seizures, but may also be used in other types of epilepsy. It may be used as an alternative to phenytoin in the treatment of status epilepticus (see below).

**Adverse effects.** They are not uncommon: drowsiness and ataxia may be troublesome and occasionally a rash resembling measles is seen. Phenobarbital, like phenytoin, is a powerful inducer of enzymes in the liver, particularly those that break down other drugs. For example, phenobarbital increases the rate of breakdown of anticoagulants and of the estrogens, which are used in oral contraceptives, and whose effects may therefore be reduced. In adults, the drug may cause sedation and mood changes, especially depression. In children, however, the reverse occurs and the drug may produce hyperactivity, aggression and insomnia. Phenobarbital can cause osteomalacia through vitamin D deficiency and megaloblastic anaemia through folic acid deficiency. Like other barbiturates, phenobarbital causes physical dependence (see also p. 291), and sudden cessation of treatment may precipitate serious withdrawal symptoms, including sometimes-fatal convulsions, especially in the elderly.

## Primidone

**Therapeutic use.** Primidone is in many ways similar to phenobarbital and is effective against tonic–clonic attacks. It is important to start treatment with a low dosage and gradually increase the dose, otherwise adverse effects such as drowsiness, vertigo and vomiting may occur. It should not be combined with phenobarbital.

## Sodium valproate and valproic acid

Sodium valproate has been available for many years, being introduced in the early 1970s. Valproic acid was introduced in the 1990s.

**Mechanism of action.** Sodium valproate has several CNS actions. It maintains levels of GABA after the neurotransmitter has been released by inhibiting enzymes that break it down, although it is not known if this is how it blocks convulsions. It also increases the breakdown of the excitatory neurotransmitter glutamate. Sodium valproate also has a weak blocking action on sodium channels in the nerve cell membrane.

**Therapeutic use.** Sodium valproate is well absorbed after oral administration and has a half-life in the circulation of about 15 hours. It is effective against both petit and grand mal epilepsy. It is especially useful for treating infants since it has relatively low toxicity and few sedative effects. It is also useful

for treating older children who may suffer simultaneously with both petit and grand mal epilepsy.

**Adverse effects.** The drug is known to cause teratogenic effects such as spina bifida. Sodium valproate fairly commonly causes a modest fall in the platelet count. Occasionally this is severe and the patient should be warned to report any bruising or bleeding. It is advisable to carry out a platelet count before major surgery. Very rarely it causes serious liver damage, particularly in those with pre-existing liver disease or in children with congenital or accidental brain damage. Drowsiness, thinning of the hair (usually reversible) and weight gain are not uncommon.

## Clonazepam and diazepam

Clonazepam and diazepam are benzodiazepine drugs. Diazepam (*Valium*) is the most well known of this group of drugs. They may produce their antiepileptic effects by enhancing the inhibitory effect of GABA. They are effective in all forms of epilepsy but cause sedation. There is also a troublesome withdrawal syndrome associated with the benzodiazepines, which can worsen epileptic seizures if these drugs are stopped. They are most useful in treating status epilepticus (see later). A newer benzodiazepine, clobazam, has been introduced (see below). The benzodiazepine **lorazepam** is useful in status asthmaticus (see below).

## NEWER DRUGS USED IN TONIC–CLONIC AND PARTIAL SEIZURES

These newer drugs are still been evaluated (see also Michael 1999c).

### Felbamate

Felbamate is chemically related to a much older anxiolytic drug called meprobamate, which is no longer in use. The mechanism of action of felbamate is not fully understood, although it is thought to act by enhancing GABA activity, inhibiting glutamate activity and blocking sodium channels.

**Therapeutic use.** Felbamate is effective over a wide range of epileptic conditions. It is particularly effective in the treatment of partial seizures, with or without secondary generalizations that do not respond to other treatments.

**Adverse effects.** Its adverse effects include insomnia and nausea, and it can cause more dangerous problems such as hepatitis and aplastic anaemia. For these reasons it was withdrawn from clinical use in the USA and in the UK is now used only on a named patient basis. Its use is therefore restricted to the treatment of one particular type of childhood epilepsy called the Lennox–Gastaut syndrome, which does not respond to other drugs.

The Lennox–Gastaut syndrome is one of the most severe forms of childhood epilepsy. It is characterized by frequent seizures of several different types. The syndrome usually starts between the ages of 3 and 5 years, but may first manifest itself in children less than 2 years of age. It is very rare for children after the age of 8 to develop this syndrome.

## Fosphenytoin

Fosphenytoin is a newer drug that has been recently introduced for use in the UK. It is a prodrug and is converted into phenytoin by the liver enzyme alkaline phosphatase. It is given by injection when phenytoin cannot be given by mouth, e.g. during status epilepticus, or seizures associated with head injuries or surgery. It causes less irritation at the injection site than phenytoin. Its adverse effects and contraindications are therefore as for phenytoin.

## Gabapentin

**Mechanism of action.**  Gabapentin was originally designed as an analogue of GABA that would pass easily through the blood–brain barrier. Surprisingly, it was discovered that gabapentin does not act as a GABA analogue, but binds instead to a widespread amino acid transporter that is present in many different cell types, and its mechanism of anticonvulsant action is unknown.

**Therapeutic use.**  Gabapentin is used to control partial and general seizures, but is no more effective than the older drugs in use. The drug is rapidly excreted unchanged, mainly through the kidneys, so three times daily dosage may be necessary. Gabapentin should therefore be used with caution in patients with renal failure, since the drug will accumulate in these patients.

**Adverse effects.**  These include (usually) sleepiness, ataxia and fatigue. There are no known serious drug interactions.

## Lamotrigine

**Mechanism of action.**  Lamotrigine inhibits the release in the brain of the excitatory neurotransmitters glutamate and aspartate, thus preventing seizures.

**Therapeutic use.**  Lamotrigine is effective in partial and tonic–clonic seizures and has been shown to be as effective as carbamazepine and better tolerated. In the UK, lamotrigine has been licensed for use in adults as add-on or monotherapy to treat partial seizures and primary and secondarily generalized tonic–clonic seizures. It is a useful addition to the range of antiepileptic drugs and may also be effective when other antiepileptics have failed. If combined with other antiepileptic drugs, dose adjustment is necessary. Higher doses may be required with phenytoin or carbamazepine and lower doses with sodium valproate. An advantage of lamotrigine is that it is well tolerated and causes little impairment of cognition.

**Adverse effects.**  Lamotrigine may cause ataxia (unsteady gait), headaches, nausea and rashes, which may be dangerous, and which occur particularly in children. It should not be used in patients with hepatic or renal impairment.

## Levetiracetam

Levetiracetam is a newer drug about which relatively little is known. In the UK it is licensed for use as an adjunctive treatment of partial seizures with or without secondary generalizations (Report 2002). It is not recommended for use in children under 16 years of age. Its adverse effects include skin rashes, nausea, dizziness, headaches, drowsiness, ataxia and occasionally anorexia. It can cause emotional problems such as aggression and nervousness. It is contraindicated or should be used with caution in cases of liver or renal disease, and in patients who are pregnant or breast-feeding.

## Oxcarbazepine

Oxcarbazepine is a prodrug that is converted in the body to an active metabolite. Its action is believed to be similar to that of carbamazepine, and it is prescribed, mainly on a named patient basis, for patients who are allergic to carbamazepine. It is licensed for use both as adjunct and monotherapy for partial seizures and for generalized tonic–clonic seizures. Several side-effects common to those for the other anticonvulsants have been reported and it must not be used by patients already on carbamazepine.

## Tiagabine

**Mechanism of action.**  Tiagabine is an example of a relatively new designer drug, introduced in 1998, and based on the structure of GABA. Like gabapentin, it was designed to pass easily through the blood–brain barrier. It acts by prolonging the action of the natural neurotransmitter GABA. Specifically, tiagabine binds to and blocks a GABA transporter on the presynaptic nerve terminal. The drug thus inhibits the normal reuptake of GABA into the nerve terminal where it is inactivated, thus prolonging GABA's action.

**Therapeutic use.** Tiagabine is used as an adjunct treatment with other agents for partial seizures that are not satisfactorily controlled with other antiepileptics.

**Adverse effects.** These include diarrhoea, dizziness, confusion, headache, depression and occasionally psychotic episodes. The drug has been reported to cause leucopenia.

## Topiramate

Topiramate is another relatively new drug with multiple actions in the brain and many side-effects. It potentiates GABA activity in the brain and also has carbonic anhydrase inhibitory activity. It is licensed for use as an add-on therapy in partial and generalized seizures and for idiopathic seizures. Its use is restricted to cases of epilepsy that do not respond to other treatments. It should not be used in pregnancy and it should not be suddenly withdrawn from the patient.

## Vigabatrin

**Mechanism of action.** Vigabatrin inhibits the breakdown in the brain of GABA, which accumulates and suppresses seizures.

**Therapeutic use.** Vigabatrin is particularly effective in partial seizures and is also used in tonic–clonic seizures. It is taken orally and, although fairly rapidly excreted, its action lasts for 24 hours, so once-daily dosage is possible. Vigabatrin is used when the older antiepileptic drugs have proved unsuccessful.

**Adverse effects.** Sedation may occur and, occasionally, gastric upsets and headaches. Behavioural problems such as irritation, aggression, hallucination and memory faults occur in about 15% of patients. Occasionally, visual field defects develop and may require withdrawal of the drug.

## OUTCOME OF TREATMENT

A single drug controls about 80% of patients with tonic–clonic seizures. When the patient has been free of seizures for 5 years, drug treatment can be slowly withdrawn. Many subjects will have no further seizures, but about 40% (rather less in children) will relapse.

**Safety note**

It is important that anticonvulsants are not discontinued too suddenly as this may precipitate seizures.

## DRUGS USED IN ABSENCE SEIZURES

### Ethosuximide

Ethosuximide was originally developed through trial and error by altering the structure of barbiturates, of which phenobarbital is an example.

**Experimental use.** Ethosuximide is the drug of choice for the treatment of absence seizures. It is well absorbed orally and has a plasma half-life of about 50 hours.

**Adverse effects.** Ethosuximide may aggravate tonic–clonic seizures and may, if necessary, be combined with a drug that controls this type of attack. Its other effects include sleepiness, gastric upsets and headaches.

### Sodium valproate

Sodium valproate (see above) is also used for the treatment of absence seizures.

## FATAL ADVERSE REACTIONS IN CHILDREN

Most of the fatal adverse drug reactions in children are attributed to anticonvulsants (see Further reading section), as reported through the Medicines Control Agency yellow card scheme.

## DRIVING

A patient may be allowed to drive a car after being free from seizures for 1 year, but not a heavy goods or public service vehicle.

## DRUG COMBINATIONS

In most patients with epilepsy, complete control can be obtained with a single drug. This is desirable as it:

- minimizes the adverse effects
- there is no problem with interactions between the drugs
- it helps to maximize patient compliance.

Sometimes, however, a combination of drugs is required to achieve better control.

## STATUS EPILEPTICUS

In status epilepticus the patient has a series of seizures, rapidly following each other. These patients require careful nursing so that they do not injure themselves. They should be nursed in the lateral semi-prone position, dentures removed and the airway established; oxygen should be given by mask. The patient should not be left unattended until the seizures have ceased.

The drugs commonly used are:

- benzodiazepines, namely diazepam, lorazepam
- phenytoin or fosphenytoin
- phenobarbital or thiopental
- paraldehyde.

The most effective drugs are diazepam or lorazepam given slowly intravenously. In young children rectal diazepam using rectal tubes (*Stesolid*) is rapidly effective and useful particularly if intravenous injection is difficult. Diazepam should control seizures within 10 minutes and if the seizures persist the dose may be repeated. Although diazepam will usually stop the seizures, relapse quite commonly occurs within the next hour. To prevent this, phenytoin, or more usually, fosphenytoin, is injected intravenously.

Phenytoin has some action on the heart and either phenytoin or fosphenytoin should be given via a central line and should be monitored by ECG and blood pressure measurements. If the seizures persist, clomethiazole should be given intravenously and the dose adjusted to produce a satisfactory therapeutic effect. Finally, if all else fails, phenobarbital or thiopental (see p. 231) can be given by intravenous injection. When these drugs are used it is essential to have an anaesthetist to help, as intubation may be necessary and the procedure is not without risk. As with other anaesthetics, there is also the risk of respiratory depression.

### Nursing point

The use of clomethiazole and thiopental requires considerable expertise and should, if possible, be carried out in an intensive care unit with expert guidance.

### Paraldehyde

Paraldehyde, an oily liquid with a pungent smell, has been used for many years. It is a CNS depressant that controls status epilepticus. It is given rectally, diluted in saline or by deep intramuscular injection; however since it is an irritant, care must be taken to avoid the sciatic nerve. Paraldehyde must be injected using a glass syringe. It is not the first-line treatment for status epilepticus, but, because it is a relatively safe drug, it can be used when facilities for close monitoring and respiratory support (if needed) are not available.

### Nursing point

The renewal of seizures or the emergence of toxicity after a period of good control may be due to poor compliance or to an interaction with a newly prescribed drug.

## FEBRILE CONVULSIONS

About 3% of infants and young children have a fit when feverish (pyrexial). Of these, only some 1% will ultimately develop true epilepsy.

The immediate treatment is to lay the child semi-prone, and most convulsions stop within a few minutes. If the seizure persists, rectal diazepam as for status epilepticus (see earlier) is the safest and easiest treatment. Hospital admission may be necessary to exclude serious infection.

### Prevention

The parents should be taught to reduce fever by removing excess clothing, keeping the environment cool, supplying cool drinks and giving paracetamol paediatric elixir. If attacks recur with fever, the alternatives are:

- To give rectal diazepam when the child develops a fever.
- To give continuous medication. Phenobarbital is effective in most children, but side-effects may limit its use and it is rarely required.
- Finally, parents will require reassurance as the majority of convulsions of this type are short-lived and cause no long-term problems.

### Answers to parents' questions

- There is a 30% chance it will happen again if the child has a fever, but attacks become rare after 4 years of age.
- Brain (cerebral) damage is very rare.

## ANTIEPILEPTICS AND PREGNANCY

There is evidence that antiepileptic drugs given during pregnancy are associated with an increased incidence of fetal malformation (see also above). If possible a single antiepileptic should be used and the dosage controlled by repeated measurement of blood levels. Most fetal abnormalities arise during the first trimester of pregnancy and women who are taking antiepileptic drugs should be advised of the risk before becoming pregnant.

Carbamazepine and sodium valproate may cause neural tube defects and phenytoin may cause a variety of abnormalities. At present, there does not appear to be an entirely safe drug. To minimize the risk, women should receive supplementary folic acid before (if possible) and throughout pregnancy.

Many antiepileptic drugs induce liver enzymes and thus increase the rate of breakdown of oral contraceptives, so the patient's method of contraception may need to be reviewed.

### Eclampsia

The control of seizures is important in the treatment of eclampsia. In the UK this has usually been attempted by using phenytoin or diazepam. It has been shown that intravenous magnesium sulphate is probably more effective. Its mode of action in these circumstances is not clear, but it may relieve cerebral ischaemia by vasodilatation or minimize cerebral damage. It is given by intravenous infusion.

## PROGNOSIS IN EPILEPSY

The prognosis with epilepsy is variable in that 70–80% of patients who develop epilepsy will at some stage become free of seizures with treatment. Treatment may be stopped in patients who have been free of seizures for 3–5 years. Approximately 50% of patients in this category who stop taking drugs will be successful in stopping drug therapy. The remaining 20–30% of patients may continue to have seizures despite treatment and may develop chronic active epilepsy. The prognosis for these patients is usually poorer and they often suffer from additional psychological or neurological problems.

The overall mortality rates for patients with epilepsy are about 3–5 times those of the general population, especially in patients with severe epilepsy and in younger sufferers. The most common causes of death include status epilepticus, accidents, suicide and tumours.

**Summary**

- In epilepsy, it is common to use monotherapy, and multiple drug regimes only in resistant cases
- Patients with epilepsy should be warned against driving vehicles, swimming and working under conditions where a seizure could produce disaster
- Doses of phenytoin should not be altered at less than fortnightly intervals
- Phenytoin is easily displaced from plasma binding sites by other drugs, and this can increase its effective concentration in the blood
- Plasma concentrations of phenytoin must be monitored regularly
- Fosphenytoin is converted into phenytoin in the body and the same precautions as for phenytoin should be observed
- Carbamazepine should be used with caution in cases of renal failure and the dose should be reduced in patients with liver disease
- Phenobarbital is potentially neurotoxic
- Phenobarbital causes physical dependence and sudden cessation of treatment may precipitate serious withdrawal symptoms, including sometimes-fatal convulsions, especially in the elderly
- Primidone should not be combined with phenobarbital

- Sodium valproate is known to cause teratogenic effects such as spina bifida
- The benzodiazepine **lorazepam** is useful in status asthmaticus
- It is important that anticonvulsants are not discontinued too suddenly as this may precipitate seizures
- A patient may be allowed to drive a car after being free from seizures for 1 year, but not a heavy goods or public service vehicle
- Paraldehyde must be injected using a glass syringe
- For febrile convulsions, parents should be taught to reduce fever by removing excess clothing, keeping the environment cool, supplying cool drinks and giving paracetamol paediatric elixir
- Carbamazepine and sodium valproate may cause neural tube defects and phenytoin may cause a variety of abnormalities. At present, there does not appear to be an entirely safe drug. To minimize the risk, women should receive supplementary folic acid before (if possible) and throughout pregnancy

# PARKINSON'S DISEASE

## INTRODUCTION

Parkinson's disease is a progressive degenerative disease of the brain. It occurs mainly in the elderly, although it can first manifest itself as early as the 40s or 50s. The onset is often gradual and insidious. It is a relatively common neurological disorder, and in the UK affects 1–2% of elderly people.

## CHIEF SYMPTOMS

- Inhibition of voluntary movements (hypokinesias), which is caused partly by inertia of the motor system and partly by muscle rigidity (see below). Inertia means that movement is difficult to initiate and difficult to stop.
- Tremor at rest, often involving the 'pill-rolling' action between thumb and forefinger, which is lessened during voluntary movement.
- Muscle rigidity, when muscles are stiff and difficult to move, using passive limb manipulation.

## OTHER CLINICAL FEATURES

The patient's face may be expressionless. Walking is difficult to initiate, and the patient may walk with rapid, small steps (called 'festination'), or with small, shuffling steps. The patient will freeze when trying to change direction when walking, and as the disease progresses the patient may fall down due to the gradual loss of postural reflexes. The resting tremor of the hands is noticeably worsened by stress. The patient's handwriting often becomes much smaller because of the difficulty performing fine motor movements. The patient sweats excessively and suffers from a greasy skin (seborrhoea). The digestive system is adversely affected. Swallowing becomes difficult and the patient may drool. Constipation occurs virtually invariably. The patient becomes depressed and may complain of difficulty with thinking (dysphrenia; cognitive impairment). In the later stages, the patient may suffer from dementia.

## CAUSES OF PARKINSON'S DISEASE AND PARKINSONISM

- Age-related degenerative changes in nerve cells in the basal nuclei of the brain
- Drug-induced brain damage
- Cerebral ischaemia
- Viral encephalitis.

Note that the term *parkinsonism* is used to describe the symptoms of Parkinson's disease, which may result, as stated above, not only from the degeneration of the nigrostriatal pathway but also from drugs or infections. The term *Parkinson's disease* is used, normally, to describe the idiopathic disease that results from the apparently spontaneous progressive degeneration of the pathway.

## DEGENERATIVE CHANGES

These are best understood in the context of the extrapyramidal system: Fine movements are controlled by the extrapyramidal system, which has its controlling centre in the brain. There is normally a fine balance between the activity of the two neurotransmitters dopamine and acetylcholine (ACh) in a part of the brain called the corpus striatum, which sends nerve impulses to the cortex and from there to the spinal cord and finally to the voluntary muscles. Dopamine is inhibitory and ACh is excitatory. The dopaminergic nerves come from an area called the substantia nigra lower down in the brain. If for any reason the inhibitory dopaminergic influence is reduced significantly, the ACh nerves in the corpus striatum are allowed too much activity, resulting in the muscle tremor and rigidity of Parkinson's disease. The system is shown diagrammatically in Figure 19.2.

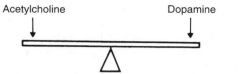

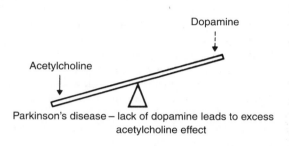

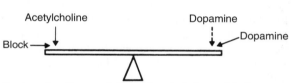

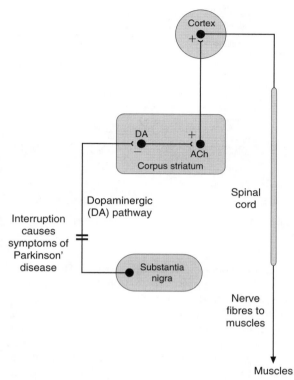

**Figure 19.2** Extrapyrimidal system simplified to show the role of the nigrostriatal dopaminergic pathway in the control of fine movement. + = excitatory, − = inhibitory.

**Figure 19.3** The use of drugs in Parkinson's disease.

It can be seen, therefore, that relief of symptoms can be achieved by reducing cholinergic activity or by increasing the amount of dopamine (Fig. 19.3).

## DRUG-INDUCED PARKINSONISM

Drugs can cause symptoms of Parkinson's disease, some temporary and others permanently. The most famous example is that of the case of a group of Californian heroin addicts who in 1982 developed a very severe form of Parkinson's disease. The cause was the presence in their drugs of a chemical called MPTP, which was a contaminant of the heroin substitute they were using. The MPTP was converted in their bodies to the active substance MPP, which was selectively taken up into the dopaminergic neurones of the nigrostriatal system and destroyed them. Strangely, the drug attacked only the dopaminergic neurones of the nigrostriatal system and nowhere else. Several other drugs in use may precipitate seizures in some patients, although this is usually a temporary adverse effect.

## TREATMENT OF PARKINSON'S DISEASE WITH DRUGS

Two main chemical approaches are used:

- reduce cholinergic activity
- enhance dopaminergic activity.

### Antimuscarinic drugs

Drugs which decrease cholinergic activity are called antimuscarinic drugs:

- benzatropine mesylate
- biperiden hydrochloride
- orphenadrine hydrochloride
- procyclidine hydrochloride
- trihexyphenidyl (benzhexol) hydrochloride.

**Mechanism of action.** These drugs antagonize the action of the excitatory neurotransmitter acetylcholine (ACh) at its muscarinic receptors in the corpus striatum, thus allowing dopamine to exert its inhibitory effect (see Fig. 19.2). Since acetylcholine is such a widely used neurotransmitter, both in the brain and elsewhere in the body, these drugs will produce many unwanted adverse effects (see below).

**Therapeutic use of antimuscarinic drugs.** Originally drugs of the belladonna group were used for this purpose but they have now been replaced by synthetic substitutes. These drugs reduce tremor, but have less effect on rigidity, which is generally more troublesome for the patient than is the tremor. They may be used in mild cases, but they have troublesome adverse effects and have been largely replaced. They are more likely to be used as adjunct therapy with dopamine agonists (see below).

**Trihexyphenidyl (benzhexol)** is given orally and the dose is gradually increased until a satisfactory response is obtained or the limit of tolerance is reached. **Orphenadrine** has the advantage of having a mood-lifting effect as well as relieving the symptoms of Parkinsonism. This is useful as these patients are often depressed. **Benzatropine** is in many ways similar to benzhexol. It is particularly useful in the excessive salivation often found in parkinsonism and in muscular rigidity. It is liable to cause drowsiness and is best given as a single dose at bedtime. They are sometimes useful if patients are also taking antipsychotic drugs.

**Adverse effects.** Nausea, constipation, giddiness, dry mouth, urinary retention and glaucoma; in overdose, confusion and hallucinations may also occur. They should be given before food if the patient complains of dry mouth.

Drugs which increase dopamine activity (see Fig. 19.4) can be subclassified as:

- Drugs that *replace dopamine*.
- Drugs that act as *dopamine agonists* (stimulate) at dopamine receptors on nerves in the corpus striatum normally supplied by dopaminergic nerves from the substantia nigra.
- Drugs that *stimulate the release of dopamine* from dopaminergic nerve terminals in the corpus striatum.
- Drugs that *block the breakdown of dopamine* after it has been released from surviving dopaminergic nerve terminals in the corpus striatum. There are at present two main types:
  - monoamine oxidase inhibitors (MAOIs)
  - drugs that block the enzyme COMT (catechol *O*-methyltransferase).

## Drugs that replace dopamine: levodopa

It is not possible to restore the deficiency in the brain by giving dopamine, as this substance will not enter

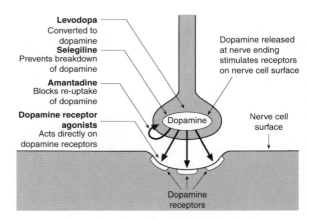

**Figure 19.4** Site of action of dopaminergic drugs used in Parkinson's disease.

the brain. Therefore **levodopa** is used. This precursor of dopamine passes freely into the brain where it is converted to dopamine. The dopamine then acts on dopamine receptors wherever they are found in the brain, including those in the corpus striatum. The drug will therefore have many central actions, resulting in sometimes-troublesome adverse effects (see below). Levodopa is particularly useful in reducing rigidity, but has less effect on tremor.

**Levodopa and a dopa decarboxylase inhibitor.** Levodopa is broken down by an enzyme called dopa decarboxylase, which is found particularly in the gut wall and liver. If this enzyme is inhibited by a drug which can be administered in combination with levodopa, the effects of levodopa are enhanced and prolonged and a much smaller dose of levodopa is required. This reduces the incidence of some side-effects. Two preparations that are widely used are:

- levodopa + carbidopa (**co-careldopa**; *Sinemet*)
- levodopa + benserazide (**co-beneldopa**; *Madopar*)

**Therapeutic use.** Adverse effects are very troublesome when levodopa is used alone, so treatment is usually started with small doses of either co-careldopa or co-beneldopa. These doses are gradually increased until a satisfactory control of symptoms is obtained, without an unacceptable incidence of adverse reactions to the drug. The intervals between the taking of doses can be critical in determining the severity of adverse effects, and will have to be chosen according to the reactions of individual patients to the drug.

The drug's efficacy falls with time of use. The patient may show slow improvement for the first

6–18 months, and this may be maintained for 1–2 years, but thereafter the drug loses efficacy. Patients may suffer from the 'on-off' effect. During the 'on' period the patient walks normally, but during the 'off' period the patient reverts to the impaired gait of Parkinson's disease. The duration of benefit of the drug often becomes shortened after prolonged use and the frequency of dosing needs to be increased, with concomitant increase in adverse effects. This is called the 'end-of-dose' effect of levodopa.

**Adverse effects.** These comprise nausea and vomiting, postural fall in blood pressure, restlessness and involuntary facial movements and constipation. Nausea and vomiting are very common but can be minimized by giving the drug in divided doses with meals. **Domperidone** (see p. 125) is a useful anti-emetic because it blocks the effect of dopamine on the chemoreceptor trigger zone (CTZ) in the brainstem, but does not interfere with the therapeutic action of dopamine at the basal ganglia. Some postural fall in blood pressure is common, but rarely causes symptoms. Blood pressure should be measured before and during treatment. A few patients become restless, and at higher dose levels involuntary movements, usually affecting the face, may occur. Constipation will require a good fluid and fibre intake.

**Drug interactions.** Levodopa/decarboxylase inhibitor combinations should not be combined with MAOIs. Concomitant use of halothane, cyclopropane or trichlorethylene carries an increased risk of cardiac arrhythmias and the drug should be stopped 8 hours before anaesthesia.

## Drugs that act as dopamine receptor agonists

- Ergot-derived dopamine receptor agonists: bromocriptine, cabergoline, lisuride, pergolide
- Ropinirole
- Pramipexole
- Apomorphine.

This group of drugs stimulates dopamine receptors in the cells of the basal ganglia. They are prescribed when treatment with levodopa is ineffective or requires supplementation, but adverse effects can limit their use (Lebrun-Frenay & Borg 2002). **Bromocriptine** and **cabergoline** are almost identical. Both drugs can cause nausea and postural hypotension and dosage requires careful adjustment. Lisuride and pergolide have similar actions, pergolide being effective for about 5 hours and lisuride for 3 hours.

There are at least three types of dopamine receptors (called $D_1$, $D_2$ and $D_3$), and the more potent agonists act on both $D_1$ and $D_2$ receptor types. **Lisuride**, which has a short duration of action, acts mainly on $D_2$ receptors. **Pergolide**, which has the longest duration of action, acts on both $D_1$ and $D_2$ receptors. **Ropinirole**, a newer $D_2$ receptor agonist (Schrag et al 2002), has been found to be useful in younger patients who may not tolerate levodopa well. **Pramipexole** acts on $D_2$ and $D_3$ receptors.

> ### Safety note
>
> There is a recent report (Editorial 2002) that dopamine receptor agonists used to treat Parkinson's disease may be associated with sudden sleep attacks. The patient falls asleep suddenly and may stay asleep for a few minutes. Clearly, if true, this has very serious implications for patient safety and that of others, e.g. when driving. Prescribers should consult the manufacturer's recommendations on driving when prescribing these drugs.

**Apomorphine** is a powerful dopamine receptor stimulant in the CTZ of the brain and has been used as an emetic. It is also sometimes prescribed to control the 'off' period associated with prolonged use of levodopa (see above). Treatment is difficult and requires close supervision and considerable patient education. Ideally, it should be initiated in hospital and domperidone is started 3 days before apomorphine to control vomiting. Apomorphine is given by multiple subcutaneous injections or by continuous subcutaneous infusion. A few patients develop postural hypotension, but the most common problem is nausea, which can be controlled by domperidone.

> ### Safety note
>
> The Committee for the Safety of Medicines has advised that all ergot-based dopamine receptor agonists should not be used until the patient has been screened for erythrocyte sedimentation rates and for urea and electrolytes, and chest X-rays and lung function tests may be advisable. This is because this class of drugs has been associated with pericardial, pulmonary and retroperitoneal fibrotic reactions.

### Drugs that may stimulate the release of dopamine from dopaminergic nerve terminals in the corpus striatum: amantadine (*Symmetrel*)

Amantadine was originally introduced as an anti-influenza treatment. It is currently believed to work by increasing dopamine release form the nerve terminal and also perhaps by blocking the reuptake of dopamine into the nerve terminal, thereby maintaining concentrations of endogenously released dopamine. Clearly, the efficacy of this type of drug will decrease with progressive loss of dopaminergic nerves.

**Therapeutic use.** Amantadine is usually introduced at an early stage of the disease as monotherapy. It is not as effective as levodopa and is useless in some patients, but can be used when that drug is contraindicated. The initial dose may be increased after 1 week if necessary.

**Adverse effects.** These include livedo reticularis (skin discoloration), blurred vision, peripheral oedema, dizziness and gastrointestinal disturbances.

**Contraindications.** The drug is contraindicated in epilepsy, renal disease, pregnancy, breast-feeding and when there is a history of gastric ulceration.

### Drugs that block the breakdown of dopamine

These consist of MAOIs such as selegiline and COMT inhibitors such as entacapone.

**Selegiline** inhibits the breakdown of levodopa in the brain by blocking the enzyme MAO type B. It is often used in combination with levodopa with or without a decarboxylase inhibitor and this allows a smaller dose of levodopa to be used and prolongs its action. It is usually given as a single dose in the morning. Adverse effects include confusion and nausea.

**Entacapone** is a drug that can be used only if levodopa is given as well, since the drug acts by blocking the action of COMT, which breaks down levodopa before it crosses the blood–brain barrier and gets into the brain. It has been found to be useful when 'end-of-dose' fluctuations in motor activity occur with levodopa (see above). Adverse effects include gastrointestinal disturbances, discoloured urine,

dyskinesias, dizziness, dry mouth and, rarely, hepatitis. Contraindications include pregnancy and breast-feeding, liver disease and phaeochromocytoma (epinephrine-secreting tumours).

## THE TREATMENT OF PARKINSON'S DISEASE

As can be seen from the preceding discussion there are a number of drugs which are useful in relieving the symptoms of this condition, but they do not prevent its progression. There is no unanimous opinion as to the order in which they should be given. In mild cases a start may be made with an anticholinergic drug such as benzhexol, especially if tremor is a problem. If this is ineffective or tolerance develops, it can be changed to amantadine or levodopa. There is no evidence that selegiline should be used early in treatment for its supposed neuroprotective action. It may indeed increase mortality. For most patients, particularly those with more severe symptoms, it is usual to start with levodopa combined with a decarboxylase inhibitor. If a very high dosage of levodopa is required to control symptoms, a dopamine receptor agonist may be added to the regime.

About three-quarters of patients with Parkinson's disease respond to drugs. Rigidity is usually most amenable to treatment and tremor less so. Unfortunately, in more than half the patients being treated by levodopa its efficacy decreases with time, so that increasingly frequent dosage is required to maintain its effect and prevent the 'on-off' phenomenon during which there are periods of weakness and loss of movement. These fluctuations can be reduced by frequent dosage or by using a controlled-release preparation. If this fails, selegiline can be added to the regime. Finally, if levodopa becomes ineffective, an oral agonist or injections of apomorphine can be used.

### Family needs in Parkinson's disease

It is highly likely that when a patient develops Parkinson's disease, a progressively greater burden will be placed on a partner, who may not be well or may be infirm through age. It is the responsibility of all health care professionals who are involved to be concerned not only about the patient but also about whether the family is coping with the problem. Specialist nurses and organizations such as the Parkinson's Disease Society and European Parkinson's Disease Society play critical and highly effective roles in this respect and the family should be put in touch with concerned groups.

---

**Nursing point**

In the UK, guidance for group protocols for variation of prescriptions by Parkinson's disease nurse specialists is available from the Parkinson's Disease Society.

# SURGICAL TREATMENTS IN PARKINSON'S DISEASE

## Neural transplantation

Great interest was generated in the 1970s when it was discovered that fetal brain tissue could be successfully transplanted into the adult brain and function normally. On this basis, several attempts have been made to transplant human fetal tissue containing dopaminergic neurones into the brains of patients with Parkinson's disease. The results have been variable, despite the proven ability of fetal grafts to be integrated into the patient's brain (Mendez et al 2002). The use of human fetal tissue has raised many problems and issues, including ethical ones. Scientists are now experimenting with stem cells and animal nerve cells that produce dopamine.

## Pallidotomy (pallidectomy)

Pallidotomy is the introduction of electrodes into the brain to destroy a particular part of the brain in an area called the globus pallidus, which contains cells that are involved in the generation of unwanted movements. It was very much a hit and miss affair and fell out of favour when levodopa was introduced. Now it is being used again because modern imaging techniques make it possible to pinpoint the cells to be destroyed with greater accuracy.

Pallidotomy is indicated mainly for patients who develop dyskinesia due to their drugs. There are risks with this procedure, including the possibility of stroke, partial loss of vision or speech, confusion and swallowing difficulties.

## Deep brain stimulation

This procedure is based on that of the cardiac pacemaker. It involves placing electrodes into specific brain areas, specifically the globus pallidus or the thalamus. As with pallidotomy, the aim is to stop uncontrollable movements. The electrodes are connected to a pacemaker-like device which the patient can switch on or off, depending on the symptoms.

## References

Editorial 2002 Sudden sleep attacks with dopamine agonists – do they exist? MeReC Extra Issue 7, November 2002

Lebrun-Frenay C, Borg M 2002 Choosing the right dopamine agonist for patients with Parkinson's disease. Current Medical Research Opinion 18: 209

Mendez I, Dagher A, Hong M et al 2002 Simultaneous intrastriatal and intranigral fetal dopaminergic grafts in patients with Parkinson disease: a pilot study. Report of three cases. Journal of Neurosurgery 96: 589

Michael T 1999a Epilepsy (1). The disease. Pharmaceutical Journal 262: 297

Michael T 1999b Epilepsy (2). Treatment – the established drugs. Pharmaceutical Journal 262: 432

Report 2002 Levetiracetam – a new drug for epilepsy. Drug and Therapeutics Bulletin 40: 30

Schrag A, Ben-Shlomo Y, Quinn N 2002 Ropinirole for the treatment of tremor in early Parkinson's disease. European Journal of Neurology 9: 253

## Further reading

Brodie M J, Dichter M A 1996 Antiepileptic drugs. New England Journal of Medicine 334: 168

Calne D B 1993 The treatment of Parkinson's disease. New England Journal of Medicine 329: 1021

Chadwick D 1994 Gabapentin. Lancet 343: 89

Dichter M A, Brodie M J 1996 New antiepileptic drugs. New England Journal of Medicine 334: 1583

Eclampsia Trial Collaboration Group 1995 Which anticonvulsant for women with eclampsia? Lancet 345: 1455

Editorial 1989 Withdrawing anti-epileptic drugs. Drug and Therapeutics Bulletin 27: 29

Editorial 1994 Epilepsy and pregnancy. Drug and Therapeutics Bulletin 32(7): 49

Editorial 1995 Selegiline in Parkinson's disease. British Medical Journal 311: 1583

Editorial 1996 Stopping status epilepticus. Drug and Therapeutics Bulletin 34(10): 73

Editorial 1999 Developments in the treatment of Parkinson's disease. Drug and Therapeutics Bulletin 37(5): 36

Freely M 1999 Drug treatment of epilepsy. British Medical Journal 318: 106

Linfear J 2002 The individual with epilepsy. Nursing Standard 16: 43

Marson A G, Kadir Z A, Chadwick D W 1996 New antiepileptic drugs: a systematic review of their efficacy and tolerability. British Medical Journal 313: 1169

Michael T 1999c Epilepsy (3). New treatments. Pharmaceutical Journal 262: 470

Neville B G R 1997 Epilepsy in childhood. British Medical Journal 315: 924

Quinn N 1995 Drug treatment of Parkinson's disease. British Medical Journal 310: 575

Rosman N P, Colton T, Labazzo J et al 1993 A controlled trial of diazepam to prevent the recurrence of febrile seizures. New England Journal of Medicine 329: 79

Valman H B 1993 Febrile convulsions. British Medical Journal 306: 1743

# Chapter 20

# CNS 3. Antipsychotics, anxiolytics and hypnotics

## Learning objectives

At the end of this chapter, the reader should be able to:

- identify some brain neurotransmitter receptors known to be important targets for drug action in psychiatry
- appreciate the special points about administering drugs to psychiatric patients in hospital
- give an account of the broad classification of antipsychotic drugs into typical and atypical with examples
- provide examples of the phenothiazines and the other classes of antipsychotic drugs, their use and adverse effects
- understand what is meant by a depot injection of drugs
- give an account of the nature and treatment of schizophrenia, and the management of the schizoid patient
- list the recommendation of NICE for the use of atypical antipsychotic drugs
- understand what is meant by the acute confusional state and its dangers for elderly patients and its treatment and patient care
- give an account of the different classifications of anxiety and know the different classifications of anxiolytic drugs
- give the names of specific benzodiazepines, their therapeutic use and adverse effects
- give an account of some of the common causes of insomnia, the nature of sleep and provide the names of the most commonly used hypnotic drugs, their therapeutic use and important adverse effects

## INTRODUCTION

Mental illness is one of the major causes of ill health. Many drugs have been produced in the hope that they would have some therapeutic effect. Certain mental illnesses, particularly depression and schizophrenia, are linked with chemical abnormalities in the brain. The nature of some of these abnormalities is known, but there are considerable gaps in our knowledge. Nevertheless, the knowledge gleaned so far from medical research has resulted in the introduction of drugs that are designed to target brain mechanisms that may mediate mental illnesses.

## TYPES OF MENTAL ILLNESS

The treatment of psychiatric disorders can be considered in terms of three main types of disorder: psychosis, anxiety and depression.

**Psychosis** is a term used to describe disorders when the patient loses contact with reality. Features of psychosis include paranoia, schizophrenia, manic behaviour, severe thought disturbance or poverty of thought. Terms such as 'delusions' and 'hallucinations' are sometimes used to describe the symptoms of psychosis.

**Anxiety** is a term used to describe a condition of generalized, all-pervasive fear. It is featured by an emotionally inappropriate response to the patient's environment and to circumstances. Traditionally patients were termed 'neurotic' but this term is no longer favoured in some clinical circles. Commonly used lay and professional terms to describe the symptoms of anxiety include 'panic attacks', generalized panic disorder and post-traumatic stress disorder. This list keeps growing due to the practice of labelling the circumstances that generate anxiety.

**Depression** is a blanket term for several disorders that are characterized by changes in mood rather than in thought or emotional response. Professionals describe depression as an **affective** disorder. Symptoms can range from extreme sadness to suicidal intent. Depression is dealt with in Chapter 21.

## BRAIN NEUROTRANSMITTERS AND PSYCHIATRIC DISORDERS

Many of the drugs that have been introduced for the treatment of psychotic disorders are known to interfere with the normal action of several of the brain neurotransmitters and their receptors. The major brain neurotransmitters that have been implicated in psychiatric disorders are:

- acetylcholine (ACh)
- epinephrine
- norepinephrine
- dopamine
- 5-hydroxytryptamine (5-HT)
- GABA (gamma-aminobutyric acid)
- neuropeptides.

The amounts of epinephrine and norepinephrine are increased in the brain by giving drugs such as monoamine oxidase inhibitors (MAOIs), which are drugs that retard their breakdown. Tricyclic antidepressants inhibit the re-uptake of catecholamines into the nerve terminals. Thus, an awakening and stimulating effect is produced, and these drugs are used as antidepressants (see Chapter 21). If the amounts of catecholamines in the brain are reduced, a tranquillizing or depressing effect is produced; 5-HT also seems to be concerned with mood, whereas GABA exerts a sedating inhibiting effect. Dopamine stimulates more than one class of receptor: it causes nausea and vomiting but also appears to be concerned with the schizoid state. In fact, the evidence suggests that the efficacy of many antipsychotic drugs can be correlated, approximately, with their ability to block dopamine $D_2$ receptors (see more below).

## ANTIPSYCHOTIC DRUGS

### ADMINISTRATION OF DRUGS TO PSYCHIATRIC PATIENTS – GENERAL POINTS

- In hospital, many people with mental health problems are not confined to bed and drugs may be administered at a central point rather than having a 'drug round'.
- Two nurses should always be concerned with drug administration.
- In psychiatric units, patient compliance may be a problem and it is necessary to ensure that medication is actually taken. For example, patients may put the tablets in their mouths, but spit them out when no longer observed by the nurse.
- In some patients, especially schizophrenics, drugs may be given by injection as depot preparations to get round the problem of non-compliance.
- Occasionally a patient's paranoia may extend to drugs they are given. They may think the staff are trying to poison them.

- Drug education for when the patient returns home is very important and relatives may have to be involved. Non-compliance is an important hazard as the patient's illness may relapse if treatment is stopped. It should also be possible for patients or relatives to have contact numbers to call for information if problems arise.
- The nurse should observe the effects of drug treatment.
- On discharge, care should be taken not to prescribe excessive quantities of drugs, particularly if there is a suicide risk.

## CLASSIFICATION OF ANTIPSYCHOTIC DRUGS

Traditionally, antipsychotic drugs such as chlorpromazine (see below) have been referred to as *major tranquillizers*, while anxiety-suppressing drugs such the benzodiazepines (see Chapter 21) have been called *minor tranquillizers*. This terminology is generally no longer in favour and will not be used here. Antipsychotic drugs are also called *neuroleptics*, and this term is still widely used. Antipsychotic drugs, because of their diverse chemical nature and wide range of pharmacological actions, are notoriously difficult to classify, but the currently favoured broad classification is into two main types:

- **classical** or **typical** antipsychotic drugs, which are generally those that have been in use for many years
- **atypical** antipsychotic drugs, which are more recent additions to the repertoire of drugs available.

This distinction is based partly on the fact that some of the newer (atypical) drugs produce fewer adverse effects on the motor system, such as tremor, and that the atypical drugs may help patients who do not respond to the older, typical drugs.

Examples of typical antipsychotic drugs:

- chlorpromazine
- flupentixol
- fluphenazine
- haloperidol
- thioridazine.

Examples of atypical antipsychotic drugs:

- amisulpride
- clozapine
- olanzapine
- risperidone
- quetiapine
- zotepine.

## MECHANISM OF ACTION OF ANTIPSYCHOTIC DRUGS

Virtually all antipsychotic (neuroleptic) drugs have so many different pharmacological actions that it is very difficult to relate any one action to a therapeutic effect. The only statement that can be made with reasonable confidence is that most, if not all, effective antipsychotic drugs share the ability to block dopamine $D_2$ receptors in the brain.

These drugs are particularly useful in controlling the states of agitation found in acute schizophrenia, mania and some other forms of delirium and in paranoia. Their exact mode of action in these conditions is not known but most of them block the action of dopamine on $D_2$ receptors in the mesolimbic system of the brain and this seems important in their sedative and antipsychotic action (Fig. 20.1). They also

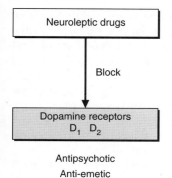

Antipsychotic
Anti-emetic
Parkinson-like symptoms

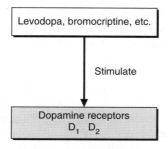

Relief of Parkinson's disease
Psychological effects
Emetic action
Bromocriptine inhibits lactation

**Figure 20.1**  Effect of drugs on dopamine receptors in the brain. The exact part played by $D_1$ and $D_2$ receptors and other subgroups is not known.

block the action of dopamine on the brain CTZ (chemoreceptor trigger zone) and are thus anti-emetic. Some, such as haloperidol (see below) block the action of the dopaminergic nerves that run from the substantia nigra to the corpus striatum. Interruption of this system causes parkinsonism (see p. 255) and so these drugs may cause various disorders of movement and posture (see later).

## THERAPEUTIC USE OF TYPICAL ANTIPSYCHOTIC DRUGS

The typical antipsychotic (neuroleptic) drugs are

- phenothiazines
- thioxanthenes
- butyrophenones
- other neuroleptics.

### The phenothiazines

**Therapeutic uses and effects.** Phenothiazines have an antipsychotic effect. Restlessness, agitation and hallucinations are reduced and this has made them especially useful for treating schizophrenia. They produce some sedation with a feeling of detachment from external worries. Many of them have some anti-emetic action. Chlorpromazine is sometimes used to control persistent hiccup. Most of the phenothiazines are well absorbed after oral dosage. They are largely metabolized in the liver to numerous breakdown substances.

The phenothiazines are used in psychiatry to reduce restlessness, anxiety and agitation in psychotic patients and to reduce the severity of hallucinations. They are thus useful for controlling schizophrenics who show these symptoms. They are sometimes used in low doses in psychoneurosis with anxiety. They are, in addition, used as anti-emetics, in severe pruritus and in association with anaesthetic agents. A number of phenothiazines are now in use; some are preferred for one type of disorder, some for another. They have been classified according to their sedative, antimuscarinic and extrapyramidal effects (Box 20.1).

The doses of these drugs are very variable and depend on the disorder being treated, and on the response and age of the patient. In long-term administration, it is not worth altering the dose more than once a week because of their variable and prolonged actions.

---

**Box 20.1    Classification of phenothiazines**

**Group 1**
- Chlorpromazine
- Levomepromazine (methotrimeprazine)
- Promazine

Sedation ++++, antimuscarinic ++, extrapyramidal ++

**Group 2**
- Pericyazine
- Pipotiazine
- Thioridazine

Sedation ++, antimuscarinic ++++, extrapyramidal ++

**Group 3**
- Fluphenazine
- Perphenazine
- Prochlorperazine
- Trifluoperazine

Sedation ++, antimuscarinic ++, extrapyramidal ++++

*Key*: ++ = few to moderate effects, ++++ = marked effects.

---

In treating psychotic patients large doses of phenothiazines are often used and may have to be continued for many months or even longer. This means that a careful watch must be kept for adverse effects, especially those involving the nervous system.

**Adverse effects of phenothiazines.** Adverse effects with phenothiazines are not uncommon and the incidence varies from drug to drug. They include:

- **Jaundice**: This occurs with chlorpromazine and is due to blocking of the bile canaliculi in the liver. It is presumed to be an allergic effect, and recovery occurs when the drug is stopped.
- **Various disorders of movement**, due directly or indirectly to a dopamine blocking action in the brain. These may occur with all neuroleptics:

  **Parkinsonism.**

  **Akathisia**, which is a feeling of restlessness with an inability to stand still.

  **Dystonia**, which is uncontrolled movements.

  **Tardive dyskinesia**, consisting of abnormal movements of the mouth and tongue and sometimes the upper limbs. It develops in about 20% of patients on longer-term neuroleptics. Its onset is usually delayed for a while. Control is difficult and it may not stop even if the drug is withdrawn.

All these symptoms may commence soon after starting treatment and require a reduction of the dose if possible. Akathisia may be helped by a benzodiazepine; anticholinergic drugs such as benztropine may help the dystonic reaction and parkinsonism.

- **Depressed leucocyte count**
- **Skin rashes**, including light sensitivity and contact dermatitis when the drug is handled. A sunscreen is advised with chloropromazine.
- **An α blocking effect** on the sympathetic nervous system, leading to a fall in blood pressure and faintness.
- **Hypothermia** in elderly patients.
- **Weight gain** and the development of gynaecomastia (breast development in men) and male impotence.
- **Dry mouth** can be troublesome.
- **Sedation**, which is greatest with chlorpromazine.
- Rarely, the **neuroleptic malignant syndrome** with hyperpyrexia, coma and muscular rigidity may develop; this requires urgent treatment.

> **Safety note**
>
> Thioridazine is a particularly effective drug, but is associated with considerable cardiotoxicity, in particular an increased risk of ventricular arrhythmias. The Committee for the Safety of Medicines has recommended that thioridazine be prescribed only for adults suffering from schizophrenia under specialist supervision. It is contraindicated in patients with cardiovascular disease who have a history of ventricular arrhythmias, Q–T interval prolongation or reduced cytochrome P450 2D6 activity.

With the present state of knowledge it is impossible to say which is the best drug of this group. Patients seem to vary in their response to individual drugs and trial and error seems to be the only way to decide which is the best for any particular patient.

> **Nursing point**
>
> Staff should avoid contact with chlorpromazine (i.e. crushing tablets, etc.) because of the risk of contact sensitization.

## The thioxanthenes

These are rather similar to the phenothiazines. They are antipsychotic and anti-emetic and are largely used in the treatment of schizophrenia. They are less sedative than the phenothiazines, but akathisia is rather common. An example is **flupentixol**, which is used as an injected depot preparation every 2 weeks or daily as tablets.

## The butyrophenones

This group of drugs has actions rather similar to those of the phenothiazines. They are less sedative, but are liable to produce extrapyramidal (parkinsonism-like) side effects. **Haloperidol** is particularly useful in the management of manic or confused patients. **Droperidol** is similar but acts more rapidly.

## Other neuroleptics

**Pimozide** is an antipsychotic drug used in the treatment of schizophrenia and manic states. It is longer acting and less sedative than chlorpromazine. Pimozide can cause adverse effects such as dangerous cardiac arrhythmias and should not be given to those who suffer from them. An ECG should be taken before starting treatment and repeated at 6-monthly intervals for those receiving high doses.

**Sulpiride** has a more specific dopamine-blocking action than the other neuroleptics but with less adverse effects. However, it can still cause various disorders of movement, and is also associated with hepatitis.

## THERAPEUTIC USE OF ATYPICAL ANTIPSYCHOTIC DRUGS

Atypical antipsychotic (neuroleptic) drugs differ from older neuroleptics in that their $D_2$ blocking action may be confined to those areas of the brain believed to be concerned with schizophrenia (the mesolimbic system); in addition, they also block serotonin (5-HT) and adrenoreceptors. The result is that they seldom cause disorders of posture and movement and may be effective when older neuroleptics fail.

**Clozapine** is used for patients who have proved resistant to neuroleptic treatment. Because of its adverse effects profile, treatment should be started in hospital under careful supervision, although in practice few people with mental problems are admitted nowadays. Its adverse effects can be serious. About 3% of patients taking this drug for 1 year develop neutropenia, so monitoring of the blood count is mandatory. Other adverse effects include seizures, hypotension, excessive salivation and sedation. It is also very expensive. Because of these problems, clozapine is at present reserved for specially selected cases.

**Risperidone** blocks several receptors in the brain, including dopamine receptors. It appears to be useful in the negative symptoms of schizophrenia, and extrapyramidal side-effects seem to be uncommon.

**Olanzapine** is similar to the above but, unlike clozapine, it does not depress the leucocyte count. It does, however, cause drowsiness and weight gain.

**Amisulpride** is indicated for schizophrenia.

At present, it is impossible to say which is the preferred drug in this group, but they appear to offer advantages over the older neuroleptics. They are considerably more expensive and their use will probably be confined to patients who run into difficulties with standard neuroleptics. Other drugs in this group are becoming available.

## DEPOT INJECTIONS

Several antipsychotic drugs are given as depot injections, including fluphenazine and flupentixol, because patients with severe mental disease often fail to take their pills regularly. Depot preparations given by deep intramuscular injection into the upper and outer part of the buttock or the lateral aspect of the thigh, using the Z technique (see p. 26), get round this problem. However, this dosage scheme is inflexible and there is difficulty if a patient develops some adverse effect. These injections may be very painful, and seepage of fluid can result in inaccurate dosage unless the injection technique is well executed. Currently, newer and more effective ways of delivering depot injections are being tested.

> **Nursing point**
>
> Do not forget the adverse effects of this group of drugs, particularly those affecting the nervous system. With long-term use careful surveillance is also required on withdrawal of treatment as the re-emergence of symptoms may be delayed for several weeks.

> **Nursing point**
>
> Special care is needed if neuroleptics are given to:
>
> 1. patients with Parkinson's disease, as symptoms may be increased
> 2. epileptics or patients with alcohol withdrawal symptoms, as fits may be precipitated
> 3. elderly patients, who may get postural hypotension
> 4. pregnant and lactating mothers.

## THE TREATMENT OF SCHIZOPHRENIA

### Introduction

Schizophrenia is a mysterious disease. It may take many forms, but the essential feature is a change of personality with disordered thought processes, which may be associated with hallucinations, delusions and withdrawal. Once schizophrenia has developed, complete recovery is unusual, although considerable improvement is possible. It usually starts in young people.

### Theories about schizophrenia

There are several theories as to its cause. It seems most likely that it is a complex biochemical disorder in the brain. The fact that symptoms can be relieved in many patients by dopamine blocking drugs supports the view that it is due to overactivity of the dopaminergic system, probably involving $D_2$ receptors in the mesolimbic system of the brain. However, not all patients respond to $D_2$ receptor antagonists and other receptors are probably involved. Although few would now support the idea that it is a disorder of personality development due to faulty inter-action with the family in early life, it is probably made worse, or even precipitated, in susceptible individuals by periods of stress and difficulty, and possibly after using drugs of abuse such as ecstasy and cannabis.

## Management of the schizophrenic patient

The total management of the schizophrenic patient has many facets but the introduction of neuroleptic drugs has greatly improved treatment, enabling many patients to take their place in the community and lead a reasonable life. Drugs alone are not enough, and very efficient social services are required to ensure that patients are properly supported.

> **Nursing point**
>
> Community psychiatric nurses play a very important role supporting patients and their families.

Decisions about dosage require individual titration for each patient, and drug treatment must be combined with support and management, especially the avoidance of stressful situations.

Drug treatment is started as soon as the diagnosis is confirmed. **Haloperidol** or one of the other standard neuroleptics is used and symptoms should remit in 2 or 3 weeks. If a patient does not respond, an atypical antipsychotic drug may be prescribed (see above). When the disorder is controlled, long-term maintenance treatment is required, either oral or by depot injection, and usually for life. Compliance may be poor and supervision is essential, otherwise relapses will occur.

> **Nursing point**
>
> A schizophrenic patient receiving appropriate drugs may well behave normally, but, if treatment is stopped suddenly, there may be a catastrophic relapse.

## National Institute for Clinical Excellence recommendations

The National Institute for Clinical Excellence (NICE) has issued recommendations for the use of atypical antipsychotic drugs (AAD) for schizophrenia, and these are given below:

- Consider the use of amisulpride, olanzapine, quetiapine, risperidone or zotepine.

- Consider the use of an AAD in acute schizophrenic episodes when it is impossible to discuss treatment with the patient.
- Consider the use of an AAD when side-effects with typical antipsychotic drugs become unacceptable for the patient, or for patients in relapse whose symptoms were not adequately controlled with typical antipsychotic drugs, or who experienced unacceptable side-effects with these.
- AADs are unnecessary for patients whose symptoms are adequately controlled with typical antipsychotic drugs, and for patients who do not experience unacceptable side-effects with these.
- Consider prescribing clozapine as soon as possible for patients whose schizophrenic symptoms are inadequately controlled despite the sequential use, each for at least 8 weeks, of two or more antipsychotic drugs. At least one of those drugs should have been another AAD.

At present, doctors make the decisions listed in the NICE recommendations above, but it is conceivable that nurses will take on some or perhaps all of these responsibilities in the not too distant future.

Diagnosis of a psychotic disorder is a specialized task and the dangers of misdiagnosis are highlighted in Case History 20.1.

## Case History 20.1

Miss M, a 15-year-old girl, who previously had been quiet, cheerful and studious, began to act irrationally at home and had a violent temper and started stealing from home and from shops. She became violent and terrorized her family. This alternated with periods of relative calm. Her parents sought medical advice and a neurologist diagnosed schizophrenia. She was placed on chlorpromazine, which sedated her and she became dull and lethargic. The family could not cope with her and she was in and out of nursing homes until the age of 20, when the family doctor retired and a new doctor took over the practice. He saw Miss M, who was now a young, attractive woman, but still subject to episodes of psychosis and unable to lead a normal life. He ordered blood tests and on the basis of these sent her to a rheumatologist who ordered brain scans and diagnosed cerebral lupus. He told the family that the disease was causing occlusion of blood flow in the brain. He prescribed heparin and the symptoms cleared up. Today Miss M is married with children and has a responsible part-time job. She continues to receive treatment for her lupus.

**Lessons**

- Psychotic behaviour may not necessarily be due to a disorder of central (i.e. CNS) origin
- Lupus can present as psychotic behaviour
- Continuing professional development is an important modern feature of clinical practice.

## MANAGEMENT OF ACUTE CONFUSIONAL STATES

Acute confusional states (ACS; called delirium by some practitioners) are states of impaired cognition, mood, and self-awareness or attention that are often superimposed on an underlying disease such as dementia or schizophrenia. They are more common in elderly people.

### Causes of ACS

Acute confusional states have many causes. They may be part of a psychiatric illness, but may also develop as a result of a serious 'organic' illness, or they may be due to drug dependence, e.g. alcohol withdrawal. The symptoms of ACS may be worsened during periods of intense stress, sleep disruption or as part of adverse reactions to antipsychotic drugs, especially in older patients. Examples of underlying conditions and drugs that cause ACS are summarized below.

Examples of underlying conditions:

- anoxia
- hyperkalaemia
- hyperparathyroidism
- hypoglycaemia
- hypokalaemia
- hypothyroidism
- metabolic acidosis
- post concussion
- postictal state (an ictus is a stroke or sudden seizure)
- transient ischaemia.

Drugs:

- anticholinergic drugs, e.g. muscle relaxants, anti-emetics, drugs for Parkinson's disease, etc.
- alcohol and CNS depressants, digoxin, antihypertensive drugs, benzodiazepines.

This list is far from comprehensive, but alerts the reader to the fact that several different types of drugs are able to cause ACS.

### Diagnosis of ACS

It is extremely important to diagnose ACS quickly and treat the underlying illness, since possibly around 20% of hospitalized elderly people who develop ACS die, and patients who develop ACS are on average hospitalized for twice as long as those who do not develop it.

The American Psychiatric Association (APA) has published the criteria for diagnosis of ACS (APA 2000) and some of the main criteria are summarized as follows:

- disturbance of consciousness with reduced attention
- altered cognition in terms of language disturbance, disorientation and memory deficit over and above symptoms of the underlying condition
- development of the symptoms of ACS over a short time (i.e. hours or days) relative to the underlying condition
- the symptoms develop during or shortly after either intoxication with drugs or during withdrawal from drugs.

The reader is referred to the manual (APA 2000) for the precise definitions, but this summary will give some indication of the circumstances that may precipitate ACS.

### Care of the patient with ACS

It is important that such patients are nursed in quiet surroundings. The nurse's approach must be calm and as much explanation given as is feasible, and the nurse should try to ascertain the patient's degree of awareness of the situation (Andersson et al 2002). Patients may be highly agitated, especially if this is a temporary and unusual experience (Fagerberg & Jonhagen 2002). If possible, drugs should be given orally. The choice lies between a benzodiazepine such as diazepam (see below) and a neuroleptic such as haloperidol. Chlorpromazine should not be given intramuscularly as it forms deposits in the muscle and may also cause hypotension. More seriously disturbed patients can be given lorazepam I.M. or droperidol I.M. Patients confused as a result of alcohol withdrawal should not be given neuroleptics owing to the risk of seizures.

## TREATMENT OF ANXIETY AND INSOMNIA

Anxiety and insomnia are, on the face of it, two different problems, and yet are treated in many cases by the same types of drugs. It is therefore logical to consider these two problems in the same chapter. This fact also highlights the problem that anxiolytic drugs such as the benzodiazepines are often sedative, and in overdose can cause respiratory depression.

### THE NATURE OF ANXIETY

Anxiety is a universal phenomenon and a certain amount is useful to the individual, acting as a stimulant and increasing efficiency. However, when it becomes disproportionate to the stimulus, an anxiety state develops, and this degree of anxiety may interfere seriously with the patient's life.

### TYPES OF ANXIETY

Anxiety has been classified into several different types, depending on the circumstances that produced its symptoms:

- **General anxiety disorder** (GAD), in which the patient feels apprehensive and tense for no particular reason, or as a result of some apparently minor problem. In addition, there may be muscle aches, nausea, sleep problems and various other symptoms.
- **Panic attacks** are unexpected attacks of anxiety, often with marked physical symptoms such as tremor, palpitation and dry mouth due to overactivity of the sympathetic nervous system.
- **Obsessive compulsive disorder** which is characterized by repetitive, anxiety-driven behaviour such as the repeated washing of hands or obsessive thoughts and doubts – for example the feeling that one needs to check things more than once, such as whether the front door was locked on going out.
- **Post-traumatic stress disorder**, which is the anxiety that follows traumatic experiences such as rape or warfare.
- **Phobic states** in which the patient fears certain situations. The commonest is agoraphobia in which the subject is frightened to go out and acute anxiety is precipitated by supermarkets or travelling on trains and buses, etc.

Various methods of treatment may be used, including counselling, relaxation techniques and cognitive and analytical therapy.

## ANXIOLYTIC DRUGS

Anxiolytic drugs comprise:

- benzodiazepines
- buspirone
- β blockers
- antidepressants.

### BENZODIAZEPINES

Benzodiazepines include:

- chlordiazepoxide
- clorazepate
- diazepam
- lorazepam.

#### Mechanism of action

It is believed that benzodiazepines act on the reticular formation and limbic system in the brain. There are specific receptor sites for benzodiazepines on the GABA receptor and they appear to enhance the action of the neurotransmitter GABA, which is produced by the brain and which depresses brain function (Fig. 20.2).

#### Therapeutic use of benzodiazepines

In addition to their use as hypnotics (see below), this group of drugs is widely used for anxiety. Benzodiazepines should only be used for acute agitation, panic attacks and for anxiety if it is severe and disabling, and the treatment should be the lowest effective dose for no more than 2 weeks and

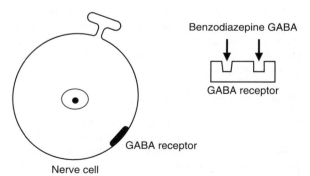

**Figure 20.2**   Gamma-aminobutyric acid (GABA) and benzodiazepine receptors are closely related. Benzodiazepines enhance the inhibitory action of GABA.

combined with other treatment. Previously, they have been used in acute emotional crises, but by preventing the patient responding to the painful situation they may delay psychological adjustment. Although the benzodiazepines are effective in relieving anxiety they have two serious disadvantages:

- They become less effective with prolonged use.
- If the drug is stopped suddenly, even after a relatively short period of use (e.g. 2–3 weeks), about one-third of patients will develop some withdrawal symptoms. These are anxiety and sleeplessness for a few days, but after prolonged and heavy dosage may include seizures, psychotic symptoms, muscle pains and twitching. They usually occur within a week of stopping the drug and earlier if it is short-acting. This suggests that dependence has developed and in severe cases patients may take some months to recover. Patients, therefore, require slow and stepwise withdrawal of the drug over several weeks.

### Other uses

Benzodiazepines have other uses:

- diazepam and clonazepam are also given intravenously for treating status epilepticus (see p. 252) and diazepam and midazolam as sedatives before various investigations
- diazepam also has some muscle relaxing properties and is used in combination with an analgesic to relieve pain and spasm in lumbago and related disorders
- dentists have used diazepam I.V. on patients when carrying out long procedures.

The benzodiazepines are metabolized in the liver and often produce further active compounds. For example, diazepam is partially converted to desmethyldiazepam, which also has a prolonged sedative action. Duration of action is also dependent on the dose and to some degree on the individual. Although the actions of these drugs are very similar the price varies considerably; diazepam is cheap and usually adequate.

### Adverse effects and interactions

The group is very safe generally. Overdose can cause marked sedation, poor coordination, memory difficulties and occasionally respiratory depression, but this is rarely serious in healthy individuals, although fatalities have been reported. Interactions with other CNS depressants (e.g. alcohol) increase sedation and can be dangerous. Diazepam is irritant when given intravenously and should be given as an emulsion (*Diazemuls*).

**Flumazenil** is a benzodiazepine antagonist. It is given intravenously and reverses benzodiazepine-induced sedation in a few minutes. It has been used in overdose and to speed recovery in patients who have been anaesthetized with midazolam. However, its effect only lasts about 1 hour so repeated doses may be required with long-acting benzodiazepines.

## BUSPIRONE

Buspirone is an attempt to produce an anxiolytic drug without adverse effects. It reacts with a group of 5-HT receptors. Buspirone appears to have no sedative action or risk of dependence; its only adverse effects appear to be occasional nausea and headache. However, its onset of action is delayed for about 2 weeks and it seems to be ineffective in treating the symptoms of benzodiazepine withdrawal.

## β BLOCKERS

β Blockers such as **propranolol** suppress the physical concomitants of anxiety (tremor and palpitations).

## ANTIDEPRESSANTS

Antidepressants are dealt with in more detail in Chapter 21, but it is worth mentioning here that both tricyclic antidepressants, and 5-HT re-uptake inhibitors such as fluoxetine (see p. 279) are also helpful in the treatment of anxiety in small doses, particularly in the case of panic attacks. Venlafaxine, a drug related to the 5-HT reuptake inhibitors, is useful for the treatment of GAD.

## INSOMNIA

Approximately 20% of the adult population consider they do not get enough sleep. This is generally a subjective opinion. Insomnia can, however, cause feelings of anxiety, inability to concentrate and general debility. Sleep requirements vary with age. Teenagers need about 10 hours sleep, adults about 8 hours and the elderly about 6 hours, but there is also considerable interperson variation.

Hypnotics are drugs which produce sleep that is comparable with normal sleep (Fig. 20.3). They do not relieve pain. Before prescribing hypnotics it is

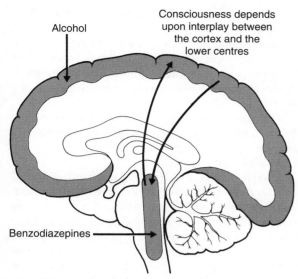

**Figure 20.3** The mode of action of hypnotic drugs and tranquillizers.

important to ascertain whether the patient is not getting enough sleep, since some people exaggerate their insomnia. It is necessary to find out if there is some reason for failing to sleep. These reasons may include:

- anxiety and stress
- depression
- physical illness, e.g. heart failure, chronic lung disease and sleep disordered breathing
- pain
- caffeine, alcohol and steroids taken before retiring.

If these problems are remedied, sleep should occur naturally. Various simple measures can be tried: for example, a walk, a bath, a rather unexciting book before retiring or a glass of milk at bedtime may be sufficient. More comprehensive programmes are detailed by Espre (1993).

Although hypnotic drugs may be required in some circumstances, for example during periods of stress or for certain chronic insomniacs, their use should be discouraged. Tolerance to their action often develops in 2–3 weeks with some degree of dependence. Withdrawal at this stage can lead to increasing wakefulness at night for a few days or longer. This is particularly important in hospitals where they are perhaps sometimes too freely prescribed and where a lifetime of habituation to these drugs may start. Patients should not as a general rule be sent home from hospital with hypnotic drugs.

## THE NATURE OF SLEEP

Sleep is not just a state into which one lapses on going to bed and from which one emerges on waking. It is a series of cycles each lasting about 90 minutes. After falling asleep the subject becomes progressively more relaxed with slow pulse and respiration rate; this phase lasts about 80 minutes and ultimately the state of 'deep sleep' is reached. Then follows a phase lasting about 10 minutes with dreaming, increased muscle tone, rapid eye movements and increased heart rate, known as rapid eye movement (REM) sleep. The whole cycle is then repeated about six times per night. It has been shown that if a subject is deprived of REM sleep he will show psychological changes during waking hours. Many centrally acting drugs and alcohol do in fact suppress REM sleep and thus do not really produce completely natural sleep.

## HYPNOTIC DRUGS

Hypnotic drugs fall into the following categories:

- chloral hydrate
- promethazine (an antihistamine)
- clomethiazole
- benzodiazepines
- zaleplon, zopiclone and zolpidem
- ethyl alcohol.

### Chloral hydrate

Chloral hydrate and its derivatives have been used as hypnotics for many years and have established a reputation for being especially useful for children. Chloral hydrate is rapidly absorbed and produces sleep in about 30 minutes, by causing interference in functioning of the brain cells. The drug is conjugated in the liver and excreted via the kidneys. Its hypnotic action lasts about 4 hours.

**Therapeutic use.** Chloral hydrate has an unpleasant taste, is a gastric irritant and can cause rashes. Although an effective hypnotic, its popularity has declined and it is no longer the hypnotic of choice, even for children. If required, its derivative, **triclofos**, is preferred, being less of a gastric irritant.

**Adverse effects and interactions.** Chloral hydrate is relatively safe but may cause gastric upset. It should be used with caution in liver or renal failure. It enhances the effects of warfarin.

## Promethazine

Promethazine is an antihistamine which is sometimes used as a hypnotic drug, especially in children. By blocking the action of histamine in the brain it produces sleep. It is not a particularly good hypnotic drug, having rather a long action with sedation next morning, and because it has an anticholinergic action it can cause a dry mouth and interfere with bladder function. It is available without prescription.

## Clomethiazole

This drug, which is related to vitamin $B_1$, is now rarely used as a hypnotic because of the risk of dependence. It can be given orally or intravenously. Its action is short-lived.

**Therapeutic use.**  Clomethiazole is used particularly in elderly subjects, for patients who are agitated and confused and for controlling withdrawal symptoms in alcoholics, although dependence on clomethiazole may develop. Clomethiazole can also be given intravenously to terminate status epilepticus or control delirium tremens. When given in this way there is a danger of respiratory depression and hypotension and the patient requires careful observation and direct medical supervision. The infusion should not usually be continued for more than 18 hours. Adverse effects are rare but some patients complain of stuffiness in the nose shortly after taking the drug.

## Benzodiazepines

Several members of this group of drugs can be given as a hypnotic. There is very little to choose between them in efficacy, their main difference being in their duration of action. Benzodiazepines with a prolonged action may produce a hangover effect the next day if given in a dose sufficient to produce sleep. They are easy to use and pleasant to take and are the most commonly prescribed hypnotic drugs.

**Nitrazepam** was the first benzodiazepine to be recommended as a hypnotic drug. Although it has been claimed that this drug is unlikely to confuse elderly patients, this is not necessarily true. In addition, some sedative effect may persist well into the following day.

**Diazepam** is more usually used as an anxiolytic drug, but it is a fairly good hypnotic drug if there is some background anxiety and sedation lasting into the next day is needed.

**Temazepam** has a shorter half-life and length of action than most other benzodiazepines and it does not produce metabolites that are also hypnotics. It is, therefore, less liable to cause drowsiness into the next day.

**Flunitrazepam** has a fairly prolonged action. Because it is tasteless, it can be added to drinks, etc., and has gained a reputation for being used when rape is intended.

**Adverse effects of the benzodiazepines.**  The benzodiazepines are remarkably free from serious adverse effects, although continued use can cause fatigue, memory problems and, rarely, behavioural disturbances. The main problem is the development of dependence. This may occur after 2 weeks or less when they are used as hypnotics. Withdrawal then results in considerable difficulty in sleeping for several days or even weeks, and the temptation is to resume taking them.

When stopping treatment with benzodiazepines, particularly if they have been taken for a long time, the dosage should be reduced stepwise, reducing it about every 14 days, depending on symptoms, and finally withdrawing it altogether.

## Zaleplon, zopiclone and zolpidem

These short-acting hypnotics, although differing in structure from the benzodiazepines, also bind to the benzodiazepine receptors and increase the sedating activity of GABA in the brain.

**Zaleplon** is indicated for short-term use. It is not recommended for patients under 18 years of age and patients should be advised not to take a second dose the same night. Contraindications include breastfeeding and patients suffering from sleep apnoea syndrome or myasthenia gravis. Adverse effects include headache, drowsiness and dizziness. The drug does cause dependence.

**Zopiclone** is rapidly absorbed and produces sleep lasting 6–8 hours. There may be some drowsiness the next morning. The available evidence suggests that tolerance may develop and dependence occurs. In general it is very similar to the short-acting benzodiazepines. A bitter metallic taste in the mouth is a fairly common adverse effect. Sometimes nausea and hallucinations and other psychological phenomena have been reported. It should not be used during pregnancy or given to children. Increased drowsiness is experienced if used with other central depressants such as alcohol or benzodiazepines.

**Zolpidem** has few after effects the next morning. The dependence potential is low but can occur. Adverse effects include drowsiness, headache and nausea.

None of these three hypnotics is ideal and whether they are preferable to the short-acting benzodiazepines (e.g. temazepam) is not clear and they are more expensive. As with the benzodiazepines, they should only be used after careful consideration and should not be taken for more than 2–4 weeks.

## Ethyl alcohol

Alcohol is occasionally used as a sedative at night, particularly in the elderly. It is not a good hypnotic and although it may help patients to get to sleep, they often waken during the night due to rebound insomnia. It is important to remember that patients who take alcohol regularly may become restless and have difficulty in sleeping if it is stopped suddenly.

## THE USE AND CHOICE OF HYPNOTICS

The first essential is to make certain that a hypnotic drug is necessary to relieve the patient's insomnia. Insomnia may be considered in three categories:

- transient insomnia
- short-term insomnia
- chronic insomnia.

## Transient insomnia

This occurs in people who usually have no sleep problem and is due to altered circumstances, i.e. admission to hospital or travel. In these cases a short-acting benzodiazepine such as temazepam is appropriate.

## Short–term insomnia

Short-term insomnia may be due to anxiety, illness, etc. Here a short-acting benzodiazepine can be used, but if anxiety is prominent, a drug such as diazepam may be more useful as its effect will last into the next day. It is important that the drug is not given for more than 2 weeks and that intermittent dosing is introduced as early as possible, as there is a definite

risk of dependence developing. The nurse has an important part to play by listening to the patient's worries and by relieving any physical discomfort if possible.

## Chronic insomnia

Careful analysis is necessary in patients with chronic insomnia. Some will be suffering from psychiatric illness, particularly depression. In other cases an excess of coffee or alcohol may be the cause. If these can be excluded, a change in lifestyle with regular exercise and reduction of stress (if possible) can be tried. Diazepam is the most suitable hypnotic drug, preferably on an intermittent basis, for a month. If this fails, trial of an antidepressant is appropriate. The long-term management of this type of patient is often difficult.

There is little indication for the use of hypnotic drugs other than the benzodiazepines, but if an alternative is required then zopiclone is probably the most satisfactory substitute.

## HYPNOTIC DRUGS IN SPECIAL CIRCUMSTANCES

**In renal failure.** Some hypnotic drugs are excreted via the kidney so that accumulation occurs in patients with renal failure. Nitrazepam does not fall into this group and is satisfactory, but small doses should be used initially.

**In liver failure.** Temazepam is satisfactory, but should be used with care.

**In respiratory disease.** All hypnotic drugs produce some depression of respiration so they must be used with great care in patients with respiratory failure and during attacks of asthma. Temazepam is as good as any.

**In the elderly.** Hypnotics should be avoided if possible. If nocturnal confusion is a problem, thioridazine is preferred.

---

**Nursing point**

1. Dependence can occur with long-term use of all hypnotics. Use the minimum dose for the minimum time.
2. Do not forget that depression can cause insomnia.

## SEDATIVES PRIOR TO MINOR PROCEDURES

Patients often require some sedation before such manoeuvres as gastroscopy, etc. Benzodiazepines are useful because they are both sedative and also produce amnesia for the event. Diazepam is often used intravenously, for example in dentistry. It is, however, irritant to the vein. A specially prepared non-irritant emulsion of diazepam (*Diazemuls*; see also above) is preferable.

Alternatively, **midazolam**, which has an action lasting about 2 hours, can be given. Following injections of this type the patient should be warned not to drive until the next day and to avoid alcohol or other depressants. With regard to adverse effects and interactions, there have been a number of reports of respiratory depression and cardiac arrest after midazolam, especially in elderly patients who do not eliminate the drug as rapidly as younger subjects. This is usually due to excessive dosage and care should be taken. The action of midazolam is increased by erythromycin.

## JET LAG

Long flights, crossing several time zones, give rise to fatigue and loss of concentration and appetite on arrival. Flights to the West lead to early wakening and to the East, difficulty getting to sleep. This is due to the body clock becoming out of phase with its local time and it may take 2 or 3 days to adjust. **Melatonin**, which is secreted by the brain, helps this adjustment and there is some evidence that, if given orally in the evening, it helps sleep and reduces jet lag. It is not licensed as a medicine in the UK but is available in the United States and elsewhere. Until its use is regulated it is probably best avoided.

### Summary

- Two nurses should always be involved when a drug is administered
- Patient compliance is a problem, e.g. patients may secretly spit out drugs
- Drugs can be given by depot injection to overcome problems of compliance, e.g. when treating schizophrenic patients
- Patients need reassuring when they are given drugs, e.g. some fear that they are being poisoned
- Antipsychotic drugs may have several adverse effects since they affect CNS neurotransmitter activity and these should be watched for as confused and fearful patients may not be able to report them
- Acute confusional states may actually be brought on by drugs
- Benzodiazepines are associated with withdrawal symptoms and patients should not use them for more than 2 weeks, and when treatment is stopped, it should not be stopped suddenly but in stepwise dose reduction
- Hypnotics will not relieve pain
- Hypnotics should not be prescribed until the probable reason for insomnia is ascertained
- Simple, harmless remedies such as stopping caffeine drinks should be tried before resorting to hypnotics
- Ideally, patients should not be sent home from hospital with hypnotics
- Care with some benzodiazepines, notably flunitrazepam, which is tasteless in drinks and has been used when rape is intended
- Nurses play a very important part in listening to patients with insomnia, reassuring them and relieving any physical discomfort if possible
- Diazepam has been used I.V. in dentistry but is irritant to veins

## References

Andersson E M, Hallberg I R, Norberg A et al 2002 The meaning of acute confusional state from the perspective of elderly patients. International Journal of Geriatric Psychiatry 17: 652

APA 2000 Criteria for diagnosis of acute confusional states. American Psychiatric Association diagnostic and statistical manual of mental disorders, 4th edition

Espre C A 1993 Practical management of insomnia. British Medical Journal 306: 509

Fagerberg I, Jonhagen M E 2002 Temporary confusion: a fearful experience. Journal of Psychiatric and Mental Health Nursing 9: 339

## Further reading

Ballinger B R 1990 Hypnotics and anxiolytics. British Medical Journal 300: 456

Behavioural emergencies 1991 Drug and Therapeutics Bulletin 29: 62

Buckley N A, Dawson A H, Whyte I M et al 1995 Relative toxicity of benzodiazepines in overdose. British Medical Journal 310: 219

Culshaw F 1994 Composition and effects of commonly used neuroleptics. Nursing Times 90: 38

Editorial 1988 Benzodiazepines and dependence. Bulletin of the Royal College of Psychiatrists 12: 107

Editorial 1988 Tardive dyskinesia. British Medical Journal 296: 150

Editorial 1994 Risperidone for schizophrenia. British Medical Journal 308: 1311

Editorial 1995 The drug treatment of patients with schizophrenia. Drug and Therapeutics Bulletin 33: 81

Gram L F 1994 Fluoxetine. New England Journal of Medicine 331: 1354

Gray R, Robson D, Bressington D 2002 Medication management for people with a diagnosis of schizophrenia. Nursing Times 98: 38

Lader M 1994 Treatment of anxiety. British Medical Journal 309: 321

Macgabhann L 1998 A comparison of two depot injection techniques. Nursing Standard 12(39): 41

Miller J L 2002 Post-traumatic stress disorder in primary care practice. Journal of the American Academy of Nurse Practise 12: 475

Pathare S R, Paton C 1997 Psychotropic drug treatment. British Medical Journal 315: 661

Quartermaine S 1995 A comparative study of depot injection techniques. Nursing Times 91(30): 36

Smith L 1995 Clozapine: indications and implications for treatment. Nursing Times 91(30): 40

# Chapter 21

# CNS 4. Antidepressants and dementias

## Learning objectives

At the end of this chapter the reader should be able to:

- list the different types of depression
- discuss brain neurotransmitters in depression
- give an account of the different groups of drugs used to treat depression and examples
- describe the adverse effects of tricyclic antidepressants
- appreciate the dangers associated with MAO drugs, particularly interactions with food and other drugs
- describe what SSRI drugs are and know examples
- provide the names of the other antidepressants mentioned
- explain what ECT is
- explain what lithium is, the preparations and when it is prescribed, and describe the dangers associated with using lithium, and the importance of monitoring blood levels of the drug
- give an account of the management of dementias and the drugs used to treat Alzheimer's disease

## DEPRESSION

Depression is a common and normal emotion and people naturally become depressed as a result of unfortunate domestic and social conditions. Sometimes, however, the depression is disproportionate to the precipitating factors or there may be no obvious cause at all. This is an illness called endogenous or psychotic depression and is commoner in older people. Some psychiatrists recognize a further type of depressive illness in which environmental factors play a more prominent part and this is sometimes called **reactive depression** or **depressive neurosis**. Sometimes depression may alternate with attacks of mania. This is known as **bipolar depression** or **manic-depressive psychosis**.

In depression the mood is at its lowest in the morning and improves throughout the day. The patient is disinterested and may be irritable and anxious. The appetite is poor and vague symptoms including headache and odd pains are common. Suicide is a special risk in depressed patients.

## BRAIN NEUROTRANSMITTERS AND DEPRESSION

The aetiology of depression is not known but there is evidence that a major factor is a reduction in the amount of neurotransmitter amines such as 5-HT (5-hydroxytryptamine; serotonin) or norepinephrine at the junctions between neurones in the brain. Many of the drugs used to treat depression increase the amount of these substances in the brain, thus providing some evidence that amines are connected with changes of mood.

The following groups of drugs are used to relieve depression:

- tricyclic antidepressants
- tricyclic anxiolytics
- selective serotonin re-uptake inhibitors (SSRIs)
- monoamine oxidase inhibitors (MAOIs)
- lithium
- other antidepressants.

## TRICYCLIC ANTIDEPRESSANTS

Tricyclic antidepressants comprise:

- amytriptyline
- clomipramine
- desipramine
- imipramine
- lofepramine
- nortriptyline
- protriptyline.

Clearly there are several tricyclic antidepressants in use and there is not a great deal of difference between them. Therefore a few representative drugs will be considered here. They are well absorbed after oral administration and undergo considerable

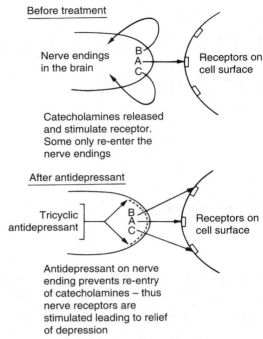

Before treatment

Nerve endings in the brain

Receptors on cell surface

Catecholamines released and stimulate receptor. Some only re-enter the nerve endings

After antidepressant

Tricyclic antidepressant

Receptors on cell surface

Antidepressant on nerve ending prevents re-entry of catecholamines – thus nerve receptors are stimulated leading to relief of depression

**Figure 21.1**  The mode of action of the tricyclic antidepressant drugs.

breakdown in the liver; some of these metabolic products are therapeutically active. It is believed that they produce their therapeutic effect by preventing the reuptake of amines at nerve endings in the brain, which thus increases the concentration of these substances available for receptor uptake (Fig. 21.1).

Some members of the group (i.e. nortriptyline and desipramine) have a greater effect on norepinephrine concentration, and others (e.g. imipramine and amitriptyline) on 5-HT concentration.

### Imipramine and amytriptyline

Imipramine was the first of these drugs to be used. Amitriptyline is very similar to imipramine but is rather more sedating. Both these drugs have a long action and need only be given once a day. If amitriptyline is given in the evening its sedative action will help sleep, which is often disturbed in depression. Imipramine is actually a prodrug and is metabolized to the active drug, namely, **desipramine** (see above).

**Therapeutic use.**  After starting treatment the sleep disorders associated with depression usually respond fairly quickly, but it is important to remember that it may take several weeks before the depression itself is relieved. Treatment should therefore be continued for 6 weeks before deciding that treatment has failed. About 80% of depressed patients will ultimately respond. Tricyclic antidepressants are also used in the treatment of pain of obscure origin such as atypical facial pain.

**Bed wetting.**   Imipramine is used for nocturnal enuresis (bed wetting) in children. It is important to explain to the child's parents that:

- the effect may be delayed for 2–3 weeks
- the tablets must be stored in a childproof place
- treatment should not usually be given for more than 3 months.

**Plasma concentrations.**   Owing to the considerable interpersonal variation in the breakdown of these drugs, plasma levels may vary widely. Extensive investigation has been carried out on the measurement of plasma levels to control treatment but it is doubtful whether this is helpful in controlling dosage.

## Adverse effects of tricyclic antidepressants

- **Anticholinergic effects**: dry mouth can be troublesome and may be mitigated by lemon juice. Elderly male patients may experience difficulty with micturition, and constipation can be a problem, particularly in depressed patients already preoccupied with their bowels. Owing to a dilating effect on the pupil of the eye, they should not be given to patients with glaucoma.
- **Postural hypotension**: this is a fall in blood pressure with occasional faintness, especially in elderly patients.
- **Increased appetite** and weight gain.
- **In epilepsy**: in patients with epilepsy, the tendency to seizures is increased and the dose of antiepileptic drugs may require alteration if tricyclic antidepressants are used.
- **Heart**: tricyclic antidepressants depress conduction in the heart, and a number of sudden deaths have been reported in patients with heart disease taking these drugs. They are therefore best avoided in this group of patients.
- **Overdose**: tricyclic antidepressants are dangerous in overdose, producing cardiovascular disturbance, seizures and coma.
- **Withdrawal symptoms** develop if the drug is stopped suddenly (see below).

## Drug interactions

Interactions with other drugs occur, including antiepileptics, sympathomimetic drugs (but not local anaesthetics) and with other antidepressants and MAOIs. They may reverse the effect of some hypotensive agents and their action is enhanced by alcohol, so care should be taken when combining tricyclics with other drugs.

## TRICYCLIC ANXIOLYTICS

**Doxepin** and **dosulepin** drugs are similar to the tricyclic antidepressants, but have a weaker antidepressant action and are particularly useful when anxiety complicates mild depression. They are also more rapidly effective than the standard tricyclics. Adverse effects are similar to those of the tricyclics but generally less marked. They are still dangerous in overdose.

**Maprotiline** is not a tricyclic drug, but is an amine re-uptake inhibitor. Its action and adverse effects profile is very similar to that of the tricyclics. It is also cardiotoxic.

### Special points for patient education

- Patients must understand that the response to treatment may be delayed by up to 6 weeks with tricyclics.
- They may be told of the possible adverse effects and how to make the best of them.
- They must be informed of the important interactions and how to avoid them.
- They must realize that most of the drugs are dangerous in overdose.

### Nursing point

Non-compliance is an important cause of treatment failure.

## SELECTIVE SEROTONIN (5-HT) RE-UPTAKE INHIBITORS – SSRIs

5-HT is concerned with mood and behaviour and a deficiency of 5-HT in the brain is believed to be a factor in depression. Several drugs have been introduced which specifically inhibit 5-HT reuptake at nerve junctions and thus raise its concentration in the brain. Those available at present are:

- **citalopram**
- **escitalopram**
- **fluoxetine**

- **fluvoxamine**
- **paroxetine**
- **sertraline**.

In relieving depression these drugs are about as effective as the tricyclics and they have also been used in anxiety states. Their advantage lies in the lack of many of the adverse effects of the older tricyclics:

- they are generally not cardiotoxic and therefore less dangerous in overdose
- they generally do not cause hypotension
- there are no anticholinergic effects
- they generally do not cause weight gain.

They do, however, have other adverse effects.

## Adverse effects

Nausea, diarrhoea, weight loss, headaches and insomnia are fairly common, especially if the patient stops the drug abruptly. Various hypersensitivity reactions can occur with fluoxetine and may herald a serious vasculitis. Blood dyscrasias are rare. Fluoxetine has been claimed to cause suicidal ideas and to produce personality changes beyond its antidepressive action, but this is a dubious point.

## Contraindications and precautions

SSRIs should not be used if a depressed patient becomes manic. They should be used with caution in epileptic patients since they can precipitate seizures, which may be prolonged with fluoxetine, particularly if the patient is receiving electroconvulsive therapy (ECT). They may precipitate adverse reactions in diabetic patients and patients with cardiac disease or angle-closure glaucoma. They should be used with caution in patients with a history of gastrointestinal bleeding or who have renal or hepatic disease.

## Drug interactions

Combination with lithium or MAOIs can cause hyperthermia, coma and seizures (serotonin-like syndrome) and an adequate gap must be left between stopping MAOIs and starting these drugs. MAOIs may increase the blood level of tricyclic antidepressants.

It seems likely that, ultimately, SSRIs may replace tricyclic antidepressants on grounds of safety, but at present they are much more expensive.

# MONOAMINE OXIDASE INHIBITORS (MAOIs)

These drugs inhibit the enzyme monoamine oxidase (MAO) and thus interfere with the breakdown of epinephrine, norepinephrine and 5-HT in the brain, which leads to an accumulation of these substances. It is tempting to link this action with the antidepressive action of these drugs, but this has not been proved. They produce a mood change with increase in cheerfulness, energy and well-being in about half of patients with depression. The main use for MAOIs is in atypical depression and phobic anxiety states. The long list of possible adverse effects limits their usefulness and they should only be prescribed by those who are familiar with the problems that may arise.

**Phenelzine** and **isocarboxazid** are *irreversible inhibitors,* which means that they bind to MAO and do not detach themselves from it, so that new enzyme has to be biosynthesized to replace it. **Moclobemide**, on the other hand, is a *reversible inhibitor;* it binds MAO and inhibits its action, but detaches itself so that the enzyme can resume its normal function of metabolizing amines. This renders it somewhat safer than the other two drugs, since there is less chance of potentiating other drugs that are amines, or interfering with the normal metabolism of amines in the diet. Nevertheless, moclobemide is associated with many and potentially dangerous adverse effects.

## Therapeutic use

All three drugs are taken orally in tablet form. They are initially usually given twice or three times daily and the dose reduced if possible, depending on the patient's response.

## Adverse effects

Monoamine oxidase inhibitors can cause, among other problems, postural hypotension, insomnia and nervousness, difficulties with micturition and, rarely, jaundice. Phenelzine can cause agitation and psychotic episodes with hypomanias. Patients may gain weight due to overeating. This is not a comprehensive list.

## Drug interactions

Interactions are important and can be dangerous:

- They may exaggerate the effects of such centrally acting drugs as the barbiturates, alcohol, cocaine, morphine and particularly pethidine (meperidine).

- They lead to overaction by vasopressors such as epinephrine and amfetamine and a number of vasoconstrictor drugs, some of which are included in widely used 'cold-cures'. The results may be headaches, hypertension, restlessness and even coma and death
- Similar effects may also occur if these MAOIs are taken with various articles of food, including cheese, meat, yeast extracts, some wines and beers, game, broad bean pods and pickled herrings. This is because these foods contain vasopressor substances that are normally broken down by MAO. If this breakdown is inhibited, the vasopressors accumulate and produce toxic effects. Therefore, the utmost care must be taken in administering these drugs and all those concerned with patients should be informed.

Hospitals often have their own cards listing restrictions. If a surgical operation is to be undertaken, when it may be necessary to give such drugs as morphine or pethidine (meperidine), the MAOIs should be stopped 2 weeks previously. It is dangerous to combine MAOIs with tricyclic antidepressants or 5-HT re-uptake inhibitors. There should be a gap of 5 weeks between treatment with fluoxetine and MAOIs.

## OTHER ANTIDEPRESSANTS

There are several other antidepressants which act by modifying the amount of amines in the brain but do not fit the above categories.

**Trazodone** has a mixed action on 5-HT receptors. It is an antidepressant and also an anxiolytic. It is not cardiotoxic and may therefore be useful for patients with cardiac disease. It is fairly sedative and, at present, much more expensive than the standard tricyclics. **Nefazodone** appears to be rather similar to trazodone.

**Venlafaxine** is a combined 5-HT and norepinephrine re-uptake inhibitor. Its main advantage is that it relieves depression more rapidly than most antidepressants. Anticholinergic side-effects are rare but nausea and rashes can be a problem. The drug may impair skilled tasks such as driving.

**Mirtazapine** increases the concentration of norepinephrine and 5-HT in the brain and, by blocking some types of 5-HT receptors, has a more specific action on depression. It appears to be about as effective as the older antidepressants with a low incidence of side-effects. Rarely, it can produce depression of the leucocyte count.

Although these drugs are effective, they are rather expensive and rarely offer any special advantage.

> **Nursing point**
>
> A persistent headache is often a warning of rising blood pressure in a patient on MAOIs.

## LITHIUM

The body treats lithium in a similar way to sodium. It is believed to modify neurotransmission in the brain.

### Therapeutic use

Lithium salts are used prophylactically, i.e. as a preventative measure for unipolar and bipolar depression (manic-depressive disorder), and for prophylaxis or treatment of mania. They are given regularly to prevent mood swings in these patients. Lithium will control acute mania, but is slow to produce a therapeutic effect and haloperidol is usually preferred in this situation. The decision to prescribe lithium is not taken lightly in view of its potential risks (see below) and specialist advice must be sought.

Before starting treatment with lithium, renal function must be checked, as retention of the drug may occur if it is impaired. The dose is adjusted to produce a blood level of 0.4–0.9 mmol/litre in a blood sample taken 12 hours after dosing. Lithium has a low therapeutic index, i.e. blood levels not much above therapeutic levels are dangerous. For example, plasma concentrations above 1.5 mmol/litre can be fatal. Plasma levels of 2 mmol/litre or more require emergency treatment.

### Preparations

The following preparations are used:

- **lithium carbonate tablets**
- **lithium citrate liquid**
- **slow-release lithium carbonate tablets** (*Priadel*).

Whatever the preparation prescribed, the dose must be adjusted to achieve a safe yet effective blood serum concentration. If the slow-release preparation (*Priadel*) is used, the tablet must be swallowed whole. Because lithium is excreted slowly it takes some days of treatment before a steady plasma level is reached and it is usual to start measuring plasma levels 1 week after starting treatment. Blood should be

**Table 21.1**    Adverse effects of lithium

| Overdose | Not dose–related |
| --- | --- |
| Weakness | Thyroid deficiency |
| Drowsiness | Increased urine secretion |
| Confusion | Weight gain |
| Coma | |

taken 12 hours after dosing and it is important not to collect it in tubes which use lithium heparin as the anticoagulant. Once a satisfactory dose is established, monitoring is only required monthly.

## Adverse effects

These can be divided into two groups – those due to overdosage and those which do not appear to be dose-related (Table 21.1).

Anything that depletes the body of sodium increases the toxicity of lithium. This includes not only diuretics (see later) but also prolonged vomiting or diarrhoea.

## Drug interactions

If a thiazide or loop diuretic is combined with lithium the excretion of lithium by the kidney is reduced and toxicity may develop. Under these circumstances the dose of lithium must be reduced and the plasma level carefully monitored. Interaction can also occur with NSAIDs, ACE inhibitors, and also with other antidepressants. Patients must be counselled and advised on how to avoid dietary regimes that unduly change sodium input or excretion, and on the importance of an adequate fluid intake.

---

### Special points for patient education

- Different preparations of lithium vary in their bioavailability and patients should receive only one preparation. They should also maintain a reasonable fluid intake.
- Record cards are available for patients taking lithium.

---

## THE MANAGEMENT OF DEPRESSION (see also Culpepper 2002)

Patients with mild to moderate depression are managed at home. Indications for hospital admission are severe depression, risk of suicide and those who cannot care for themselves. All patients need support and encouragement.

The main physical methods of treatment are drugs and ECT. There is considerable debate as to whether the tricyclic or the 5-HT re-uptake antidepressants should be the drug group of choice. They are equally effective and both have adverse effects, but those of the tricyclics are rather more unpleasant than those of the 5-HT re-uptake group. The tricyclics are certainly more dangerous in overdose. However, the 5-HT re-uptake drugs are much more expensive. If tricyclics are used, amitriptyline is preferred in patients with sleep problems as it is fairly sedative; otherwise, imipramine is satisfactory. The other members of this group are used in special circumstances. Because of their long half-life, once daily dosage, usually before retiring, is sufficient. Sleep problems respond promptly, but it may take several weeks for the depression to lift.

Patients who are at special risk from tricyclics such as elderly patients with bladder or eye problems or those with heart disease should be given a 5-HT re-uptake inhibitor. Some authorities think that the use of 5-HT re-uptake inhibitors should largely replace tricyclics. In severe depression, especially if there is a serious risk of suicide or antidepressants have failed, ECT (see below) is often used.

In depressive neurosis when environmental factors are significant factors, MAOIs are sometimes used and can be combined with a benzodiazepine. Tricyclic antidepressants must not be combined with MAOIs as this may cause excitement and pyrexia. Normally there should be a 2-week gap when changing from one type of antidepressant to another (5 weeks following fluoxetine).

Treatment for depression is usually continued for at least 4 months after recovery. Shorter periods of treatment increase the risk of relapse. The drug should then be phased out over about 6 months, otherwise withdrawal symptoms may ensue. These consist of anxiety, diarrhoea, insomnia and restlessness, or relapse may occur.

In bipolar depression (manic-depressive illness) the manic phase can be controlled by a neuroleptic (usually haloperidol) and the depressive phase by a tricyclic antidepressant. The long-term use of lithium to prevent the mood changes has revolutionized the treatment of this condition. Sometimes it is more effective if carbamazepine is combined with lithium.

## ELECTROCONVULSIVE THERAPY

ECT is the passing of electric current through the brain, which actually causes a convulsion or seizure. The modern method is to pretreat the patient with a muscle relaxant and apply general anaesthesia so that the patient is not conscious during the procedure and the violence of the spasm is avoided. Electrodes are placed on the brain and the current applied. The patient may experience headache, confusion and loss of memory afterwards, but these effects usually pass off soon. ECT is used for clinical depression and occasionally for mania or schizophrenia. Applying the electrodes unilaterally to the non-dominant hemisphere of the brain can reduce these after-effects.

The combined use of drugs and ECT is illustrated in Case History 21.1.

### Case History: 21.1

Mr G, aged 55, was made redundant by his company. He had been a highly energetic and successful executive, but was the casualty of a takeover by another company. He tried to get another job but was consistently unsuccessful. He gradually sank into a depression and one evening while watching a tense film experienced a panic attack and had to stop watching. He and his wife went to their doctor, who diagnosed clinical depression. The doctor prescribed imipramine, a tricyclic antidepressant, and told them it would take several weeks to have any effect. He also prescribed temazepam, a short-acting benzodiazepine hypnotic drug, to help Mr G get some sleep. The panic attacks became more frequent and the doctor referred Mr G to a psychiatrist. The psychiatrist advised Mr G to start seeing a psychotherapist regularly. In the meantime, the panic attacks became worse and more frequent and the tricyclic antidepressant appeared to precipitate paranoia, when Mr G became convinced that he was the target of terrorist organizations and of his next-door neighbour. The psychiatrist prescribed a phenothiazine, trifluoperazine (*Stelazine*), to treat the paranoia and several sessions of electroconvulsive therapy (ECT). Thanks to the support of his family and the coordinated efforts of his doctor, a psychiatrist and a psychotherapist, Mr G gradually came through this trying period, and after about a year after the first panic attack became well enough to set up his own consultancy business. To date there has been no occurrence of the panic attacks and the psychotherapist recently advised Mr G that he no longer needed sessions with her.

**Lessons:**
- Family and community support are possibly more important than drugs in helping people recover successfully from nervous breakdowns.
- Psychoactive drugs may cause further problems and exacerbate existing ones and cannot be expected to solve problems such as those of Mr G without psychiatric help and psychotherapy

## DEMENTIA

Dementia is the progressive loss of cognition and normal brain function. The most common cause of dementia is Alzheimer's disease. Other forms of dementia are alcohol-related dementias, Lewy body dementia, Pick's disease and vascular dementias (including multi-infarct dementia). All these diseases damage and kill neurones and other CNS cells.

In **Alzheimer's disease**, a protein called amyloid forms plaques and filaments in the neurone and forms what are termed tangles. The cause of Alzheimer's disease is unknown. Some forms of Alzheimer's disease that affect people under 65 may be inherited. The build-up of amyloid protein in the brain may be inherited.

Dementias can also result from strokes. The most common vascular dementia is **multi-infarct dementia**, when strokes (or infarcts) damage small areas of the brain.

### SYMPTOMS OF DEMENTIA

The symptoms of dementia are not invariable, and will reflect the area of the brain that is damaged. In Alzheimer's disease, for example, the degenerative changes seem to target brain areas responsible for short-term memory, while initially sparing long-stored memories. Thus, patients may not remember something that has just happened, but will be able to retrace their steps to an address they had lived in 30 years ago. As the disease progresses, so memories fade progressively. Patients lose track of time and date and become confused and frightened. Gradually they lose the ability to reason and to function at home and outside of it.

Personality changes occur and these can be devastating for those nearest to the patient, who becomes more and more difficult to manage, and the primary carer is very often an elderly and perhaps frail partner. As time goes by, so the patient will gradually lose the ability to perform simple everyday functions such as dressing, eating, washing and attending to their personal toilet. The disease can place unbearable strains on the home for perhaps 10 years or more. Eventually the patient has to be hospitalized.

There seems little doubt with the increased life span of modern Western life that dementia is going to become a much more prevalent problem. Alzheimer's disease, for example, affects about one-quarter of those over 85 years. The health care system faces a large incipient demand on resources to treat the growing population of dementia sufferers, to assist those who have to care for patients at home and to provide inpatient care when these patients reach the point when they need permanent hospitalization (Cummings et al 2002, Hake 2002). This makes the development of treatments and research into dementias a very high priority.

## DRUG TREATMENTS IN ALZHEIMER'S DISEASE

The only clue that has led to a treatment with some modest alleviation of symptoms (see below) was the discovery that Alzheimer's disease is associated with the loss of acetylcholine neurones (the cholinergic system) in parts of the brain associated with memory.

There are no satisfactory or effective drugs for this disease. The only drugs that seem to have any palliative effect are the anticholinesterases (Camps & Munoz-Torrero 2002), which inhibit the breakdown of the neurotransmitter acetylcholine at its site of action at the synapse between neurones. The anticholinesterase inhibitors currently used include:

- **donepezil**
- **galantamine**
- **rivastigmine**
- **tacrine**.

Donepezil was introduced in the UK and tacrine in the United States. Both inhibit cholinesterase and both therefore produce the adverse effects associated with the inhibition of the cholinesterase system (see p. 54). These drugs seem to help about 40% of sufferers and the improvement is moderate only, and the drugs are unlikely to help significantly once the cholinergic systems are destroyed.

Antidepressants, anxiolytics and atypical antipsychotic drugs are sometimes prescribed for patients with Alzheimer's disease, but these should be given with caution and only under the care of a specialist physician. Some of these drugs can actually be dangerous: for example, the use of antipsychotic drugs in patients with Lewy body dementia (Swanberg & Cummings 2002).

The big breakthrough will possibly be the still-awaited discovery of a drug that slows down or stops altogether the formation of amyloid plaques, and of the genes responsible for the disease, since this information may yield treatments as well.

## Summary

- Suicide is a special risk in depressed patients
- If amitriptyline is given in the evening its sedative action will help sleep, which is often disturbed in depression
- It may take several weeks before depression is relieved by antidepressant drugs and treatment should therefore be continued for 6 weeks before deciding that it has failed.
- Imipramine is used for bedwetting in children and patients should be advised on the use and storage of this drug
- Antidepressants with anticholinergic effects must not be given to patients with glaucoma
- Elderly patients on antidepressants may fall due to hypotension
- In patients with epilepsy, the tendency to seizures is increased and the dose of antiepileptic drugs may require alteration if tricyclic antidepressants are used
- Tricyclics are best avoided in patients with heart disease
- Tricyclics have interactions with many other drugs; they can reverse the action of some antihypertensive drugs
- Alcohol enhances the action of tricyclic antidepressants
- Selective 5-HT re-uptake inhibitors (SSRIs) generally have less adverse effects and are less dangerous in overdose than the older tricyclic antidepressants; they do, nevertheless, have adverse effects
- SSRIs should not be used if a depressed patient becomes manic
- SSRIs must be used with caution in patients with a history of gastrointestinal bleeding or who have renal or hepatic disease
- Cheese and other substances that contain tyramine are absolutely contraindicated with

- monoamine oxidase inhibitors (MAOIs), as the combination can cause a fatal hypertensive crisis
- The plasma levels of lithium must be monitored regularly

- ECT has proved to be of benefit in the treatment of depression
- The family of a patient with dementia needs a great deal of practical and emotional support and the community nurse plays an invaluable role

## References

Camps P, Munoz-Torrero D 2002 Cholinergic drugs in pharmacotherapy of Alzheimer's disease. Mini Reviews in Medicinal Chemistry 2: 11

Culpepper L 2002 The active management of depression. Journal of Family Practise 51: 769

Cummings J L, Frank J C, Cherry D et al 2002 Guidelines for managing Alzheimer's disease: Part II. Treatment. American Family Physician 65: 2525

Hake A M 2002 The treatment of Alzheimer's disease: the approach from a clinical specialist in the trenches. Seminars in Neurology 22: 71

Swanberg M M, Cummings J L 2002 Benefit–risk considerations in the treatment of dementia with Lewy bodies. Drug Safety 25: 511

## Further reading

Editorial 1996 Three new antidepressants. Drug and Therapeutics Bulletin 34(9): 65

Editorial 1997 Donepezil for Alzheimer's disease. Drug and Therapeutics Bulletin 35(10): 75

Editorial 1999 Acetylcholinesterase inhibitors for Alzheimer's disease. British Medical Journal 318: 615

Edwards J G 1994 Selective serotonin re-uptake inhibitors in the treatment of depression. Prescribers Journal 34: 197

Gram L F 1994 Fluoxetine. New England Journal of Medicine 331: 1354

Henry J A, Alexander C A, Sener E K 1995 Relative mortality from overdose of antidepressants. British Medical Journal 310: 221

Jefferson J W 1998 Lithium. British Medical Journal 316: 1330

Song F, Freemantle N, Sheldon T A et al 1993 Selective serotonin reuptake inhibitors: meta-analysis of efficacy and acceptability. British Medical Journal 306: 683

Tyrer P 1988 The Nottingham study of neurotic disorder. Lancet ii: 235

Chapter **22**

# CNS 5. Drug dependence (drug addiction)

## Learning objectives

At the end of this chapter, the reader should be able to:

- explain the meanings of the terms psychological and physical dependence on drugs
- give theories to explain why some people become dependent on drugs
- list the risks associated with heroin dependence
- describe the drugs used to treat opioid dependence
- give an account of the effects of cocaine, amfetamines and ecstasy, and the dangers associated with their use
- give an account of the use of cannabis and hallucinogens and the dangers associated with solvent sniffing
- describe the effects of alcohol and the relationship between blood concentration and effects
- describe the effects of chronic alcoholism
- explain what 'safe' levels of alcohol consumption means and the dangers of alcohol and driving
- recognize the association between cigarette smoking and disease
- describe what treatments are used to aid people to give up smoking
- list some commonly used foods that contain caffeine

## INTRODUCTION

Drug dependence may be defined as a state resulting from the interaction of a person and a drug in which the person has a compulsion to continue taking the drug to experience pleasurable psychological effects and sometimes avoid discomfort due to its withdrawal. Drug abuse is the use of a drug for recreational rather than medical reasons, often in excessive quantities.

There are several groups of drugs of dependence:

- opioids
- cocaine
- amfetamines and ecstasy
- barbiturates
- cannabis
- volatile solvents (glue sniffing)
- hallucinogens
- alcohol
- nicotine
- caffeine.

## TYPES OF DRUG DEPENDENCE

Dependence is usually divided into **psychological** and **physical** dependence.

In psychological dependence, the patient exhibits compulsive drug-seeking behaviour. The drug often produces a pleasant feeling, often relaxation, freedom from worry, or heightened awareness and increased energy and sexual drive. The patient suffers mental anguish when it is withdrawn.

In physical dependence, repeated administration produces biochemical changes in the subject taking the drug. If the drug is withdrawn, very unpleasant symptoms and signs of a physical nature develop which may last for a varying period, but will finally disappear. During this period there is an intense craving for the drug, which, if given, will temporarily relieve the unpleasant symptoms. Thus, after the establishment of physical dependence, the patient's drug-seeking behaviour is motivated chiefly by fear of the withdrawal symptoms.

## TOLERANCE TO DRUGS

Tolerance is a phenomenon whereby more of a drug is needed to produce the same response. This often develops with drugs causing dependence, especially morphine and heroin. Tolerance usually (but not always) develops to the central but not peripheral effects of a drug. Morphine and heroin cause euphoria (central) and constipation (peripheral). Thus, with heroin or morphine, tolerance to the central effects develops invariably, and the user will have to keep increasing the dose to get the euphoria, but will not develop tolerance to the drug's effect in

causing constipation and will be severely and chronically constipated.

## REASONS FOR DRUG ABUSE AND DRUG DEPENDENCE

Drugs may be used intermittently for social or emotional reasons – for example, to relieve a stressful situation. Those who are truly dependent, take drugs continually and may reach a state in which their whole life centres round obtaining and using drugs. Dependence may not be confined to one drug or group of drugs. It is common to find dependent subjects who have escalated from minor drugs (for example, cannabis) to hard drugs (for example, heroin) and some subjects may alternate or combine drugs; for example, cocaine and morphine would produce alternating stimulation and relaxation.

### Why do people become dependent?

This is a very difficult question and the answer is still incomplete. It appears that there is no single cause for drug dependence and no single set of circumstances. There is some evidence to support the theory that there are some special types of personality which render the person more susceptible to becoming dependent. Among the motives which may be important are:

**Curiosity and wanting to belong.** Many young people start taking drugs because they want to know what it feels like. Pressure from peer groups may also play a part, particularly with drugs such as alcohol and cannabis, which are to some degree socially acceptable. This in turn may be tied up with the wish to belong to a group who have a common interest in drug taking and there may be an element of rebellion against accepted values. This need to achieve social acceptance may well be symptomatic of an underlying character disorder so that there are both social and psychological factors at work.

**Chemical props and escapism.** Some people take drugs to relieve mental tension and worries or to give themselves more energy and confidence. Most people have to face difficulties from time to time and some look for a prop to help them. This may include advice from a friend, religion, a holiday or the development of a psychiatric illness. The dependent person has taken what may be termed the 'chemical way out' and by altering his or her psychological state with drugs has partially escaped from reality. Unfortunately, this method brings only temporary relief as it does not solve anything and brings in its train further problems, which are both physical and psychological.

**Biological make–up.** It has long been suggested that people who become drug dependent differ in their genetic or biochemical make-up from those who show no interest in drugs. This has been particularly suggested in alcoholism, which might be regarded as a disease of metabolism, one facet of which is craving for alcohol. This is an attractive hypothesis because it takes the 'sin' out of dependence and puts it in a medical setting, but so far there is little evidence to support it.

**Availability.** There is little doubt that the availability and price of drugs of dependence influence both the amount and pattern of dependence. For example, countries where alcohol is cheap, such as France and South Africa, have a high incidence of alcoholism, cirrhosis of the liver, etc.

**Pressure of work.** It has long been known that those who have to work long hours and do arduous jobs may turn to certain drugs to give them energy. In South America, for example, the natives who were pressed into service in the silver mines by the Spanish chewed coca leaves to give themselves energy. The use of cocaine among workers in high-pressure financial institutions and in the modern entertainment industry is well known. Doctors and nurses through the stresses and pressures of their vocation have a long history of being particularly susceptible to the temptations offered by the use of stimulant drugs, especially given the long hours they have to work and the accessibility of drugs. The emotional involvement that comes with working with the very ill has driven many a health worker to the use of opioids at one time or another. Nowadays, access to these drugs is very strictly controlled and their use is (or should be) documented meticulously. The records are inspected regularly and those who seek to remove these drugs from stock risk heavy penalties, not least de-registration and loss of their career.

## OPIOIDS

- **Heroin (diamorphine)**
- **Morphine**.

There are probably more than 100 000 people dependent on opioids in the UK at present and the number is increasing. Most members of the opium group of drugs are to a greater or lesser extent drugs of dependence. The most frequently used is heroin, which is extremely potent. Heroin passes through the blood–brain barrier much more readily than does morphine, and in the brain it is converted into morphine. The user thus gets a larger dose than if the equivalent doses of morphine were used, and the duration of the effect is shorter than with morphine.

## WITHDRAWAL AND OTHER RISKS OF DEPENDENCE

Heroin may be injected intravenously, taken orally or smoked and produces a feeling of euphoria and relaxation. Dependence is both psychological and physical, and a few hours after withdrawal of the drug the person develops a craving for a further dose, combined with increasing restlessness, anxiety and distress. After 48 hours, physical withdrawal symptoms such as nausea, vomiting and muscle cramps become prominent. Gooseflesh may develop ('cold turkey') and the patient may be pyrexial with a raised pulse rate and blood pressure. The withdrawal symptoms last for about a week.

In addition to the hazards of withdrawal the patient runs further risks:

**The possibility of overdosage:** The drug is often adulterated with other powders and preparations may vary considerably in potency. In addition, the development of tolerance will increase the dose required for the desired effect.

**Sepsis.** There is a frequent occurrence of sepsis due to injection under non-sterile conditions. This may take the form of septicaemia or endocarditis. In addition, the sharing of injection needles greatly increases the risk of being infected with the virus of hepatitis B or C or the HIV causing AIDS. A high proportion of intravenous drug users are carrying the HIV and will eventually develop AIDS.

**Effects on baby.** Babies born to an addict may have a low birth weight and, in addition, will suffer acute withdrawal symptoms after birth with a mortality of 50%.

**Crime.** An addict may go to any length, even serious crime, to obtain further supplies of the drug.

## MANAGEMENT – A PRACTICAL SUMMARY

Addicts must be registered and may then receive a supply of their drug from approved doctors. Sometimes patients present to the A and E Department with opioid withdrawal symptoms. Hospitals vary in their approach to this problem, but the main points include:

- Confirm that the patient is dependent and is genuinely experiencing withdrawal symptoms (e.g. by getting in touch with the patient's doctor and looking for needle marks: a urine sample is useful for screening).
- Minor withdrawal symptoms can be managed symptomatically with anti-emetics, antidiarrhoeals and minor tranquillizers.
- Severe withdrawal symptoms are treated with oral methadone mixture (1 mg/ml). If after 6 hours the symptoms are not relieved, the dose should be repeated. In the long term, methadone should only be given once or twice daily as it has a long half-life.
- Liaison with a specialist unit is essential.
- The Home Office must be informed of subjects who are believed to be opioid or cocaine addicts.

## TREATMENT OF OPIOID DEPENDENCE WITH DRUGS

The basic aims of treatment are to keep the craving for drugs and the unpleasant withdrawal symptoms at bay so that the patient does not seek to obtain heroin or morphine illegally.

The drugs used to treat opioid dependence are:

- methadone
- buprenorphine
- naltrexone
- clonidine
- lofexidine.

### Methadone

Methadone has already been mentioned (see p. 137). Methadone is used orally as a substitute for morphine or diamorphine in the treatment of drug dependence. When taken orally, the drug prevents the severe symptoms of withdrawal from heroin while not producing the euphoria. It is rarely required more frequently than every 12 hours in the management of opioid withdrawal (see also p. 137). Methadone is potentially a drug of abuse and should be prescribed only to patients who are dependent on opioids.

### Safety note

Patients treated with methadone liquid for treatment of heroin dependence have been known to inject the liquid, when the drug produces the euphoric effect. In order to discourage this, opioid antagonists such as naloxone (see below) have in the past been added to the formulation and the patient advised of this. The naloxone is ineffective if taken orally, but if injected would immediately precipitate withdrawal symptoms, which all heroin addicts fear (see p. 289). The wisdom of this drastic strategy is, however, debatable, and the formulation is no longer used.

### Buprenorphine

Buprenorphine has already been mentioned on p. 139. It is a partial agonist that is used as a substitute for heroin in patients who are considered to be only moderately dependent on opioids. It is inadvisable to use buprenorphine in patients who are severely dependent on heroin as the drug may precipitate withdrawal symptoms due to its antagonist effects. It is administered as a sublingual tablet.

### Naltrexone

Naltrexone is an orally active opioid antagonist. It is inadvisable to give antagonists to very dependent patients as this will precipitate withdrawal symptoms. It is more important to supply patients who have been withdrawn from heroin for at least 7–10 days with naltrexone, as this helps to prevent relapse into heroin use. Naltrexone is supplied as oral tablets.

### Clonidine

Clonidine blocks presynaptic $\alpha_2$ adrenoceptors on adrenergic nerve terminals, thus reducing the release of the neurotransmitter norepinephrine, and thereby reducing blood pressure. Clonidine prevents the rise of norepinephrine in the brain which occurs when opioids are withdrawn and which is responsible for many of the unpleasant withdrawal symptoms. Its use in these circumstances requires careful monitoring, combined with full support. It is important to tell the patient that the relief of symptoms may be delayed for 12–24 hours.

### Lofexidine

Lofexidine is similar, but does not lower blood pressure.

Whichever method of opioid withdrawal is used, the main problem is to prevent relapse and a great deal of support is needed.

Case History 22.1 gives a representative example of the presentation of opioid overdose and both emergency and longer-term treatment.

## Case History 22.1

Her boyfriend brought Miss L, a young woman of 21 years old with a known dependence on heroin, into A and E. She was comatose, pale and her breathing was shallow. Her fingers and fingernails were blue and she had abscesses on both arms. She was immediately intubated to assist her breathing and given an injection of an opioid antagonist to block the action of any heroin still in her body. After she had regained consciousness she was admitted as an inpatient and prescribed methadone liquid to prevent the occurrence of withdrawal symptoms. Fortunately, she was HIV-negative despite her admission that she had shared needles with other addicts. After discharge, she was referred to a specialist clinic where she was treated to ensure that she was opioid-free. Once the team were satisfied she had been opioid-free for at least 2 weeks, they prescribed naltrexone tablets, an opioid antagonist, to help her prevent a relapse, and warned her not to try and overcome the block produced by naltrexone, as she would suffer another heroin overdose.

## COCAINE

Cocaine dependence is still on the increase. The drug produces a feeling of elation and appears to temporarily increase physical capacity. In South America the leaves of the coca tree, which contain cocaine, are chewed for this purpose. Cocaine can be given orally; also it is absorbed through mucous membranes and may be sniffed, which can produce ulceration of the nasal septum. More rapid effects are obtained by giving cocaine intravenously, when it may be mixed with heroin. Crack is the free 'base' of cocaine. If this is vaporized and the fumes inhaled the drug is absorbed through the lungs, producing a rapid and intense effect. Because the action of cocaine is short-lived it often is taken in repeated doses every 30 minutes or so and there is risk of dangerous overdose. Dependence is largely psychological and withdrawal symptoms are depression, sleepiness and increased appetite.

## AMFETAMINES AND ECSTASY

For many years amfetamines were used as appetite suppressors and to treat mild depression, and many people, mainly middle-aged women, became mildly dependent on them. In large doses amfetamines are powerful stimulants, producing feelings of confidence, but also, sometimes, hallucinations and other mental disturbances. There is considerable psychological dependence, but the withdrawal symptoms are not severe. Except for special circumstances (see p. 51), amfetamines are now rarely used in medical practice.

**Ecstasy (MDMA)** is an amfetamine derivative that produces a feeling of elation, 'togetherness' and boundless energy. In the UK it is used largely as a dance drug at 'rave' parties. It is manufactured illegally and the strength of tablets is variable. The lethal dose also varies considerably, depending on the individual. The danger is that with vigorous dancing, hyperpyrexia, dehydration and electrolyte disturbances can develop, and a person who has taken ecstasy runs the risk of seizures, collapse, renal failure and death. In addition, it can cause nausea and bruxism (spasm of the jaw muscles). Ecstasy appears to have a low addictive potential, but long-term use may cause some cerebral damage. It is a far from safe drug.

## BARBITURATES

Until some time after the Second World War barbiturates were the most commonly used hypnotic and sedative drugs. It is now realized that prolonged use, particularly in large doses, can lead to dependence. The drug abuser on barbiturates is drowsy, ataxic and examination frequently shows nystagmus. Sudden withdrawal produces well-marked symptoms with anxiety, vomiting and epileptic seizures that can be fatal in the elderly.

## CANNABIS (MARIJUANA)

Cannabis is a resin obtained from a plant that is widely grown in America, Africa and Asia. It is usually smoked. It produces mild excitement combined with a feeling of relaxation and peace. Perception of time is distorted and the passage of time is slowed ('spaced-out') and the subjects may be hungry ('the munchies'). The conjunctivae appear red due to vasodilatation.

Substances related to cannabis (cannabinoids) have been used as anti-emetics for patients who are being treated with cytotoxic drugs. Cannabis is illegal in the UK, but whether it is more addictive and socially more undesirable than alcohol is a matter of debate. Some main arguments against its legalization are:

- Repeated use, particularly in high doses, can reduce motivation and interfere with the subject's life.
- Rarely, it can cause a psychotic state with hallucinations and disorientation.
- The use of cannabis may lead a person on to take more seriously addictive drugs such as heroin. Although this happens infrequently, most heroin addicts have passed through a phase of using cannabis.
- Cannabis is a drug of dependence in that there are withdrawal symptoms (anxiety and sleeplessness) and tolerance develops.

The argument has also been put forward that cannabis destroys personal motivation in society and the user 'opts out'.

Unfortunately, many so-called recreational drugs are resorted to as remedies for symptoms produced by others, and Case History 22.2 illustrates the plight of an otherwise healthy individual who experimented with these drugs.

## Case History 22.2

Miss C, a 26-year-old receptionist, complained to her doctor about chest palpitations, anxiety, insomnia, depression and loss of appetite. The doctor questioned her about her lifestyle and it became apparent that she was using an array of drugs.

Apparently, Miss C had been out clubbing with friends regularly on Friday nights. In order to be able to enjoy the music and dancing and to forget about stress and problems at work she took a couple of amfetamine capsules. Later the same evening, when the effect of the drug eased off, she took more amfetamines and ecstasy pills to restore her energy and make her feel good. When she got hot and thirsty she drank beer. At the end of the night, in order to calm down and relax she shared a joint (cannabis cigarette) with a friend. Afterwards at home, when she could not sleep, she smoked another joint to fight against an upcoming depression.

The doctor explained that the cocktail of drugs had affected her and caused insomnia and anxiety. The amfetamine and ecstasy tablets had the short-term effect of her feeling more energetic and confident. Ecstasy caused sweating and a dry mouth and throat, and it also encouraged her to drink: in her case alcohol. Alcohol intensified the effects of the substances taken. Once the body's energy supplies were exhausted, the predominant feelings in her case were anxiety, confusion,

depression and restlessness. In order to combat these unpleasant feelings, she self-medicated with alcohol and cannabis in order to be able to relax and cheer herself up.

The doctor explained that mixtures of different drugs, particularly when coupled with alcohol, intensify the effect of the individual substances. This makes it difficult to control the effect of substance use. Insomnia and loss of appetite over several days debilitate the body and make it vulnerable to diseases: for example, catching colds, flu and infections. Usually, when the effect of the substances subsides, the symptoms also subside. He advised her to cease taking all so-called recreational drugs and moderate her intake of alcohol. He warned her that experimentation with drugs could lead to eventual dependence on harder drugs such as cocaine and heroin. He arranged for her to visit a herbalist, who prescribed detoxifying teas and an acupuncturist for treatment to calm her down. He also arranged for periodic visits by a community nurse.

**Lessons learnt:**
- The substance use behaviour of Miss C is very similar to other young people on a night out clubbing
- Substances used as mood enhancers can increase existing feelings of depression and anxiety
- When substances are taken as a cocktail of drugs, particularly when coupled with alcohol, the effect of the individual drug is stronger. Substance use therefore is likely to get out of control
- Energy retrieved through the use of amfetamines or ecstasy is only borrowed energy. The body usually needs days to recover and restore its energy levels
- Insomnia and loss of appetite over several days debilitates the body and makes the user vulnerable to diseases and infections
- Substance use can lead to panic attacks, anxiety, confusion and drug-induced psychosis. Mostly, these symptoms cease when substance use is stopped
- The nurse can give information on the effects on substance use and/or refer to specialist drug treatment services.

## VOLATILE SOLVENTS

Various substances contain organic solvents which are volatile and highly fat-soluble and therefore easily penetrate the brain causing depression of the cerebral function with euphoria and occasional hallucination. The problem of 'glue sniffing' has become serious among teenagers and is difficult to control, as the use of these solvents has become more widespread and these preparations are widely available.

In the UK the sale of inhalable products to young people is under statutory control. The Intoxicating Substances Supply Act, which was passed in 1985, makes it an offence in England and Wales to supply to a young person under 18 a substance which the supplier has reason to believe will be 'used to achieve intoxication'. Nevertheless health workers who deal with solvent abuse are aware that many users are adults. Between 1971 and 1991 there were in the UK over 1000 recorded cases of death by inhalation of solvents, and more than two-fifths were over 18 years old.

## HALLUCINOGENS

### LYSERGIC ACID DIETHYLAMIDE (LSD)

LSD is a synthetic derivative of lysergic acid, which occurs naturally in ergot (see p. 57). It produces vivid hallucinations that disorientate the taker, causes heightened appreciation of colours and sounds, and the taker may experience a feeling of complete detachment from the body. It can produce so-called 'bad trips' that consist of highly terrifying images and experiences and can lead to suicide attempts, although successful suicides from LSD are rare. It can produce autonomic effects such as sweating and digestive upsets. The drug is believed to exert its effects mainly as an agonist at central 5-HT$_2$ receptors. It is illegal to possess, use or distribute the drug except under a Home Office licence.

### PSILOCYBIN (MAGIC MUSHROOMS)

These are mushrooms that produce hallucinations and unusual sensations rather like those produced by LSD, although not as powerfully, nor for as long. The chief danger with harvesting these from the wild is the very real possibility of picking the wrong mushroom and poisoning oneself. It is not illegal to pick any mushroom, but it does become illegal if the mushroom is dried, crushed, boiled or cooked to make what is legally termed 'another product'.

### MESCALINE

Mescaline is a chemical found in the dried tops of certain Mexican cactuses, including one called *Lophophora williamsii*. It produces vivid hallucinations and a condition that resembles inebriation (drunkenness). It has no therapeutic value.

## ALCOHOL

### INTRODUCTION

Alcohol presents a special problem, as moderate amounts are taken for social reasons by many people and may, in fact, even be beneficial. Dependence on alcohol is very common and its management is a difficult medical and social problem. It occurs most often in those countries where alcoholic drinks are cheap, for instance the United States and France. Not only does it frequently lead to moral and financial breakdown for the patient but also it is a tragedy for his family.

### EFFECTS OF ALCOHOL

Alcohol causes both acute and chronic disorders. Acute consumption of excessive amounts of alcohol produces a deterioration of brain function, with changes in behaviour progressing through slurred speech and unsteady gait to unconsciousness.

The relationship between plasma concentration and effect is given in Table 22.1.

There is considerable interpersonal variation.

One half-pint of beer or one glass of wine or one single of spirits raises the plasma alcohol level to about 10–20 mg/100 ml. Normally, alcohol is rapidly absorbed from the gastrointestinal tract, though food may slow absorption. Peak blood levels are reached in about 1 hour. It is largely metabolized in the liver, though small amounts are excreted in the urine and breath.

Given the same dose of alcohol, women have a higher blood level and appear more prone to develop alcohol-related diseases. This is partly because they

Table 22.1 Plasma concentration and effect of alcohol

| Plasma level (mg/100 ml) | Effect |
|---|---|
| 20 | Relaxed |
| 30 | Talkative |
| 50 | A little uncoordinated (knocks over glass) |
| 100 | Fall about, vomiting |
| 300 | Stupor |

are generally smaller than men so the volume of distribution is less, but also because, in women, less alcohol is broken down as it passes from the gastrointestinal tract via the liver to the circulation (greater bioavailability).

## Hangovers

Hangovers follow excessive intake of alcohol, although there is considerable interpersonal variation in their severity. The symptoms of headache, thirst, anxiety and nausea are familiar. To some degree they depend on the type of alcoholic beverage consumed. Brandy is the worst culprit and vodka is the least likely to provoke symptoms. This is because brandy contains substances, other than alcohol, which are toxic. Other factors involved are dehydration, hypoglycaemia, tachycardia, gastric irritability, excessive smoking and lack of sleep.

## Chronic alcoholism

Chronic alcoholism damages several organs:

In the **CNS**, abuse leads to tremor, failure of memory and confusion with ultimate dementia and peripheral neuritis. Some of these changes are linked to vitamin B1 deficiency.

**The liver** may be damaged (Stewart et al, 2001), leading ultimately to cirrhosis. The **stomach** may develop gastritis and alcohol can affect the **heart muscle** resulting in atrial fibrillation and cardiomyopathy. In addition, high alcohol consumption raises **blood pressure** and may be a factor in precipitating strokes. Chronic alcoholics are especially prone to infection and have a high incidence of **tuberculosis**.

It is now recognized that excessive consumption of alcohol during pregnancy causes the fetal alcohol syndrome with mild mental retardation, small head, turned-up nose and other facial abnormalities.

## Alcohol intake

The intake of alcohol is usually measured in terms of units per day or per week:

One unit = Half pint of beer
One glass of wine
One glass of sherry or port
One measure of spirits

Each of these contains about 8 g (10 ml) of alcohol.

A 'safe' level of daily alcohol consumption is very difficult to establish, but a frequently quoted figure is three units per day for a man and two units per day for a woman* and there is now considerable evidence that moderate consumption of alcohol protects against coronary artery disease. It should, however, be remembered that even if the average intake of alcohol is within the safe range, a bout of high intake is associated with an increased risk of accident and injury.

## Treatment

Withdrawal of alcohol from a dependent person leads to tremor, anxiety tachycardia and vomiting.

Sedation is best achieved with diazepam. Clomethiazole is excellent at relieving symptoms, but has its own dependence risk. It is common practice to give large doses of vitamins in the early stages of treatment, as deficiency of the vitamin B group may play a part in producing symptoms.

## Delirium tremens

Delirium tremens is a more serious withdrawal disorder with hallucination and disorientation and the patient may be violent. The mortality is around 5%. In these circumstances diazepam (in the form of *Diazemuls*) may have to be given I.V. and repeated as required. Alternatively, clomethiazole can be given by infusion. Because it is normally broken down in the liver, reduced dosage may be required in alcoholics. Vitamins should be given as above and fluid and electrolytes corrected as necessary.

Most alcoholics should give up drinking completely and this requires considerable supportive treatment. Occasionally giving **disulfiram** may help them. This drug inhibits the breakdown of alcohol, producing toxic substances, which cause flushing, nausea and headaches, and thus the patient is discouraged from further drinking. Alternatively, **acamprosate**, a centrally acting drug that modifies the gamma-aminobutyric acid (GABA) system, can be used. It reduces the risk of relapse and is started immediately after withdrawal and continued for 1 year.

## Alcohol and driving

Increasing doses of alcohol produce a progressive deterioration in physical and mental performance. This is particularly important as it may cause road traffic accidents. Drunk in charge of a car is a serious

---

*The Department of Health has recommended four units daily for men and three units for women. Some experts consider this to be too high.

offence, but the definition of drunkenness is difficult. In the UK it is an offence to have more than 80 mg of alcohol per 100 ml of blood while in charge of a car. There are currently several techniques available for monitoring the levels of alcohol in the blood (Sharpe 2001).

## NICOTINE

### INCIDENCE OF DISEASES, MORTALITY AND WITHDRAWAL

Nicotine is a constituent of tobacco smoke. It stimulates the autonomic nervous system (raised blood pressure and pulse rate) and has a mild cocaine-like stimulant action on the brain. It causes both psychological and physical dependence. Unfortunately, its use is associated with an increased incidence of several diseases, most notably:

- **cancer of the lung, lip and tongue**
- **chronic bronchitis and emphysema**
- **coronary artery disease**
- **peripheral vascular disease.**

**The death rate** among smokers is about twice that of non-smokers and the figure is higher for heavy smokers, whose life expectancy is reduced by about 5 years. There is a progressive improvement in prognosis after giving up smoking.

**Withdrawal symptoms** include craving for nicotine, constipation and increased appetite.

### TREATMENT

- *Nicorette*
- **Bupropion**.

Treatment is difficult and requires high motivation on the part of the patient. Subjects vary in their method of withdrawal, some preferring to stop suddenly, others to slowly reduce the number of cigarettes smoked. Various aids such as nicotine chewing gum *(Nicorette)*, skin patches or hypnosis may be used. The success rate at 1 year is about 25%. The success rate is higher if drug treatment is combined with counselling, which is available in many smoking cessation clinics, including specialist services and others run by primary health teams.

### Bupropion

Bupropion is a drug that was originally introduced as an antidepressant. It has been found useful as an aid to help smokers give up the habit. It is taken orally in tablet form. Its mechanism of action, both as an antidepressant and for giving up smoking, is unknown. Its use is associated with some dangers and contraindications.

**Adverse effects of bupropion.** The drug has several adverse effects, the most common being insomnia, rashes, urticaria and depression.

**Contraindications.** Bupropion lowers the seizure for thresholds. This makes it dangerous for epileptics or anyone who has ever had a seizure for any reason. Other contraindications are for patients:

- concomitantly receiving monoamine oxidase inhibitors (MAOIs)
- with bulimia or anorexia nervosa
- who are withdrawing from alcohol or benzodiazepines
- with a CNS tumour
- who are pregnant or breast-feeding.

NICE (National Institute for Clinical Excellence) has published guidelines for treatment with nicotine replacement therapy and these are published in the *BNF*.

## CAFFEINE

Although caffeine is not a serious drug of addiction, transient symptoms of headaches, sleepiness and general depression occur when it is withdrawn from the diet. It is perhaps not generally realized that most people are taking caffeine regularly because not only is it found in coffee but also in other dietary components such as tea, chocolate, cocoa and some proprietary colas.

Occasionally, exclusion of caffeine from the diet will cure sleeplessness, anxiety and palpitations.

**Summary**

- Opioid users become tolerant to the central but not to the peripheral actions of the drugs, and the continual increases in dose means they will suffer from chronic constipation
- It is not unusual for opioid dependence to develop because the user has escalated to opioids from more minor drugs such as cannabis
- Peer group pressure is a powerful stimulus to taking drugs

- Tension, job pressure, chronic illness and domestic upheaval are important factors in drug misuse
- Overdose is a continual danger with street buying of drugs, which have unknown potency
- Injection under non-sterile conditions is an important source of sepsis among drug misusers
- Shared needles is an important cause of the rise in HIV infection
- Babies born of opioid addicts are dependent on opioid and will suffer acute withdrawal symptoms after birth
- Opioid users may try to inject methadone which is prescribed for oral administration to suppress withdrawal symptoms

- Ecstasy can and has proved fatal due to variable tablet quality of manufacture and consequent unpredictability of dose
- Taking large amounts of alcohol during pregnancy may result in the birth of a mentally retarded baby with a small head and facial deformities
- Smoking cessation clinics are widely available and do increase the success rate in giving up smoking
- Bupropion is a drug used to aid giving up smoking, but it does lower the seizure threshold in epileptics and must not be used by them; neither should it be used by anyone with bulimia, anorexia nervosa, alcohol dependence or withdrawal or during pregnancy and breast-feeding

## References

Sharpe P C 2001 Biochemical detection and monitoring of alcohol abuse and abstinence. Annals of Clinical Biochemistry 38: 652

Stewart S, Jones D, Day C P 2001 Alcoholic liver disease: new insights into mechanisms and preventative strategies. Trends in Molecular Medicine 7: 408

## Further reading

Benowitz N L 1997 Treating tobacco addiction; nicotine or no nicotine. New England Journal of Medicine 337: 1230

Ecstasy (MDMA) 1995 Alerting users to the dangers. Nursing Times 91: 30

Editorial 1989 Cocaine and crack. British Medical Journal 299: 338

Farrell M et al 1994 Methadone maintenance treatment in opiate dependence. British Medical Journal 309: 997

Friedman G D, Khatsky A L 1993 Is alcohol good for your health? New England Journal of Medicine 329: 1882

Hall W, Solowij N 1998 Adverse effects of cannabis. Lancet 352: 1611

Hall W, Zador D 1997 The alcohol withdrawal syndrome. Lancet 349: 1897

Henningfield J E 1995 Drug therapy: nicotine medications for smoking cessation. New England Journal of Medicine 333: 1196

Interdepartmental Working Group 1995 Sensible drinking. Department of Health, London.

O'Connor P G, Schottenfield R S 1998 Patients with alcohol problems. New England Journal of Medicine 338: 592

Percival J 2002 Strategies for smoking cessation. Nursing Times 98: 66

Preston A 1992 Substance abuse: pointing the risk. Nursing Times 88(13): 24

Rassool G 2002 Substance abuse and mental health: an overview. Nursing Standard 16: 47

Sievewright N A, Greenwood J 1996 What is important in drug misuse treatment? Lancet 347: 373

Swift R M 1999 Drug therapy for alcohol dependence. New England Journal of Medicine 340: 1482

White I R 1996 The cardioprotective effects of moderate alcohol consumption. British Medical Journal 312: 1179

Woodrow P 1998 The effects of 'ecstasy'. Nursing Standard 12: 39

Chapter **23**

# Antibacterial drugs

At the end of this chapter, the reader should be able to:

- explain how the bacterial cell wall is a target for antibiotics
- define the terms Gram-positive and Gram-negative bacteria
- discuss how an antibiotic is chosen
- distinguish the different classes of antibiotics and give important examples of each
- give an account of what TB is, how it is diagnosed and treated with drugs, and about immunization
- describe resistance to antibiotics, and how it happens with penicillins
- explain how antibiotics are used to treat common infections
- appreciate the practicalities and precautions of antibiotic handling and administration

## INTRODUCTION

Antibacterial drugs have revolutionized the treatment of infection, and many diseases such as bacterial meningitis, which previously were often fatal, are now usually curable, but it must be realized that the battle against pathogenic bacteria is by no means over. Many organisms have become resistant to antibacterial drugs and this requires a continuing search for new drugs and modification of those already in use. It also means that they should not be used unnecessarily.

It should be remembered that even with powerful antibacterial drugs the patient's natural resistance plays an important part in combating infection. The nurse will note that patients with impaired immunity, due to prolonged illness, old age or perhaps the use of cytotoxic or immunosuppressive drugs, respond poorly to antibacterial drugs and the infection is much harder to eradicate.

## HOW ANTIBACTERIAL SUBSTANCES WORK

Antibiotics exert their effects in two main ways:

- bactericidal agents kill bacteria rapidly (e.g. aminoglycosides, polymyxin)
- bacteriostatic agents prevent bacteria from replicating, but do not kill them (e.g. sulphonamides, tetracyclines, chloramphenicol)

The distinction between these two categories is not clear. Many antibiotics that operate principally as bacteriostatic agents can become bactericidal under favourable circumstances. Factors affecting the mode of action include the concentration of the drug and the number and type of organisms. When relatively modest numbers of bacteria are present and the drug is given in high doses to highly sensitive organisms, a normally bacteriostatic agent such as penicillin may become bactericidal.

## ANTIBIOTICS AND THE BACTERIAL CELL WALL

Each of the main groups of antibiotics has a different molecular structure and this is the factor that determines its mode of action. Many antibiotics exert their effects directly on the bacterial cell wall or must pass through it before disrupting bacterial metabolism at the intracellular level. The cell walls of all bacteria are composed of layers of protein molecules bound together by cross-linkages, resulting in a large, complex chemical aggregate, but their fine structure depends on whether they are Gram-positive or Gram-negative. The fine structure of the cell wall influences susceptibility to the different groups of antibiotics. For example, erythromycin is able to penetrate the cell walls of Gram-positive bacteria and is effective in the treatment of some staphylococcal or streptococcal infections, but has no effect on Gram-negative bacteria. Some of the diverse ways in which the different groups of antibiotics exert their effects are illustrated in Figure 23.1.

## GRAM-POSITIVE AND GRAM-NEGATIVE BACTERIA

With few exceptions, bacteria may be classified as Gram-positive or Gram-negative, according to a staining technique used in laboratory identification. Generally, Gram-positive bacteria are able to withstand desiccation better than Gram-negative bacteria and many form spores that resist drying. Gram-negative species multiply rapidly in the presence of moisture even when provided with minimal nourishment. Several Gram-positive and Gram-negative bacteria have had a long association with hospital infection and, because they can be carried on the hands, may be spread by cross-infection in any health care setting (Table 23.1).

**Anaerobes.** This term refers to bacteria that can live and multiply in the absence of free oxygen. In the

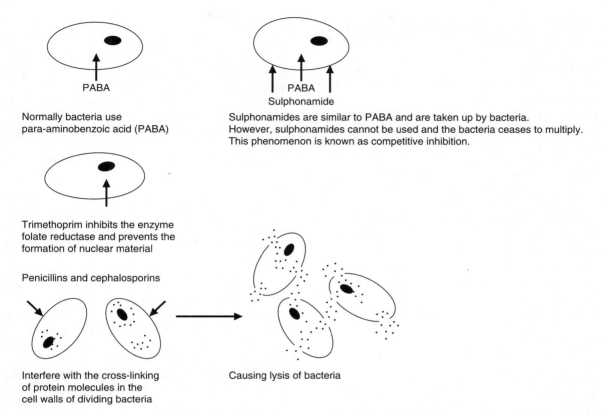

Normally bacteria use para-aminobenzoic acid (PABA)

Sulphonamides are similar to PABA and are taken up by bacteria. However, sulphonamides cannot be used and the bacteria ceases to multiply. This phenomenon is known as competitive inhibition.

Trimethoprim inhibits the enzyme folate reductase and prevents the formation of nuclear material

Penicillins and cephalosporins

Interfere with the cross-linking of protein molecules in the cell walls of dividing bacteria

Causing lysis of bacteria

Tetracycline, aminoglycoside and chloramphenicol interfere with protein synthesis within the cell. In normal cells RNA is bound to ribosomes which are essential for protein synthesis. This group of antibiotics binds onto the ribosomes, excluding the RNA and preventing protein synthesis. Thus bacteria do not multiply.

**Figure 23.1**   Some of the modes of action of antibacterial drugs.

**Table 23.1    Gram-positive and Gram-negative organisms in hospitals**

| Gram–positive | Gram–negative |
|---|---|
| Staphylococcus aureus | Haemophilus (H.) influenzae |
| Streptococcus pyogenes | Neisseria (N.) gonorrhoeae (Gonococcus) |
| Streptococcus viridans | Neisseria (N.) meningitidis (Meningococcus) |
| Streptococcus pneumoniae (Pneumococcus) | Escherichia (E.) coli |
|  | Proteus |
|  | Pseudomonas |
|  | Klebsiella |

laboratory they require special conditions before they will grow in culture, but they are able to cause severe infections given the correct circumstances. Anaerobic bacteria naturally inhabiting the gut may cause severe sepsis following abdominal surgery. If

*Clostridium tetani* gains access to a penetrating wound that is free of oxygen the organism multiplies and produces a toxin that causes tetanus.

## CHOOSING AN ANTIBIOTIC

When faced with a patient with an infectious disease, the first consideration is whether an antibiotic is required. Many infections (e.g. a mild sore throat) get better quickly without specific treatment. If antibiotic treatment is needed the following points should be considered:

- The infecting organism: this is often suspected from the nature of the disease and initial treatment is usually based on this guess. If possible, the nature of the organism should be confirmed by culture of blood, sputum, urine, etc., although in practice this is not always possible.
- The correct antibiotic to eradicate the infection.

• The ability of the antibiotic to penetrate the site of infection (for example, in meningitis not all drugs enter the cerebrospinal fluid).

• The route of administration: some antibiotics are ineffective orally and injection may also be required for rapid action.

• A drug history is essential (as always) to ensure that the patient has not previously had an adverse reaction to the chosen antibiotic, or that the antibiotic will not compromise any other drug being used, e.g. rifampicin and the Pill (see below).

• Possible complicating factors such as pregnancy, renal or hepatic failure.

• In these difficult times, the cost of the drug, although this decision should not jeopardize the patient's safety or return to health.

Note that *antibiotic* is a term used to describe any substance produced by or derived from an organism which inhibits the growth of or destroys another organism, usually a bacterial or fungal infection.

Case History 23.1 gives an example of the procedures used.

## Case History 23.1

Miss B, aged 27, developed a cough which produced phlegm and she bought a proprietary cough mixture, which didn't stop the cough. She also became troubled by shortness of breath, especially when she lay on her back, and a severe headache; therefore, she decided to visit her GP. The GP, who listened to her chest and said there was nothing untoward except a slight sound on one side, diagnosed a bacterial infection. A sputum specimen was taken and sent away for analysis. There was indeed a bacterial infection and a course of clarithromycin was prescribed to treat the chest infection; Miss B was told to complete the full course of treatment. Salbutamol, an $\alpha_2$ agonist, was prescribed for the shortness of breath, together with a spacer to help deliver the full dose of salbutamol. It was also recommended that Miss B take aspirin for the headache.

## THE SULPHONAMIDES

This is one of the oldest groups of antibacterial agents. They differ to some extent in the range of organisms they attack, but most of their pharmacological properties are similar. They have been largely replaced because of the development of bacterial resistance and adverse side-effects, and most have

Table 23.2    Available sulphonamides

| Drug | Important features |
| --- | --- |
| Sulfadimidine | Well absorbed orally |
| Sulfasalazine | Used in ulcerative colitis. It is particularly useful for long-term maintenance treatment |
| Silver sulfadiazine | Applied locally as a cream to prevent infection in severe burns |

disappeared from use. They are, with few exceptions, well and rapidly absorbed from the intestinal tract. They circulate widely in the body fluids and cross the meningeal barrier to enter the cerebrospinal fluid (CSF).

After absorption, the liver begins to acetylate the sulphonamides. The acetylated drugs together with unaltered sulphonamide are excreted in the urine. The acetylated sulphonamides are very poorly soluble and therefore there is a danger that they will precipitate in the urine unless an adequate flow is maintained. Most of the sulphonamides are effective against a fairly wide range of bacteria. Unfortunately, certain of these bacteria have become resistant. Table 23.2 gives a number of available sulphonamides.

## THERAPEUTIC USE OF SULPHONAMIDES

### Sulfadimidine and Sulfasalazine

Sulfadimidine is still used occasionally in urinary infections provided that the infecting organism is susceptible. Sulfasalazine is given in the long-term treatment of ulcerative colitis and Crohn's disease (see p. 114). Sulfasalazine can also be used in the treatment of rheumatoid arthritis.

### Adverse effects

• Nausea can be troublesome and with sulfasalazine may be relieved by giving small and more frequent doses

• Rashes of various types, sometimes with fever

• Blood dyscrasias: polyarteritis nodosa is a rare, but dangerous, complication

• The sperm count is reduced by sulfasalazine, but recovers on stopping the drug

• Precipitation in the urinary tract causing obstruction; the patient should be given 2–3 litres of fluid daily to maintain a good urinary flow when receiving sulfadimidine.

## Co-trimoxazole–trimethoprim and sulfamethoxazole

**Mechanism of action.** Sulphonamides affect bacteria by interfering with their use of para-aminobenzoic acid (PABA), a precursor of folic acid, which is ultimately essential in cell division (see Fig. 23.1). Trimethoprim interferes with folic acid metabolism, at the phase when folic acid is changed to folinic acid to build up the cell nucleus. This requires the action of an enzyme, and, by combining with that enzyme, trimethoprim stops the reaction and the cell dies. The combination of a sulphonamide with trimethoprim is particularly effective in preventing bacterial cell division and is also bactericidal. Co-trimoxazole is effective against *S. pyogenes*, *S. pneumoniae*, *E. coli*, *H. influenzae*, *salmonella* and *Pneumocystis carinii* (in large doses).

**Therapeutic use.** The combined tablet of cotrimoxazole–trimethoprim plus sulfamethoxazole has been widely and successfully used in exacerbations of chronic bronchitis and in urinary infections. It also has a place in the treatment of the more severe salmonella and other infections. Unfortunately, its adverse-effect profile has led to its use being largely confined to pneumocystis pneumonia. In large doses it is used to treat pneumocystis infection of the lung, a disease which occurs in patients whose immunity has been suppressed, often as a result of cancer chemotherapy or HIV.

**Adverse effects.** These are largely those of the sulphonamides, namely nausea and vomiting, and occasionally blood disorders. More serious is the occasional development of the Stevens–Johnson syndrome with a bullous rash, mouth ulceration and fever, which can be fatal.

## Trimethoprim

Trimethoprim can also be used alone. At present it is largely used to treat urinary infection. It can also be used to treat bronchitis.

**Adverse effects.** These include nausea, rashes and, rarely, depression of the blood count.

**Contraindication.** It should not be used in the first 3 months of pregnancy.

## THE NITROFURANS

This group of chemotherapeutic agents has been investigated sporadically for over 30 years. The only one currently used is **nitrofurantoin**.

Nitrofurantoin has a fairly wide antibacterial spectrum and is considerably concentrated in the urine. It is used in the treatment of urinary tract infections, or as a prophylactic. Nausea sometimes occurs but can be minimized by giving the drug after food. Other adverse effects include rashes and fever. It should not be used in patients with renal failure, as accumulation will occur.

## THE QUINOLONES

The quinolones comprise:

- **ciprofloxacin**
- **levofloxacin**
- **nalidixic acid**
- **norfloxacin**
- **ofloxacin**.

This group of antibacterial drugs is increasingly important; several are available already and more will probably be introduced in the next few years. They interfere with an enzyme necessary for the cell division of bacteria.

## Ciprofloxacin

**Therapeutic use.** Ciprofloxacin acts against a wide range of organisms, but is not very effective against some Gram-positive organisms, particularly pneumococci. It is given orally twice daily or by infusion, which is very expensive. At present, its use should be confined to patients for whom older antibacterial drugs are unsatisfactory, particularly for typhoid, urinary infection and gonorrhoea. It is the preferred drug in adults as a prophylactic for close contact with meningococcal meningitis.

**Adverse effects.** These include gastrointestinal upsets and rashes. It should be avoided, if possible, in patients with epilepsy as it has a potential to cause seizures, and in children it may cause damage to developing weight-bearing joints. It can also cause pain and inflammation of tendons, especially in older people.

**Drug interactions.** Ciprofloxacin raises the blood levels of theophylline. The action of warfarin is increased.

There has been a large increase in resistance to ciprofloxacin in recent years.

**Ofloxacin** is similar to ciprofloxacin. **Levofloxacin** is more active against *S. pneumoniae* and can be used in community-acquired pneumonia but offers no real advantage over the usual antibiotics.

**Norfloxacin** and **nalidixic acid** are effective in uncomplicated urinary tract infections and are used when the infecting organism is resistant to the older antibacterial drugs. For an uncomplicated infection a 3-day course is adequate, but prolonged treatment is required for severe or recurrent infections. They should be avoided in children and pregnancy, in cases of porphyria and renal impairment.

## β LACTAM ANTIBIOTICS

The β lactam antibiotics can be divided into:

- the penicillins
- the cephalosporins
- others.

The β lactam antibiotics all contain the β lactam ring, which is a chemical structure essential for their antibacterial activity. The family of β lactams is summarized in Figure 23.2.

## THE PENICILLINS

The penicillins comprise:

- ampicillin
- azlocillin
- amoxicillin
- benzylpenicillin
- co-amoxiclav
- flucloxacillin
- phenoxymethylpenicillin
- piperacillin
- pivampicillin
- ticarcillin.

The penicillins were the first antibiotics to be isolated. Over the years their structure has been repeatedly modified to deal with the problem of resistance to penicillin and to extend their antibacterial range. They are still probably the most widely used family of antibiotics.

### Benzylpenicillin

Benzylpenicillin was the first penicillin to be used clinically. It is usually given by deep intramuscular injection, which is painful, and if a large single dose is needed it should be given intravenously. It enters the circulation rapidly and spreads through the body; it does not, however, cross into the CSF in any great quantity, although this may be increased if the meninges are inflamed.

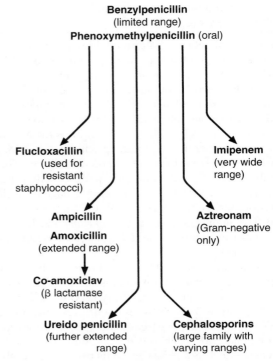

Figure 23.2    The β lactam family of antibiotics.

**Elimination of penicillins.** All penicillins are excreted by the kidneys, partially through the glomeruli but the major part via the renal tubules. The excretion is rapid and blood levels fall nearly to zero 4 hours after injection. If benzylpenicillin is given orally it is partially broken down by the gastric acid and is not now given by this route.

**Range of benzylpenicillin.** Benzylpenicillin is effective against a fairly wide range of organisms. Table 23.3 lists the most common.

Penicillins are bacteriostatic and in higher doses are bactericidal. When treating infection it is ideal to maintain the blood level of penicillin continually at bactericidal levels, and this requires injections every 4 hours. In milder infections, however, it is often adequate to give less frequent injections. Even after the blood levels of penicillin have dropped below bactericidal or bacteriostatic levels, the organism may take some time to recover and by that time the blood level of penicillin has risen again following a further injection.

### Procaine benzylpenicillin

Numerous attempts have been made to prolong the action of benzylpenicillin after injection by slowing

**Table 23.3**    Main uses of benzylpenicillin

| Organisms | Disease |
| --- | --- |
| *Streptococcus pyogenes* | Tonsillitis, scarlet, fever, septicaemia |
| *Streptococcus viridans* | Subacute bacterial endocarditis |
| *Staphylococcus aureus*[a] | Carbuncles, osteomyelitis, septicaemia, boils |
| *Streptococcus pneumoniae* | Pneumonia |
| *Neisseria gonorrhoeae* | Gonorrhoea |
| *Neisseria meningitidis* | Meningococcal meningitis |
| *Treponema pallidum* | Syphilis |
| *Clostridium perfringens* | Gangrene |
| *Clostridium tetani* | Tetanus |
| *Actinomyces* | Actinomycosis |

[a] Note that a high proportion of staphylococci found in hospital are now resistant to benzylpenicillin.

down its release from the injection site. A successful method is to combine benzylpenicillin with procaine. The combination is called procaine benzylpenicillin and will maintain a satisfactory blood level for at least 12 hours. This preparation is, however, rather slow to produce a satisfactory blood level, so that if a rapid effect is required, benzylpenicillin should be given as well.

The action of penicillin can be augmented and prolonged by slowing down its excretion. This can be done by giving **probenecid**, a drug that blocks the tubular secretion of penicillin, thus allowing the drug to accumulate in the body.

### Penicillin resistance: penicillinase and the β lactam ring

Certain organisms develop resistance to the action of penicillin. Organisms which were originally sensitive appear to adapt themselves to the penicillin by producing an enzyme called **penicillinase,** which inactivates penicillin by attacking part of the penicillin molecule known as the **β lactam ring**. This structure is an essential part of penicillins and cephalosporins, and the family of enzymes involved is sometimes known as the **β lactamases**. This is particularly so in the case of staphylococci and strains of this organism which are resistant to penicillin and other antibiotics are a serious clinical problem. There is now a considerable degree of alarm because of the rapidly reducing number of effective antibiotics, and there is growing realization

that we may be in danger of entering a period analogous to that before antibiotics were originally introduced.

### Other penicillins

These comprise:

- phenoxymethylpenicillin
- flucloxacillin
- broad-spectrum penicillins
- extended-spectrum penicillins (ureidopenicillins).

There are a number of penicillins that are similar to benzylpenicillin but are effective by mouth. Some of the examples given below are not destroyed by the acid in the stomach and are fairly well absorbed from the intestinal tract.

**Phenoxymethylpenicillin.** Adequate absorption with a satisfactory therapeutic response usually occurs with oral penicillin but it is important that it is taken 30 minutes before a meal. The patient must be carefully observed in case the drug is ineffective due to vomiting or inadequate absorption. Penicillin must then be given by injection.

**Flucloxacillin.** The elucidation of the structure of the penicillin nucleus has made it possible to produce penicillins which are not broken down by penicillinase and are therefore effective against organisms, particularly staphylococci, which have become resistant to benzylpenicillin. Flucloxacillin is a commonly used example. It is used almost exclusively for treating staphylococcal infections.

Strains of staphylococci have emerged which are resistant even to flucloxacillin. They are called **methicillin-resistant** *Staphylococcus aureus* (**MRSA**) and respond only to **vancomycin** or **teicoplanin** (see p. 309).

**Broad–spectrum penicillins.** These include ampicillin, amoxicillin and pivampicillin.

**Ampicillin** is effective against a number of bacteria, including salmonellae, *E. coli, Shigella* and *H. influenzae*, which are little affected by benzylpenicillin. It has proved particularly useful in chronic bronchitis, urinary infections and typhoid. It can be given orally or by injection.

**Amoxicillin** is very similar to ampicillin, but is better absorbed so a smaller dose is required. For this reason it is perhaps to be preferred to ampicillin.

**Pivampicillin** consists of ampicillin linked to another molecule that facilitates absorption. As it passes through the gut wall it is split and ampicillin is released. It therefore has no advantage over ampicillin except that it is better absorbed.

**Co-amoxiclav**: Some bacteria produce β lactamases capable of breaking down both ampicillin and amoxycillin together with other antibiotics. Antibiotics can be combined with a substance called clavulanate, which prevents this breakdown and thus enables it to destroy β lactamase-producing bacteria. The combined preparation of amoxicillin and clavulanate is called co-amoxiclav.

**Extended–spectrum penicillins (ureido penicillins).** These include azlocillin, piperacillin and ticarcillin. This group of extended-spectrum penicillins ureido penicillins) have much the same antibacterial spectrum as ampicillin but are also effective against *Pseudomonas aeruginosa* and *Proteus morganii*. They are, however, inactivated by some β lactamases and are therefore not active against penicillin-resistant staphylococci and, in addition, are not very effective against other Gram-positive organisms (e.g. *S. pneumoniae*). They are not absorbed from the gut and must be given by injection. They are reserved for serious infections with pseudomonas or when the causative organism is not known. In this case, due to deficiencies in their antibacterial spectrum, they are usually combined with an aminoglycoside, *but must not be mixed in the same infusion or syringe*. They are very expensive.

**Azlocillin** is the most effective of the three against pseudomonas, but is not so effective against other microorganisms. **Piperacillin** has good all-round activity. **Ticarcillin** is available combined with clavulanic acid.

As these drugs are excreted via the kidney, the dose should be reduced in renal failure.

### Adverse effects of penicillins

Considering the wide use of penicillin, it is remarkably free from toxic effects. Pain and rarely abscess formation may be seen at the site of injection. More commonly, sensitization rashes occur either as a result of contact with the drug during or after systemic administration. The rash is often urticarial and is sometimes resistant to treatment. With ampicillin or amoxicillin the rash is sometimes erythematous and is particularly liable to occur if they are given to a patient with glandular fever or lymphoma. It may also appear after the drugs have been stopped. Rarely, penicillin causes an acute anaphylactic reaction with collapse, which can be fatal.

> **Nursing point**
>
> Always ask about previous drug reactions before giving a patient a penicillin, cephalosporin, or for that matter, any other drug.

Other adverse effects include diarrhoea, and penicillins may reduce the efficacy of the contraceptive pill. Co-amoxiclav can cause jaundice.

> **Safety point**
>
> It is advisable to ask an outpatient to stay at the surgery for half an hour after giving an injection of penicillin, especially if there is anything in the patient's history to suggest allergy to drugs or certain foods such as eggs, because of the risk of anaphylaxis. The same precaution, incidentally, applies when giving a 'flu' vaccination which has been raised in eggs.

## THE CEPHALOSPORINS

This is a large group of antibiotics that structurally bear some relationship to the penicillins in that they both contain a β lactam ring. They have a wide spectrum of antibacterial activity, although there are differences in this respect between the older cephalosporins and the newer introductions. Most of them can be given only by injection. Although they are efficient antibiotics they are rarely the drugs of first choice, as for many infections there are cheaper, effective substitutes.

They can be divided into three groups:

- the older cephalosporins
- the recently introduced cephalosporins
- oral cephalosporins.

### The older cephalosporins

The older cephalosporins (Table 23.4) are active against:

- *Staphylococcus aureus* (including some strains resistant to penicillin)
- *Streptococcus pyogenes*
- *Streptococcus pneumoniae*
- *E. coli* (most strains)
- *Klebsiella* (most strains)
- *Proteus* (most strains)
- *H. influenzae* (variable).

Table 23.4    The older cephalosporins

| Drug | Important features |
| --- | --- |
| Cefazolin | Some biliary excretion so used before surgery on the bile duct |
| Cefradine | Fairly β lactamase-stable |

This group is being superseded.

They may be inactivated by β-lactamases and are excreted by the kidneys.

## The newer cephalosporins

These are an improvement on the older members of the group. They are more β-lactamase-resistant and are therefore effective against some resistant strains.

In general, they act against:

- *Streptococcus pyogenes*
- *Staphylococcus aureus*
- *H. influenzae*
- *N. meningitidis*
- *E. coli*
- *Proteus.*

Some of them also have activity against pseudomonas and *Bacillus fragilis*, which are important organisms in abdominal infection. The latest introductions do, however, show some falling off in their activity against certain Gram-positive organisms. There are now so many of this group available that only a selection is shown in Table 23.5.

The main uses for these new cephalosporins:

- to treat severe infection (septicaemias, etc.) when the causative organism is not known or other antibiotics are contraindicated
- cefotaxime and ceftriaxone penetrate well into the cerebrospinal fluid and are effective in meningococcal meningitis

Table 23.5    The newer cephalosporins

| Drug | Important features |
| --- | --- |
| Cefuroxime | Good all-round activity |
| Cefamandole | Effective against staphylococci |
| Cefoxitin | Active against *B. fragilis* |
| Cefotaxime | Good all-round activity against Gram-negative organisms |
| Ceftizoxime | Similar to cefotaxime |
| Ceftazidime | Useful in pseudomonal infection |
| Ceftriaxone | Long-acting |
| Cefpirome | Good all-round activity |

- possibly in hepatobiliary or abdominal sepsis
- very rarely in resistant urinary infections
- cefuroxime is effective in most chest infections even by Gram-positive organisms, i.e. *Streptococcus pneumoniae*.

Most of this group are expensive.

## Oral cephalosporins

**Cefadroxil** is given every 12 hours and has a similar antibacterial range to the older cephalosporins. It can be used in urinary and respiratory infections. **Cefixime** is similar but rather long-acting and more effective against *H. influenzae*. Although **cefuroxime** is ineffective if given orally, a compound of it (**cefuroxime axetil**) is absorbed from the gastrointestinal tract and is now available. **Cefpodoxime** is used in respiratory infections.

## Cross–sensitivity with penicillin

Approximately 10% of patients who are allergic to penicillin will also be allergic to a cephalosporin. In general, this excludes the use of cephalosporins in penicillin-sensitive patients, although exceptions may be made in special circumstances.

## OTHER β LACTAMS

**Aztreonam** has a relatively narrow spectrum of antibacterial action. It can be used against infections caused by *N. gonorrhoeae* and *H. influenzae*, but is ineffective against the common Gram-positive organisms. It is given by injection.

**Imipenem with cilastatin** has the widest antibacterial range of any antibiotic, including not only the usual Gram-positive and Gram-negative bacteria, but also pseudomonas and anaerobes. It is administered either via an I.V. infusion, or by deep I.M. injection. It is excreted via the kidney and is inactivated in the renal tubule by an enzyme; the urinary concentration is therefore very low. Combining imipenem with cilastatin, which inhibits the enzyme, prevents this. At present, its use is confined to patients in whom older antibiotics are contraindicated or ineffective.

Both aztreonam and imipenem can show cross-sensitivity with penicillin.

**Meropenem** is similar to the other two drugs, but is not broken down by the kidneys and therefore does not need to be combined with cilastatin. It is given by injection.

## THE AMINOGLYCOSIDES

Aminoglycosides comprise:

- amikacin
- gentamicin
- neomycin
- netilmicin
- spectinomycin
- streptomycin
- tobramycin.

This group of antibiotics interferes with protein synthesis in the bacteria and they are bactericidal; i.e. they kill the bacteria rather than preventing them from multiplying. They have a fairly wide antibacterial range and one of them (streptomycin) is effect-ive against *Mycobacterium tuberculosis* (Table 23.6).

## EFFECTIVENESS OF AMINOGLYCOSIDES

They have a number of common properties:

- they are all given by injection if a systemic effect is required
- the kidneys excrete them all and accumulation occurs with impaired renal function
- they are all, to a greater or lesser degree, ototoxic (they impair hearing and/or balance) and nephrotoxic
- their antibacterial spectrum differs a little, but they are generally active against a fair range of organisms.

**Table 23.6**   Main uses of aminoglycosides

| Organism | Disease |
| --- | --- |
| *Staphylococcus aureus* | Septicaemia, abscesses |
| *Streptococcus viridans* | Endocarditis |
| *H. influenzae* | Pneumonia, meningitis |
| *Brucella abortus* | Abortus fever |
| *E. coli* | Renal and other infections |
| *Proteus* | Various infections, largely abdominal |
| *Pseudomonas* | |
| *Klebsiella* | Chest infection |
| *Mycobacterium tuberculosis*[a] | All forms of tuberculosis; they are not particularly effective against *Streptococcus pneumoniae* or *Streptococcus pyogenes*. |

[a] Streptomycin only.

## Gentamicin

**Therapeutic use.**   This antibiotic is widely used, especially in treating severe infection by staphylococci and by various Gram-negative organisms. It is given intravenously or intramuscularly. Excretion, which is via the kidneys, is fairly rapid so that it is usually given three times daily.

It is important to maintain a correct blood level, which should be measured every 48 hours, or more often if necessary. The peak blood level half an hour after injection should be between 5 and 10 mg/litre and the trough level (just before injection) should be below 2 mg/litre. The dose is adjusted to produce these levels. If the blood level is too low the antibiotic may not be effective, but if it is above 10 mg/litre for long, ototoxicity will result. It should be remembered that toxicity depends not only on the blood level but also upon the length of treatment.

Increasing interest is being shown in the once daily administration of aminoglycosides. Blood levels are measured once or twice daily and the dose adjusted accordingly.

**Excretion.**   Gentamicin is excreted via the kidneys, and accumulation and toxicity will occur if the drug is given to patients with impaired renal function. In these circumstances a lower dosage will be required and information is available which relates the dose necessary to the degree of impairment of renal function. Reduced dosages are usually given also to elderly patients.

> **Nursing points**
>
> 1. It is essential to monitor the blood levels of gentamicin, etc. Renal function may deteriorate in the course of a serious illness and, if impaired, accumulation and toxicity will occur.
> 2. Gentamicin reacts with many drugs *in vitro*; therefore it should be given as a bolus or separate injection.

**Drug interactions and adverse effects.**   Renal damage may occur if gentamicin is combined with furosemide (frusemide). Gentamicin is ototoxic, causing disorders of balance and hearing, which are dose-related. Gentamicin augments the action of curare-like neuromuscular blocking agents. It should be avoided during pregnancy, as it is ototoxic to the fetus.

Tobramycin, amikacin and netilmicin are very similar to gentamicin; however, they are sometimes effective against Gram-negative organisms that are resistant to gentamicin. They should only be used in this situation, as they offer no other advantage. Side-effects are similar, except that netilmicin is perhaps a little less toxic.

Spectinomycin has only one use, namely the treatment of gonorrhoeal infection due to organisms that have become resistant to penicillin. Adverse effects include rashes and vomiting.

## Neomycin

Neomycin is an antibiotic that is bactericidal against a wide range of Gram-positive and Gram-negative organisms and against *Mycobacterium tuberculosis*. It is very poorly absorbed from the intestinal tract and because of toxicity is not given systemically. It is chiefly used to sterilize the gut before surgery. It can also be applied locally as ear or eye drops.

Extensive local application to areas such as burns should be avoided, as enough absorption can occur to cause ototoxicity.

## Streptomycin

Streptomycin is derived from one of the actinomyces group of fungi.

**Therapeutic use.** Streptomycin is usually given by intramuscular injection. The maximum concentration in the blood is reached after about 1–2 hours and excretion is not completed for 24 hours or more. Streptomycin is excreted in the urine. It is not absorbed after oral administration so this route is not used except for treating gut infections. Streptomycin is now rarely used for infections other than drug-resistant tuberculosis. It may be combined with doxycycline in the treatment of brucellosis.

**Resistance.** The development of resistance to streptomycin is relatively common. Combining streptomycin with some other chemotherapeutic agent or antibiotic to which the organism is sensitive may largely prevent this. With such treatment the development of resistance is delayed or even prevented altogether.

## THE TETRACYCLINES

Following the discovery of penicillin (which was originally discovered in a fungus) and streptomycin, a large-scale investigation was carried out into substances that were produced by various fungi.

Three important antibiotics, namely the tetracyclines, were discovered. They are very similar in chemical structure and toxic effects and are effective against the same wide range of organisms. They are:

- **chlortetracycline**
- **oxytetracycline**
- **tetracycline**.

The properties of these drugs are so similar that they may be considered together.

## PROPERTIES OF MAIN TETRACYCLINES

### Administration

They are usually given orally, are quite well absorbed from the intestinal tract and 6-hourly dosage is satisfactory. Tetracycline hydrochloride may also be given by I.V. injection. It is, however, very irritating to the vein and is best given by continuous I.V. infusion. The absorption of tetracyclines from the gut is delayed or reduced by antacids, milk and various salts, e.g. calcium, zinc, aluminium, iron and magnesium.

### Distribution and excretion

After absorption, the tetracyclines spread widely through the body. The penetration across the meningeal barrier into the CSF is variable, being greatest in the case of tetracycline itself. The greater part of these drugs is excreted in the urine; the fate of the remainder is unknown.

### Therapeutic use

The tetracyclines have a very wide antibacterial range, which includes not only true bacteria but also some of the larger viruses and some other groups of organisms. However, with some bacteria, resistant strains have emerged which limit their use. The main uses for the tetracyclines at present are shown in Table 23.7.

**Table 23.7**    Main uses of tetracyclines

| Organism | Disease |
| --- | --- |
| *H. influenzae* | Bronchitis |
| *Streptococcus pneumoniae* | Bronchitis |
| *Mycoplasma* | Pneumonia |
| *Chlamydia* | Non-specific urethritis |
| *Rickettsia* | Typhus, Q fever, etc. |
| *Brucella abortus* | Abortus fever |

They are also used over long periods in the treatment of acne. Whether their efficacy in this disorder is due to their antibacterial action or is due to some other factor is not known. Chlortetracycline is now available only as an ointment or as eye drops.

> **Nursing point**
>
> Tetracycline tablets should be swallowed whole with the patient sitting or standing and washed down with plenty of water. Absorption is reduced by concurrent administration of iron, calcium or magnesium compounds (including milk).

## OTHER TETRACYCLINES

These comprise:

- **demeclocycline**
- **doxycycline**
- **lymecycline**
- **minocycline**.

Demeclocycline is similar to the others in the group, but rather smaller doses are required and its action is more prolonged. Doxycycline is similar to the older tetracyclines, but is excreted slowly so that only one dose is required daily. The other important difference is that, unlike tetracycline, it can be used when renal function is impaired (see below). It is also used in the prevention of malaria. Minocycline has a broader spectrum than the other tetracyclines have, and is active against *Neisseria meningitidis*.

## ADVERSE EFFECTS OF THE TETRACYCLINES

- A certain amount of nausea, vomiting and epigastric disturbance due to a direct irritant effect often follows administration of the tetracyclines.
- Because of their wide antibacterial spectrum the tetracyclines cause considerable changes in the bacterial flora both in the intestine and elsewhere. This often results in diarrhoea, which usually recovers quickly when the drug is stopped. Occasionally, they may cause serious enteritis due to the multiplication of a resistant organism, usually a staphylococcus. Candida is the other troublesome organism that may emerge in those receiving tetracyclines, causing 'thrush' in the mouth or vaginal candidiasis.
- Tetracyclines damage and discolour developing teeth and should be avoided if possible from the fourth month of pregnancy until the child is 12 years old.
- Other toxic effects are rare, but include skin rashes and other sensitization phenomena.

**Contraindications.** Tetracyclines (except doxycycline) should not be given when renal function is impaired as they cause increased tissue breakdown with a subsequent rise of breakdown products in the blood, and exacerbation of the renal failure.

## CHLORAMPHENICOL

Chloramphenicol is a broad-spectrum antibiotic closely related in its action to the tetracyclines. It has, however, serious but rare toxic effects on the bone marrow; this limits its use to those patients who cannot obtain benefit from any other form of treatment.

### Therapeutic use

Chloramphenicol is given by mouth and is rapidly absorbed from the intestine. It diffuses widely and crosses the meningeal barrier into the CSF. It is excreted via the kidneys. Like the tetracyclines it is effective against a wide range of organisms with the important addition of *Salmonella typhi* and the paratyphoid group.

Bone marrow toxicity limits its use but it can be used for meningitis and acute epiglottitis due to *Haemophilus influenzae*. It is also very effective in typhoid and paratyphoid fevers, although resistant strains are emerging and ciprofloxacin may be preferred. It is also commonly used in solution as eye and eardrops.

### Adverse effects

The most serious toxic effects of chloramphenicol are on the bone marrow. Although they are rare, they are nearly always fatal when they occur. The most common effect is aplastic anaemia; the other reported change is depression of white leucocytes and platelets.

Toxic effects are more common after prolonged or repeated courses of chloramphenicol and their appearance may be delayed for up to 2 months after receiving the drug.

In newborn infants, chloramphenicol is less rapidly broken down so that accumulation may occur, producing the so-called 'grey syndrome' with circulatory collapse and shock.

## THE MACROLIDES

These comprise:

- erythromycin
- clarithromycin
- azithromycin.

### ERYTHROMYCIN

Erythromycin was first introduced in 1952. It is absorbed rather erratically after oral administration and diffuses widely, but does not enter into the CSF very well. It is bacteriostatic and acts against a wide range of organisms, including:

- *Streptococcus pyogenes*
- *Staphylococcus aureus*
- *Mycoplasma pneumoniae*
- *Legionella pneumophila*, which causes legionnaires' disease.

It is not, however, always effective against *Haemophilus influenzae*, a common cause of respiratory infection.

#### Resistance

Bacteria fairly readily become resistant to erythromycin, but do not show cross-resistance to other antibiotics.

#### Therapeutic use

Erythromycin has a similar range of activity to penicillin and is used instead of that drug in those who are sensitive to penicillin. It is used for various respiratory diseases, including *Mycoplasma pneumoniae* and legionnaires' disease. To reduce nausea it is best taken with food. Erythromycin can be given by infusion as the preparation **erythromycin lactobionate**.

#### Adverse effect

These are rare and include diarrhoea and vomiting and rarely jaundice, if injected. Intravenous administration is liable to cause thrombophlebitis.

### CLARITHROMYCIN

Clarithromycin has a similar antibacterial spectrum to erythromycin, but higher concentrations are found in the tissues and it has a greater effect against *Haemophilus influenzae* than erythromycin. It is also used for the eradication of *Helicobacter pylori* (see p. 112). Gastrointestinal upsets are less frequent.

### AZITHROMYCIN

Azithromycin appears to be similar, but with a long half-life; one daily dose is adequate.

#### Drug interactions

Erythromycin and clarithromycin interfere with the breakdown of certain drugs. They should not be combined with terfenadine or cisapride.

## MISCELLANEOUS ANTIBIOTICS

### Clindamycin

Clindamycin is effective against many Gram-positive organisms and can be used to treat infections by anaerobic organisms, particularly those that complicate bowel surgery. It is well absorbed when taken orally and appears to penetrate into bone. This makes it particularly useful for treating infection in bone.

**Adverse effects.** These are not common; diarrhoea may be a problem and rarely takes the form of a serious colitis (pseudomembranous colitis).

### Polymyxin

Polymyxin is effective against a wide range of Gram-negative organisms. It is particularly useful when applied locally for resistant infections by such organisms as pseudomonas; for example, otitis externa.

### Sodium fusidate

Sodium fusidate is effective against resistant staphylococci. When used, it is usually combined with other antibiotics in the treatment of severe staphylococcal infections. It is relatively free of side-effects, although high doses may cause jaundice, which recovers when the drug is stopped.

### Vancomycin

Vancomycin is particularly useful for treating severe staphylococcal infections resistant to other antibiotics. It is also given orally in the treatment of pseudomembranous colitis, which occasionally follows the use of antibiotics and is due to infection of the colon with *Clostridium difficile*. It is given by slow I.V. infusion and blood levels are measured to control the dose.

**Adverse effects.** It is ototoxic and nephrotoxic and is often given into a central vein as it can cause venous thrombosis.

## Teicoplanin

Teicoplanin is similar, but with considerably less adverse effects and a longer action. It is indicated for potentially serious infections such as *Staphylococcus aureus*, and for dialysis-associated peritonitis and endocarditis. It is also useful in orthopaedic surgery where there is a risk of infection with Gram-positive organisms.

**Adverse effects.** Several adverse effects have been reported, including angio-oedema, anaphylaxis, various blood disorders and mild hearing loss and injection site abscesses. Both liver and kidney function should be assessed during treatment. Contraindications include pregnancy, breast-feeding and renal impairment. If a patient has adverse effects with vancomycin, then teicoplanin should be used.

## Linezolid

Linezolid is a newer type of antibiotic that interferes with protein synthesis in the bacteria. It is effective against *Staphylococcus aureus* and *Streptococcus pneumoniae*, and in the treatment of pneumonia and soft-tissue infections caused by Gram-positive bacteria. It is given orally or intravenously and has a relatively short half-life. It is also a monoamine oxidase inhibitor (MAOI), and patients should therefore be warned about taking the drug together with other MAOIs or with cheese or other tyramine-containing foods.

**Adverse effects.** These include disturbances of taste, tongue discoloration, hypertension, tinnitus and various blood dyscrasias.

**Contraindications.** These include breast-feeding and, as mentioned above, other MAOIs. The Committee for the Safety of Medicines (CSM) has published guidelines for the use of linezolid, particularly with respect to its effects on the blood (see the *BNF*).

## Colistin and polymyxin B

Colistin is an example of a polymyxin antibiotic active against Gram-negative bacteria such as *Pseudomonas aeruginosa*. It is a toxic substance that is not absorbed when taken orally, and is used, usually together with the antifungal nystatin (p. 325), for bowel sterilization in neutropenic patients. It should not be used to treat gut infections. Polymyxin B is another antibiotic potent against Gram-negative bacteria; it is used in topical applications for the eye and ear infections.

## Dalfopristin with quinupristin

This is a mixture of two so-called streptogramin antibiotics to treat Gram-positive infections and has only recently been licensed for use. The preparation is recommended only for patients who have failed to respond to any other antibiotics or who cannot take any others. It is indicated for serious infections such as soft-tissue and skin infections, infections caused by vancomycin-resistant *Enterococcus faecum* and some forms of hospital-acquired pneumonia. It is ineffective against *Enterococcus faecalis*.

The preparation consists of a powder for reconstitution to give a mixture of quinupristin/dalfopristin and is administered via an intravenous infusion into a central vein.

**Adverse effects.** These include myalgia, rashes, pruritus, nausea and vomiting, blood dyscrasias and electrolyte disturbances.

**Contraindication.** It is contraindicated in severe liver disease and should be used with caution in patients with renal or heart disease, and during pregnancy and breast-feeding.

The antibacterial activity of some of the major antibiotics is summarized in Table 23.8.

## TUBERCULOSIS

In former times tuberculosis (TB) was a common and frequently fatal disease. In the UK in the first half of the last century its incidence declined rapidly, due to improved living conditions and effective drug treatment. However, where the resistance of the population is lowered by poverty, malnutrition and, more recently, by HIV, it is becoming a major health problem again.

Tuberculosis is an infectious bacterial disease caused by *Mycobacterium tuberculosis*. It may be caught by inhaling the aerosol from an infected person's sneezing or coughing, but is caught usually only after prolonged close proximity with an infected person. It is more often spread by contaminated hands. According to World Health Organization (WHO) estimates, about a third of the world's population is infected with TB, mainly in Africa and Asia, where incomes and standards of living are poor, coupled with genetic susceptibility. The most at risk are:

- alcoholics and drug misusers
- immunocompromised people, e.g. HIV sufferers

**Table 23.8** The antibacterial activity of antibiotics and chemotherapeutic agents

| Organism | Diseases | Macrolides | Benzyl–penicillin | Gentamicin | Ampicillin, Amoxicillin | Others |
|---|---|---|---|---|---|---|
| Staphylococcus aureus | Purulent infection | ++ | ++[†] | ++ | ++[†] | Vancomycin ++<br>Erythromycin ++<br>Flucloxacillin ++<br>Sodium fusidate ++ |
| Streptococcus pyogenes | Tonsillitis, scarlet fever | ++ | ++ | 0 | ++ | |
| Streptococcus viridans | Infective endocarditis | ++ | ++ | + | ++ | |
| Streptococcus pneumoniae | Pneumonia | ++ | ++ | 0 | ++ | |
| N. meningitidis | Meningitis | 0 | ++ | 0 | ++ | Newer cephalosporins ++ |
| N. gonorrhoeae | Gonorrhoea | 0 | ++ | ++ | ++ | Spectinomycin ++<br>4-quinolones ++ |
| E. coli | Urinary tract infection | 0 | 0 | ++ | ++ | Trimethoprim<br>Nitrofurantoin ++ |
| Shigella | Dysentery | 0 | 0 | + | ++ | Ciprofloxacin ++ |
| Salmonella typhi | Typhoid | 0 | 0 | + | ++ | Chloramphenicol ++<br>Trimethoprim ++ |
| Haemophilus influenzae | Meningitis and pneumonia | + | 0 | + | ++ | Chloramphenicol ++ |
| Treponema pallidum | Syphilis | ++ | ++ | 0 | 0 | |
| Pseudomonas aeruginosa | Various infections, septicaemia | 0 | 0 | ++ | 0 | Ureido penicillins ++<br>some new<br>Cephalosporins + |
| Chlamydia | Non-specific urethritis | ++ | 0 | 0 | ++ | Doxycycline ++ |

Very effective, ++; sometimes effective, +; little or no action, 0.
[†] Owing to resistance – flucloxacillin, ++

- doctors, nurses and other health workers in continual contact with patients who have pulmonary TB, unless protected by immunization (see below)
- patients on immunosuppressive chemotherapy
- populations in overcrowded conditions
- patients suffering from debilitating diseases such as diabetes, or those recovering from serious surgery, e.g. operations on the gastrointestinal tract.

## COMMON SYMPTOMS OF TUBERCULOSIS

These include swollen lymph glands, especially in the neck, loss of weight and appetite, tiredness, chronic non-productive cough, pleurisy, sweating at night and, in advanced TB, haemoptysis (coughing up blood).

## TESTING FOR TUBERCULOSIS

The tuberculin test consists of the injection into the skin of very small amounts of the tuberculin protein, which is extracted from cultures of M. tuberculosis. A strong patch of inflammation on the skin about 48–72 hours later indicates a positive reaction. There may be a mild reaction, which is not unusual, but does not necessarily signify TB. The test is called the Mantoux test, and a positive skin reaction is confirmed by testing a sample of sputum.

## IMMUNIZATION

Large-scale immunization of a population can control the spread of TB. In the UK, the BCG (bacille Calmette-Guérin) vaccine is used. It is administered at birth in high-risk situations, or to children between the ages of 10 and 14. The vaccine is not recommended for those over the age of 45 unless there is a high risk of infection. Immunization usually lasts for at least 15 years. Concerns have been expressed about the possibility of TB transmission through air travel. There is no evidence for infection on the journey; it is more likely that the disease is being imported by people who were infected abroad.

## MAIN DRUGS USED IN TUBERCULOSIS

Antituberculons drugs include:

- **isoniazid**
- **rifampicin**
- **rifabutin**
- **ethambutol**
- **capreomycin**
- **pyrazinamide**
- **cycloserine**
- **streptomycin**.

### Isoniazid

**Therapeutic use.** Isoniazid is bacteriostatic and possibly bactericidal to *M. tuberculosis*. It is rapidly absorbed from the intestine and largely excreted by the kidneys. It diffuses widely through the body and it crosses the meningeal barrier to the CSF in amounts adequate to inhibit the growth of *M. tuberculosis*.

Isoniazid is metabolized in the liver. It is possible to divide people into two groups: those who break isoniazid down rapidly and those who break it down slowly. As a result of this the rapidly inactivating group will have lower concentrations of the drug in their blood than the slow inactivators. In the dosage schemes used in the UK this is of no importance, but in less developed countries where the drug may be given less frequently to save cost, rapid inactivators are in danger of getting less than a full therapeutic effect from the drug.

**Adverse effects.** Neuropathy can develop in slow inactivators who are given large doses and in those at special risk of nerve damage (patients with diabetes, alcoholics). Giving pyridoxine can prevent this.

### Rifampicin

Rifampicin is effective against several Gram-positive and Gram-negative organisms and in particular against *M. tuberculosis*. Its use is largely confined to tuberculosis but it can also be used in legionnaires' disease and to prevent infection in subjects who have had close contact with meningococcal meningitis. It is well absorbed orally and is taken once daily before breakfast. It is mainly excreted in the bile. It is useful in the treatment of tuberculosis, but must be combined with other antituberculous drugs to prevent resistance developing.

**Adverse effects.** These are uncommon, but it should not be used in patients with liver disease as it can cause changes in liver function tests and, rarely, severe liver damage. It may cause red discoloration of the urine and sputum. By increasing the rate of breakdown of estrogen, rifampicin may reduce the effectiveness of oral contraceptives.

### Rifabutin

Rifabutin is similar to rifampicin.

### Ethambutol

Ethambutol is usually satisfactory, but is now rarely used unless there is a possibility of resistance to other antituberculous drugs. The most important side-effect is damage to the optic nerve, leading to deterioration of visual acuity and colour vision. Correct dosage reduces this risk, but vision should be tested before starting treatment and at 6-monthly intervals.

### Pyrazinamide

Pyrazinamide is powerful and effective with good penetration into tuberculous lesions and the CSF. Its use is limited by adverse effects but is justified, particularly in tuberculous meningitis, provided that the correct dose is given and the course lasts no longer than 2 months. During treatment, liver function tests should be performed and alcohol avoided.

**Adverse effects.** These include liver damage with jaundice, light sensitization (use a barrier cream) and attacks of gout.

### Combined preparations

Preparations that combine isoniazid, rifampicin and pyrazinamide are available and they improve compliance. Streptomycin is very effective against *M. tuberculosis*, but resistant strains develop in about 6 weeks if it is used alone. This is prevented if it is combined with other antituberculous drugs. It is given by injection once daily. Because it has to be injected and adverse effects can be troublesome, it has now been largely replaced by other drugs.

**Adverse effects.** These are not uncommon with streptomycin. The most important are those affecting the eighth nerve. The symptoms include high-pitched tinnitus and vertigo. This may be followed by varying degrees of deafness. Sensitization phenomena also occur with streptomycin. These may affect not only the patient but also the person injecting the drug. Swelling of the eyelids is an early sign. Care should be taken when giving the drug to avoid contamination of the hands and face, which may occur when the syringe is held at eye level to measure the exact dose. The wearing of plastic gloves and a mask is advisable for those who handle large quantities of streptomycin

## DRUG REGIMES FOR THE TREATMENT OF TUBERCULOSIS

There are now a number of drugs that are effective against *M. tuberculosis*. It is important, however, that:

- at least two drugs are used at the same time to prevent the emergence of resistant organisms
- Treatment is continued for a long time to eradicate the infection completely.

The choice of drugs is determined by the sensitivity of the infective *M. tuberculosis* bacillus.

Ethambutol is only used if resistance is a possibility.

Variation in the drugs used is due to their differing penetration of tissue, their effectiveness against dividing organisms and their ability to sterilize a lesion. The excellent penetration of isoniazid and pyrazinamide into the CSF makes them particularly useful in meningeal tuberculosis. Resistance by *M. tuberculosis* to one or other drug may require a change of regime.

Although the discovery of these drugs has revolutionized the treatment of tuberculosis, it must be realized that they form only part of the treatment. The basic measures of rest, good food and good nursing are as important as ever. The barrier to treatment is poor compliance, especially among those of no fixed abode. Outreach teams play an important role in reaching this part of the community and can help by providing opportunities to obtain nourishing food and dietary supplements.

## BACTERIAL RESISTANCE TO ANTIBIOTICS

Resistance may be produced in several ways. In any population of bacteria there may be a few organisms that are resistant to an antibiotic and when all the sensitive organisms have been killed

off, the resistant ones are left to flourish and multiply. These resistant organisms have often been produced by mutations (changes in their genetic make-up). It has also been shown that certain bacteria can transmit resistance to each other and even to different types of bacteria by incorporating foreign DNA, which induces resistance. It follows therefore that wherever antibiotics are widely used, resistant strains will appear. To reduce resistance to a minimum certain precautions should be taken.

- Antibiotics should only be used when really necessary.
- Antibiotics should be given in adequate doses.
- The use of antibiotics prophylactically is generally to be deplored as it breeds resistant strains. There are exceptions to this rule, i.e. the use of penicillin to prevent tonsillitis in patients who have had rheumatic fever and to prevent endocarditis when those with damaged heart valves have dental treatment or before major surgery when sepsis is a risk.
- In certain circumstances, i.e. the treatment of tuberculosis, the use of several antibiotics together may prevent resistant strains developing.
- The use of antibiotics by farmers to promote animal growth should be strictly controlled as it has led to the emergence of resistant strains of bacteria.

## ANTIBIOTIC POLICIES

Policies have been developed to encourage the efficient, safe and economical use of antibiotics. One of their chief aims is to reduce the emergence of antibiotic-resistant strains. In most hospitals a local formulary is drawn up to reserve the use of particular drugs. Most local policies adopt the following general format:

- A section that includes a single member of each of the main groups of antibiotics. Each of these can be prescribed without formality. These drugs are held as ward stock.
- A reserve section containing alternatives, including the most newly developed antibiotics. These are not usually prescribed without liaison with the infection control team and are not held as ward stock.
- Policies need regular updating.

## MULTIDRUG RESISTANCE

In recent years the problem of patients infected with *M. tuberculosis* which are resistant to one or more antibiotics has emerged. This happens most often in patients who have relapsed as they may have received inadequate treatment. Patients infected with HIV disease have poor resistance to infection (Chapter 24); this makes treatment difficult and may add to the number of resistant organisms. Such patients require individually designed combinations of drugs and the treatment is prolonged. Among the drugs used are streptomycin, capreomycin, cycloserine and clarithromycin.

The aminoglycosides, for example capreomycin, kanamycin and amikacin, and the newer quinolones,

---

**Special points for patient education**

It is very important that patients realize the importance of taking their medication regularly as directed. Poor compliance or failure to finish the course of treatment is common in tuberculosis and is a major factor in the emergence of resistant strains.

---

**Nursing points**

- Patients with tuberculosis should cease to be infectious after 1 week of treatment provided that the organism is sensitive.
- When nursing patients with open tuberculosis, nurses must be careful to avoid open infection. This is particularly important if the patient has a multidrug-resistant infection, when the infectious period may be prolonged.

---

for example ciprofloxacin and ofloxacin, are used only in patients who are resistant to other drugs. Combinations of a β lactam antibiotic with a β lactamase inhibitor appear to improve the effectiveness of treatment. An example of the disturbing growth of resistant strains is a recent report from a Public Health Laboratory Service Surveillance Programme of an increase in ciprofloxacin resistance to gonococcal infections (Editorial 2002).

## ANTIBIOTIC DRUGS IN THE TREATMENT OF SOME COMMON INFECTIONS

### THE COMMON COLD

The treatment of the common cold is the relief of symptoms with NSAIDs, paracetamol, antihistamines

and inhalations. The value of vitamin C is still undecided. Although antibiotics are often prescribed, they are usually of no value in healthy adults; they are expensive and increase the risk of resistant organisms emerging. Various antiviral agents have been tried, including interferons, but as yet there is no evidence that they are of special benefit.

### SORE THROAT

Minor sore throats are usually viral and do not require antibiotic treatment, but streptococcal throat infection should be treated with phenoxymethylpenicillin four times daily for 10 days. If vomiting is a problem, benzylpenicillin should be given by injection. This drug is also used in smaller doses over long periods to prevent throat infection in those who have had rheumatic fever and thus decrease the chance of recurrence.

### BRONCHITIS

A mild attack of acute bronchitis in an otherwise healthy adult does not usually require antibiotic treatment and is frequently due to a viral infection. A severe attack or an acute exacerbation of chronic bronchitis is best treated with amoxicillin three times daily or doxycycline as the infection in these circumstances may be due to *Haemophilus influenzae*, *Streptococcus pneumoniae* or *Moraxella catarrhalis*.

### PNEUMONIA

The problem with pneumonia is that various bacteria with different antibiotic sensitivities may cause it. Sputum and blood cultures may help the correct choice of antibiotic when results are available. Penicillin-resistant *Streptococcus pneumoniae* has appeared, and in the future this may alter the choice of antibacterial treatment.

### URINARY INFECTIONS

Urinary infections are usually due to *E. coli* and respond satisfactorily to trimethoprim every 12 hours for 5 days. It should, however, be avoided in the first 3 months of pregnancy. A 3-day course of cefadroxil can also be used. In some areas the organism has become resistant to these antibacterial drugs and norfloxacin twice daily is an alternative. In serious infections cefuroxime can be added to the regime. It is sometimes necessary to use antibacterial drugs prophylactically, particularly in children. Trimethoprim at night or on alternate days is usually adequate.

## MENINGITIS

Meningitis may be caused by a variety of organisms and its treatment is complicated because certain antibiotics penetrate poorly into the CSF. Drugs that penetrate poorly have been given intrathecally (Table 23.9).

### Meningococcal meningitis

This should be treated with a dose of benzylpenicillin intravenously, every 4–6 hours. Enough penicillin will diffuse through the inflamed meninges to eradicate the infection. If the bacterial diagnosis is in doubt, ceftriaxone should be used as it has a wider antibacterial spectrum. Immediate treatment is important as sometimes a very dangerous state of shock develops.

**Prevention.** Those in close contact with patients with meningococcal meningitis should be given rifampicin twice daily for 2 days for children, or ciprofloxacin as a single dose for adults.

### Meningitis in neonates

This is usually due to Gram-negative organisms and is treated either with gentamicin and ampicillin, or with a new cephalosporin such as ceftriaxone or cefotaxime.

### *Streptococcus pneumoniae* meningitis

This does not usually respond so well as meningococcal infection. The usual treatment is with cefotaxime as some strains of *Streptococcus pneumoniae* are penicillin-resistant.

Table 23.9    Drug penetration

| Good penetration | Poor penetration |
| --- | --- |
| Sulphonamides (particularly sulfadiazine) | Penicillin |
| | Streptomycin |
| Chloramphenicol | |
| Tetracycline | |
| The newer cephalosporins | |

### *Haemophilus influenzae* meningitis

Ceftriaxone I.V. followed 24 hours later by I.V. treatment daily for 5 days.

## INFECTIVE ENDOCARDITIS

This is an infection of damaged heart valves, usually with *Streptococcus viridans*. Because the organisms are buried in the thick vegetation on the valves, they are difficult to reach and kill with antibiotics, so that prolonged treatment with high doses is needed. Usually, benzylpenicillin and gentamicin are given together for 2 weeks and penicillin continued for another 2 weeks. If the organism is less sensitive, benzylpenicillin and gentamicin should be continued for 4 weeks. Other organisms may require other regimes and the management should be worked out with the infection control team. If a 'butterfly' needle is used to give the antibiotics intravenously, it is necessary to change the site of the cannula regularly or local infection will occur.

**Prevention.** The trauma of dental treatment often releases microorganisms into the blood. If the patient has damaged heart valves, the organism settles on the valve and sets up an infection. Giving an antibiotic to cover dental treatment can prevent this. A single oral dose of amoxicillin given 1 hour before treatment is easy to give and is usually most satisfactory.

## STAPHYLOCOCCAL INFECTIONS

These cover a wide range, including boils and carbuncles and extending to severe and sometimes fatal septicaemias, pneumonias and osteomyelitis. Mild infections used to respond to phenoxymethylpenicillin, but they are now resistant and in addition the severe infections are often due to organisms that have also become resistant to penicillin. In these circumstances flucloxacillin four times daily by mouth or by injection is given. Other useful antibiotics in staphylococcal infections are gentamicin, erythromycin, clindamycin, sodium fusidate and vancomycin or teicoplanin. One or other of these is often combined with flucloxacillin.

Infection due to methicillin-resistant *Staphylococcus aureus* (MRSA) will require special infection control precautions in line with local policy. A high degree of hygiene should be maintained. Wounds will require cleaning and the local application of antibacterial agents such as *Iodosorb*. In addition, an appropriate antibiotic (usually vancomycin) will be employed.

Many hospitals will have their own protocols to deal with this difficult problem.

## CHLAMYDIAL INFECTION

Organisms of the chlamydia group can cause various infections. *Chlamydia trachomatis* is responsible for most cases of non-specific urethritis and cervicitis, which are the most common sexually transmitted diseases in the Western world. Acute infections may lead to chronic pelvic sepsis in women and prostatitis in men. Treatment is with doxycycline twice daily for 2 weeks or azithromycin as a single dose. Both sexual partners must be treated.

## INTESTINAL INFECTIONS

Intestinal infections can be caused by various organisms, the most common in the UK being salmonellae and shigellae. Although these organisms are sensitive to a number of antibiotics it has been found that their use does not hasten recovery and may lead to an increased number of chronic carriers of these infections. Antibiotic treatment is usually not indicated, therefore, except in the dangerous systemic infection by *Salmonella typhi* (typhoid or paratyphoid fever) or severe gut infection, which is treated with ciprofloxacin.

## SEPTICAEMIAS

Septicaemias are becoming a major problem, particularly in ill and/or immunosuppressed patients. Various bacteria may be implicated and initial treatment aims at a wide antibacterial effect until the nature of the infection becomes clear as a result of blood cultures. Gentamicin combined with flucloxacillin and metronidazole is frequently used, but there are many other possibilities. Gram-negative septicaemia in particular affects those who have undergone extensive surgery or have depressed immunity. It is a very dangerous infection, leading rapidly to organ failure. It should be treated as early as possible with a combination of antibiotics.

## PREVENTION OF SURGICAL SEPSIS

Antibacterial agents are now commonly given before surgery involving the gut and orthopaedic procedures to prevent postoperative sepsis. Opinions differ as to the best drugs to use, but the drugs show in Table 23.10 are popular. Prophylaxis is most effective if antibiotics are given within 2 hours before surgery.

## PRACTICAL POINTS IN THE ADMINISTRATION OF ANTIBIOTICS

- Oral penicillins and tetracyclines should be given 30 minutes before meals to facilitate absorption. Erythromycin, sodium fusidate and metronidazole should be given with or after food to minimize nausea.
- In general, intravenous antibiotics should be given as a bolus. A few, e.g. piperacillin, are given as short-term infusions. If long-term infusions are used, remember that some antibiotics are unstable in certain solutions and rapidly lose their potency. Among the most important are:
  - ampicillin – loses activity in dextrose solutions
  - gentamicin – unstable in solution and inactivated if combined with penicillins.

**Table 23.10**  Antibiotic treatment in surgery

| Surgical procedure | Treatment |
| --- | --- |
| Acute appendicitis (anaerobes, coliforms) | Metronidazole suppository inserted 2 hours before surgery. Cefuroxime I.V. at induction |
| Large bowel surgery (anaerobes, coliforms) | Metronidazole as above + cefuroxime at induction followed by doses at 8 and 16 hours |
| Biliary surgery | Not required in elective surgery; otherwise, cefuroxime as above at induction and then at 8 and 16 hours |
| Amputation of ischaemic limb (staphylococci, clostridia) | Metronidazole as above + flucloxacillin I.V. at induction and every 8 hours for 48 hours |
| Hip replacement | Cefuroxime at induction and every 8 hours for 48 hours |

- Do not as a rule mix drugs in an infusion bottle and, if this is necessary, check their compatibilities with the pharmacist.
- Do not mix **ureido penicillins** with **aminoglycosides** in the same infusion or syringe.
- When making up solutions for injection avoid contamination of hands, etc., due to the risk of contact dermatitis. Hands should be washed after as well as before giving injections and gloves should be worn for I.V. injections due to risks of contaminated blood. When patients are taking antibiotics at home, compliance must be assured by full explanation of its importance, particularly with reference to taking the full course prescribed.

## Reference

Editorial 2002 Ciprofloxacin resistance is on the increase, latest PHLS data show. Pharmaceutical Journal 269: 733

## Further reading

Angel J 1992 The modern management of pulmonary tuberculosis. Prescribers Journal 32: 144

Begg E J, Barclay M L 1995 Aminoglycosides – 50 years on. British Journal of Clinical Pharmacology 39: 597

Classen D, Evans R S, Pestotnik S L et al 1992 The timing of the prophylactic administration of antibiotics and the risk of surgical wound infection. New England Journal of Medicine 326: 281

Editorial 1999 Tackling antimicrobial resistance. Drug and Therapeutics Bulletin 37(2): 9

Gold H S, Moellering R C 1997 Antimicrobial drug resistance. New England Journal of Medicine 335: 1445

Griffith G, Krishna S 1998 Infectious diseases. Journal of the Royal College of Physicians, London 12: 306

House of Lords Select Committee on Science and Technology, 7th Report. Resistance to antibiotics and other antimicrobial agents. Stationery Office, London, 1998

Mossad S B 1998 Treatment of the common cold. British Medical Journal 317: 33

Rodvold K A, Danzinger L H, Quinn J P 1997 Single daily doses of aminoglycosides. Lancet 350: 1412

Smith J M, Seymour H E, Snider K, Hollyoak V 2000 Impact of national recommendations on antibiotic prescribing in an NHS region. Pharmaceutical Journal 259: R51

Stamm W E, Hooton T M 1993 Management of urinary infection in adults. New England Journal of Medicine 329: 1328

Standing Medical Advisory Committee. Report of sub-group on antimicrobial resistance. The path of least resistance. Department of Health, London, 1998

Taylor D, Littlewood S 1998 Pneumonia. Nursing Times 94(7): 48

Taylor D, Littlewood S 1998 Tuberculosis. Nursing Times 94(11): 51

Tunkel A R, Scheld W M 1995 Acute bacterial meningitis. Lancet 346: 1675

Walters J 1993 How antibiotics work. Professional Nurse 8(12): 788

Chapter **24**

# Antifungal and antiviral agents: treatment of HIV disease

## Learning objectives

At the end of this chapter, the reader should be able to:

- explain how cytomegalovirus is treated
- list the names of important drugs used to treat HIV disease and explain how they work
- describe what is meant by reverse transcriptase inhibitors and give examples
- appreciate the importance of combined therapy for HIV disease
- recognize the danger of needle-stick injuries and provide examples of drugs that are used to try to prevent infection with HIV after a needle-stick injury
- give an account of fungal infections and explain that they may be superficial or systemic
- list the names of antifungal drugs and some of their uses
- give an account of the treatment of candidiasis
- discuss the growth in incidence of systemic fungal infections due to AIDS and organ and tissue transplantation

## ANTIVIRAL AGENTS

Antiviral agents include:

- amantadine
- aciclovir
- famciclovir
- foscarnet
- inosine pranobex
- tribavirin
- valaciclovir.

Viruses cause a number of diseases, some of which are serious and potentially fatal, although most are of minor importance (e.g. the common cold). In subjects who are immunosuppressed – e.g. by the human immunodeficiency virus (HIV) or treatment with cytotoxic drugs – a relatively benign viral infection may become virulent.

It is difficult to produce effective antiviral agents for several reasons:

- Viruses live within human cells and they use processes in those cells to multiply. They are not therefore readily accessible.
- They are very sophisticated structures and are not easy to kill.
- Furthermore, a great deal of virus replication occurs before the patient develops symptoms.
- Viruses mutate rapidly and this can render vaccines and many drugs useless. Many viruses, e.g. influenza virus, are subject to antigenic drift.

## Aciclovir

This agent is effective against the herpes viruses. It enters the infected cells where it is changed into a powerful antiviral agent.

### Therapeutic use

- It can be applied as a 3% ointment five times daily to treat ulceration of the cornea due to the herpes simplex virus and should be continued for 3 days after healing.
- Given orally five times daily for 5 days it accelerates the healing of genital herpes. Very severe attacks may require parenteral treatment.
- A 5% cream of aciclovir is only effective in labial herpes if used in the prodromal period when there is only a local burning sensation.
- In generalized herpes simplex infection in immunosuppressed patients or in herpes meningoencephalitis it is given by intravenous infusion. This may cause an apparent deterioration of renal function, which should be monitored. Patients with impaired renal function will require smaller doses.
- Aciclovir is prescribed for herpes zoster (shingles); if the ophthalmic branch of the trigeminal nerve is affected, this may be followed by prolonged neuralgia and damage to the eye and aciclovir should be given for 7 days. It should be started within 48 hours of the onset of symptoms.
- It also shortens the course of varicella (chickenpox), but its use in this disorder should be confined to those at special risk (i.e. immunosuppressed patients).

**Adverse effects.** These include rashes, nausea and vomiting.

**Contraindication.** Pregnancy.

**Famciclovir** and **valaciclovir** are similar and are given orally to treat herpes simplex and herpes zoster (shingles). They have the advantage of only needing to be administered two or three times daily.

**Amantadine** (see also p. 257) has some action against the influenza virus. **Tribavirin** is used in the treatment of respiratory tract viruses, particularly respiratory syncytial virus, which causes bronchiolitis in infants. It is given by nebulizer or aerosol inhalation.

## Cytomegalovirus

**Ganciclovir** is used specifically for the treatment of serious infections by the cytomegalovirus. The disease is usually mild, except in immunosuppressed patients (e.g. those with AIDS) and as a risk to the fetus in pregnancy. It is given by intravenous infusion.

The most serious adverse effect is suppression of the white cell count and of the platelets, which usually recover when the drug is stopped. It is contraindicated during pregnancy, and patients should be warned to take effective contraceptive measures during treatment. Men should take contraceptive measures during treatment and for at least 90 days afterwards.

**Valganciclovir** is a prodrug of ganciclovir. It is used for the treatment of cytomegalovirus retinitis in AIDS patients. The precautions for use are as for ganciclovir.

**Foscarnet** is reserved for cytomegalovirus infection in immunocompromised patients. It is given by intravenous infusion and is highly nephrotoxic.

**Cidofovir** is prescribed for the treatment of cytomegalovirus retinitis in AIDS patients when the use of other antiviral agents is not appropriate. It should not be used in patients with impaired renal function. It is a nephrotoxic drug.

## ACQUIRED IMMUNODEFICIENCY SYNDROME (AIDS)

There are at least 30 million people worldwide who are infected with HIV at present, and this number is likely to rise. So far, no cure is available but treatment is becoming more successful and the progression of the disease can be successfully halted. There are three known forms of the HIV virus: namely, $HIV_1$, $HIV_2$

and HIV$_3$. HIV$_1$ and HIV$_3$ seem to be the ones that are plaguing Africa and India, whereas HIV$_2$ is more prevalent in Europe and the United States.

## THE DISEASE

After infection there is a latent period when the patient is symptom-free. During this time the virus enters the cells of the immune system (CD4 T cells) and, using the host cells' metabolic processes, multiplies and finally kills the cells, releasing further viruses. When the immune system has been sufficiently depleted of T cells, the patient becomes susceptible to a variety of opportunistic infections that ultimately prove fatal (Fig. 24.1). The median latency between infection with HIV and the onset of these opportunistic infections is about 10 years in the UK.

## TREATMENT

The aim of treatment is to reduce the numbers of virus particles as much as possible for as long as possible. This creates two problems: the patient will take toxic drugs for a long time and the virus develops resistance to the drugs. The use of single agents against the HIV leads to the emergence of resistance and failure of treatment. It is now apparent that using several antiviral agents simultaneously, particularly

if they affect different phases in the viral life cycle, is more effective.

Antiviral treatment is indicated if:

- the patient has significant symptoms related to HIV infection
- the CD4 cell count is less than 350/mm$^3$
- the viral load is greater than 30 000 (bDNA) or 55 000 (PCR) copies/ml
- the patient acquired HIV infection within the prior 6 months.

Drugs are used to block two key steps in viral replication:

- the conversion of viral RNA into viral DNA in the host cell, catalysed by the viral enzyme reverse transcriptase. Drugs called reverse transcriptase inhibitors can block the action of this enzyme
- the action of viral proteins called proteases.

There are three main types of inhibitors:

- nucleoside reverse transcriptase inhibitors (NRTIs)
- non-nucleoside reverse transcriptase inhibitors (NNRTIs)
- protease inhibitors (PIs).

### Nucleoside reverse transcriptase inhibitors

These drugs are similar in structure to the cellular chemicals used as building blocks by the viral enzyme reverse transcriptase when it makes viral DNA from its own viral RNA in the host cell. The enzyme is 'fooled' into trying to incorporate the drug into the strand of growing viral DNA. Once the drug is incorporated into the DNA it stops the reaction from going any further, and the virus can no longer replicate itself in the host cell. Examples are:

- abacavir
- didanosine
- lamivudine
- stavudine
- tenofovir
- zalcitabine
- zidovudine.

**Zidovudine (AZT).** An analogue of thymidine, zidovudine is the most widely used drug of this group. It can be given orally or intravenously. It is converted to a triphosphate and then used by the virus to try and make viral DNA. The drug may

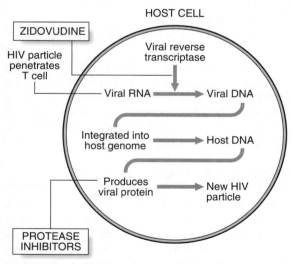

**Figure 24.1** Intracellular cycle of an HIV virus particle and site of action of zidovudine which inhibits the enzyme reverse transcriptase and protease inhibitors which prevent the formation of new virus particles.

become ineffective with prolonged use, as the HIV virus mutates and one consequence is a reduced conversion of zidovudine to the triphosphate. Also, in the later stage of the disease, the viral load increases dramatically due to the failure of the immune system, and this, too, reduces the efficacy of zidovudine (and other antiviral agents).

**Adverse effects of zidovudine.** These include nausea, headache and muscle pains and, rarely, bone marrow suppression.

## Non-nucleoside reverse transcriptase inhibitors

Non-nucleoside reverse transcriptase inhibitors, efavirenz and nevirapine, are newer synthetic drugs that interfere with the action of viral reverse transcriptase.

**Therapeutic use.** Both drugs are used together with other agents. For example, efavirenz may be used in combination with an NRTI such as zidovudine. Efavirenz is also sometimes prescribed with one or more protease inhibitors (see below). Efavirenz is given in a once daily oral dose, and nevirapine is started as a once daily dose, and if after 14 days there is no rash, it is increased to twice daily dosage.

**Adverse effects of efavirenz and nevirapine.** The most common side-effects of efavirenz are rash, abnormal dreams, dizziness, impaired concentration and insomnia. These symptoms are more frequent early in treatment and generally resolve within 3–4 weeks. Rashes should be reported to the doctor immediately. Less frequent side-effects include vomiting, depression, raised serum cholesterol and elevated liver enzymes, particularly if the patient is seropositive for hepatitis B or C.

Nevirapine has similar side-effects, especially in terms of rashes, especially in the first 8 weeks of treatment. Liver toxicity is a problem and has to be monitored closely. Treatment should be stopped if significant liver impairment is observed.

**Contraindications for efavirenz.** These include breast-feeding, and the drug should be used with caution in cases of hepatic impairment and pregnancy. Nevirapine is contraindicated in breast-feeding and when there is severe hepatic impairment.

## Protease inhibitors

These comprise:

- amprenavir
- indinavir
- lopinavir
- nelfinavir
- ritonavir
- saquinavir.

These drugs act at a later stage in the formation of virus particles by inhibiting viral proteases, which are necessary for the formation of viral proteins.

**Therapeutic use.** Lopinavir is usually prescribed together with ritonavir. All of these drugs are to be used in combination with other antiviral drugs. Ritonavir is prescribed specifically in advanced HIV infection together with NRTIs.

**Adverse effects.** These include nausea, vomiting and diarrhoea. All carry the risk of hepatic impairment, and hepatic function must be monitored closely in patients who take protease inhibitors. Patients taking indinavir should have a high fluid intake, as there is a risk of renal stone formation. All of these PIs should be used with caution in patients with renal problems.

**Contraindications.** All PIs are contraindicated in breast-feeding patients, and ritonavir is contraindicated in patients with hepatic impairment.

---

**Nursing point**

Two or three drugs are given together (nucleoside analogue + protease inhibitor) and most experts believe that it is best to start treatment when the infection is first diagnosed rather than when symptoms develop. Although it is too early to talk of a cure, active life can be prolonged and complications minimized.

---

Antiviral agents are expensive and considering the widespread nature of HIV infection, much of it in the Third World, the cost of treatment will be enormous. In addition, when the disease is controlled, some maintenance treatment may be necessary to prevent relapse.

## NEEDLE-STICK INJURIES

Accidental infection of health professionals is very rare but the possibility of becoming HIV positive after a needle-stick injury is about 1 : 400. For those thought to be seriously at risk, a recommendation is to give (zidovudine + lamivudine + indinavir) for 4 weeks and treatment should be started within 2 hours of exposure. This will greatly reduce the chance of infection. Occupational health departments in hospitals develop protocols in line with the infection control team.

## HEPATITIS B AND HEPATITIS C VIRUS

Two other viral infections to which nurses and other health care workers may be exposed in their occupation are of particular concern. These are:

- **hepatitis B virus (HBV)**
- **hepatitis C virus (HCV).**

Transmission is usually via contaminated blood or blood products, and other body fluids may be involved because these are so often contaminated with blood. Infection occurs most commonly by needle-stick injury. Often it is through a break in the skin or via a mucous membrane. It does not occur through intact skin, but even a minute abrasion will let in the infection.

### Prevention and management

The most important preventative measure is avoidance of risk and scrupulous techniques when dealing with possible sources of infection. Active immunization is available against HBV, but not against HCV. If exposure to the virus has occurred, the following steps are advised, though it is possible that advances may alter these procedures:

- **Hepatitis B:** determine the immune status of the exposed subject – if susceptible, give HBV hyperimmune globulin and immunize with vaccine.
- **Hepatitis C:** there is no effective protection yet, but the subject must be followed up for evidence of infection, as there is a chance of developing chronic active hepatitis, as there is with HBV as well.

## MOTHER-TO-INFANT TRANSMISSION OF HIV

Treating both the pregnant mother and the newborn infant with zidovudine can considerably reduce mother-to-infant transmission of HIV from an infected mother to the fetus during pregnancy.

## MONITORING TREATMENT

It is important to measure the extent of HIV infection in a patient in order to decide on optimal treatment and to assess progress. This can be achieved by:

- counting the number of CD4 T cells in the blood – the lower the count, the more advanced the disease
- measuring the concentration of RNA derived from the HIV in the plasma (viral load) – the higher the load (which is a measure of viral multiplication), the more active the disease.

## COMPLICATIONS OF HIV INFECTION

*Pneumocystis carinii* pneumonia is common and is treated by high-dose co-trimoxazole or by intravenous pentamidine. Relapse can be prevented by long-term treatment with co-trimoxazole, inhaled pentamidine or dapsone. Patients with HIV disease are also susceptible to various fungal and viral infections and to tuberculosis.

**Summary**

- The aim of treatment of HIV disease is to reduce the numbers of virus particles as much as possible for as long as possible
- It is generally considered better to start treatment as soon as HIV is diagnosed
- Occupational hazards associated with the HIV and hepatitis can be minimized using scrupulous techniques when dealing with possible sources of infection
- Personnel should be immunized against HBV
- If a worker is exposed to HBV, HBV hyperimmune globulin should be given and the worker vaccinated
- Mother-to-infant transmission of HIV can be considerably reduced during pregnancy by treating the infected mother with zidovudine
- The extent of HIV infection can be assessed by counting the numbers of CD4 T cells in the blood and by monitoring HIV RNA in the blood (the viral load)

## THE INTERFERONS

This is a family of protein-like substances produced by various cells in the body in response to viral infections. Interferons have the ability to act on cells and increase their resistance to viral infections and may also modify the immune response. In addition, they control the growth and differentiation of cells.

Interferons can now be produced synthetically and have been used in both neoplastic and infective disease in humans. Their main success has been in treating leukaemias, particularly the hairy-celled types, and to a lesser degree in some other forms of cancer. In the control of viral infections their usefulness is limited but they are used with some success in hepatitis B and C infections.

**Interferon B** is now being used in the relapsing/remitting form of multiple sclerosis with some benefit. It is given by intramuscular injection. Adverse effects are fever and nausea.

A steroid that has been reported possibly to help sufferers with multiple sclerosis is estriol, which is one of the estrogens secreted in large amounts during pregnancy, that is also used for HRT. A small number of patients given oral estriol for 6 months were reported to have a significant reduction in the size and number of lesions in their brains (Editorial 2002).

## ANTIFUNGAL AGENTS

## INTRODUCTION

Fungi are simple organisms that lack chlorophyll; they were originally considered as plants. Fungi include mushrooms, moulds, yeasts and rusts. Some live commensually with a human, which means that neither organism harms the other. Some, however, cause disease when they infect. Fungal infections, at least in temperate countries, do not usually pose serious threats to health, and have largely been superficial in nature. The most common problems have been, for example, athlete's foot and vaginal or oral thrush.

Systemic fungal infections in the UK were rare, but are now on the increase, as exemplified by Case History 24.1. This is due to the widespread use of broad-spectrum antibiotics, which destroy the non-pathogenic bacteria, especially in the gut, which compete with ingested fungi for food. Another exacerbating factor is the higher incidence of patients with reduced immune competence, due to diseases such as HIV disease and the use of immunosuppressive treatments such as irradiation and anti-cancer drugs.

## CLASSIFICATION OF FUNGAL INFECTIONS

Fungal infections are collectively called **mycoses**. They can be classified for convenience as superficial infections and systemic infections.

### Superficial infections

Superficial infections have not been traditionally serious in nature. They involve skin, mucous membranes, scalp and nails. They can be classified as candidiasis (thrush) and dermatomycoses.

**Candidiasis** infections are caused by a yeast-like fungus that infects mouth, skin and vagina.

Fungi called **dermatophytes** cause dermatomycoses infections. A dermatophyte feeds on keratin. The most common and therefore best known are the tinea fungi, which cause what is commonly called ringworm:

- tinea capitas is ringworm of the scalp
- tinea pedis is athlete's foot
- tinea cruris affects the thighs and groin
- tinea barbae affects the skin under a beard.

### Systemic infections

In the UK, systemic candiasis is the most common fungal infection. Examples of others are:

- cryptococcal meningitis (endocarditis) – the yeast is commonly found in pigeon droppings
- pulmonary aspergillosis
- invasive pulmonary aspergillosis, which is an important cause of death in patients who have received bone marrow transplants (see explanation of aspergillosis below)
- rhinocerebral mucormicosis (*Mucor* is a genus of fungus found on decaying organic matter).

These conditions are still comparatively rare in the UK (but see Case History 24.1).

Aspergillosis refers to infection with the fungal genus *Aspergillus*, usually *A. fumigatus*. Infection occurs quite often in patients with pre-existing lung disease and three forms occur:

- an allergic reaction in asthma
- a colonizing form that forms a fungus ball in a lung cavity, e.g. a healed tuberculous cavity
- a form that may spread from the lungs to the rest of the body, usually in patients with compromised immune systems (e.g. in HIV patients or after bone marrow transplants).

# DRUGS USED TO TREAT FUNGAL INFECTIONS

These include:

- amphotericin
- clotrimazole
- fluconazole
- flucytosine
- griseofulvin
- itraconazole
- ketoconazole
- metronidazole
- miconazole
- nystatin
- terbinafine

Many of these preparations can be sold without the need for a prescription and the pharmacist will advise.

**Nystatin** binds to the wall of the fungus, disrupting its integrity. It is very poorly absorbed after oral administration and is therefore used to treat infections of the intestinal tract or is applied locally. It is particularly used in *Candida* infections. Oral infections respond to nystatin pastilles dissolved in the mouth four times daily. It is very effective in treating vaginal candidiasis, one pessary being inserted daily for 14 days. Nystatin cream may be applied to the penis of the sexual partner over the same period, although it is not much used nowadays as it takes so long to work.

**Clotrimazole** and **miconazole** are most effective if applied locally as pessaries in the treatment of vaginal candidiasis. Miconazole is available as a gel for treating oropharyngeal infection. Both can be applied to the skin as a 1% or 2% ointment for dermatophytoses.

**Ketoconazole** is largely used in severe candidiasis and other systemic fungal infections. It can be given orally and is well absorbed. The most important adverse effects is jaundice, when internal use of the drug must be stopped; others include nausea, drowsiness and, rarely, adrenal suppression.

**Itraconazole** is used in systemic candidiasis and dermatophyte infections. The dose is variable and the capsules should be taken immediately after food to ensure maximum absorption. It should not be used in patients with liver disease.

**Fluconazole** is effective in candidiasis and cryptococcus. Serious adverse effects, particularly liver damage, have been reported. For vaginal candidiasis and for oropharyngeal infections a single oral dose is adequate.

**Griseofulvin** is administered orally in the treatment of various fungal infections. It is used in most types of fungal infection of the skin, particularly in ringworm of the scalp where local treatment is inadequate. It is slow-acting and may be continued for several weeks. As regards adverse effects, gastrointestinal upsets may occur when it is used, and griseofulvin may enhance the action of alcohol taken at the same time as the drug.

**Terbinafine** is given orally for tinea infections of the skin or nails. It is applied locally over long periods (6–12 months) for fungal infection of the nails.

**Amphotericin** is used in systemic infection with fungal organisms, namely systemic candidiasis, cryptococcal meningitis and histoplasmosis. After an initial test dose, it is given by intravenous infusion, the dose being increased gradually. **Amphotericin B** is now available enclosed in liposomes for use intravenously. This renders it easier to use and less toxic. It is also used in lozenges that are given four times daily in the treatment of oral candidiasis. Adverse effects that may limit the dose are nausea, vomiting and fever. Some renal damage may occur.

**Flucytosine** is an antifungal agent effective against *Candida albicans* and cryptococcus. It is given orally, four times daily. The kidney excretes it and therefore reduced dosage may be required in patients with impaired renal function. Side-effects are rare, but depression of the blood count has been reported.

## CANDIDIASIS

Candidiasis is a common and troublesome problem. It can occur for no apparent reason but is particularly common in:

- ill or immunocompromised patients, particularly those receiving broad-spectrum antibiotics
- those receiving drugs which suppress immunity (i.e. cytotoxic drugs and steroids)
- patients with HIV disease
- patients with diabetes
- infants
- pregnancy
- healthy women taking the Pill.

It may affect the mouth (thrush), the vagina or other mucous membranes. Rarely, it enters the bloodstream and becomes a systemic infection.

## Treatment

### Oral candidiasis

- Acute: nystatin pastilles or amphotericin B tablets sucked every 6 hours after food
- Oropharyngeal: fluconazole or itraconazole daily for up to 14 days
- Children: miconazole gel

### Oesophageal, intestinal or systemic candidiasis

- Fluconazole

### Vaginal candidiasis

- Fluconazole, a single oral dose or itraconazole twice daily for 1 day
- Clotrimazole vaginal pessaries, one inserted at night as a single dose.

### Nursing points

1. In oral candidiasis remove dentures (if any) during treatment. They should be soaked in sodium hypochlorite overnight and rinsed before being worn again.
2. In vaginal candidiasis do not forget to treat the partner (if any) with a cream preparation.

## SYSTEMIC FUNGAL INFECTIONS

These are increasing problems because of the large number of immunocompromised subjects due to HIV, cancer chemotherapy and other causes. Until fairly recently, amphotericin and flucytosine were the only drugs available, but recent introductions, including fluconazole and itraconazole, are equally, and sometimes more, effective. The correct drug for a particular fungal infection is still being studied and the choice of treatment requires expert guidance.

**Metronidazole** is useful for eradicating some protozoan parasites such as *Trichomonas vaginalis*, bacteroides infections and in amoebiasis and giardiasis (see p. 354).

The use of antifungal agents to treat systemic infections is illustrated in Case History 24.1.

### Case History 24.1

Miss K, a 19-year-old woman from Ghana went to her doctor complaining of feeling feverish and chest pains and a dry cough. She reported that the sputum had traces of blood in it. Her temperature was slightly raised and during auscultation the doctor heard marked crackling on the left side. Miss K had been treated several years before for tuberculosis and the doctor suspected the presence of an aspergilloma (a ball of fungus that has formed in a lung cavity formed by healing of a lesion, e.g. in tuberculosis). She was sent for an X-ray, which showed up a small opacity in the superior segment of the left lower lobe, surrounded by a horseshoe-shaped crescent of air. A sputum test confirmed the diagnosis and she was prescribed oral clotrimazole and aerosolized amphotericin B.

### Summary

- Systemic fungal infections are on the increase because of widespread use of broad-spectrum antibiotics
- Nystatin is particularly useful in *Candida* infections
- Clotrimazole and miconazole are most effective if applied locally in the treatment of vaginal candidiasis
- Ketoconazole is well absorbed after oral administration and is useful to treat systemic fungal infections
- Fluconazole can cause serious liver damage
- Griseofulvin is administered orally for treating ringworm of the scalp
- Terbinafine is useful by oral administration for treating tinea skin or nail infections and can be administered topically to the nails over long periods
- Amphotericin B is available in liposomes, which renders it less toxic
- The dose of flucytosine should be reduced in patients with impaired kidney function

## Reference

Editorial 2002 Phase 1 clinical trial shows oral estriol may offer hope to women with multiple sclerosis. Pharmaceutical Journal 269: 474

## Further reading

Barry M G, Back D J, Breckenridge A M 1995 Zidovudine therapy in HIV infection: which patients should be treated and when? British Journal of Clinical Pharmacology 40: 107

Brenner B G, Turner D, Wainberg M A 2002 HIV-1 drug resistance: can we overcome? Expert Opinion in Biological Therapy 2: 751

Como J A, Dismukes W E 1994 Oral azole drugs as systemic antifungal therapy. New England Journal of Medicine 330: 263

De Clercq E 2002 Highlights in the development of new antiviral agents. Mini Reviews in Medicinal Chemistry 2: 163

Editorial 1996 Interferon Beta-1B – hope or hype. Drug and Therapeutics Bulletin 34: 9

Editorial 1997 Major advances in the treatment of HIV-1 infections. Drug and Therapeutics Bulletin 35: 25

Editorial 1997 Postexposure treatment of HIV. Taking the risk for safety's sake. New England Journal of Medicine 337: 1542

Gerberding J L 1995 Management of occupational exposure to blood-borne viruses. New England Journal of Medicine 332: 444

# Chapter 25

# Sera and vaccines

## Learning objectives

At the end of this chapter, the reader should be able to:

- list the basic components of the immune system
- explain humoral and cell-mediated immunity
- explain active and passive immunization
- describe how these immunizations are achieved
- appreciate the dangers and precautions associated with the administration of serum
- understand what is meant by antiserum
- give an account of immunization against hepatitis A and B

## THE IMMUNE REACTION

The human body is continually subjected to the risk of infection by microorganisms (bacteria, viruses, fungi) and to damage by toxins produced by bacteria. These foreign substances are known collectively as antigens.

The cells that recognize and react to antigens are called lymphocytes. They are distributed throughout the body in blood, lymph and lymphoid tissues (spleen, lymph nodes, tonsils and adenoids). All lymphocytes originate in the bone marrow, but there are two main groups, the B and T cells, which mature differently and help to defend the body against foreign antigens in different ways (Fig. 25.1).

### HUMORAL IMMUNITY

Humoral immunity is a property of the B lymphocytes, which mature in the spleen and lymph nodes

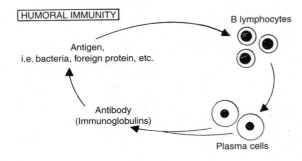

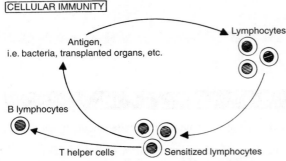

**Figure 25.1** The sequence of events in the production of humoral and cellular immunity.

after they leave the bone marrow. B lymphocytes are specific for particular antigens and the body can produce hundreds, possibly thousands, of types of B lymphocytes, each able to respond to a different microorganism. When an antigen gains access to the tissues the B lymphocytes become activated, dividing many times to form a clone of identical plasma cells. The plasma cells release proteins called immunoglobulins, which are also known as antibodies. Antibodies circulate in the blood and react with antigens to neutralize their effects and destroy them. Once the antigens have been removed most of the plasma cells disappear, but a few persist as memory cells. If a second exposure occurs the memory cells multiply rapidly and release antibodies even more swiftly than during the first exposure. This establishment of 'memory' by the B lymphocytes forms the basis of active immunization against bacteria and the harmful toxins they produce (see later).

## CELL-MEDIATED IMMUNITY

Cell-mediated immunity is a property of the T lymphocytes, which mature in the thymus gland before they enter the circulation. T lymphocytes do not produce antibodies, but are an essential component of the immune response, as B lymphocytes require them to function properly. Some T lymphocytes (T helper cells) appear to play an important part by 'switching on' the immune response when antigens invade, while others 'switch off' the immune response when the body no longer requires it. Cell-mediated immunity is especially important in the rejection of foreign materials such as transplanted organs, and in chronic infections such as tuberculosis. People whose cell-mediated immunity is impaired by HIV infection, which destroys the T helper cells, become very prone to fungal and protozoan infections, which T lymphocytes usually keep in check.

## ACTIVE IMMUNIZATION

The principle of this method is to promote the production by the patient of antibodies or sensitized lymphocytes to bacteria or toxins produced by bacteria before infection occurs. If the patient then becomes infected, the antibodies are quickly produced and are capable of rapidly dealing with the infecting organism or its toxin and thus preventing or minimizing the disease.

Antibodies are usually produced by injecting the patient with killed or modified bacteria, which, although harmless, are still capable of producing antibodies. These organisms are known as a vaccine. A good example of this method is the widespread immunization against poliomyelitis by the Sabin vaccine, which is a live virus that has been attenuated (rendered harmless).

Similarly, bacterial toxins may be modified to produce toxoids which are no longer harmful but which are capable of acting as antigens. They are then injected and protect against future damage from the particular toxin. Good examples of toxoids are the various diphtheria toxoids that produce immunity to the very dangerous toxin produced by the diphtheria organism (*Corynebacterium diphtheriae*).

Following injection of the antigen, whether vaccine or toxoid, there is usually an interval of a few days before antibodies appear. These antibodies may then persist for varying periods, from a few months up to many years. It is often the practice to give two or more booster injections of the antigen to produce a higher level of immunity.

Active immunization is used in the prevention of the following diseases:

| | | |
|---|---|---|
| measles | rubella | tuberculosis |
| rabies | diphtheria | cholera |
| pneumococcal | whooping | yellow fever |
| infections | cough | smallpox (rare) |
| anthrax | tetanus | hepatitis A and B |
| meningitis | typhoid | varicella |
| influenza | (not often) | |
| mumps | typhus | |

Active immunization may take several weeks before enough antibodies are produced to be effective. This is satisfactory as a prophylactic measure, but is not much good to treat established disease. Under these conditions passive immunization is used.

## PASSIVE IMMUNIZATION

In this method of immunization the appropriate antibody against the invading organism or toxin is injected. In the past, this antibody was produced on a large scale in animals by injecting an antigen, either vaccine or toxoid, until a high blood level of antibody was obtained. Some of the blood was then removed and the antibody extracted and stored until required. Following the injection of antibody, immunity will last about 2 weeks. This method suffers from the disadvantage that it is not possible to purify the antibodies produced completely and there is therefore a risk of a hypersensitivity reaction. Nowadays, genetic engineering and cloning procedures mean that antibodies can be grown *in vitro*.

Certain types of antibody can be obtained from human blood, either after the subject has been actively immunized or has suffered a particular infection. These antibodies, usually called human immunoglobulins, are safer and rarely produce a serious reaction, although there may be discomfort at the injection site.

Common examples of animal- and human-derived antibodies are, respectively, diphtheria antitoxin, which was obtained from horse serum, and antitetanus immunoglobulin injection from human blood.

## ADMINISTRATION OF SERUM

Antitoxin raised in animals, often called antiserum, carries a real risk of a hypersensitivity reaction. This is particularly liable to occur in patients who have had previous serum injections or who suffer from allergic disorders (e.g. asthma). The reaction occurs because the antibody in the serum reacts with antigens already present in the patient, releasing histamine and other substances. Serum reactions take two forms:

- **Immediate or anaphylactic reaction**: within a few minutes of injection the patient collapses with difficulty in breathing, low blood pressure and, sometimes, widespread urticaria. Rarely it can be fatal.
- **Serum sickness** occurs about a week after injection of serum. This is a delayed reaction. The patient is pyrexial with a rash and arthritis. It clears up in a few days.

### Nursing point

Sera and vaccines should be kept in a refrigerator at the correct temperature. Guidelines are given in *Immunization against infectious diseases* (HMSO 1996).

## PRECAUTIONS WHEN INJECTING SERUM

Ask the patient:

- Have you had serum before?
- Have you had asthma or eczema?
- Do you suffer from allergies?

If all answers are negative, give a test dose of serum subcutaneously and if there is no reaction in 30 minutes the rest may be given and the patient kept under observation for a further 1 hour.

These precautions may well be unnecessary if human immunoglobin is used, but are mandatory for diphtheria antitoxin, which is raised in animals.

### Safety note

Whenever serum is injected by any route a syringe containing 1 : 1000 of epinephrine, an antihistamine and hydrocortisone hemisuccinate should be ready at hand in case of immediate reaction.

## ANTISERA

**Diphtheria antitoxin** is an antiserum raised in animals and there is a real risk of a hypersensitivity reaction.

Dose: Prophylactic – erythromycin + vaccine
Therapeutic – Not less than 10 000 units of antitoxin intramuscularly or intravenously

**Tetanus antitoxin** is an immunoglobin prepared from human sources, with little or no risk of a hypersensitivity reaction. Following injury, immunized patients require a booster dose of vaccine to stimulate immunity. Penetrating and contaminated wounds may need, in addition, tetanus immunoglobin plus antibiotic cover. Non-immunized patients require 250 units of tetanus immunoglobin and a course of tetanus vaccine should be started. These should not be given in the same syringe or into the same site. This should be combined with antibiotic cover.

## VACCINES

Vaccines comprise:

- adsorbed diphtheria vaccine
- adsorbed tetanus vaccine
- *Haemophilus influenzae* type B (Hib)
- Diphtheria, tetanus and pertussis (DTP) vaccine
- Typhoid vaccine
- bacille Calmette-Guérin (BCG) vaccine
- poliomyelitis vaccine
- rubella vaccine
- measles, mumps and rubella (MMR) vaccine
- meningococcal A & C vaccine
- pneumococcal vaccine
- influenza vaccine.

**Adsorbed diphtheria vaccine** for adults and adolescents is prepared by adsorbing toxoid onto aluminium phosphate. In addition to single vaccines, combined vaccines stimulating immunity to diphtheria, whooping cough and tetanus are available and are routinely used for immunizing infants.

**Hib** is a vaccine against *H. influenzae* type b. Immunization is not required after the age of 4 years as infection is much less likely. Protocols for the immunization of children are shown in Table 25.1.

Table 25.1  Immunization of children

| Age | Vaccine | Note |
| --- | --- | --- |
| During first year of life | Triple (diphtheria tetanus and pertussis) + polio + Hib | First dose at 2 months 3 doses at 4-weekly intervals |
| During second year of life | MMR Hib | One dose if not previously given |
| At school entry | Diphtheria, tetanus + polio MMR | |
| At 10–14 years | BCG | If tuberculin test is negative |
| On leaving school | Diphtheria, tetanus + polio | |

Smallpox vaccination is not now given as a routine unless the subject is going to a country which still requires a certificate of vaccination despite the elimination of the disease! It should also be offered to laboratory workers at special risk.

*H. influenzae* is the most common cause of meningitis in the under 4s.

People at risk from **tetanus** should receive a booster dose of toxoid every 5 years. For **typhoid**, both oral and injected vaccines are available for those visiting a high-risk area. They are effective for about 3 years.

The controversy over the use of **pertussis (whooping cough) vaccine** has waxed and waned over the last 30 or so years over the issue that pertussis was suspected of causing brain damage. In the 1970s many parents in the UK (over 50%) opted to omit the pertussis component of the diphtheria, tetanus and pertussis (DTP) vaccine and, consequently, several thousand children were admitted to hospital and over 100 died of whooping cough. In countries such as Sweden and Hungary, which actively adopted a strategy to drop the pertussis vaccine, childhood deaths from pertussis rose 10–100 fold. Most countries have now dropped anti-pertussis campaigns. An article published in the *Lancet* (Gangarosa et al, 1998) is the source of the information given here.

Nevertheless, controversy continues and, unfortunately, children's issues are very emotive, and fears can be raised that may result in unwise measures. The recent fears over MMR vaccine provide another example of the difficulty that is caused by extreme responses to sometimes ill-advised publication of emotive research reports, particularly those which do not have sufficient hard data to support their theses.

**Nursing point**

- Children who develop a fever after receiving the MMR vaccine can be given paracetamol (see p. 150), which can be repeated once if necessary, after 4–6 hours.
- In the past there have been fears that brain damage might, rarely, follow the use of pertussis vaccine and, although the frequency was difficult to assess, a figure of less than 1 : 80 000 was given. More recently, even this risk is considered unlikely. The dangers attached to having whooping cough, especially in infancy, are considerably greater.

**BCG vaccine** is a suspension of living bacilli that will produce tuberculosis antibodies. **Poliomyelitis vaccine** may be either inactivated poliomyelitis viruses type 1, 2 and 3 (Salk vaccine) or attenuated live virus (Sabin vaccine); the latter is to be preferred as it avoids injections, provides a more prolonged immunity and by producing antibodies in the intestine it prevents the spread of infection.

**Rubella vaccine** should be offered to seronegative women of childbearing age. It is important to exclude pregnancy when giving the vaccine and to avoid it for 1 month thereafter.

**Nursing point**

Nurses should ensure that they are immune to rubella. All nurses should be immunized if necessary.

The combined **measles, mumps and rubella (MMR) vaccine** should be given as a single dose by intramuscular or deep subcutaneous injection to children aged 12–15 months and 4–5 before starting school. It occasionally produces malaise, fever, a rash and parotid swelling about 1 week after injection. Meningitis due to the mumps component occurs in about 1 in 1 000 000 doses. There is no hard

evidence that MMR vaccine is a cause of autism or bowel disease (Editorial 2002a).

**Meningococcal vaccine** is effective only against the A and C strains of the organism, which do not predominate in the UK. It should be given to travellers to tropical zones, where meningitis is common.

**Pneumococcal vaccine** is given to people who are at special risk from pneumococcal infection, including those with chronic lung and heart disease, diabetes, patients who have had a splenectomy, and those who are immunosuppressed or have sickle cell disease.

**Influenza vaccine** protects against the 'flu' viruses, which are changing continually. WHO recommends which strains of virus should be included in the vaccine for a particular year. The vaccine only protects about 70% of subjects for about 1 year and its use is confined to those at special risk, e.g. the elderly, those with heart, lung or renal disease and patients with diabetes. There may be some local discomfort, but systemic reactions are rare.

**Nursing point**

**Vaccines and safety.** Vaccination is one of the most successful methods of preventing disease. Vaccines should be safe as they are given to large numbers of healthy people and, often, to very young children. They certainly have side-effects but these are usually minor and transient, such as a short bout of fever. From time to time an adverse effect of a serious nature is reported, which ultimately turns out to be very rare or based on insecure evidence. Meanwhile, the public become confused and anxious, the rate of immunization falls and the incidence of the disease in question may rise.

It is therefore very important for nurses, especially those involved in immunization programmes, to be familiar with the adverse effects of vaccines and to distinguish between those caused by the vaccine and those which are coincidental. No vaccine is absolutely safe but the patient (or parent) should consider the risk against the benefit.

A new antiviral influenza drug called Oseltamivir (*Tamiflu*) has been introduced. It is not a vaccine. It has been found to reduce the incidence of 'flu' significantly in some patients in nursing homes, and to reduce its duration, if the patient does get 'flu'. It is not recommended as a replacement for vaccines (Editorial 2002b).

## IMMUNIZATION AGAINST VIRAL HEPATITIS

**Hepatitis A virus** is spread by poor hygiene, and infection is usually due to contaminated food and water. A vaccine is now available and is given as a single injection with a booster dose after 6 months. It appears to be very effective in preventing hepatitis A, but the duration of protection is not yet known. There may be local soreness at the site of injection. Alternatively, normal human immunoglobulin, given by I.M. injection, confers passive immunity for up to 2 months.

---

### Nursing point

A doctor may delegate the responsibility of immunization to a nurse provided that:

1. the nurse is willing to be accountable for the work
2. the nurse has received training in the subject
3. the nurse has been trained in the diagnosis and treatment of anaphylaxis. Consent must always be obtained before immunization.

**Anaphylaxis** is very rare with active immunization but treatment should be immediately available (see above).

#### Contraindications to immunization
1. Acute illness.
2. Live vaccines should not be given to those who have reduced immunity to:
   (a) high doses of steroids or cytotoxic drugs
   (b) active lymphomas, including Hodgkin's disease
   (c) other causes of reduced immunity
3. Pregnancy. Rarely the risk of infection outweighs this precaution.
4. HIV-positive subjects should receive BCG, yellow fever or oral typhoid vaccine. Their response to immunization may be reduced.

Immunization programmes are constantly reviewed and altered from time to time. In case of doubt, nurses are referred to *Immunization against infectious diseases* (HMSO 1996) or to the current edition of the *British National Formulary*.

---

**Hepatitis B** viral infection is of particular importance to the health professional as it can be spread by infected body fluids (blood and saliva) and precautions should be enforced when nursing all patients, as it is impossible to predict who are carriers from the patient's history alone.

A vaccine prepared from the surface antigen of the virus is available (H-B-Vax). Three injections are given into the deltoid muscle; the first and second are given 1 month apart, and the third after 6 months. Immunity persists for at least 2 years. Passive immunization is also possible using a special serum containing large amounts of antibody against the hepatitis B virus.

## DRUGS THAT BLOCK THE IMMUNE REACTION

The immune response can be blocked either:

- **by interfering with the effects of immunity with drugs, or**
- **by suppressing cells involved in cellular or humoral immunity (immunosuppression).**

These effects, particularly suppression of the cells involved in cellular and humoral immunity, are extremely important when considering the treatment of cancer, which is covered in Chapter 26.

---

### Summary

- Active immunization can protect the patient for years
- Active immunization will not be used to treat an established disease, whereas passive immunization is sometimes used
- Passive immunization does not last long (usually, perhaps weeks or a few months at most)
- Antitoxins (antiserum) raised in animals carry the risk of a hypersensitivity reaction
- Patients must be questioned about previous hypersensitivity reactions and about any allergies before injecting serum into them
- Even if answers are negative, inject a small test dose first, and if there is no reaction by 30 minutes, the rest may be given, and the patient should be kept under observation for another hour
- Whenever injecting serum into a patient by any route, always have ready a syringe with 1 : 1000 epinephrine, an antihistamine and hydrocortisone hemisuccinate for emergency use
- Keep antisera refrigerated at the correct temperature

- Smallpox vaccine should be offered to laboratory workers at special risk
- Children may be given paracetamol if they develop fever after receiving MMR vaccine
- Although there is controversy, there is no convincing evidence at the time of writing that MMR vaccine causes autism in children (Editorial 2002a)
- All nurses should ensure that they are immunized against rubella, especially if they are working in an obstetric role
- Rubella vaccine should be offered to seronegative women of childbearing age, but to exclude pregnancy first, and to avoid pregnancy for at least 1 month after receiving the vaccine
- Nurses should be familiar with the adverse effects of vaccines
- For the nurse's own protection, precautions must be taken when nursing all patients since it is not possible to ascertain from the patient's history alone which patients may be carriers of hepatitis B
- Epinephrine is very effective in acute anaphylaxis

## References

Editorial 2002a No correlation between MMR vaccination and autism. The Pharmaceutical Journal 266: 209

Editorial 2002b Use Tamiflu for prevention not treatment of flu, says *DTB*. Pharmaceutical Journal 270: 6

Gangarosa E J, Galazka A M, Wolfe C R et al 1998 Impact of anti-vaccine movements on pertussis control: the untold story. Lancet 351: 356

HMSO 1996 Immunization against infectious disease. HMSO, London

## Further reading

Coppola J, Johnston R 1998 Cold comfort. Nursing Times 94(11): 72

Editorial 1998 MMR vaccination and autism. British Medical Journal 316: 715

Lockhead Y J 1991 Failure to immunise children under five years. Journal of Advanced Nursing 16: 130

Steimle D, Aston R, Van Damme P 2002 Immunisation information for parents. Nursing Standard 16: 40

Thakker Y, Woods S 1992 Storage of vaccines in the community. British Medical Journal 304: 756

# Chapter 26

# Drugs used in the treatment of malignant disease

## Learning objectives

At the end of this chapter, the reader should be able to:

- describe the main stages of the cell cycle
- explain how the main classes of drugs for cancer are classified
- give some examples of each class and which cancers they are used for
- give an account of the important general adverse effects of anticancer drugs, e.g. myelosuppression
- describe the advantages of combination chemotherapy
- define palliative and adjuvant therapy
- appreciate the problems of administering drugs, e.g. extravasation and dangers to staff
- give an account of the nurse's involvement in cancer chemotherapy and in patient counselling and care

## INTRODUCTION

A great deal has been discovered about normal cell function and cell division, but after many years of research it is still not known exactly why malignant cells behave as they do. The pattern of their behaviour is familiar. Instead of differentiating in an orderly fashion to take their place in the formation of some tissue, they multiply in a haphazard way showing little, if any, attempt at differentiation and, further, instead of remaining in their organ of origin they invade neighbouring structures. Cell emboli from new growths are swept in the blood or lymphatic circulation to distant parts of the body, take root and set up further tumours known as secondary deposits or metastases.

## NUCLEAR DIVISION AND CYTOTOXIC DRUGS

The cells of the body vary enormously in appearance and function, but all share some common characteristics. With very few exceptions (e.g. erythrocytes), cells consist of a nucleus surrounded by cytoplasm. The most vital component of the nucleus is deoxyribonucleic acid (DNA), which consists of two chains of molecules arranged into a double helix. DNA contains the code which, through production of messenger RNA, determines the types of proteins that are made by the cell and thus ultimately how the cell functions.

Most cytotoxic drugs interfere with DNA or RNA and thus they have a profound effect on cells and their functions. Unfortunately, these actions are not confined to the malignant cells, but affect normal cells as well.

Some cells in the body divide frequently to replace those that have become worn out, particularly the cells of the bone marrow, the lymphatic system and the lining of the intestinal tract, and these are particularly sensitive to the action of cytotoxic drugs.

## THE CELL CYCLE

The cell goes through the following phases:

- $G_1$ phase
- S phase
- $G_2$ phase
- mitotic phase.

During its life the cell passes through a series of changes. The newly formed cell enters the **$G_1$ phase,** which is a period of protein synthesis and intense metabolic activity. This may last for a variable time, from a few hours to many years. Many cells remain in this phase throughout the life of the organism, but some undergo division and enter the **S phase**. This phase is short and is concerned with DNA and RNA synthesis so that the DNA strands may split when cell division occurs. It is a period of great metabolic activity. The **$G_2$ phase** which follows is a short period of consolidation before cell division occurs. In the **mitotic phase** the DNA spiral splits longitudinally so that each daughter cell has its full complement of DNA, which is exactly the same as that in the parent cell (Fig. 26.1). A proportion of the cells in a cancer are in a resting phase, sometimes called the **$G_0$ phase,** when they are not dividing.

This is important because at this stage they are very resistant to chemotherapy.

### Drugs and the cell cycle

Some cytotoxic drugs will affect cells at any phase in their life cycle; others will only act at a single phase of the cell cycle, usually when the cell is dividing, and are called **phase specific**. It follows therefore that when using phase-specific drugs repeated dosage is necessary if the maximum effect is to be achieved.

The term *neoplastic growth*, incidentally, refers to any new and abnormal growth, which may be either benign or malignant.

## TREATMENT WITH DRUGS

### Current aims of chemotherapy

The aim of treating neoplastic disease with drugs is to find a drug that will kill the neoplastic cells while leaving the normal cells of the body unharmed. However, the metabolic process of the neoplastic cells is so very similar to or perhaps even the same as that of normal cells that so far it has been impossible to reach this ideal. Nearly all drugs that have so far been discovered, although having a marked toxic effect on neoplastic cells, have some adverse effect on the normal cells of the body, especially those of the bone marrow. The best that can be done is to give the cytotoxic drug or drugs at repeated intervals so arranged that the recovery of normal cells can occur, but little recovery of cancer cells is possible. It may then be possible progressively to reduce the number of malignant cells without unduly reducing the normal cells until ultimately all the malignant cells are eradicated (Fig. 26.2).

There are now, however, newer types of drugs on the market that are designed to target certain cells more specifically. It has long been the dream of the drug designers to design the successful 'magic bullet' – the drug that affects only the cancer cell. In practical terms, this involves attaching a cytotoxic drug to another chemical that will bind only to some marker on the surface of a cancer cell, and kill it while sparing normal dividing cells that do not have the marker. This dream has not yet been realized, although so-called biologic drugs have been developed that target specific antigens on the cancer cell and block the production of growth factors that promote cancer cell proliferation (see, for example, trastuzumab below).

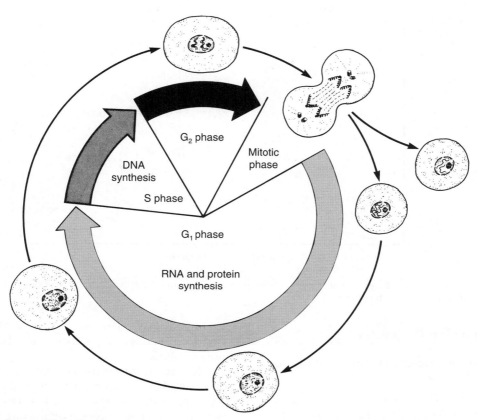

**Figure 26.1**   Phases of the cell cycle.

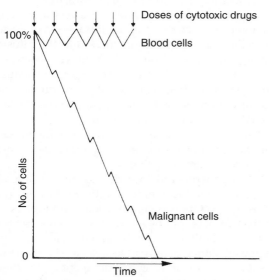

**Figure 26.2**   Progressive reduction in the number of malignant cells produced by repeated doses of a cytotoxic drug, with recovery of the normal blood cells. An ideal therapeutic response.

## THE NATURAL HISTORY OF CANCER

The growth rate of tumours varies considerably and the development of clinical symptoms and signs occurs at a late stage in the disease process (Fig. 26.3). Note particularly the long subclinical period and, that after chemotherapy, although the patient is apparently in full clinical remission, a small amount of tumour may remain.

As a result of these considerations and a large amount of work on animal models of cancer, certain general principles and features of treatment have emerged:

- cytotoxic drugs are usually given in intermittent high-dose treatments over long periods
- the smaller the mass of tumour treated, the better the result because small tumours have less resting cells which are insensitive to chemotherapy
- suppression of the bone marrow is very common, as cytotoxic drugs have to be given at the maximum tolerated dose.

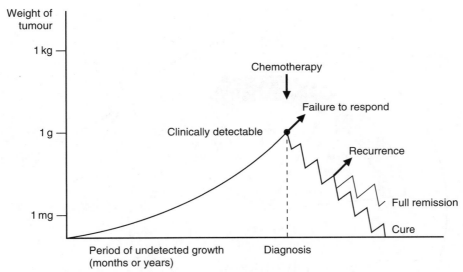

**Figure 26.3** Tumour growth and possible responses to chemotherapy. Modified from Ritter et al, A textbook of clinical pharmacology, 3rd edn, Edward Arnold, London.

## MAIN CLASSES OF DRUGS

There are several different classes of drugs for the treatment of cancer:

- cytotoxic drugs
- sex hormones and hormone antagonists
- drugs affecting the immune response
- other immunomodulating drugs.

## CYTOTOXIC DRUGS

Drugs in this group kill dividing cells and are therefore toxic not only to cancer cells but also to healthy dividing cells in the body. It is, nevertheless, perhaps the most widely used group, and there are several different types of drug within this group:

- alkylating agents
- cytotoxic antibiotics
- antimetabolites
- topoisomerase I inhibitors (campothecins).

### Alkylating agents

These are chemically very active substances that combine with the DNA in the cell nucleus and thus damage or kill the cell. Unfortunately, although these substances have a marked effect on certain types of malignant cells, they also damage normal cells, particularly those of the bone marrow and gastrointestinal tract, which have a high rate of division. There are a number of alkylating agents now available.

**Chlormethine (mustine)** is related to mustard gas and is used in the treatment of neoplastic diseases of the lymphoreticular system such as Hodgkin's disease, and with less success in certain carcinomas such as those of the ovary and bronchus. Because of toxicity its use is decreasing and it is now rarely used.

*Therapeutic use.* Chlormethine (mustine) is given by intravenous injection, and as it is very irritant it is common practice to set up an intravenous infusion of saline and inject chlormethine into the infusion tubing and flush it through the vein with saline.

*Adverse effects.* Most patients experience nausea and vomiting for some hours after treatment. Bone marrow suppression is an ever-present risk, usually affecting the white cells and platelets.

Chlormethine (mustine) may also be injected into malignant effusions and may either slow down or prevent their formation.

**Cyclophosphamide** was developed in an attempt to improve the therapeutic effectiveness of this type of drug. Cyclophosphamide itself is non-toxic, but in the liver it is split by enzymes which release cytotoxic metabolites. It can be given orally or intravenously, either daily or weekly and is frequently combined with other cytotoxic agents. The therapeutic effect is usually delayed for a week or more.

*Adverse effects.* These include depression of the bone marrow and (alopecia) loss of hair. A metabolite called acrolein is excreted in the urine which can cause severe cystitis. This may be avoided by giving a high fluid intake (4 litres a day) or combining it with the drug **mesna**, which binds to acrolein and neutralizes it (see also later).

**Ifosfamide** is closely related to cyclophosphamide, from which it differs slightly in efficacy. It is less likely to depress the blood count than cyclophosphamide, but is more likely to damage the kidneys and bladder. To prevent this adverse effect it is, like cyclophosphamide, combined with mesna.

**Chlorambucil** is a useful drug of the chlormethine group. It is effective by mouth and although depression of the bone marrow can occur, vomiting is unusual.

*Therapeutic use.* Chlorambucil is given orally over long periods. It is one of the few cytotoxic drugs that is used continuously rather than as high-dose intermittent treatment. It has been used on an outpatient basis but community chemotherapy is now being introduced. Nevertheless, the patient should have regular blood counts and if severe bone marrow suppression occurs recovery may be slow. It is effective against various forms of Hodgkin's disease and non-Hodgkin lymphoma and is probably the drug of choice in chronic lymphatic leukaemia.

**Busulfan** is used particularly in chronic myeloid leukaemia where it has a selective depressing action on the abnormal white cells. Excessive dosage will produce dangerous depression of normal white cells and platelets.

*Therapeutic use.* Busulfan is given orally. Treatment is continued over weeks or months and is modified by the response of the patient.

*Adverse effects.* In addition to bone marrow depression it can cause pigmentation and fibrosis of the lungs.

**Melphalan** is used particularly in multiple myelomatosis. It is usually given daily for a week, and may be repeated if the blood count is satisfactory. Melphalan is a powerful depressant of white cells and platelets.

**Lomustine (***CCNU***)** is similar in many ways to the alkylating agents and, although its mode of action is different, it is effective against the same types of cancer. It is given orally as a single dose and should not be repeated for 4 or preferably 6 weeks as depression of white cells and platelets may be delayed.

*Adverse effects.* Nausea and sometimes vomiting is common for about 12 hours after dosage.

**Carmustine** is similar to lomustine.

**Estramustine** is a combination of chlormethine and an estrogen. It is an example of the magic bullet approach. The drug is meant to be concentrated in tissues that have estrogen receptors and both the estrogen and the cytotoxic chlormethine attack the cancer cell. Unlike many other cytotoxic agents estramustine does not destroy the DNA.

*Therapeutic use.* Estramustine is used in some cases of prostate cancer, for which estrogens have long been used. It is administered orally in capsule form.

*Adverse effects.* These include gynaecomastia because of the estrogenic effect, and heart and liver toxicity. The drug is contraindicated in heart and liver disease, and in patients with peptic ulcer.

## Cytotoxic antibiotics

This is also a group of very widely used anticancer drugs. They are drugs derived from microorganisms and they work mainly by preventing cell division either through a direct action on the DNA itself or by blocking the enzymes involved in DNA replication, or through both actions. Some important ones are:

- doxorubicin
- mitoxantrone (mitozantrone)
- epirubicin
- daunorubicin
- bleomycin
- dactinomycin
- mitomycin
- idarubicin.

**Doxorubicin** (*Adriamycin*) is probably the most widely used cytotoxic antibiotic. It has been used successfully to treat lymphomas, leukaemias and solid tumours. It has two actions: it binds to the DNA itself, thus preventing both DNA and RNA synthesis; more importantly for this drug, it inhibits the action of an enzyme called topoisomerase II that allows DNA to be reproduced (see also below).

*Therapeutic use.* It is given by intravenous injection, every 3 weeks, usually in combination with other cytotoxic drugs. It can be instilled directly into the bladder.

*Adverse effects.* It can depress bone marrow and this occurs about 2 weeks after treatment, rather later than with most cytotoxic drugs. It is toxic to heart muscle and this requires regular ECG monitoring. Toxicity is dose-related. Other effects are nausea, vomiting and hair loss.

**Mitoxantrone** and **epirubicin** are both structurally related to doxorubicin. Mitoxantrone (mitozantrone) is given as a single injection at 3-weekly intervals.

It is used in a variety of cancers. The incidence of adverse effects is relatively low and it is useful in controlling the disease, particularly on an outpatient basis. It does, however, cause bone marrow suppression and has a dose-related cardiotoxicity. Epirubicin is less cardiotoxic than is doxorubicin. **Idarubicin** has similar properties to those of doxorubicin and may replace it. It is indicated for acute leukaemias and advanced breast cancer. It is given by mouth or intravenously. Like many of the cytotoxic antibiotics it is cardiotoxic. **Daunorubicin**, too, has similar properties to those of doxorubicin and is used to treat acute leukaemias. It is administered by intravenous infusion. There is a liposomal preparation of daunorubicin that is licensed for use in treating HIV-related Kaposi's sarcoma.

**Bleomycin**, another antibiotic with relatively weak anticancer effects, is used in combination to treat lymphomas and testicular cancers. However, unlike all the drugs already discussed, it does not depress the bone marrow. It is usually injected at weekly intervals, and a spike of fever may follow injection. Prolonged use leads to lung fibrosis.

> ### Nursing point
>
> Cytotoxic drugs, especially antibiotics, can be necrotic to local tissue if they leak into extravascular compartments. Therefore when given I.V. only specially trained staff should administer them (see also p. 350).

## Antimetabolites

These agents resemble substances used by the cells for their metabolic processes. They thus become incorporated in the cells and because they cannot be metabolized they normally cause the cell to die. Malignant cells often have a very rapid metabolic turnover and thus incorporate antimetabolites more rapidly than normal cells. It is thus possible to kill the majority of malignant cells without interfering too drastically with normal cells. Excessive dosage will inhibit normal cell production, particularly in the bone marrow. Many antimetabolites resemble the purines or pyrimidines, which are the building blocks of DNA. They become incorporated in the growing strand of DNA and stop the process. Examples include:

- methotrexate
- mercaptopurine (purine analogue)
- fluorouracil (pyrimidine analogue)
- capecitabine
- raltitrexed
- tegafur
- tioguanine (purine analogue)
- cytarabine (pyrimidine analogue)
- fludarabine (purine analogue)
- cladribine (purine analogue)
- gemcitabine (pyrimidine analogue).

**Methotrexate** is similar in structure to folic acid and it blocks one of the chemical processes necessary for the production of cell nuclear material from folic acid.

*Therapeutic use.* Methotrexate can be given orally, intravenously or intrathecally, but large doses are not well absorbed from the intestine and must be given by injection. Dosage schedules depend on the type of cancer being treated. It is excreted via the kidney and it is essential that renal function is measured before starting treatment. With impaired function the dose is reduced. The drug is prescribed together with folic acid as a supplement.

In certain types of malignant disease, a very large and potentially lethal dose of methotrexate is given; then, after 24 hours, giving folinic acid reverses the action of the drug. It is extremely important that this is carried out precisely. This method is known as folinic acid rescue.

*Adverse effects.* In addition to bone marrow suppression methotrexate can cause liver damage and mouth ulceration (Van Outryve et al 2002).

Methotrexate in low doses is also used as an immunosuppressant in rheumatoid arthritis and psoriasis (see p. 155).

**Mercaptopurine** is closely related chemically to adenine and hypoxanthine, two substances used in the formation of the cell nucleus. It is believed that mercaptopurine replaces these substances in the nucleus of cells and thereby prevents their further division. It is used in combination with other drugs in the treatment of acute leukaemia, a disease where the bone marrow is rapidly overgrown by very malignant white cells. Mercaptopurine can also be used in chronic myeloid leukaemia.

*Therapeutic use.* Mercaptopurine is given daily by mouth, and the course of treatment is determined by the response of the patient. Excessive or prolonged treatment will produce depression of normal white cells.

**Fluorouracil** is another antimetabolite that is used with some benefit in a wide variety of tumours, including those of the gastrointestinal tract. It is given by intravenous infusion or as a bolus; the dose varies with circumstances. It can also be applied locally to certain skin cancers. It produces leucopenia and in particular ulceration of the mouth.

**Cytarabine** is a drug that interferes with the nuclear function in the malignant cell and is used in acute leukaemia. It can cause bone marrow depression.

**Raltitrexed** blocks one of the enzymes involved in DNA synthesis, namely thymidylate synthetase. It is administered intravenously to treat advanced colorectal cancer when drugs such as fluorouracil cannot be used. It is usually well tolerated by patients, but can cause gastrointestinal upsets and myelosuppression (a reduction in blood cell production by the bone marrow).

## Plant and animal-derived drugs

These drugs can be divided into:

- vinca alkaloids
- etoposide
- trastuzumab
- taxanes
- campothecins.

Vinca alkaloids comprise

- vinblastine
- vincristine
- vindesine
- vinorelbine.

**Vinblastine** is an extract of periwinkle. It is believed to act at the stage of cell division (mitosis) and is therefore phase specific. Vinblastine is useful as part of a cytotoxic drug regime in treating certain lymphomas and is given in a single weekly injection. It can cause a leucopenia which is, however, usually short-lived.

> **Nursing point**
>
> Vinca alkaloids should be given intravenously and, under no circumstances, intrathecally.

**Vincristine**, which is related to vinblastine, is also given intravenously, at intervals. It is used as an initial drug in acute leukaemia to induce a remission and is also useful in treating lymphomas and other cancers. It is less likely to cause leucopenia, but may also damage peripheral and autonomic nerves, producing constipation with abdominal distension and tingling and numbness in the limbs.

**Vinorelbine** is a newer, semi-synthetic vinca alkaloid. It is used for advanced breast cancer when other treatments have failed, and for advanced non-small lung cancer.

Etoposide is related to podophyllin, an extract of mandrake, which can be applied locally in the treatment of warts. Its action is to prevent cell division. Etoposide can be given orally or intravenously and is usually used in combination in the treatment of a wide range of malignancies.

*Adverse effects.* These include bone marrow depression and vomiting in a small number of patients.

**Taxanes** – **paclitaxel (***Taxol***)** and **docetaxel** – are obtained from yew. They inhibit cell division in the $G_2$ and M phase (see Fig. 26.2) and are used to treat ovarian and breast cancer when other regimes have failed. They are given by intravenous infusion. They both depress the blood count and there is a risk of hypersensitivity reactions with flushing, rashes, dyspnoea and collapse. To prevent this, patients are given a steroid and an antihistamine before infusion.

## Campothecins

**Irinotecan** and **topotescan** are derivatives of an extract from tree bark and are chemically related to the taxanes. They inhibit cancer cell growth by inhibiting topoisomerase I, an enzyme concerned with DNA replication. Irinotecan is licensed to be used for metastatic colorectal cancer together with fluorouracil and folinic acid or on its own if the combined treatment with fluorouracil fails. Topotescan is used for metastatic ovarian cancer when other therapies have failed. Both drugs are administered by I.V. infusion. Both cause gastrointestinal upsets and a dose-related myelosuppression.

**Trastuzumab** is a newer drug and is one of the so-called biologic remedies. It is a monoclonal antibody protein that binds to and inactivates a receptor called the human epidermal growth factor receptor 2 (HER2). HER2 is overexpressed in many cancers, especially breast, lung, ovarian and prostate, and overexpression of HER2 is associated with a poor prognosis. HER2 is normally involved in cellular growth, cell proliferation and survival.

*Therapeutic use.* Trastuzumab is used for patients with breast cancer who are known to overexpress HER2, and in whom other approaches have failed. It may be used either alone or in combination with paclitaxel (see above). It is administered by I.V. infusion under medical supervision.

*Adverse effects.* Several have been reported, including infusion-related symptoms such as fever, chills and hypersensitivity reactions, given that a protein is being administered. Delayed reactions include gastrointestinal upsets, such as severe diarrhoea, hypotension, headache, chest pains and cardiotoxicity.

*Contraindications.* These include breast-feeding and dyspnoea at rest. The use of trastuzumab together with the cytotoxic anthracycline antibiotics such as doxorubicin is associated with cardiotoxicity.

Note that the suffix – *mab* usually denotes that the drug is a *m*onoclonal *a*nti*b*ody.

## Miscellaneous drugs

**Procarbazine** is used in the treatment of lymphomas. Nausea is less likely if the drug is given after meals and it may have to be combined with an anti-emetic. If alcohol is taken at the same time as the drug it may produce a reddish flush.

**Dacarbazine** is largely used in treating Hodgkin's disease and melanomas. It has to be given intravenously and is highly irritant so it must be injected very slowly into a fast running drip. It also causes considerable vomiting and severe myelodepression.

**Cisplatin** is based on the metal platinum. It is effective in a number of cancers, but has found a particular use in regimes designed to treat cancer of the testicle and ovary and has proved very successful.

*Therapeutic use.* Cisplatin is given intravenously and usually in combination with other anticancer agents at 3–4 week intervals. Certain precautions must be observed:

- a diuresis is essential when the drug is given or it will damage the kidneys
- hearing should be tested regularly as cisplatin damages the inner ear
- vomiting is usually very troublesome and treatment for this should be at hand when administering the drug.

It follows, therefore, that this drug should only be given by those who are aware of the complications that can occur, such as trained oncology nurses.

**Carboplatin** is similar and is used in ovarian carcinoma. It is not, however, as nephrotoxic as cisplatin.

## SEX HORMONES AND HORMONE ANTAGONISTS

Various hormones will produce a temporary remission in malignant disease. Their mode of action is not clear, but it is believed that certain malignant tumours – for example some types of breast cancer – are in part dependent on hormones. By removing these hormones (i.e. by removing the endocrine glands where the hormones originate) or by suppressing their release by giving other hormones, the stimulus to growth is removed from the malignant cells and they regress.

## Estrogens

**Diethylstilbestrol** is one of the older synthetic estrogens in use. It was used to treat prostate cancer but is now rarely used for this purpose because of its adverse effects, although it is occasionally used in postmenopausal women with breast cancer. It is taken orally in tablet form.

*Adverse effects.* These include sodium retention and oedema, nausea, gynaecomastia and impotence in men, and venous and arterial thrombosis. It can cause bone pain and hypercalcaemia when used for breast cancer.

**Ethinylestradiol** is a very powerful synthetic estrogen and is widely used in oral contraceptives (see p. 217). It is occasionally prescribed for breast cancer.

*Adverse effects.* These are similar to those of diethylstilboestrol.

**Fosfestrol** is a prodrug. After administration it is converted in the body to diethylstilbestrol by the enzyme acid phosphatase. It is used to treat prostate cancer. It is administered either orally or by slow I.V. injection.

*Adverse effects.* These are the same as for diethylstilbestrol.

## Progestogens (progestins)

These comprise:

- gestonorone caproate
- medroxyprogesterone acetate
- megestrol acetate
- norethisterone.

These compounds imitate the action of the hormone progesterone and are used in endometrial cancer, renal cell carcinoma and as second- or third-line therapy for breast cancer. Progestogens are not used for prostate cancer. Medroxyprogesterone and megestrol are the most popular and are given orally. There are few adverse effects, and these include occasional nausea, weight gain and fluid retention.

## Androgens

These comprise:

- **testosterone**
- **testosterone esters:**
     **testosterone enantate**

**testosterone propionate**
**testosterone undecenoate**
**mesterolone**.

Androgens are still used occasionally as second- or third-line treatments for breast cancer. Testosterone is administered as a patch, the undecenoate and mesterolone orally, and the other esters either by intramuscular injection or as depot preparations. Their uses are associated with several problems and contraindications. They cause hirsutism, increased libido, electrolyte disturbances, acne, male-pattern baldness and precocious puberty in children. They can actually precipitate prostate cancer (but see Patterson et al 2002). They are contraindicated in pregnancy, breast-feeding, hypercalcaemia, nephrosis (degenerative changes in kidney tubule epithelium), prostate cancer, breast cancer in men and in patients with a history of primary liver tumours.

The sex hormones are necessary for fertility, but they are a two-edged sword in that they are also potent carcinogens and they are able to accelerate cancers of certain organs. Estradiol can exacerbate breast cancer (see Clamp et al 2002), and testosterone can prove fatal in patients with prostate cancer. Traditionally, before the introduction of hormone antagonists, the gonads were routinely removed in patients with breast or prostate cancer. Today we have drugs that can block the action of the sex hormones or which block their production.

Hormone antagonists block the actions of the sex hormones estradiol and testosterone at their receptors. Aromatase inhibitors are drugs that block the action of the aromatase enzymes that catalyse the production of the estrogens. Gonadorelin (GnRH, gonadotrophin hormone-releasing hormone; see also p. 172) is the hormone from the hypothalamus of the brain that enables the anterior pituitary gland to synthesize and release the gonadotrophins, which in turn promote both ovarian and testicular function.

## Hormone antagonists

Tamoxifen and toremifene are estrogen receptor antagonists, whereas cyproterone acetate, flutamide and bicalutamide are androgen receptor antagonists.

**Tamoxifen** has been used for over 20 years to treat women with advanced breast cancer. It is also used to prevent recurrences among women with early breast cancer. The drug works by competing with the body's estrogen for its receptor sites, thus blocking the accelerating effects of estrogens on the disease.

Recent large trials with tamoxifen have provided strong evidence that it can actually prevent breast cancer among healthy women who are considered at high risk for breast cancer.

More than one trial has found evidence that tamoxifen is associated with a two- to three-fold increase in the risk of endometrial cancer and a two- to three-fold increase in the risk of thromboembolism. Nevertheless, tamoxifen remains probably the most widely used drug for breast cancer chemotherapy and it is generally considered that the benefits outweigh the risks (Editorial 2002a).

*Therapeutic use.* Tamoxifen is prescribed for women whose breast cancer shows positive for the presence of estrogen receptors. Some tumours are estrogen receptor-negative, and tamoxifen is not considered effective in these cases. About 60–65% of women with estrogen receptor-positive tumours respond to initial tamoxifen treatment, while less than 10% of patients with estrogen receptor-negative tumours will respond. Tamoxifen is supplied in tablet form for oral administration to be taken daily for breast cancer.

Tamoxifen is also prescribed for anovulatory sterility, when the drug is taken on days 2, 3, 4 and 5 of the menstrual cycle.

*Adverse effects and contraindications.* Adverse effects are mild and include occasional nausea, oedema, flushing and bone pain and a slightly increased risk of endometrial cancer. The drug is contraindicated in breast-feeding, and should be stopped before planned pregnancy, and advice should be sought as well (Editorial 2002b).

*Drug interactions.* Tamoxifen increases the anticoagulant effect of warfarin.

**Toremifene** is another estrogen receptor antagonist. It is chemically similar to tamoxifen (it is a chlorinated analogue). It is used to treat hormone-dependent metastatic breast cancer in post-menopausal women. It is, like tamoxifen, taken orally.

*Adverse effects.* These are similar to those of tamoxifen. It is associated with hypercalcaemia, especially if there are metastases to bone.

*Contraindications.* It is contraindicated in pregnancy, breast-feeding, in patients with a history of liver or thromboembolic disease and when there is endometrial hyperplasia.

There is sometimes confusion over the terms hyperplasia and hypertrophy. *Hyperplasia* is the increased production and growth of more normal cells in any organ or tissue, e.g. benign prostatic hyperplasia in older men. Breast enlargement during pregnancy is also hyperplasia. *Hypertrophy* is the enlargement of the cells themselves without necessarily an increase in cell number. The increase in muscle size following exercise or 'pumping iron' is an example of hypertrophy.

## Aromatase inhibitors

Aromatase inhibitors block the production of estrogens and are therefore used in breast cancer.

**Aminoglutethimide** has been used for many years. It inhibits steroid synthesis in the adrenals and also suppresses estrogen and androgen production in the peripheral tissues. For this reason it is used in the treatment of prostate cancer and advanced breast cancer. It can also be used to control the overproduction of adrenal steroid hormones in Cushing's disease. It is, however, no longer the treatment of choice for advanced breast cancer. It is administered orally in tablet form.

*Adverse effects.* Aminoglutethimide can cause adrenal insufficiency since it suppresses cortisol production. This is particularly important in conditions of acute illness, surgery or stress. Patients may need supplemental glucocorticoids. Other important adverse effects include allergic alveolitis, when the drug should be withdrawn immediately, cholestatic hepatitis, agranulocytosis, leucopenia, hyperkalaemia, and a host of other, more minor problems.

*Contraindications.* These include breast-feeding, pregnancy and porphyria.

**Anastrozole** and **letrozole** are non-steroidal aromatase inhibitors and they prevent the production of estrogens. They are more specific than aminoglutethimide since they do not suppress adrenal cortisol production. They are used in the treatment of advanced breast cancer in postmenopausal women.

*Adverse effects* are usually minimal but they can cause thrombotic episodes.

**Exemestane** is a steroidal aromatase inhibitor. It is used for advanced breast cancer in postmenopausal women in whom tamoxifen has failed.

**Treatment of prostatic carcinoma with drugs.** Androgen receptor antagonists and GnRH agonists are used.

Prostatic carcinoma carries a poor prognosis with metastases, especially to bone, and traditionally the testes were removed to remove testosterone from the system (orchidectomy). Patients were also given the synthetic estrogen diethylstilbestrol, but this is associated with several adverse effects (see p. 344).

Subcapsular bilateral orchidectomy is still sometimes performed, but more recent developments in the understanding of pituitary function and the introduction of androgen receptor antagonists have brought newer drug treatments for this disease. Instead of orchidectomy, the patient may be given synthetic analogues of the hypothalamic hormone GnRH (gonadorelin), which normally stimulates luteinizing hormone (LH) release from the anterior pituitary (see also p. 172). If, however, GnRH is given as a continuous treatment, it shuts down the production of LH and therefore of testosterone (see McArdle et al 2002).

**Cyproterone acetate**, **flutamide** and **bicalutamide** block the actions of the male sex hormones (androgens) at their receptor sites. They are licensed to be used alone or with other treatments for prostate cancer. They should be prescribed before treating patients with GnRH agonists (see below), since GnRH agonists cause an initial large release of testosterone from the testes before shutting them down, and this burst of testosterone can exacerbate the cancer and even prove fatal for the patient.

*Adverse effects.* Androgen receptor antagonists can cause gynaecomastia and other problems associated with androgen lack, such as decreased libido and weight changes. Cyproterone acetate has been reported to cause direct hepatic failure in some patients after prolonged use, and patients should have blood counts and tests of hepatic function before and during treatment with these drugs. Other unwanted effects include hirsutism due to partial agonist activity, and nausea, vomiting and changes in appetite.

*Contraindications.* There are at the time of writing no contraindications for the use of cyproterone acetate in prostate cancer. With all three drugs, hepatic and adrenal impairment might pose problems and the patient should be tested for adrenal hepatic function before and during treatment.

For summaries of the hormonal treatment of prostate cancer see Debruyne (2002), Denis & Griffiths (2002) and Samson et al (2002).

## GnRH analogues

As mentioned above, these substances shut down pituitary production of luteinizing hormone, thus effectively shutting down testosterone production. Some are prescribed not only for prostate cancer but also for early estrogen receptor-positive breast cancer and advanced breast cancer.

*Therapeutic use.* **Buserelin** is administered as an injection or as a nasal spray. **Goserelin** is administered as an implant which is injected subcutaneously into the anterior abdominal wall. **Leuprorelin** is supplied as a microsphere powder for reconstitution and subcutaneous or intramuscular injection. **Triptorelin** is supplied as a microsphere powder for reconstitution and intramuscular injection.

---

### Safety note

As mentioned earlier, before these substances are administered to men with prostate cancer, the patient should first be given an androgen receptor antagonist such as flutamide or cyproterone acetate, for at least 3 days before the GnRH analogue. This is to prevent the sometimes fatal flare up that may result from the initial testosterone release caused by the GnRH analogue.

---

*Adverse effects.* The GnRH analogues all produce the typical effects of gonadectomy. In women these effects include the symptoms of menopause – hot flushes, sweating, vaginal dryness, changes in breast size and anorexia – and in men there may be gynaecomastia. In both sexes there may be sleep disorders and mood swings.

## IMMUNOTHERAPY

Several approaches to cancer chemotherapy involve drugs that affect the immune response. These include:

- **corticosteroids and other immunosuppressants**
- **interferons and interleukins.**

### Corticosteroids and other immunosuppressants

**Prednisolone** is a synthetic corticosteroid (a glucocorticoid) whose properties and adverse effects have already been discussed elsewhere in this book (see p. 205). This steroid has been and still is used to suppress the immune response in several autoimmune diseases, including rheumatoid arthritis, lupus, psoriasis and multiple sclerosis.

It is also used to suppress organ transplant rejection. It is useful in cancer because it causes tumour regression in some cancers, including hormone-responsive breast cancer, Hodgkin's disease, non-Hodgkin's lymphomas and lymphoblastic leukaemia.

Prednisolone is also useful as part of palliative care in end-stage malignant disease as it lifts the patient's mood and to some extent restores appetite.

**Ciclosporin** is a peptide originally isolated from a fungus, and is a very powerful immunosuppressant. Its discovery transformed organ transplantation since it significantly reduced both rejection and morbidity. It suppresses the immune system by binding to an intracellular protein called an immunophilin, and this reaction inhibits another intracellular protein called calcineurin, which normally activates the immune response.

*Therapeutic use.* Ciclosporin is administered either orally or by intravenous infusion. Absorption after oral administration is variable and sometimes poor.

*Adverse effects.* The drug is not myelotoxic but is toxic to the kidney (nephrotoxic). It may cause hypertension and hepatic toxicity. Other unwanted effects include hirsutism, gum hypertrophy, paraesthesia, which is a tingling sensation and tremor.

*Contraindications.* It is contraindicated in uncontrolled malignancy, infection or hypertension, and patients on ciclosporin should be monitored for renal function.

**Tacrolimus** is an antibiotic with a similar mechanism to that of ciclosporin in that it inhibits calcineurin and is also toxic to the kidneys. It is administered orally or by intravenous infusion. It can cause cardiomyopathy (any chronic disorder involving heart muscle). Patients on ciclosporin should be warned about driving a car as ciclosporin impairs performance.

**Sirolimus** is an immunosuppressant which does not inhibit calcineurin; it works by blocking the action of an important early mediator of the immune response called interleukin 2 (IL-2). It is used for renal transplantation. It is administered orally either in tablet or liquid form and the oral solution should be taken with at least 60 ml of water or orange juice, followed by another 120 ml in the same container to ensure the full dose is taken. Sirolimus is sometimes prescribed in conjunction with ciclosporin.

*Adverse effects* include hyperlipidaemia, arthralgia, acne, abdominal pain and diarrhoea.

*Contraindications* include pregnancy and breast-feeding, and it should be used with caution in patients with hepatic disease.

**Basiliximab** and **daclizumab** are both monoclonal antibodies directed against T lymphocytes, preventing them from proliferating. They are examples of the rapidly growing collection of biologic drugs that target the immune system. Both are administered by I.V. infusion, and, as with other infused proteins, patients need to be medically supervised during and for a while after infusion.

**Rituximab** and **alemtuzumab** are both monoclonal antibodies that block the lysis of B lymphocytes. Rituximab is used to treat diffuse large B cell non-Hodgkin's lymphoma in conjunction with other chemotherapeutic agents, and advanced follicular lymphoma that is resistant to other chemotherapies. Alemtuzumab is prescribed for patients with chronic lymphocytic leukaemia who have failed to respond to other treatments. Both drugs are administered by intravenous infusion under medical supervision, and patients may experience chills, fever, nausea and vomiting, and other infusion-related adverse effects. Prior to infusion, patients may be given antihistamines, analgesics and possibly also a corticosteroid, especially with rituximab. Rituximab should be used with caution in patients with heart disease.

### Interferons and interleukins

**Interferons** are substance produced by cells that are infected by viruses and they have the ability to suppress viral growth. There are three types of human interferon: alpha (from white blood cells), beta (from fibroblasts) and gamma (from lymphocytes). Interferon alpha has proven to be of some use in the treatment of cancer, rare hairy-celled leukaemia and certain solid tumours.

**Interleukins** are a family of proteins that are part of the control mechanisms of the immune response; a well-known example is IL-2 (see above). IL-2 is used clinically and is called **aldesleukin**, which is IL-2 prepared using recombinant DNA technology. It is used to treat metastatic renal cell carcinoma and is administered by subcutaneous injection. It is extremely toxic to several organs, including the thyroid, bone marrow, liver, kidney and brain.

## COMBINATION TREATMENT IN CANCER

In most forms of malignant disease which can be treated successfully by drugs, better results with less toxicity are achieved if several cytotoxic agents are combined in the course of treatment. Most regimes consist of repeated courses given at intervals of 1–2 weeks and extending over 6–12 months or even longer. This enables the malignant cells to be attacked at different stages in their cell cycle; also careful timing enables the normal cells of the body to recover while the malignant cells remain suppressed. Treatment is usually carried out in day units. As an example of a treatment which has been used for widespread lymphomas, the CHOP regime is shown below:

cyclophosphamide days 1 and 8
doxorubicin day 1
vincristine days 1 and 8
prednisolone daily for 5 days

The course is given in cycles of 3–4 weeks and repeated about six times.

Many combination regimes are being used in the treatment of various types of cancer. Among the malignant diseases which can nearly always be improved and quite often cured by chemotherapy are:

- various leukaemias, particularly acute lymphoblastic in children
- Hodgkin's disease
- non-Hodgkin's lymphomas (some types)
- testicular cancer
- ovarian cancer
- retinoblastoma
- chorioncarcinoma.

Other types of cancer can often be improved without effecting a cure; these include carcinoma of the breast and prostate, and myeloma. Chemotherapy may be combined with surgery or radiotherapy and the management of a patient is often an integral operation.

Although much cancer is still treated in general hospitals, it is preferable for this to be carried out in special units experienced in this type of work and such units are being widely established. In terms of nursing organization it requires frequent short-term admissions or special outpatient facilities and careful checks on the general health of the patient and the blood count. Oncology nurses are very highly trained to play an important role in specialist and non-specialist units.

## ADJUVANT TREATMENT

It is common experience that, although a malignant growth appears to have been totally removed, a recurrence may occur somewhere else in the body at a later date. This must mean that at the time of operation there was already a seedling deposit, and the object of adjuvant treatment is to give cytotoxic drugs after operation even if there is no evidence of spread to eradicate hidden small deposits which are particularly susceptible to drug treatment. For example, over half the women who have operative treatment for carcinoma of the breast will ultimately die from metastases, although these were not apparent at the time of operation. Results of trials in this condition have made it clear that adjuvant treatment improves the long-term prognosis in all age groups. The type of chemotherapy is determined by the age of the patient, the nature of the cancer cells and whether the axillary nodes are involved. It varies from tamoxifen given alone to postmenopausal low-risk patients, to polychemotherapy, perhaps combined with ovarian ablation, for high-risk younger patients. It must be remembered, however, that adjuvant treatment results in some patients receiving chemotherapy who in fact have no metastases and which is therefore unnecessary. This presents a difficult ethical problem. A similar strategy, which is being investigated, is to give chemotherapy before operation (primary treatment).

## PALLIATIVE CHEMOTHERAPY

In some types of advanced cancer, chemotherapy can relieve symptoms and prolong life, but is not curative. Most regimes have some side-effects and before embarking on palliative chemotherapy it is very important to weigh possible benefits against disadvantages. This will require a compassionate discussion with the patient and ascertaining the views of relatives, doctors and nursing staff and others who are involved. As with all chronic diseases much supportive care will be necessary, and, generally, such treatment should be given in specialist oncology units.

It is impossible to discuss the palliation of all the cancers in which this treatment is an option, but the group includes:

- carcinoma of the breast
- small cell carcinoma of the lung
- carcinoma of the ovary and cervix
- colorectal carcinoma
- carcinoma of the bladder
- head and neck cancer
- various lymphomas
- malignant melanoma.

## SOME PRACTICAL POINTS

### STORAGE OF DRUGS AND PREPARATION OF SOLUTIONS

Oncology units should have a pharmacist with special experience and expertise in handling cytotoxic drugs to advise and supervise others. Solutions for injection should be prepared in a designated area by:

- nurses who have received special training
- pharmacists
- medical staff.

Some of these substances are very irritant, and, in addition, can be highly dangerous if absorbed.

> **Nursing point**
>
> Although some cytotoxic drugs can be used for some time after the solutions have been prepared, it is usually best to discard all unused remnants at the end of the treatment session.

**The following precautions should be observed:**

- Wear plastic gloves and a plastic apron when making up solutions. If any of the drug splashes onto the skin it should be washed off immediately. Some of the drugs are irritant and there is always the risk of an allergic reaction.
- Wear protective spectacles to protect the eyes. If the drug comes into contact with the eyes, they should be washed out with water and further advice should be sought.
- Care should be taken to avoid absorbing the drug either systemically or by inhalation. Hands should be washed after preparing a drug (even when gloves are worn). Although at present there is no evidence that those who handle cytotoxic drugs are more liable to suffer long-term ill-effects, there are certainly no grounds for complacency and every care must be taken.
- Pregnant staff should not prepare cytotoxic solutions.
- If spillage occurs, it should be mopped up with absorbent paper, which must be disposed of properly, and the whole area washed down thoroughly.
- Waste material should be disposed of safely.

## ADMINISTRATION OF CYTOTOXIC DRUGS

In view of the possible danger when giving cytotoxic drugs, the following authorization should be applied and a **practical summary** is given below:

- Oral – no special restriction.
- I.M. or I.V. infusion: may be by a pump – nurses with special training.
- Intravenous bolus – nurse with special training or medical staff.
- Intrathecal or intra-arterial – medical staff.
- Never use the brachial vein for vesicant drugs.
- Use a No. 23 butterfly or a cannula (22–24) for intravenous administration.
- Vesicant drugs should be given into a fast-running infusion over at least 5 minutes. For patients with difficult veins or when frequent injections are given, a Hickman catheter/Portacath may be used.

## EXTRAVASATION OF CYTOTOXIC DRUGS ON INJECTION

Even if great care is taken, some leaking of the injected drug may occur around the vein and this can cause problems. **Vesicant drugs** carry a high risk of severe tissue necrosis if they extravasate. They are:

| | |
|---|---|
| chlormethine (mustine) | vinblastine |
| melphalan | doxorubicin |
| dactinomycin | vincristine |
| mitomycin | epirubicin |
| daunorubicin | vindesine. |

Bleomycin and ifosfamide are irritant drugs which cause pain but do not lead to tissue damage. For vesicants the following **practical summary** of the full extravasation procedure is given below:

1. The needle should be left *in situ*, the infusion stopped and as much as possible of the extravasated fluid removed.
2. The needle can now be removed.
3. Ice packs should be applied to the area.
4. The area should be kept cool for the next 24 hours and 1% hydrocortisone cream applied twice daily.
5. The episode and subsequent progress should be recorded in the patient's notes.
6. An expert should be consulted.
7. The area should be inspected after 24 hours and as often as necessary thereafter.

Policies may vary in different units and local policies and procedures should be available and strictly followed (see Pattison 2002).

Occasionally, necrosis occurs despite all the measures, and skin grafting may be required.

## VOMITING WITH CYTOTOXIC DRUGS

Many cytotoxic drugs cause the patient to vomit a few hours after administration (Table 26.1).

There is as yet no complete remedy for this troublesome adverse effect. A variety of regimes may be tried in an attempt to mitigate the symptoms and patients vary in their preference. It is usual to give cytotoxic drugs in the late evening so that the patient may sleep as much as possible through the period of nausea. For mildly or moderately emetic cytotoxic drugs, dexamethasone, prochlorperazine, domperidone or low-dose metoclopramide can be used. Combinations are often more effective and intravenous dexamethasone and metoclopramide initially, followed by both orally, is useful.

It is believed that the most severely emetic drugs (e.g. cisplatin) stimulate the 5-HT$_3$ receptors in the gastrointestinal tract and brainstem. Ondansetron, a 5-HT$_3$ antagonist, combined with dexamethasone given intravenously, immediately before treatment and followed by further doses of ondansetron, either orally or intravenously, or by dexamethasone with domperidone is the most effective anti-emetic for this type of cytotoxic drug.

Some patients, particularly towards the end of their course of treatment, become anxious and tense before treatment and may indeed vomit before receiving their drugs. This is a difficult problem. Lorazepam an hour before coming to hospital may be tried and sometimes psychiatric support with a desensitization programme helps.

**Table 26.1** Vomiting with cytotoxic drugs

| Severe | Moderate | Mild |
|---|---|---|
| Cisplatin | Cytarabine | Bleomycin |
| Cyclophosphamide (high dose) | Etoposide | Busulfan |
| Dacarbazine | Procarbazine | Chlorambucil |
| Daunorubicin | Vinblastine | Fluorouracil |
| Doxorubicin | | Melphalan |
| Lomustine | | Mercaptopurine |
| Chlormethine (mustine) | | Methotrexate |
| | | Vincristine |

## CARE OF THE MOUTH

Mouth ulceration may occur with many cytotoxic regimes. This is partially due to the direct effect of the drugs on the mucous membrane of the mouth. Also the general suppression of immunity, particularly of the leucocytes, encourages infection. This unpleasant complication can be minimized and a **practical summary** is given below:

• Before starting treatment, the patient should be seen by a dentist or dental hygienist and have any infections treated.

• If the white blood cell count drops or the mouth becomes sore, the patient should have nystatin pastilles (for candida) every 6 hours and *Corsodyl* mouth washes twice daily. Some units use fluconazole systemically.

• If ulceration develops, the pain can be relieved by *Difflam Oral Rinse*, which contains benzydamine, a local anaesthetic. The mouth is rinsed out every 3 hours with the undiluted solution. Lidocaine gel can also be applied to the painful area.

## ALOPECIA

Hair loss may occur with many cytotoxic drugs (particularly doxorubicin, etoposide and ifosfamide). It will recover, but causes embarrassment to patients. With doxorubicin ice-cold water caps applied to the scalp during treatment may decrease the loss, otherwise wigs may help, while other patients will prefer to put up with it. It is important to warn the patient of this problem before treatment is started.

## BONE MARROW SUPPRESSION AND INFECTION

Cytotoxic drugs (except bleomycin and vincristine) depress bone marrow function. This leads to a low white blood cell count and, sometimes, to low platelet and red blood cell counts usually after 7–10 days. As a result, immunity is suppressed and the patient is liable to develop an infection or to bleed. In addition to those caused by the usual bacteria, infections may be due to fungi, viruses and even organisms which do not normally cause disease in healthy people. Attempts have been made to diminish the risk of infection by isolating the patients, but this is difficult and, if strictly implemented, very expensive. In most cases it appears to be sufficient to avoid obvious sources of infection. Those caring for these people should always watch for signs of infection and the patients should be told to report any suspicious symptoms. Immunosuppressed patients often respond poorly to antibacterial treatment and the infecting organism may be obscure, so a combination of antibiotics is often used.

The extent and duration of the low blood count can be minimized by giving haemopoietic growth factor and this has proved a useful adjunct to the more intense courses of chemotherapy.

Sometimes very large doses of cytotoxic drugs are given in an attempt to eradicate a tumour which is poorly sensitive to chemotherapy and this will destroy the blood-forming cells in the bone marrow. In these circumstances, bone marrow is removed from the patient before starting treatment, or stem cells, which can form bone marrow, are harvested from the patient's peripheral blood and stored. After the chemotherapy is finished the stored cells are injected back into the patient to multiply and restock the bone marrow. This is a rather high-risk procedure with an appreciable morbidity and mortality, but potentially will extend the range of cancers which can be controlled or cured.

## LONG-TERM RISKS OF THE USE OF CYTOTOXIC DRUGS

Most cytotoxic drugs interfere in some way or other with the structure of the cell nucleus and this can have serious long-term implications.

### Second malignancy

These drugs may induce changes in normal cells so that they ultimately become malignant. This means that although the original cancer is eradicated, a different malignancy may develop at a later date. Second malignancies are more common after certain cytotoxic drugs and if drugs are combined with radiotherapy. It is necessary to put this risk in perspective, as the chance of dying from the initial cancer, if untreated, is much greater than that of developing a further cancer. Some information is now available as to the risk of second malignancies with various cytotoxic drugs and the situation is becoming increasingly well defined. This risk will be one factor to be considered when choosing a suitable regime.

### Gonadal damage

Many cytotoxic drugs damage the gonads. In men permanent sterility may result; in women amenorrhoea is common but periods usually return after stopping treatment. It is possible to store a man's sperm before treatment in case gonadal function is permanently suppressed.

## Teratogens

Most cytotoxic drugs are potentially teratogenic, especially in early pregnancy. If pregnancy is avoided during and for 6 months from the end of treatment, there does not seem to be an increased risk of an abnormal infant being born.

## THE ROLE OF THE NURSE IN CANCER CHEMOTHERAPY

The establishment of units specializing in oncology has enabled nurses to receive advanced training which is of direct benefit to patients and their families. A multidisciplinary approach is important in the treatment of cancer and the team will consist of nurses, doctors, pharmacists and social workers. In most centres part of the work will be concerned with therapeutic trials and this will require ancillary staff.

The management of malignant disease may be by chemotherapy alone or may involve surgery or radiotherapy. In this book only the problems of chemotherapy are considered. In addition to technical knowledge the nurse will have a most important role in patient support. The distress and fear of having cancer is enough to shake the stoutest heart and, indeed, chemotherapy is usually prolonged and often unpleasant.

In the initial assessment nurses should try to establish what patients know about malignant disease and their beliefs, if any, about treatment. They will appeal to the nurses for information and this provides an opportunity to dispel myths and at the same time explain what treatment will entail. Patient education is multifaceted and can take the form of booklets, videos, question and answer sessions and group discussions so that sufferers can gain support from others in similar circumstances. Patients usually attend oncology units at regular intervals for treatment and follow-up so it is possible for the nursing staff to build up a supportive relationship with those who know and trust them.

A good deal of research is in progress by oncology units to mitigate the unpleasantness of chemotherapy and one of the key areas that has been examined is the use of self-help measures at home.

## References

Clamp A, Danson S, Clemons M 2002 Hormonal risk factors for breast cancer: identification, chemoprevention, and other intervention strategies. Lancet Oncology 3: 611

Debruyne F 2002 Hormonal therapy of prostate cancer. Seminars in Urology and Oncology 20 (3 Suppl 1): 4

Denis L J, Griffiths K 2000 Endocrine treatment in prostate cancer. Seminars in Surgical Oncology 18: 52

Editorial 2002a Tamoxifen is treatment of choice for preventing breast cancer recurrence. Pharmaceutical Journal 268: 705

Editorial 2002b Tamoxifen prevents breast cancer, but are side effects outweighing benefits? Pharmaceutical Journal 268: 419

McArdle C A, Franklin J, Green L et al 2002 Signalling, cycling and desensitisation of gonadotrophin-releasing hormone receptors. Journal of Endocrinology 173: 1

Patterson S G, Balducci L, Pow Sang J M 2002 Controversies surrounding androgen deprivation for prostate cancer. Cancer Control 9: 315

Pattison J 2002 Managing extravasation. Nursing Times 98: 32

Samson D J, Seidenfeld J, Schmitt B et al 2002 Systematic review and meta-analysis of monotherapy compared with combined androgen blockade for patients with advanced prostate carcinoma. Cancer 95: 361

Van Outryve S, Schrijvers D, van den Brande J et al 2002 Methotrexate-associated liver toxicity in a patient with breast cancer: case report and literature review. Netherlands Journal of Medicine 60: 216

## Further reading

Editorial 1994 Immunosuppressing drugs and their complications. Drug and Therapeutics Bulletin 33: 66

Royal College of Nursing 1998 Practice Guidelines. The administration of cytotoxic chemotherapy

Chapter **27**

# Treatment of tropical and imported diseases; anthelmintics

## Learning objectives

At the end of this chapter, the reader should be able to:

- discuss the impact of modern air travel on the spread of tropical diseases
- describe the symptoms and treatment of tropical diseases that affect the gastrointestinal tract
- give an account of the cause and treatment of leprosy
- give an account of the cause, symptoms and use of drugs to suppress and treat malaria, and the limitations of treatment
- give an account of the protozoan infections such as leishmaniasis
- describe the treatments for the various worm infestations
- describe the precautions to take in order to reduce the chances of being bitten by flying insects, and provide sensible bite avoidance strategies

## INTRODUCTION

Tropical diseases, like their background, are inclined to be dramatic and florid. The majority are infective or due to dietary deficiency and in former times, and to some degree today, great epidemics have caused widespread disease with a very high death rate.

During the last 50 years the causative organisms of nearly all these diseases have been discovered and drugs have been devised which are capable of dealing with them. The problem of treating tropical disease is further complicated by the primitive conditions which prevail in many parts of the tropics and the lack of proper medical and nursing facilities. However, in spite of these difficulties, immense progress has been made in this sphere.

In recent years, air travel has brought tropical diseases much nearer home (Ryan et al, 2002). It is possible to catch malaria in Central Africa and not be taken ill until after arrival in London. Some knowledge of these disorders is therefore necessary even if the nurse does not intend to work in tropical countries. In this chapter, the consideration of tropical disease will be carried out under headings of the disease rather than the drug.

## THE DISEASES AND INFESTATIONS

### TRAVELLERS' DIARRHOEA

A holiday in tropical or subtropical countries is often interrupted by an attack of diarrhoea, colic and vomiting, which, although rarely severe, interferes with a few days' pleasure. It is believed that there is usually an infective cause and the organism most often implicated is an unusual variant of *Escherichia coli*.

Prevention should include care over drinking water and washing uncooked foods such as fruit and vegetables in chlorinated water. The prophylactic use of antibiotics is not recommended except for those at special risk (e.g. bowel disease) or if for social or business reasons diarrhoea must be avoided. In these cases **trimethoprim** or **doxycycline** are satisfactory. For the developed attack, **fluid replacement** with added **glucose** and **electrolytes** (e.g. *Dioralyte* or a similar preparation) is important. Symptoms can be improved with **loperamide,** which should not be given to children under 4 years. In severe cases trimethoprim twice daily or **ciprofloxacin** as a single dose is effective.

### AMOEBIC DYSENTERY

Amoebic dysentery is an infection of the lower bowel by an organism called *Entamoeba histolytica* and is characterized by chronic diarrhoea. Sometimes the infection spreads outside the bowel, particularly to the liver, where it causes an abscess.

The chief drug used in this infection is **metronidazole**, which is now the first choice in treating amoebic infection of the bowel and abscess

of the liver. A 5-day course is often sufficient (metronidazole is also used to treat the protozoan parasite *Trichomonas vaginalis*). Vomiting can be troublesome at the dose levels used to treat amoebic dysentery.

Metronidazole can be combined with **diloxanide furoate**, which is active against organisms in the bowel lumen, but not in the tissues. The combination appears to be even more efficient at eradicating the infection.

### GIARDIASIS

Giardiasis is due to the organism *Giardia lamblia*, which affects the intestine and causes distension, gas and frothy stools. Infection can occur in many parts of the world, and symptoms often develop on return from a holiday abroad. **Metronidazole** daily for 3 days is an effective treatment.

### BACILLARY DYSENTERY

This may be caused by a variety of organisms of the *Shigella* group. In mild cases, symptomatic treatment only is required and there is no evidence that antibiotics produce a more rapid cure. In severe cases the organism should be cultured and its sensitivity to antibiotics defined. If there is no time for culture, treatment may be started with **trimethoprim** twice daily. **Ciprofloxacin** is used if trimethoprim resistance is a problem. **Fluid** and **electrolyte** replacement is important.

### CHOLERA

Cholera is due to an organism, *Vibrio cholerae* which invades the intestine, producing severe and copious diarrhoea and vomiting. This leads to intense dehydration and sodium and potassium deficiency and is often fatal. The most important part of treatment is to replace the lost water and salts orally or by intravenous infusion.

The cholera vibrio is sensitive to **tetracycline** and **ciprofloxacin**, which can be used to eradicate the infection and shorten the course of the illness.

In developing countries, where this disease reaches epidemic proportions, large-scale intravenous infusion may be difficult. An important advance has been the discovery that if glucose is added to the electrolyte replacement solution and given orally, water and electrolytes are well absorbed and

I.V. infusion is less often required. The oral replacement solution contains:

sodium chloride 3.5 g
sodium citrate 2.9 g
potassium chloride 1.5 g
glucose 20 g
made up to 1 litre.

The volume given is titrated against the loss in the stools and by vomiting. Some authorities claim that a most readily available and suitable alternative fluid in all countries, provided no other alternatives are available, is in the form of proprietary diet colas such as *Coca-Cola* or *Pepsi-Cola*. (*Tip*: stay away from sugar when suffering from diarrhoea; sugar acts as a laxative.)

A cholera vaccine is available, but is of little use.

## LEPROSY

Leprosy is a disease of great antiquity and is referred to in the Bible. It is caused by the bacterium *Mycobacterium leprae*; these bacteria cause chronic infection of the skin, visceral nerves and other parts of the body. Leprosy has long resisted treatment, but in recent years the introduction of new drugs has made the outlook more hopeful.

*Mycobacterium leprae* can become resistant to the drugs used in treatment; therefore at least two antibacterial drugs should be given together to prevent this. Three drugs are used in leprosy at present: dapsone, clofazimine and rifampicin.

**Dapsone** is widely used. It is given orally, usually over long periods.

*Adverse effects* are uncommon, but include headaches, cyanosis, anaemia and blood dyscrasias.

**Clofazimine** is useful in treating leprosy and is combined with other agents. It is given orally over long periods.

*Adverse effects* are rare, but it may cause pigmentation of the skin.

**Rifampicin** is also effective against *Mycobacterium leprae*, although resistance may develop.

| Nursing point |
| --- |
| See the *BNF* for regimes to be followed for multibacillary leprosy. |

## MALARIA

Malaria has been known for thousands of years and is one of the most widespread diseases which attack humans. Although it is largely confined to tropical and subtropical zones, air travel has led to its increased frequency in this country. Malaria is most active in the broad band between the tropics. Increasing tourism to such areas has resulted in malaria presenting as a significant risk. Every year about 2000 travellers from the UK contract malaria and up to a dozen deaths occur as a result of infection. Over a third of such cases occur in those from ethnic groups resident in Britain who have returned to their country of origin for a visit.

Malaria is caused by a small organism called a plasmodium (Goodyer 2000b). There are three varieties of plasmodia which produce the commonly found varieties of human malaria. They are:

- *Plasmodium vivax*, which causes benign tertian malaria
- *Plasmodium malariae*, which causes quartan malaria
- *Plasmodium falciparum*, which causes malignant tertian malaria.

These plasmodia are injected into the bloodstream of its human victim by the mosquito. They are carried to the liver where they go through a stage of division known as the exo-erythrocyte stage. After a short period some plasmodia enter the red cells of the bloodstream. Here they divide in a simple asexual fashion to form more plasmodia, which rupture the red cells and then re-enter further red cells: the breaking up of the red cells corresponds with the rise of temperature with rigor and later sweating which is so characteristic of the disease.

Other plasmodia which have entered the red cells form male and female gametes. These may be sucked out by the mosquito when it bites, and they then continue the cycle in the infected mosquito. The cycle is shown graphically in Figure 27.1.

### Drugs used to treat malaria

The drugs which are effective in treating malaria may be divided into two groups:

- drugs which act on the asexual stage of the malarial parasite in the blood – quinine, chloroquine, proguanil, halofantrine, mefloquine and pyrimethamine
- drugs which act on the exo-erythrocyte stage in the liver and the gametocytes – primaquine.

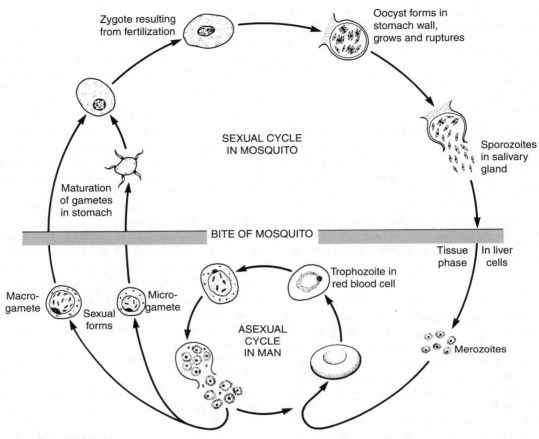

**Figure 27.1** The malarial cycle.

**Quinine** is described first, because it was the first effective remedy. It is one of the alkaloids obtained from the bark of the cinchona tree and has been known to be effective against 'fever' for several hundred years.

For some years it was largely replaced by newer antimalarial drugs, but is now proving very useful in *Plasmodium falciparum* infection when it is resistant to other drugs.

Quinine is given either orally or intravenously. It is well absorbed from the intestine. It suppresses the multiplication of the plasmodia in the bloodstream. It does not, however, have any effect on the gametes or exo-erythrocyte stages of the malarial life cycle and thus symptoms may recur when quinine is stopped.

Quinine has a number of other actions. It has a depressing action to the heart similar to that of quinidine; it is also said to cause contraction of the uterus and should, therefore, be avoided in pregnancy. It is sometimes used in the treatment of muscle cramps.

*Adverse effects* are common with quinine; the syndrome produced is known as cinchonism. This may occur with large doses. Some people, however, are hypersensitive to the drug and develop toxic effects after small amounts; the chief symptoms are vertigo, tinnitus, deafness and visual disturbances. In addition, it can cause delirium, haemolytic anaemia, thrombocytopenia and renal failure.

### Nursing point

If quinine is given intravenously, which is required in fulminating malignant tertiary malaria, it should be given as quinine dihydrochloride.

**Chloroquine** is a most useful drug to treat malaria, but resistant strains of *P. falciparum* are common.

It can be given orally, intramuscularly or intravenously. It is rapidly absorbed and is stored in various organs of the body, part being destroyed and part excreted in urine. It is effective against the asexual forms of the plasmodia in the bloodstream, but has no effect on the gametes or on the exo-erythrocyte stages. Strains of malaria resistant to chloroquine have appeared in South-east Asia, South America and Central and East Africa.

*Adverse effects* are rare, but include nausea and headaches, and, as chloroquine may cause fetal damage, it should not be used during pregnancy.

**Mefloquine** is effective against chloroquine-resistant *P. falciparum* and is used in parts of the world where this is common. It is excreted very slowly so a single or divided doses once weekly, but not for more than 1 year, is used.

*Adverse effects* of nausea and giddiness are fairly common. Psychotic disturbances, including hallucinations, panic attacks and depression, can occur and the patient should be warned of this possibility. Mefloquine should not be used during pregnancy or in people with epilepsy.

**Halofantrine** can be used to treat resistant infection due to *P. falciparum* but, owing to adverse effects, it has fallen from favour.

**Artemisinin** and its derivatives are obtained from sweet wormwood; they originated in China. They appear to be rapidly effective in treating severe *P. falciparum* infections, either alone or combined with other antimalarials, and are given by injection, although oral and rectal routes are possible. They are not yet generally available in the UK.

**Atovaquone** acts against the three types of malaria, but if used alone relapses are common. However, when combined with proguanil it is effective both in treating *P. falciparum* malaria and also as a prophylactic.

**Proguanil** is given by mouth. It is rapidly absorbed but disappears rapidly from the bloodstream. It is effective against the bloodstream asexual phase of the plasmodia and also has some action against the gametocytes and against the exo-erythrocyte stage of *P. falciparum*. It is, however, slower at relieving an acute attack of malaria than chloroquine and, furthermore, resistant strains of plasmodia have been encountered. Toxicity is very low.

Proguanil is very slow in its antimalarial action and it is therefore largely used as a suppressant.

**Doxycycline** is effective against resistant *P. falciparum* and has been used with success in the Far East. It should be taken after meals with copious fluids.

**Pyrimethamine** is effective against the asexual bloodstream phase of the malarial parasite but is too slow to be used in treating an acute attack. Owing to the emergence of resistant strains it is now only used in combination, e.g. pyrimethamine + sulfadoxine (*Fansidar*).

It can be seen that all the drugs so far described, with the possible partial exception of proguanil, while effectively suppressing the asexual bloodstream phase of the malaria organism and relieving acute symptoms, are ineffective against the exo-erythrocyte stage in the liver and against the gametocytes. This is particularly important when the malaria is caused by *P. vivax* or *P. malariae*, as a relapse may occur on stopping treatment. In these types of malaria the initial treatment should be followed by a drug which acts against the parasites in the exo-erythrocyte stage.

**Primaquine** is effective against the exo-erythrocyte stage and against the gametocytes. It is not free from toxic effects and may produce nausea and vomiting. It is not used alone in the treatment of the acute malarial attack, but may follow treatment of *P. vivax* with chloroquine, when it is particularly valuable in eradicating benign tertian malaria. Relapses will not occur unless there is re-infection.

Before starting treatment it is important to test the patient for G6PD deficiency, an inherited disorder of the red blood cells which results in severe haemolysis with primaquine and some other drugs.

### The treatment of malaria

It is impossible to give precise instruction as to the best drug or drugs in the treatment of malaria as this is always changing and may also vary with different forms of malaria infection.

It must be realized that there are two possible ways in which malaria may be attacked by drugs:

- suppressive
- treatment of established disease.

**Suppressive\*.** Suppressive treatment means the regular administration of a drug to prevent the clinical manifestation of the disease.

The best drug for this purpose varies in different parts of the world. This is because the widespread use of antimalarial drugs has led to the development of resistant strains of *P. falciparum*, particularly in South-east Asia, but also in South America and

---

\* Full details are given in the *British National Formulary*.

parts of Africa. It is wise to obtain up-to-date advice before travelling.

The chosen drug must be started 1 week (2 weeks for mefloquine) before entering the malarial area and continued for 1 month after leaving it. In addition, precautions should be taken against mosquito bites, including the use of nets at night, as drug prophylaxis is not totally effective (see also below). Travellers in highly malarious areas who are likely to be remote from medical care should take an emergency treatment kit.

**Treatment of established disease.** The really dangerous type of malaria is caused by *P. falciparum*, which may prove fatal unless treated rapidly. Strains from many parts of the world are resistant to one or more antimalarial drugs and it is safest to regard all *P. falciparum* infections as chloroquine-resistant.

Recommendations for prevention and treatment are always changing and nurses are advised to seek up-to-date advice from the Travel Clinic of the Hospital for Tropical Disease: Tel (020) 7388 9600.

## LEISHMANIASIS (KALA-AZAR)

There are several varieties of kala-azar caused by closely related organisms. These organisms may invade the spleen, liver, lymph glands and bone marrow, producing a generalized disease with constitutional symptoms or a local ulcerative lesion. It may complicate HIV infection.

Leishmaniasis is caused by a small protozoan organism transmitted by the bite of a sandfly. It is found in Africa, South America and the Mediterranean. It is often missed by physicians who are unused to meeting the condition. Relatively few cases are reported annually in travellers from the UK.

The most useful drugs for treating leishmaniasis are those which contain antimony. They are believed to interfere with enzymes within the parasite.

**Sodium stibogluconate** given intravenously for 20 days is usually adequate. Sometimes it may be necessary to repeat courses at intervals of 2 weeks. The patient usually responds within 2 weeks and should be restored to full health within 2 months.

*Adverse effects* include irritation at the site of injection, muscle aches and cardiotoxicity with arrhythmias.

**Paromomycin**, an antibiotic, is also effective, either alone or combined with sodium stibogluconate.

*Adverse effects* are uncommon but include ototoxicity.

## SCHISTOSOMIASIS (BILHARZIASIS)

This disease is caused by flukes which inhabit the veins of the bladder and the lower bowel, leading to haematuria and rectal bleeding.

**Praziquantel** has now emerged as the most useful drug. It is effective against all types of the disease and, unlike formerly used drugs, it appears free from serious adverse effects.

## ANTHELMINTICS

Anthelmintics are drugs which are used to treat worm infestations. Although such infestations, with the possible exception of threadworms, are not common in this country, they may occur in immigrants, being endemic in some regions of the world, and are of great medical and economic importance. The anthelmintics are a diverse group of substances with widely differing properties and they will be described under the headings of the type of infestation they are used to treat.

## THREADWORMS

Threadworms (*Enterobius vermicularis*) appear like short lengths of thread. They live in the caecal region of the gut and the females migrate to the anus, where they lay eggs and provoke intense itching. The resulting scratching leads to the hands becoming contaminated with eggs, which may then be transferred to food, and thus further infestation occurs.

General cleanliness and scrubbing of the nails before meals is important in treating this disorder.

It must be remembered that the whole family of an infected patient must be examined for infestation as it is common to find several members of a family harbouring worms, and re-infection will occur unless the worms are eradicated from the whole family.

**Mebendazole** as a single dose is effective. It should not be given to children under 2 years or during pregnancy and, rarely, it causes nausea and diarrhoea. A second dose can be given after 3 weeks as re-infection is common. It is available without prescription.

**Piperazine** is effective in treating threadworm infections and is not liable to produce side-effects. It is conveniently prepared as an elixir. A dose should be given for a week followed by a week's rest and then a further week's treatment if necessary.

*Pripsen* sachets containing piperazine and sennosides are also available.

*Adverse effects* are rare, but it should not be used in patients with epilepsy, during pregnancy or in patients with peptic ulcers. It may cause gastrointestinal upsets and rashes.

## STRONGYLOIDES STERCORALIS

This worm, which is common in the tropics, lives in the intestines. The larvae of *Strongyloides stercoralis* can penetrate the anal skin and thus reinfect the host, so infection can last for a long time. Usually they only cause mild intestinal symptoms, but if the patient is immunosuppressed (i.e. given large doses of steroids or has HIV disease) widespread penetration of the bowel occurs, which may be fatal.

**Tiabendazole** twice daily for 3 days is effective, but side-effects of nausea and drowsiness are common. It should not be used during pregnancy.

## TAPEWORMS

There are two common types of tapeworm, *Taenia solium* and *Taenia saginata*. Both these worms inhabit the small intestine of humans where they may reach several feet in length. They consist of a head which is embedded in the wall of the intestine and a body consisting of a large number of segments. These segments, which contain eggs, are shed and pass out in the faeces.

The eggs may then infect an animal host, which is the pig in the case of *Taenia solium* and the bullock in the case of *Taenia saginata*. In the animal's gastrointestinal tract the larval form is released and migrates via the bloodstream throughout the body where it remains until the animal is killed; the meat is eaten by humans and reinfection occurs.

There are several drugs which can be used to treat tapeworms, the most effective being **niclosamide**. No preparation is required. In the morning the drug is chewed and swallowed on an empty stomach. After 1 hour the dose is repeated. This is followed 3 hours later by a saline purge. In *Taenia solium* infestation a more powerful purge should be used as it is important to clear all the ova from the gut. Treatment may be preceded by **metoclopramide** to minimize the risk of vomiting.

The drug appears very free of side-effects and acts by actually killing the worm.

Alternatively, a single dose of **praziquantel** is effective.

## ROUNDWORMS

The roundworm (*Ascaris lumbricoides*) is similar to a pale-coloured earthworm. It lives in the small intestine and its eggs are passed out in the faeces. If reinfection occurs, the larval forms are liberated in the gastrointestinal tract and pass via the bloodstream to the lungs. They then migrate up the trachea to the pharynx and are swallowed, thus completing the cycle.

**Piperazine** is useful for treating roundworms. It paralyses the muscle of the worm, which is passed through the faeces alive via the rectum. A single dose of the elixir for an adult is effective and should be repeated after 14 days. Alternatively, one *Pripsen* sachet (containing piperazine + sennosides) may be used, the purgative helping to clear the bowel of worms.

**Mebendazole** twice daily for 3 days is an alternative.

## HOOKWORM

The hookworm, although not seen in this country, is extremely common in tropical and subtropical countries in both the Old and New World.

This worm lives in the small intestine of humans; the fertilized eggs are passed out in the faeces and develop into larvae in the soil. The larvae penetrate the skin and pass via the bloodstream to the lung. Here they enter the bronchial tree and migrate to the intestinal tract via the trachea. Severe infestation can cause iron deficiency anaemia.

**Mebendazole** twice daily for 3 days is effective. It should not be used during pregnancy or for children under 2 years old.

## FILARIASIS

The parasitic worms *Loa Loa*, which cause subcutaneous swellings, and *Wuchereria bancrofti*, another filarial parasite which causes elephantiasis, may be eradicated by diethylcarbamazine.

## PREPARATIONS AND BITE AVOIDANCE
### (See also Goodyer 2000a,c)

Sensible precautions can be taken to minimize contraction of disease transmitted through drinking water, food and insect bites, especially if one knows some of the habits of the insects whose bite one wishes to avoid. In general:

● Prepare for the trip by getting all necessary vaccinations, and if a trip to a malaria-infested area is planned, take the necessary drugs. Take medical advice well before the trip.

● Take water-purifying tablets to countries whose water is likely to be contaminated, and drink only bottled water if available.

● Ascertain whether rivers, dams and pools have bilharzias before swimming, especially in Africa.

● Reduce exposure to insects through knowledge of their behaviour and what attracts a bite.

● Use insect repellents on the skin.

● Use insecticides impregnated into materials clothing, tents and nets.

● Use contact insecticides, i.e. knock-down sprays or burners/mats.

## MOSQUITOES

● Don't wear dark clothing, which attracts mosquitoes.

● Powerful perfumes and other strong smells attract mosquitoes.

● *Anopheles* mosquitoes carry malaria, and are most active in the early evening and at night.

● Wear long-sleeved, loose-fitting clothing, especially at and after sunset.

● Apply insect repellents to the skin.

● Be aware that women are bitten more than men.

● Ensure that mosquito nets are not torn and are sprayed with an insect repellent.

● Some guides insist that a cut tomato placed in the sleeping area at night draws mosquitoes away from human targets.

## SANDFLIES

● Sandflies can pass through mosquito nets, so the nets should be treated with an insecticide.

● Sandflies fly low, so it is best to sleep high up, e.g. on the upper floors.

## References

Goodyer L 2000a Bite avoidance. The Pharmaceutical Journal 264: 298
Goodyer L 2000b Malaria. The Pharmaceutical Journal 264: 405
Goodyer L 2000c Tropical disease and the traveller. The Pharmaceutical Journal 264: 812

Ryan E T, Wilson M E, Kain K C 2002 Illness after international travel. New England Journal of Medicine 347: 505

## Further reading

Bergquist N R 2002 Schistosomiasis: from risk assessment to control. Trends in Parasitology 18: 309
Driver C 2002 What is malaria? Nursing Times 98: 34

Hainsworth T 2002 Travel health: reducing the risks. Nursing Times 98: 35

# Chapter 28

# Drugs and the eye

## Learning objectives

At the end of this chapter, the reader should be able to:

- reproduce the drawing of the eye given here
- list the different types of local preparations used in the eye
- recognize that antibiotics are used in the eye and list some of the more common infections treated
- recognize that antiviral agents are used in the eye and list some of the infections treated
- explain what is meant by protozoan infections and how they are treated
- list some steroids used topically in the eye
- explain what is meant by mydriasis and miosis and give examples of drugs that produce these, and their uses in the eye
- describe the types of glaucoma and how it is treated with drugs
- give an account of the local anaesthetics used in the eye
- recognize that stains are used in the eye and explain why they are used
- explain how some commonly prescribed drugs can have adverse effects on the eye

## STRUCTURE OF THE EYE

The structure of the eye and orbit are shown in Figure 28.1.

## TYPES OF DRUGS USED

The following types of drug are in frequent use in the treatment of eye disorders:

- antibiotics
- steroids and other anti-inflammatory drugs
- those which affect pupil size
- those used in the treatment of glaucoma
- local anaesthetics
- stains
- miscellaneous preparations.

Drugs can be administered to the eye either by local or systemic routes.

## LOCAL USE OF DRUGS ON THE EYE – TYPES OF APPLICATIONS

The following preparations are used in the local treatment of eye diseases:

- eye lotions
- eye drops
- eye ointments
- subconjunctival injections
- ampoules for injection into the anterior chamber at operation.

Whenever administering local preparations to the eye it is of paramount importance to ensure that the eye to receive treatment is clearly designated. Often only one eye is to be treated or the two eyes are to be treated differently. For example, after an operation for angle closure glaucoma in one eye it

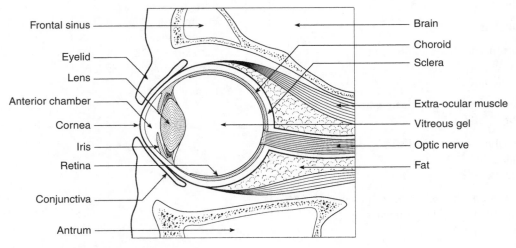

**Figure 28.1** Cross-sectional anatomy of eye and orbit.

Labels: Frontal sinus, Eyelid, Lens, Anterior chamber, Cornea, Iris, Retina, Conjunctiva, Antrum, Brain, Choroid, Sclera, Extra-ocular muscle, Vitreous gel, Optic nerve, Fat

may be necessary to dilate the pupil with drugs called mydriatics. Such treatment given to the other eye could be disastrous.

## EYE LOTIONS PRESCRIBED AS COLLYRIUM

These are used to wash foreign material from the eye and some have a mild antiseptic action. They are applied from an undine, which is a small glass container with a fine spout and which resembles a miniature chemistry retort. In an emergency, however, if a little jug is at hand it will serve as well and may save vital minutes in treating a contaminated eye.

The patient should lie back or sit in a chair with the head extended. The lotion should be warmed to 35°C (95°F), and before washing the eye the lotion should be run up the cheek into the medial canthus, the lids being firmly separated by the fingers and a small basin held by the patient close to his face to catch the effluent. This is less unpleasant than pouring the lotion directly onto the cornea. The lotion should be steadily poured from the undine, the patient being instructed to move the eyes in all directions.

There are many types of lotion, but simple normal saline is satisfactory for the removal of foreign material or dirt from the eye. In emergency cases, however, as in chemical contamination, it is better to use cold tap water than to lose time in starting the treatment.

In cases of contamination by lime or cement an irrigation with dihydrogen sodium versenate is recommended. This substance is a chelating agent and converts an insoluble heavy metal salt such as calcium hydroxide into a soluble complex anion which can be removed in solution.

## EYE DROPS PRESCRIBED AS GUTTAE

A number of drugs can be applied to the eyes by means of drops which should be instilled into the lower conjunctival sac. The patient is told to look upwards away from the dropper and the lower lid is held down with the finger. One drop only is instilled into the lower fornix and the patient is then told to close their eye for a short while and the excess is wiped away.

All drops and ointment should be sterile when supplied and once opened can no longer be considered so. There is an increasing tendency for them to be dispensed in single dose containers which can be discarded after use. This is particularly useful for patients who require medication over long periods and who may develop sensitivity to benzalkonium chloride, the preservative present in most eye drops.

---

### Nursing point

Drugs or preservatives in eye drops may become absorbed into hydrophilic contact lenses and cause irritation. Therefore, lenses should be removed before eye drops are instilled and not worn again until the treatment is finished. Similarly, contact lenses should not be used with eye ointments.

---

## EYE OINTMENTS PRESCRIBED AS OCULENTUM

These can be applied similarly either on a glass rod or from a single dose container; the lower lid is pulled down and the ointment is placed in the lower fornix. About half an inch of ointment as squeezed from the tube should be used at each application. This should be delivered onto the end of a sterile glass rod or a prepacked plastic spatula. A separate applicator should be used for each eye if both are to be treated.

## SUBCONJUNCTIVAL INJECTIONS

This method of application is used to obtain immediately a high concentration of a drug in the anterior chamber. This would be appropriate in the treatment of an acute intra-ocular infection. This treatment is painful and the eye must first be thoroughly anaesthetized by the instillation of several drops of local anaesthetic. Injection is made with a hypodermic syringe and a fine needle. Some drugs are manufactured in a depot form and are bound to a base substance from which they are released slowly. For example *Depo-Medrone* (methyl prednisolone acetate) can be used as a steroid preparation for the local treatment of iridocyclitis (inflammation of the iris and ciliary body). It is given as a subconjunctival injection and its action is continuous over a period of 3–4 days.

## INTRACAMERAL ADMINISTRATION

In certain disorders, it may be desirable to achieve high therapeutic concentrations of antibiotic drugs with a minimum of delay. This calls for delivery of the drug directly into the globe of the eye, either into the anterior chamber or the vitreous cavity.

**Anterior chamber administration** is frequently used during cataract operations when, to constrict the pupil, the iris is irrigated directly with *Miochol-E*, which is an acetylcholine preparation. In severe intra-ocular infections – for example, postoperative endophthalmitis (inflammation within the eye, usually due to infection) – it may be necessary to remove a sample of the vitreous humour for bacteriological examination. It is then expeditious to inject the vitreous cavity with broad-spectrum antibiotics. Several modern antibiotics can be used in this way, although care is needed to avoid any toxic effects on the delicate intra-ocular structures such as the retina. Consequently, the injections need to be carefully prepared and used only in the recommended dosage, and administration should generally be under sterile theatre conditions.

## ANTIBIOTICS USED IN THE EYE

The following antibiotics are used:

- chloramphenicol
- ofloxacin
- tetracyclines
- penicillins
- sodium fusidate
- vancomycin
- ceftazidime
- amikacin
- amphotericin
- cefazolin
- ciprofloxacin.

Antibiotics are used to treat a wide range of eye infections and they may be administered in three ways:

- Drops are satisfactory for superficial inflammation such as conjunctivitis, but rapid dilution occurs because of the tears. The drops should be instilled at 2-hourly intervals at least if a reasonable concentration of antibiotic is to be maintained.
- Ointments release the antibiotic more slowly and their action is helped by the eye being covered.
- Subconjunctival injection is the best way of ensuring a rapid and high concentration of antibiotic within the anterior ocular segment. The maximum volume which can be injected at one time is 1.0–1.5 ml.

Although, owing to the accessibility of the eye, diseases of the anterior segment can usually be effectively treated by means of the local administration of drugs, for those diseases which affect the posterior part, or the deeper intra-ocular structures, systemic administration is generally necessary.

Eye infections may be due to a variety of agents, both bacterial and viral. The correct antibiotic can be selected as a result of clinical observation and bacterial or viral studies.

The aminoglycosides and chloramphenicol are widely used in the treatment of superficial eye infections. They are active against a broad spectrum of bacteria and are particularly suitable for local administration as this avoids systemic toxicity. They include:

- **chloramphenicol 0.5% drops or 1.0% ointment**
- **fusidic acid eye drops 1% in gel base**
- **neomycin 0.5% drops and ointment**
- **gentamicin 0.3% drops**
- **ampoules of gentamicin sulphate 40 mg/ml for subconjunctival injection**.

These drugs are active against both Gram-positive and Gram-negative organisms.

> **Nursing point**
>
> The use of chloramphenicol has been questioned on account of its tendency to cause blood dyscrasias when given systemically. The evidence that these can arise as a result of local administration to the eye is still far from conclusive. Chloramphenicol remains in general use as it is by far the most effective drug for short-term use in bacterial infections of the eye and for prophylaxis. Fusidic acid, which is used as a substitute, can be effective, especially against staphylococci.

**Ofloxacin**, a member of the quinolone group, has a broader spectrum of antibacterial action than chloramphenicol and other commonly used antibiotics. It has fewer local side-effects than gentamicin and appears to have a similar spectrum of activity. It rivals chloramphenicol as a general prophylactic antibiotic.

**The tetracyclines** are wide-spectrum antibiotics against bacteria which also show activity against certain viruses and *Rickettsia*, particularly those causing trachoma. Tetracycline is available as a 1% ointment and its use together with systemic administration has helped to bring this widespread and blinding condition under control.

Two ocular disorders which respond well to prolonged administration of systemic tetracycline in low dosage are chronic staphylococcal blepharitis (inflammation of the eyelid margins) and ocular involvement in cutaneous acne rosacea.

**Contraindications.** Tetracyclines are contraindicated in young patients before eruption of the second dentition as the permanent teeth can be discoloured. The same caution must apply in administration during pregnancy.

Antibiotics of the **penicillin** group are rarely, if ever, used as local eye applications as they have a marked tendency to cause allergic reactions. However, they have an important place in the treatment of spreading infections of the eyelids, which are commonly of staphylococcal origin (provided the infection has not developed resistance). In such cases the infection is deep in the tissues, requiring systemic rather than local administration. In general, a broad-spectrum penicillin is best, but if the infection is acquired in hospital one of the penicillinase-resistant types is preferable.

**Sodium fusidate** is particularly active against penicillin-resistant staphylococci. It has the property of being concentrated in bone and other connective tissues, including the sclera of the eye and the vitreous, and is therefore useful in treating intra-ocular infections, especially those acquired in the operating theatre, which can often be due to resistant organisms. Fusidic acid is also used as eye drops in gel which liquefies on contact with the conjunctiva for a variety of superficial infections. Frequently after major intra-ocular operations, antibiotics are injected subconjunctivally.

Prophylaxis against postoperative infection is gaining importance in the face of a growing trend for major surgery, in particular for cataract, to be performed on an outpatient basis. For this purpose **gentamicin** is often used. This drug, however, causes a degree of toxic damage to the periocular tissues. **Cefuroxime** has recently proved less troublesome in this respect.

## BACTERIAL CONJUNCTIVITIS

Conjunctivitis is a common complaint with various causes. The bacterial infection is usually by *Streptococcus pneumoniae* or, more rarely, staphylococci.

Treatment is with chloramphenicol eye drops, every 4 hours, but more florid infections may require more frequent application. Chloramphenicol ointment may be used at night. The alternative is fusidic acid eye drops twice daily.

## ACUTE INTRA-OCULAR INFECTIONS

In acute bacterial infection of the eye much of the damage occurs as a result of the inflammatory response rather than the direct activity of the bacteria. Consequently, it is important to use steroids at the same time as effective antibiotics.

A particular problem exists in severe intra-ocular infections such as those following eye surgery. It is essential that vigorous antibiotic and anti-inflammatory treatment is started without delay. Otherwise, if the eye is not completely destroyed, it may well lose all useful vision. As time cannot be allowed to obtain the results of bacterial investigations before commencing treatment, a combination of broad-spectrum antibiotics and steroids can be used by both subconjunctival and systemic routes and even by direct intravitreal injection, together with a mydriatic (a drug that causes the pupil to dilate). The ophthalmologist should be consulted for the combinations and doses to be used.

Systemic administration of antibiotics can be either orally or by injection. Their use may be indicated in spreading infections involving the eye, the eyelids and ocular adnexa (adnexa means adjoining parts) such as the lacrimal sac. Sepsis around the eye, in particular in the vicinity of the internal angular vein, is of particular clinical importance as it may lead to a septic cavernous sinus thrombosis.

## OTHER ANTIBIOTICS*

In certain severe cases of intra-ocular infection the following antibiotics have been used successfully when injected directly into the vitreous. Preparations of a suitable strength for intraocular injection are not available yet and the following method of dilution has been devised at Moorfields Eye Hospital.

**Vancomycin** is effective against Gram-positive bacteria. The injection should contain 1.0 mg dissolved in 0.05 ml of injectable saline and should be prepared as follows. A vial containing 500 mg vancomycin is reconstituted in 8 ml normal saline. The entire contents are then withdrawn and made up to

---

*Some of these antibiotic preparations are only available in specialist units and hospitals.

10 ml, giving a concentration of 50 mg/ml. A volume of 2 ml of this solution is returned to the vial and is further diluted by the addition of 3 ml of normal saline, resulting in a concentration of 20 mg/ml. The therapeutic volume of 0.05 ml, containing 1 mg, is withdrawn into an insulin syringe for intravitreal injection.

**Ceftazidime** is active against Gram-negative organisms and can be used simultaneously with vancomycin. The therapeutic dose is 2 mg in 0.1 ml, which is the same concentration as for vancomycin and the injection is prepared similarly.

**Amikacin** treats infections from a wide spectrum of Gram-negative organisms, but its toxicity to the intra-ocular tissues precludes more than one injection.

**Amphotericin** is used to treat fungal infections such as *Candida*.

Several more recently developed antibiotics have been used systemically to supplement the effect of those given by intravitreal injection: chief among these is **cefazolin**, which, with few exceptions, is effective against Gram-positive organisms that are sensitive to methicillin.

**Ciprofloxacin** is used to treat a wide range of Gram-negative organisms and is similarly effective against many Gram-positive types.

## ANTIVIRAL AGENTS

Antiviral agents comprise:

- idoxuridine
- idoxuridine in dimethyl sulfoxide (*Herpid*)
- aciclovir
- trifluorothymidine (F3T).

Many eye infections are due to a virus. To mention some of the more common ones, herpes simplex, adenovirus and herpes zoster are all infections that are frequently seen clinically.

**Idoxuridine** was the first generally available antiviral agent and it was and still is effective against the herpes simplex virus that causes dendritic ulceration of the cornea. This drug was available for ocular application under the name of *Kerecid* but is now withdrawn.

A similar preparation called **Herpid** is available for general cutaneous treatment, for example in herpes zoster (shingles). One warning, however: *Herpid* contains dimethyl sulfoxide, which aids cutaneous absorption, but which causes cataracts if applied in the region of the eye. It must therefore never be used to treat the eyes or eyelids.

Idoxuridine acts as a competitive inhibitor in that it competes with other nucleosides used to build viral genetic material, and synthesis is halted. For this reason to be effective the concentration in the conjunctival sac has to be maintained at a high level. Prolonged use of idoxuridine has led to unwanted toxic effects on the corneal epithelial cells and although it is still mentioned in the *BNF* its value is considered dubious.

As a treatment for ocular herpes simplex infections, the more recently developed **aciclovir** has become the drug of choice. It is highly effective when applied in the form of a 3% ointment five times daily and has minimal, if any, toxic effects. Its action can be supplemented by oral administration and this may well be helpful in cases of herpes simplex keratitis which have been previously treated in error with preparations containing steroids, which greatly reduce the rate of healing.

**Herpes zoster** may affect the eye, especially when it involves the naso-ciliary branch of the ophthalmic division of the trigeminal nerve. Provided that treatment is commenced at the first appearance of the vesicular rash, aciclovir can significantly reduce the severity of this distressing disorder. For this purpose, however, higher doses are required. When successful, it shortens the time before cutaneous healing occurs and materially reduces the pain in the acute stage and also the post-herpetic pain which often lasts for many years after healing has taken place.

As an antiviral drug **trifluorothymidine** shows good activity against herpes simplex. Its main use, however, is against the adenovirus which causes an unpleasant and prolonged acute conjunctivitis, often with corneal involvement which to some extent affects vision, albeit temporarily. In these cases it is the drug of choice as none of the other antiviral drugs has an effect on this virus. It is not readily available, but can often be obtained from the pharmacy of specialist eye hospitals. It is not a particularly stable preparation and must be freshly prepared and kept refrigerated.

## ANTIPROTOZOAN DRUGS

### ONCHOCERCIASIS

Onchocerciasis is a protozoan infection of the eye which is not uncommon in some tropical countries in Africa and South America. This disease is spread by flies which transfer the microfilariae from one human host, who harbours the adult worms in cutaneous nodules, to another individual in whom they spread throughout the body. In the eye they set up inflammation in both the superficial and deeper tissues. Typically they can be seen with a microscope, swimming in the aqueous humour. The drug of choice for treating this disorder is **ivermectin**, which is a semi-synthetic macro-cyclic lactone. At the time of writing it is still available only from the manufacturer on a named-patient basis.

## ACANTHAMOEBA KERATITIS

Since the generalized use of hydrophilic (soft) contact lenses, especially those of the non-sterilizable or disposable type, infections of the cornea with *Acanthamoeba* keratitis, a sight-threatening condition, have occurred more often. This amoeba occurs in soil and contaminated water. Diagnosis is made by microscopic examination of deep corneal scrapings and treatment is with the drug **polihexanide (polyhexamethylene biguanide)**. This is a sterilizing agent. It is chemically related to **chlorhexidine**, which has also been used to treat acanthamoeba. Both drugs are made up in 0.02% strength and are applied as eye drops. Neither preparation is generally available and at present can only be obtained from the pharmacy of certain specialized eye units.

## STEROIDS AND OTHER ANTI–INFLAMMATORY DRUGS

The most commonly used steroid for local ophthalmic application is **betamethasone disodium phosphate** (*Betnesol*). This can be used in 0.1% drops or ointment. In some preparations the steroid is combined with an antibiotic: for example, *Betnesol-N* contains neomycin. Application can be as frequent as hourly and drugs of this type are used to suppress a wide variety of inflammatory processes within the eye. Steroids should not be used indiscriminately as their improper use may be followed by serious complications. This is particularly so for infective processes which may spread rapidly if steroids are given without a suitable antibacterial agent. For similar reasons they are rarely applied to virus infections of the eye and never in the presence of active herpes simplex (dendritic ulcer).

Administration of dilute steroid eye drops is, on the contrary, often beneficial in the treatment of herpetic corneal infection. This, however, is when corneal stromal opacification threatens and when the viral activity has already been contained. For this purpose **prednisolone** eye drops of 0.1% administered two or three times daily can, by suppressing the antibody–antigen reaction in the deeper layers of the cornea, prevent serious loss of vision. For local administration in the form of eye drops, **dexamethasone** (*Maxidex*) is often used. This drug has good penetration into the eye and is useful in the routine treatment of inflammatory disorders such as iritis. It is available in 1% solution and may be combined with neomycin and polymyxin B sulphate, when it is marketed as *Maxitrol*. In severe ocular inflammation a subconjunctival injection of **methylprednisolone acetate** (*Depo-Medrone*) produces a continuous level of steroids in the anterior chamber for several days.

In inflammation of the posterior uvea (choroiditis) it is necessary to administer steroids systemically as local applications do not readily reach the site of the disease. Here prednisolone may be used and is generally given in a very high dosage for a short period, followed by a rapid reduction at first, which is tailed off more slowly.

All steroid drugs, whether administered locally or systemically, can result in a rise in intra-ocular pressure. A steroid more recently developed and named **fluorometholone** can be used for local administration. It has been shown to be relatively free of the unwanted side-effects that are characteristic of other steroid drugs. It has proved particularly useful in the management of chronic allergic conjunctival inflammations.

For superficial inflammation of allergic origin such as vernal conjunctivitis, a histamine antagonist such as **sodium cromoglicate** is often useful. To be effective the concentration in the conjunctival sac must be maintained at a high level, necessitating frequent or continuous administration. This must be done over the entire period of exposure to the antigen, i.e. throughout the pollen season.

The value of NSAIDs for ocular use lies in their anti-prostaglandin effect. In cataract surgery, prostaglandins are liberated as a response to tissue trauma. These mediators of inflammation can cause constriction of the pupil with consequent surgical difficulties. **Diclofenac sodium**, as a preservative-free 0.1% solution marketed as *Voltarol Ophtha*, seems to protect against this effect. There is also evidence that patients who receive NSAIDs preoperatively show a lower incidence of macular oedema following cataract removal.

## DRUGS WHICH AFFECT PUPIL SIZE

These can be divided into:

- those which enlarge the pupil (mydriatics)
- those which constrict it (miotics).

## MYDRIATICS

Mydriatics are of two sorts:

- *antimuscarinic drugs* – these cause paralysis of the muscular sphincter of the iris; the sphincter muscle is innervated by the parasympathetic nervous system (see also p. 41)
- *sympathomimetic drugs* – these stimulate contraction of the radial dilator pupillae muscle, which is sympathetically innervated (see also p. 43).

### Antimuscarinic drugs

**Atropine.**   One of the earliest known drugs of this type, atropine is the active principle in the poisonous berry of the deadly nightshade plant. Its mydriatic properties have been known for centuries and in the Middle Ages it was used as a cosmetic, hence the name belladonna (Italian for beautiful woman). Today one of its main uses is to dilate the pupil in patients with iritis, where the inflamed iris goes into spasm and adheres to the lens of the eye, causing blindness. Because the ciliary muscle has the same nerve supply as the sphincter muscle of the iris, atropine can be used to paralyse the focusing of the eye (accommodation) for sight testing young children.

*Therapeutic use.* It is commonly used as eye drops of 1% or 0.5% strength and in the form of ointment. The action of this drug lasts for 18 days and it is not reversible by means of miotics. It is, therefore, unsuitable for dilating the pupil for fundal examination.

*Adverse effects.* Atropine can be dangerous as it can cause acute angle closure glaucoma in patients with narrow anterior chamber angles. This will not respond to miotic treatment and will almost certainly require an emergency operation.

**Homatropine.**   For most purposes a mydriatic with a shorter duration of action is appropriate.

Homatropine, which is a homologue of atropine, can be used in 1% or 2% strengths. This has a rapid action, producing pupillary enlargement in 5–10 minutes and its effect rarely lasts for more than 24 hours and can be reversed with miotics.

**Cyclopentolate.**   A synthetic drug, cyclopentolate is now commonly used as a mydriatic and also as a cycloplegic for sight tests in young children, in whom it is necessary to abolish their accommodation. It has a very short duration of action (about 4 hours). Its action is reversed by **physostigmine** eye drops.

**Tropicamide.**   This is another short-acting mydriatic which, although it is a rapid pupillary dilator, is a weak cycloplegic and causes less blurring of vision. It is therefore useful for clinical fundal examination as it has only a slight effect on the patient's ability to read afterwards.

### Sympathomimetic drugs

A typical drug is **phenylephrine**, which is used as eye drops in 10% strength. **Ephedrine** is another and also **cocaine**, which can be combined with homatropine to make up 'guttae H and C'. The cocaine is used at a concentration of 2% which is sufficient for it to be a controlled drug.

Sympathomimetic drugs can be used synergistically to assist those of the antimuscarinic group in cases where dilatation is difficult.

## MIOTICS

Miotic drugs all act on the sphincter muscle of the iris, either directly or indirectly constricting the pupil.

**Pilocarpine** is used to treat chronic glaucoma. It is available in strengths of 1–4% in the form of eye drops.

**Ecothiopate** is a synthetic miotic which has been widely used when strong pupillary constriction is required. Unfortunately, with prolonged use it produces cysts of the iris epithelium which may largely occlude the small, miotic pupil, thereby severely reducing vision. It can now only be used under expert supervision.

**Acetylcholine** is used during intra-ocular surgery such as cataract extraction, where a rapid miosis may be required. This can be achieved by the injection of acetylcholine directly into the anterior chamber. It is marketed as *Miochol-E*, a dry powder in a sterile ampoule containing its own diluent fluid. Mixing is done by breaking an inner seal but, as the preparation has limited stability, it should be made up just before use. Its effect is dramatic but short-lived. After the insertion of an iris-supported acrylic lens replacement, a longer-acting miotic is often advisable.

## DRUGS USED IN THE TREATMENT OF GLAUCOMA

Primary glaucoma is of two types:

- chronic open angle type
- acute angle closure.

These are two entirely different diseases, but the one common factor is that the eye pressure is raised above normal by the failure of the aqueous humour to pass through the outflow channels. The continuous secretion of aqueous by the ciliary body causes a build-up of pressure within the eye.

Drugs used in the treatment of glaucoma can be divided into two groups:

- those which facilitate the outflow of the aqueous humour
- those which reduce its production by the ciliary body.

In angle closure, the draining of aqueous into the canal of Schlemm through the trabecular meshwork is obstructed by the root of the iris. To treat this disorder miotics are used to constrict the iris sphincter muscle and pull the root of the iris centrally, thus relieving the obstruction. In patients with shallow anterior chambers and therefore narrow angles, both mydriatics and strong miotics can precipitate acute glaucoma. These are termed either mydriatic glaucoma or, in the case of miotics, paradoxical glaucoma. In such subjects both groups of drugs should be used with extreme caution.

## DRUGS MODIFYING THE AUTONOMIC NERVOUS SYSTEM

In acute angle closure glaucoma, intensive administration of 4% pilocarpine eye drops is often the first part of the treatment. This means giving one drop a minute for 5 minutes, one every 5 minutes for half an hour and quarter-hourly thereafter. If this is successful in re-opening the angle, the pupil will become small and the corneal oedema will clear in an hour or so.

It is easy to see why miotics are effective in angle closure glaucoma as they help outflow by relieving the obstruction of the drainage angle. It is more difficult to understand why they should work in glaucoma of the open angle type. It has, however, been shown that they act by speeding up the passage of aqueous humour through the trabecular meshwork, which is the band of specialized tissue which separates the anterior chamber from the canal of Schlemm, thus increasing the facility of outflow. In chronic open angle glaucoma **pilocarpine** is frequently used in strengths of between 1% and 4% applied four times a day as it is only effective for 6 hours.

A useful innovation to improve absorption is known as a prodrug in which the drug is modified chemically so that it passes more readily into the eye. After absorption it is split, releasing the active constituent; an example is **dipivefrine hydrochloride**, which is converted by intra-ocular enzymes to epinephrine.

**Guanethidine monosulphate 1%** has also been used in open angle glaucoma. Its effect in lowering the pressure is often disappointing when used by itself. However, it has been found that when combined with neutral epinephrine there is a striking reduction of ocular pressure and a much weaker concentration of epinephrine can then be used (0.2%). This helps to avoid the unwanted side-effects of the epinephrine. Problems with prolonged use include conjunctival fibrosis with secondary corneal changes. If the preparation is used, the conjunctiva and cornea should be examined at least every 6 months.

**Timolol** is another drug which, acting as a β blocker, causes a reduction in aqueous secretion. This is marketed under the name of *Timoptol* in 0.25 and 0.5% strengths. It reduces the amount of aqueous humour that is formed and thereby lowers intra-ocular pressure. It has the advantage that it does not cause unwanted changes in pupillary size and is, therefore, a very useful drug in the treatment of open angle glaucoma. For this reason, however, it is not suitable for glaucoma of the closed angle type unless a miotic is used simultaneously. Another advantage of timolol is that, so far, it has been found not to have any irritative effects on the eye in strengths of 0.5% or less.

*Adverse effects.* Timolol can, however, be absorbed systemically to an extent that it may produce an unwanted fall in blood pressure in some subjects, resulting in dizziness or even collapse. It is also contraindicated in patients with known asthma and care is needed in those with chronic obstructive airways disease.

**Betaxolol** is similar, but is less likely to produce systemic effects. It seems to be less effective than timolol in lowering the intra-ocular pressure. There is, however, some evidence that its absorption via the conjunctiva results in a systemic effect which may increase the blood supply to the optic nerve.

**Brimonidine tartrate** (*Alphagan*) is available as 0.2% eye drops. It is an $\alpha_2$-stimulant and can be used when β blockers are contraindicated; for example, in patients with asthma.

## PROSTAGLANDINS

**Latanoprost** (*Xalatan*), another pressure-reducing agent, is a prostaglandin analogue whose action is to increase the aqueous outflow. It is used in patients whose glaucoma is resistant to other drugs or who are allergic to them.

## CARBONIC ANHYDRASE INHIBITORS

### Acetazolamide

Acetazolamide (see also p. 167) has the action of inhibiting the enzyme carbonic anhydrase, which is necessary for the secretion of aqueous humour. In acute glaucoma the drug is very useful, as by reducing the aqueous production the intra-ocular pressure can be at least temporarily lowered, and this may have the effect of allowing better penetration of locally applied anti-glaucoma treatment.

Acetazolamide may also be used to avoid having to operate on a hard and inflamed eye. It does, unfortunately, have some unwanted side-effects and its diuretic action may be inconvenient. It almost always causes paraesthesia of the extremities. Neither of these effects is permanent. Gastric irritation, nausea and depression are, however, more serious and if they occur the drug should be discontinued.

Acetazolamide is available in tablets and also as a sustained-release capsule. The sustained-release capsule produces a more even action and, as it is absorbed in the intestine, avoids the gastric side-effects.

### Dorzolamide

Dorzolamide (*Trusopt*) is a carbonic anhydrase inhibitor which can be administered locally in the form of eye drops. This is of value in view of the great reduction in side-effects. It can also be given in combination with other anti-glaucoma drugs, and is best used in this way.

## DEHYDRATING AGENTS

Another method of reducing the pressure in acute glaucoma before surgery involves the intravenous infusion of certain hypertonic solutions, which include such substances as **urea** and **mannitol**. These have the effect of producing a vigorous diuresis and cause dehydration of the bodily tissues, including the eye, and at the same time produce an inhibition in the secretion of aqueous.

## LOCAL ANAESTHETICS

These comprise:

- tetracaine (amethocaine)
- oxybuprocaine (*Benoxinate*)
- lidocaine (lignocaine)
- bupivacaine.

Because the eye is a surface organ and covered with mucous membrane it is particularly amenable to topically applied anaesthetics which produce good operative conditions.

Cocaine has been in use for over a century, its application to ophthalmic surgery being first described in 1884. Although still one of the most effective drugs of its kind, it is no longer widely used owing to the advent of highly successful synthetic homologues. Also, as an unfortunate result of its frequent abuse, the stringent regulations – which, of necessity, apply to all its legitimate clinical applications – have reduced its popularity. In addition, it causes clouding of the corneal epithelium. Nevertheless, the impact it had on ophthalmic surgery when first introduced will be appreciated if a moment's thought is given to the experience of an eye operation without anaesthesia of any kind! For surface anaesthesia – that is, of the cornea and the conjunctival sac – tetracaine (amethocaine) in a 1% solution produces rapid anaesthesia which lasts for up to 20 minutes. It does, however, cause stinging when first instilled and for this reason **oxybuprocaine** (*Benoxinate*) may be preferred, especially in children. The action of this drug is rapid, but less well sustained, which makes it very useful for accident and emergency work as corneal sensitivity is regained relatively soon.

## INJECTION OF LOCAL ANAESTHETICS

### Retrobulbar injection

For the performance of eye operations under local anaesthesia, an injection is often given behind the eyeball and within the cone of muscles that surround the optic nerve. This is known as retrobulbar injection and may only be given by someone who is medically qualified and trained to do so. For this purpose lidocaine 1% can be used, up to a total volume of 2–4 ml. When a prolonged period of analgesia is required, a mixture of lidocaine and bupivacaine is effective. All these anaesthetic agents can be combined with epinephrine, but these combinations are usually avoided by ophthalmic surgeons in view of the danger of injecting directly into an orbital vein.

### Peribulbar anaesthesia

A more recent technique involves the injection of local anaesthetic into the tissue space surrounding the globe and extra-ocular muscles of the eye, rather than directly into the muscle cone. This is known as peribulbar anaesthesia and is less likely to cause the embarrassing and highly inconvenient, if rarely dangerous, complication of a retrobulbar haemorrhage.

For this procedure a larger volume injection is given amounting to 8 or 10 ml. As a preliminary, the conjunctiva is anaesthetized using a few drops of tetracaine (amethocaine). A mixture of lidocaine and bupivacaine is used and a diluted fraction is injected into the medial and lateral angles and, after a minute or so, the remainder of the main injection is given into the peribulbar space, half medially and half laterally. Such a volume does cause an excessive pressure on the outside of the eye for intra-ocular surgery to be safely performed. A balloon is therefore secured onto the front of the closed eyelids with a *Velcro* strap and is inflated to a pressure of 40 mmHg.

After 5 minutes all the excess fluid will have been dispersed from the orbit and the effect of the anaesthesia and akinesia (absence of movement) will be complete. To ensure rapid spread of the local anaesthetic agent, a proteolytic enzyme called hyaluronidase (*Hyalase*) is often included in the injection.

## STAINS USED IN OPHTHALMOLOGY

### FLUORESCEIN

Fluorescein is applied locally to the eye to stain ulcers and abrasions of the cornea and thus allow them to be easily seen. It is usually dispensed dry in the form of impregnated paper strips, as in solution it tends to form a culture medium for infecting bacteria, especially *Pseudomonas*.

It can also be used in photographic investigations of patients with retinal diseases. Here it is injected rapidly intravenously using 5 ml of a 5% or 10% solution. As it passes through the retinal blood vessels it causes them to fluoresce and any leakage through blood vessel walls as, for instance, may occur in diabetic retinopathy, can be vividly demonstrated.

### ROSE BENGAL

This is a stain of carmine hue which is taken up actively by injured or infected cells. It is thus very useful for detecting an active virus infection of the corneal epithelium: for example, in herpes simplex.

## MISCELLANEOUS PREPARATIONS

There are many different eye drops designed to replace moisture when the tear film is deficient, as in Sjögren's syndrome. These all contain a water-binding substance, often a higher molecular weight organic sugar such as **hydroxyethylcellulose**, **hypromellose** eye drops being a typical product. As this preparation drips, leaving a white deposit, one containing polyvinyl alcohol may be preferred.

Another highly effective preparation to treat 'dry eye' is an ophthalmic gel, marketed as *Viscotears*. Its main constituent is polyacrylic acid.

**Fluorouracil**, the cytotoxic drug, has found a place in eye surgery as it exerts a delaying effect on the healing of scleral wounds. This is useful after drainage operations for glaucoma. The drug is given as a subconjunctival injection into the lower fornix, taking care that the bleb does not abut on the cornea. A 0.2-ml volume containing 5 mg is injected daily for 5 days. This dose is so small that serious side-effects are avoided.

## DRUGS WITH ADVERSE EFFECTS ON THE EYE

Many drugs in general use have an unwanted and often disastrous effect on the eye. Nurses in charge of patients receiving these drugs should be aware of the likely problems, as their early recognition may help to avoid permanent ocular damage and possibly total blindness. It should be remembered that where a drug is being administered systemically both eyes may be at risk. Some of the more important drugs are now described.

### CHLOROQUINE

Chloroquine was first used as an antimalarial drug and now plays a part in the management of rheumatoid disorders and tropical diseases. It can cause opacities in the cornea and has a toxic effect in the retinae. The corneal disorder is reversible when the treatment is stopped, but that in the retina is permanent and visual loss can be severe. All patients receiving this drug should be under regular ophthalmic supervision.

### DRUGS AFFECTING THE AUTONOMIC NERVOUS SYSTEM

A variety of drugs have a sympathomimetic or anticholinergic action as their primary or secondary effects. These include bronchodilators such as ephedrine and others used in asthma and bronchitis, antidepressants of the tricyclic group and drugs used for parkinsonism such as trihexyphenidyl (benzhexol) or levodopa.

All these drugs have dangers when used in patients with glaucoma, but here a distinction must be made between the open and the closed angle types of disease. A patient with open angle glaucoma may merely show a relative increase in the resistance to aqueous outflow, with the result that the ocular pressure becomes more difficult to control. One with narrow filtration angles, however, may suffer an acute attack which can be bilateral, resulting in rapid and perhaps complete blindness. In the open angle type the use of such drugs may be justified provided the risk is recognized and the glaucoma treatment suitably adjusted. In patients with narrow angle filtration these drugs should be avoided unless they are essential. When in doubt an ophthalmic opinion should be sought.

## CORTICOSTEROIDS

Corticosteroids which are widely used to suppress the inflammatory response can have serious side-effects on the eye. They are also used as immunosuppressants in the longer term following organ transplantation. Such patients are subject to three major side-effects on the eye:

- **corneal infection**
- **open angle glaucoma**
- **cataracts**.

Steroids can, as previously mentioned, precipitate a corneal infection with herpes simplex, but with prolonged administration they can induce glaucoma of the open angle variety and can cause cataracts. The two latter effects can be produced by either local or systemic administration.

### ETHAMBUTOL

This antituberculous agent can cause inflammation of the optic nerve with some visual disturbance. Fortunately, these effects regress spontaneously when treatment is discontinued.

### AMIODARONE

Amiodarone is very effective in treating some types of cardiac arrhythmias. It does, however, produce corneal deposits similar in appearance to those caused by chloroquine. Fortunately, retinal side-effects are absent and the corneal changes do not affect vision.

### TAMOXIFEN

This drug, used in carcinoma of the breast, has been reported to cause blurring of vision as the result of changes in the cornea, lens and retina. This occurs mainly after high doses.

### CHEMICAL TOXICITY

Ocular irritation may result from substances contained in ophthalmic preparations: either the active principle, the preservative or greasy base of ointments. Prolonged use can cause chronic and sometimes permanent pathological changes in the conjunctiva. This effect can also be seen with the proprietary cleaning and sterilizing fluids used in the care of hydrophilic contact lenses.

## Summary

- Ensure that the eye to be treated is clearly delineated
- Warm lotions to 35°C (95°F) before applying them to the eye
- Contamination of the eye by lime or cement can be removed by dihydrogen sodium versenate
- Antibiotics used as drops are rapidly diluted by tears, and ointments release antibiotics more slowly

- Topical use of penicillins in the eye is associated with allergic reactions
- Any intra-ocular infections following eye surgery must be tackled promptly and aggressively
- Be aware of the dangers of infection with *Acanthamoeba* associated with disposable hydrophilic contact lenses
- Infective processes can spread rapidly if topical steroids are used alone without the inclusion of an antibacterial agent
- Steroids are never applied to the eye in the presence of active herpes simplex

Guidance for use of ophthalmic preparations in hospital and care homes

*Introduction*   This circular encompasses the review of HSC(IS)122 undertaken by a working group established by the Royal Pharmaceutical Society in 1999. The guidance herein should help to ensure the safe and pragmatic use of topical ophthalmic preparations in hospitals and care homes. This guidance excludes the presentation and use of contact lens solutions.

*Presentation of single and multiple-application ophthalmic preparations*   All ophthalmic preparations used in hospitals and nursing homes for direct application to the **eye** should be supplied in a sterile condition. Both single application and multiple application packs should have tamper-evident closures and packaging.

Formulation of **eye**-drops and **eye** ointments should comply with the criteria stated in the British and European Pharmacopoeias.

The working group endorses the principal of colour coding of **eye**-drop preparations, but feels that such an issue needs to be pursued at a European Union forum.

*Labelling*   The small size of **eye**-drop and **eye** ointment containers may limit the amount of printed information with which a preparation is labelled.

At the time of dispensing, labelling of containers should specifically include: the words "for use in the **eye** only"; the name and concentration of the active ingredient(s); a statement to confirm the presence or absence of a preservative; directions for use; an "in-use" expiry date; any particular storage requirements; patient's name; and date of dispensing.

*Methods of use of eye-drops*

*(a) In the wards (inpatients) and nursing homes* – All patients should receive a fresh supply of **eye**-drops on admission to hospital or nursing home. A separate bottle for each **eye** should only be supplied if both **eyes** require treatment and the patient has an open **eye** infection and/or medical opinion thus dictates. It is recommended that the period of use of each bottle should not exceed 14 days. This may include both inpatient and post-discharge use. (*Br J Ophthalmol* 1998; 82: 4735). A fresh supply of **eye**-drops should be provided after any **eye** surgery. If a fresh container of **eye**-drops is supplied on discharge from hospital this may be apportioned a "user life" of 28 days.

*(b) In outpatient departments* – Single application containers should be used whenever possible. Every patient who has undergone outpatient surgery and has evidence of current or recent ocular infection should be given a fresh supply of **eye**-drops after the operation, a separate bottle being supplied for each **eye** if both require treatment.

*(c) In eye disease clinics, operating theatres and ophthalmic accident and emergency departments* – These environments possess greater risk of transferring viral **eye** infections, notably epidemic keratoconjunctivitis and epidemic haemorrhagic conjunctivitis. There would appear to be a significant danger of transferring infection between patients in the handling of multiple-application **eye**-drop bottles. It is therefore essential that single application containers should be used whenever possible. Furthermore, every container, which is used, whether single application or multiple application, should be discarded after being used for each patient.

*Extemporaneously prepared, preservative-free eye-drops*   It is recognised that these preparations are widely used in hospital practice and that although they should be discarded immediately after single use, in practice they are given an in-use life of one to seven days. This is an issue which requires urgent investigation.

**Figure 28.2**   Guidance for use of ophthalmic preparations in hospital and care homes. Reproduced from *The Pharmaceutical Journal* 2001; 267: 307 by kind permission of the Pharmaceutical Press; a revised version of guideline originally published as Department of Health guidance in Health Service Circular HSC(IS) in March 1999.

The Royal Pharmaceutical Society has produced a pamphlet giving guidelines for the use of ophthalmic preparations in hospitals and care homes (see Further reading) and these are given in Figure 28.2.

## References

Guidance for use of ophthalmic preparations in hospital and care homes 2001. Pharmaceutical Journal 267: 307

## Further reading

Alward W L M 1998 Medical management of glaucoma. New England Journal of Medicine 339: 1298

Fraunfelder F T, Hampton R F 1980 Current ocular therapy. W B Saunders, Philadelphia.

Fraunfelder F T 1996 Drug-induced ocular side-effects. Williams & Wilkins, Philadelphia.

Wiholm B E, Kelly J P, Kaufman D et al 1998 Relation of aplastic anaemia to use of chloramphenicol eye drops in two international case–control studies. British Medical Journal 316: 666

Chapter **29**

# Application of drugs to the skin, nose and ears

## Learning objectives

**Topical preparations**
At the end of the chapter the reader should be able to:

- list the different bases used for topical preparations
- identify the relevant base to use for a medication depending on the acuteness of the skin condition
- identify the main treatments for common skin diseases
- list the potential sensitizers used in topical preparations
- describe the action of the different potencies of topical corticosteroids

**Application of skin preparations**
At the end of the chapter the reader should be able to:

- demonstrate the correct way to apply the different forms of topical medications
- describe the recognized methods for applying the prescribed amounts of corticosteroids
- identify the drugs that may cause a reaction on the skin

**Lessons**
- Itchy skin can be symptomatic of a problem elsewhere in the body
- When oily substances for skin are added to the bath it makes the bath slippery and potentially dangerous, especially for older patients
- The nurse specialist has an important follow-up role

## THE SKIN

When drugs are applied to the skin, the term *topical treatment* is often used. A topical application generally consists of an active application, the drug, in a base or vehicle. The type of topical application that is used depends on the type and stage of the skin disease, and it is just as important to use the correct base as it is to use the correct active agent. The base consists of one or more of the following: powder, water and grease. The most commonly used bases or vehicles are as described in the following sections.

## OINTMENTS

The distinction between modern ointments and creams is no longer so obvious because of the wide range of bases that are used for both ointments and creams. Ointments are generally more 'greasy' and creams are thinner and consist of emulsions of various types.

Ointments are of three types:

- **Water soluble ointments**: these bases have the advantage that they do not stain.
- **Emulsifying ointments**: these emulsify with water. An example is lanolin (hydrous wool fat), which is still very commonly used. Prolonged use of non-medical grade lanolin in some patients can lead to sensitization to the lanolin. These bases are useful for retaining active agents in contact with the skin for as long as possible.
- **Non-emulsifying ointments**: these do not mix with water. The paraffins form the basis of most of the very greasy ointments. With the addition of a suitable active agent they are a good treatment of chronic, dry skin disorders such as chronic atopic eczema, psoriasis, ichthyosis (dry skin with fish-like scales) and for common disorders such as chapping of the hands.

## CREAMS

Creams are emulsions which are either water dispersed in oil (i.e. oily cream) or oil dispersed in water (i.e. aqueous cream). The latter are generally very acceptable to patients cosmetically and are used to moisten and soften the skin surface. Appropriate active agents can be added. Barrier creams protect the skin against physical agents such as water or sunlight.

## PASTES

Pastes can be greasy or drying and they contain a large amount of powder. They are particularly useful for localized lesions: for example, in psoriasis. In this disorder it is particularly important that the active agent should not be applied to the normal skin and therefore a paste is used for the abnormal areas. Pastes can also be used to protect inflamed or excoriated skin and can be applied very freely. A good example is compound zinc paste.

## LOTIONS

Water lotions are used to cool acutely inflamed skin and may have to be frequently reapplied. Potassium permanganate lotion is very helpful for acute exuding lesions of the hands and feet. Lotions should generally not be used when the acute phase has subsided.

Lotions cool by evaporation and leave an inert powder on the skin surface. They are useful and safe for subacute lesions. Calamine lotion is a good example.

## DUSTING POWDERS

These are drying agents and increase the effective evaporating surface. They are particularly useful in the folds of the skin. Talc, starch and zinc oxide are commonly used powders. Active agents can be added as needed – for example, antiseptics for bacterial infections and antifungal agents for athlete's foot (tinea pedis).

## INGREDIENTS IN PREPARATIONS

### THE BASE

When formulating a skin preparation, the first decision to make is the type of base that will be used. This will depend on the acuteness of the lesion. Many lesions in fact often derive more benefit from the base than from the active agent. A decision on the active ingredient to be added generally implies a diagnosis of the skin disorder. It is no longer useful to remember detailed prescriptions because the common ones can be found in the *British National Formulary* or equivalent publications. Ointments prepared by pharmaceutical companies have complicated formulae, but

**Table 29.1**   Potential skin sensitizers in topical preparations

| Preparations | Sensitizer |
| --- | --- |
| Beeswax | Isopropyl palmitate |
| Benzyl alcohol | Polysorbates |
| Butylated hydroxyanisole | Propylene glycol |
| Chlorocresol | Sorbic acid |
| Edetic acid (EDTA) | Wool fat and related |
| Ethylenediamine | substances including lanolin |
| Fragrances | (development of purified |
| Hydroxybenzoates (parabens) | versions of wool fat have |
|  | reduced the problem) |

**Table 29.2**   Topical corticosteroid potencies

| Potency | Examples |
| --- | --- |
| Mild | Hydrocortisone 1% |
| Moderately potent | Clobetasone butyrate 0.05% |
| Potent | Betamethasone valerate 0.1%, |
|  | Mometasone furoate 0.1% |
| Very potent | Clobetasol propionate 0.05% |

it is very important to know the active ingredients and their strength in these preparations.

It is also important to check for additives in topical preparations which may be associated with sensitization (Table 29.1).

## ACTIVE INGREDIENTS

### Local corticosteroids

These are probably the most widely prescribed and useful ingredients to be added to the various bases. For this reason they are often overprescribed and in particular *they should not be used alone where the cause of the skin disease is a bacterial, fungal or viral infection as they may cause spread of the infection by lowering local resistance.* They are very useful for acute and subacute disorders such as the eczemas and they are excellent for itching (pruritus).

Topical corticosteroids are classified according to their potency (Table 29.2).

The choice of a topical corticosteroid should be the least-potent preparation at the lowest strength which is effective.

**Hydrocortisone ointment** (0.5–1%) is the most useful, standard preparation. Nothing stronger than this should ever be used in infants or on the face. (In certain cases a short course of a more potent preparation may be prescribed under strict supervision of the dermatologist.) These ointments need not be applied more than twice a day.

**More potent corticosteroids** (e.g. betamethasone valerate) can achieve a much more intense effect than hydrocortisone, but this may not be an advantage and can lead to atrophy of the skin. They are valuable for thick, dry skin disorders, such as the chronic eczemas, or with some special disorders such

as lupus erythematosus. The absorption of these preparations is enhanced by occlusive dressings – for example, if they are covered with polythene. However, there is great danger of secondary infection with this method.

Sometimes corticosteroids are combined with an antibacterial or antifungal agent and used to treat dermatoses with superimposed bacterial or fungal infections.

### Coal tar

Coal tar applied to the skin is an antimitotic and anti-inflammatory agent. A tar is the product of the destructive distillation of organic substances and coal tar is in many valuable preparations, although their use has been superseded by the corticosteroid preparations. For disorders such as psoriasis and chronic eczema they are preferred because there are fewer side-effects. Cosmetically acceptable preparations are now available and a liquid form can be added to the bath for the treatment of some patients with psoriasis. The *British National Formulary* calamine and coal tar ointment contains the equivalent of 0.5–1.0% of tar. Coal tar pastes are also often used in eczemas. A useful preparation for psoriasis is betamethasone valerate ointment with liquor picis carb (tar) in yellow soft paraffin.

Dithranol is widely used to treat psoriasis (Case History 29.1). It is an irritant and application must be limited to the psoriatic areas as it burns normal skin, particularly if the skin is fair or has previously been treated with steroids. It should not be used if there is evidence of infection.

### Clinical note

Psoriatic arthritis has been found to respond dramatically to treatment with the newer drug infliximab, a drug given systemically by intravenous infusion to treat rheumatoid arthritis (see p. 156).

## Case History 29.1

Several months after his retirement Mr T developed such an itchy skin that he was unable to avoid persistent scratching. He went to the doctor who observed that Mr T had generalized dryness and scaling and complained of pruritus. He was referred to the dermatologist who examined his skin. Eczema, psoriasis, contact dermatitis or any infestation were excluded as causes of the pruritus. Blood tests and a skin biopsy were arranged to exclude any other possible cause of the itching such as iron deficiency, renal, liver or thyroid disease, or a malignancy. Mr T's diagnosis was pruritus of the elderly (senile pruritus) and he was prescribed *Eumovate* (clobetasone), a topical corticosteroid ointment, for 5 days to relieve the acute itching as well as regular emollient therapy. He was referred to the nurse specialist who showed him how to apply the ointment and a range of samples of different emollients to discover which would be the most suitable for him and which he would prefer to use. Mr T then commenced an emollient regime that included aqueous cream as a soap substitute and an emollient containing an anti-pruritic (*Balneum Plus*) to use in his bath. He was advised to use a non-slip mat in the bath. As a regular moisturizer a fragrance-free, hydrating gel containing liquid paraffin (*Doublebase*) was prescribed for him to be applied after the bath and frequently during the day. Follow-up appointments were made with the nurse specialist to monitor progress and in case of an underlying lymphoma or systemic disease.

## Antibacterial agents

If a bacterial infection is suspected it is important to send a swab to the laboratory for culture and sensitivity tests first. In addition, many infections of the skin are best treated with systemic rather than topical antibacterial agents. The prolonged use of most antibacterial agents (e.g. neomycin) on the skin carries a very high risk of sensitization to the agent so that a bacterial infection may be replaced by a contact dermatitis! Chlortetracycline is probably the best to add to an ointment. If topical antibacterial agents are used the treatment should be determined by the sensitivity of the organism. Sulphonamides and penicillin should never be used on the skin owing to the high risk of sensitization.

## Antifungal agents

Skin scrapings to identify the fungus are best taken before commencing treatment. Systemic treatment is used for widespread, unresponding fungal infections and for nail (Tinea unguium) and scalp ringworm. **Griseofulvin** is the drug of choice for widespread or intractable fungal infections of the skin. It is more effective in the skin than in the nails and needs to be continued for some months.

Topical treatments are usually adequate for most localized infections.

An acute fungal infection may need to be treated by **potassium permanganate lotion 0.01%** for the first few days. An ointment with salicyclic acid and benzoic acid is known as **Whitfield's ointment** and is widely used, but tends to be cosmetically unacceptable. Effective preparations which are commonly used are the imidazoles **clotrimazole, econazole** and **miconazole**. The **undecenoates** and **tolnaftate** are less effective in the treatment of ringworm infections. **Terbinafine** is now also available in the form of a cream. **Amorolfine** is an antifungal which is available as a cream for fungal skin infections and as a lacquer for fungal nail infections.

Lotions and creams are usually the vehicle of choice. As ointments have occlusive properties they should be avoided on moist areas. Dusting powders are therapeutically ineffective in the treatment of fungal infections and liable to cause skin irritation and should be avoided except for toiletry purposes.

Infections with *Candida albicans* are common in patients with diabetes mellitus and those who have been treated with antibiotics and immunosuppressive drugs. Treatment may be with the broad-spectrum antifungal imidazoles. **Nystatin** is also equally effective and must be applied to the affected area, either as an ointment or a lotion.

## Antiviral agents

**Aciclovir** cream is the treatment of choice for herpes simplex of the skin. It is extremely important that the cream should be applied as early as possible, five times a day, for 5 days.

## Emollients

These are used for dry skin (xeroderma) and especially for dry, scaly skin (e.g. ichthyosis, when the scale can be removed). They soothe and smooth the skin and a simple preparation such as aqueous cream is often a good treatment. **Zinc cream** is a traditional remedy and *E45* a more recent one. With hyperkeratotic (i.e. thickened) and scaly conditions it is important to hydrate the skin first with a bath or shower.

The emollient should be applied immediately afterwards to keep the skin hydrated.

> **Nursing point**
>
> In order to encourage regular use, patients should be offered a choice of appropriate emollients (often referred to as moisturizers) so that they may select the one that they prefer.

## Miscellaneous

Many other agents can be applied to the skin for different, but sometimes very common, disorders.

For example:

- **Scabies**: permethrin or lindane is used for the treatment of scabies.
- **Sunscreen preparations** containing substances such as aminobenzoic acid to protect the skin against ultraviolet B radiation (UVB) and sunburn. The sun protection factor (SPF) provides guidance on the degree of UVB protection offered by the preparation (e.g. using one with an SPF of 15 should enable a person to remain in the sun 15 times longer without burning). Protection against UVA and the associated effects of long-term skin damage is offered by preparations containing reflective substances such as titanium dioxide.
- **Cleansing agents** such as cetrimide are useful for removing adherent crusts or ointments.
- **Rosacea**: metronidazole is used in rosacea.
- **Acne and blackheads**: preparations containing benzoyl peroxide or azelaic acid are used in the treatment of acne with comedones (blackheads) and inflamed lesions. Tretinoin, a vitamin A derivative, and its isomer, isotretinoin, may be used to treat acne.
- **Callosities,** e.g. **corns**: salicylic acid may be used to soften callosities, such as corns in the feet. These agents are called keratolytics.
- **Aluminium chloride (20% lotion)** is an antiperspirant, often effective in the treatment of hyperhidrosis (excessive sweating), at any site. It is also used in many commercially available deodorants.
- **Barrier creams** contain water-repellent substances such as dimeticone and may be used to protect the skin in such areas as around the stoma. Barrier creams are also sometimes used in industry to try and prevent damage to the skin; however, most have been shown to be ineffective. Emollient creams, however, may be effective if used properly (wear gloves when applying).

- **Mild-to-moderate psoriasis**: calcipotriol and tacalcitol are vitamin D derivatives used in the treatment of mild-to-moderate psoriasis. Calcipotriol is available as a cream or ointment and in a scalp solution; it is applied twice daily to the affected areas. A combination of calcipotriol with betamethasone is a recent advance in the treatment of mild-to-moderate psoriasis. Tazarotene is the first topical retinoid (vitamin A derivative) available to treat mild-to-moderate plaque psoriasis. Tazarotene gel should be applied thinly, once daily to the affected skin only, avoiding healthy skin and the skin folds.
- **Atopic eczema**: tacrolimus (FK 506) and ascomycin derivative SDZ ASM 981 are topical immunosuppressive drugs that are a recent development in the treatment of atopic eczema.

## APPLICATION OF SKIN PREPARATIONS

**Use of gloves by nurses.** It must be remembered that drugs can be absorbed through the intact skin. It is therefore very important that the nurse wears gloves when applying any preparation to the skin, particularly one containing active ingredients.

**Patient education.** Many patients will be required to apply their skin preparations over long periods so that it will be necessary that they are taught the correct technique. Adverse effects, such as redness and soreness and relapse, may require a change of treatment.

**Wet wraps.** Wet wraps are warm, wet occlusive dressings made up from elasticated viscose stockinette. They are used for children in the treatment of atopic eczema to rehydrate the skin using emollients, treat inflammation with appropriate corticosteroids, cool the skin and promote skin healing. The dressings are usually applied daily for about a week. The procedure for use is as follows:

1. Lengths of the tubular bandage are used to make two body suits. They are measured and cut to fit the patient.
2. The prescribed medication is applied to the skin.
3. The first layer is soaked in warm water, squeezed out and applied to the body while still warm and wet.
4. The second dry layer is applied over the wet layer.
5. The child then can put on normal clothing.
6. The process is repeated after 24 hours

### Nursing point

Wet wraps should not be used on infants under 6 months because of the risk of hypothermia. Children and parents need support and education from specially trained nurses when using wet wraps on the children.

### Medicated baths

- The bath water should be approx. 36°C.
- Stir in the medication and mix well to ensure an even concentration.
- The patient should soak for about 10 minutes.

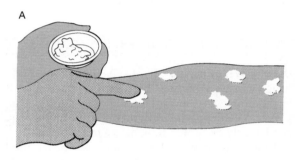

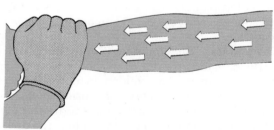

**Figure 29.1** Application of creams and ointments: smooth on in the direction of the hair fall.

**Figure 29.2** Measuring ointment/cream.

### Creams and ointments

- Apply sparingly.
- Do not rub unless specifically prescribed.
- Smooth the preparation on gently in the direction of the hair fall (see Fig. 29.1).
- A 10 cm strip of cream or ointment from a standard nozzle of a tube of medication is the equivalent of 2 g (see Fig. 29.2).

### Steroid application

- Steroids are best applied to hydrated skin.
- Apply an emollient 20 minutes before the steroid to increase its effectiveness.
- Care should be taken to apply only the prescribed amount of corticosteroid to avoid potential side-effects. The rule of nines is a recognized method for assessing the quantity of the preparation to be applied (see Fig. 29.3).
- Patients may also be advised on how to use the 'fingertip method' to apply their topical preparations in safe quantities (see Fig. 29.4).

### Dithranol application

- Apply to affected areas only.
- Palpate skin lesions (psoriatic plaques) to identify the edges of the lesion before applying dithranol.
- Dithranol in Lassar's paste is applied to the lesions with a spatula.
- Starch powder or talc is patted on to dithranol in Lassar's paste to prevent spread of medication onto normal skin. The medication is removed with vegetable oil.
- Dithranol in cream or ointment base is rubbed into the skin lesion with a gloved hand (powder is not used).
- Dithranol in cream in a lipid-stabilized base is removed with plenty of lukewarm water only.
- Short contact treatment – dithranol is left on the skin for 20 minutes or the prescribed time and then removed.

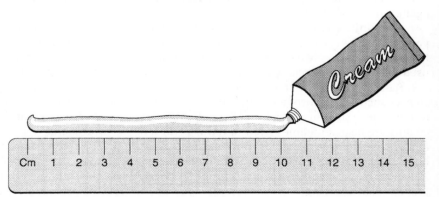

**Rule of Nines**

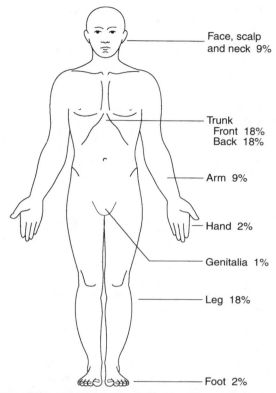

Face, scalp
and neck 9%

Trunk
Front 18%
Back 18%

Arm 9%

Hand 2%

Genitalia 1%

Leg 18%

Foot 2%

**Figure 29.3** This shows the percentage of the total body surface area made up of the various parts of the body. It can be seen that the percentages are usually 9% or a multiple of 9%. In general, no more than 2 g of steroid ointment per 9% of body surface should be applied at any one time, i.e. 4 fingertip units per 9% of body surface (measured by the male finger) or 5 fingertip units per 9% of body surface (measured by the female finger).

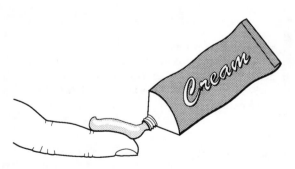

1 g ointment/cream = 2 fingertip units (males)

2.5 fingertip units (females)

**Figure 29.4** Fingertip unit.

## DRUG ERUPTIONS

A skin eruption due to drug treatment is now so commonly seen that this cause must always be considered whenever a patient is seen with an unusual rash. In addition, patients are often receiving more than one drug so that it is difficult or impossible to determine which one is responsible. All that can be done is to give an assessment of the possibilities.

The skin can only react in a certain number of ways, which are known as reaction patterns. A good example is urticaria, which can be provoked by a number of different drugs. If, however, the patient is taking aspirin or its derivatives, this is by far the most likely drug to provoke this reaction pattern. However, in practice, some drugs so commonly cause a particular eruption that this drug can be strongly suspected to be the cause if the patient is seen with a specific rash. For example, furosemide (frusemide) can cause a purpuric rash, glutethimide a generalized erythema and sulphonamides a measles-like rash.

Some drugs can cause many different types of skin eruption. Gold can provoke a generalized exfoliative erythroderma, which may be fatal, or a rash resembling pityriasis rosea or just a nondescript erythema associated with a stomatitis. Penicillin usually causes a severe erythema, and this may be so marked that a diagnosis of erythema multiforme may be considered.

In a few cases, adverse drug reactions including Stevens–Johnson syndrome and toxic epidermal necrosis (TEN) may be so severe that they become life-threatening (Table 29.3).

> **Nursing point**
>
> With the advent of nurse prescribing, care should be taken to ensure that any preparation being prescribed for or recommended to a patient does not include any ingredients to which that patient is sensitive.

**Table 29.3** Drugs most frequently associated with Stevens–Johnson syndrome and TEN

| | |
|---|---|
| Sulfadoxine | Barbiturates |
| Sulfadiazine | Phenylbutazone |
| Sulfasalazine | Piroxicam |
| Co-trimoxazole | Allopurinol |
| Phenytoin | Aminopenicillins |
| Carbamazepine | |

**Table 29.4**   Common allergens in contact dermatitis

| Allergen | Sources |
|---|---|
| Balsam of Peru | Perfumes, citrus fruit |
| Colophony | Sticking plaster, collodion |
| Neomycin | Topical medicaments |
| Benzocaine | Topical anaesthetics |
| Parabens | Preservatives in creams and cosmetics |
| Wool alcohols | Lanolin, creams and cosmetics |
| Imidazolidinyl urea | Preservatives in creams and cosmetics |
| Formaldehyde (aqueous) | Cosmetics, clothing, glues, paper |

**Table 29.5**   Drugs causing photosensitivity reactions

| Phototoxic | Photoallergic |
|---|---|
| Topical | |
| Coal tar preparations, e.g. dithranol | Halogenated salicylamides |
| Psoralens | |
| Furocoumarins, e.g. bergamot oil | |
| Systemic | |
| Demeclocycline | Sulphonamides |
| Doxycycline | Phenothiazines |
| Chlorpromazine | Griseofulvin |

## CONTACT DERMATITIS

Contact dermatitis is an eczematous eruption produced by external agents, including some drugs (Table 29.4). Some emollients and paste bandages contain preservatives and many preparations have fragrance additives, both of which are known sensitizers. The *British National Formulary* and pharmaceutical company data sheets list additives in preparations.

> **Nursing point**
>
> Medicated agents such as antiseptics can cause contact dermatitis. This is an occupational health hazard in nursing and may increase the risk of contracting parenteral viral infections such as HIV due to the production on the skin of micro-abrasions.

## LIGHT SENSITIZATION

Some drugs sensitize the skin to ultraviolet light. A skin eruption occurs when the photosensitive person has taken or applied the medication and then been exposed to sunlight. Two subtypes of reactions occur, phototoxic and photoallergic (Table 29.5).

Phototoxic reactions develop a few hours after exposure to sun and often resemble severe sunburn. In photoallergic reactions the onset is delayed and the rash is eczematous in nature. Table 29.6 lists other agents causing photosensitivity.

## TREATMENT

Treatment is generally simple in that all drugs which are the likely cause should be withdrawn.

**Table 29.6**   Other agents causing photosensitivity

| Agent type | Examples |
|---|---|
| Drug reactions | |
| Antibiotics | Sulphonamides, tetracycline |
| NSAIDs | Azapropazone |
| Hypoglycaemics | Chlorpropamide, glibenclamide |
| Sedatives | Chlorpromazine |
| Diuretics | Amiloride, thiazides |
| Contact sensitivity | |
| Drugs | Chlorpromazine |
| Sunscreens | Para-aminobenzoic acid (PABA) |
| Cosmetics | Perfumes, especially musk ambrette |
| Plants | Chrysanthemum and other compositae |

Symptomatic treatment for symptoms may be called for, with calamine cream for pruritus or systemic antihistamines to make the patient more comfortable. It should be noted that the topical application of antibiotics, antihistamines and local anaesthetics should be avoided as they often cause sensitization rashes.

> **Nursing point**
>
> Photosensitive patients, including those with disorders such as systemic lupus erythematosus, porphyria and chronic actinic dermatitis, must be advised to wear sunscreens and protective clothing when outdoors.

## CONCLUSION

From this brief review it will be seen that practically anything can be applied to the skin and often is! Patients may have used a variety of unsuitable remedies before they see a doctor or nurse and one's first duty is to apply a remedy that will not do any harm. This is why many dermatologists are very conservative in the treatment that they prescribe. Like any other part of the body, when it is inflamed the skin must be allowed to rest. If there is an external cause for the trouble then this must be removed and it is as well to remember that this may be an ointment which has been prescribed. If there is an infection it must be treated. The topical application of a suitable base may be all that the skin requires. The active agents, or drugs, should only be added if there is a definite indication for their use.

## SKIN CARE

There is no doubt that good skin care needs soap and water daily. Some individuals may prefer to use a soap substitute, such as an emulsifying ointment. The patient's preferred emollient or moisturizer should be applied regularly to maintain skin hydration and help prevent dryness and scaling. Make-up should always be removed at night. The skin should always be protected from excessive exposure to the sun and, if possible, excessive use of perfumes, hair dyes and so on. When it is said someone looks healthy, this means the skin is in good condition and looks normal.

## THE NOSE

Drugs may be instilled into the nose. It must be remembered, however, that their effect is very transient; the cilia lining the nasal cavities completely remove them in about 20 minutes. Furthermore, medication with strong solutions of antibiotics or vasoconstrictors will paralyse the cilia and thus impede rather than help the clearance of infected material from the nasal cavities.

### APPLYING NOSE DROPS

Nose drops are best given as follows: The patient should lie back on a couch or bed with his or her head extended over the end. About 5 ml of the appropriate drops are instilled into each nostril, the patient being instructed to breathe through the mouth, thus closing the back of the nose and holding the nose drops in the nasal cavities. This position should be maintained for 3 minutes. This method of administration may be too strenuous for

elderly patients. There are a number of nose drops in use; among the most useful is ephedrine nose drops.

### EPHEDRINE NOSE DROPS

Ephedrine nose drops are useful in sinus infection because the ephedrine causes shrinkage of the swollen and inflamed mucosa and thus clears the nasal airway and allows proper drainage from the nasal sinuses. Overuse, however, may damage the delicate ciliated epithelium lining the nasal passages and the drops should not be used for more than a week.

### Drug interactions

Ephedrine nose drops should not be given to patients taking monoamine oxidase inhibitors (MAOIs) or within 2 weeks of stopping these drugs, owing to the risk of a hypertensive crisis. Corticosteroids (betametasone 0.1%) can be given as nose drops two or three times daily or beclometasone is available as a nasal spray, the dose being two sprays into each nostril twice daily. Sodium cromoglicate can be given as a nasal spray, as drops or as an insufflation.

### ALLERGIC RHINITIS

Allergic rhinitis can be treated locally with preparations which relieve congestion or by oral antihistamines. Local steroids appear to be the most effective.

**Azelastine,** which is an antihistamine, can also be given as a nasal spray.

Local antibiotics have little place in the treatment of nasal infections, but a cream containing chlorhexidine and neomycin (*Naseptin*) can be applied locally in patients who are carriers of staphylococcus, especially MRSA. This is a wise procedure in these patients before they undergo surgery since it may reduce the risk of cross-infection to other patients.

**Mupirocin** or *Polyfax* ointments are used for the eradication of MRSA.

## THE EAR

Although the instilling of drops into the ear may be useful in relieving symptoms, it is often done without any consideration of the underlying disease and thus proves fruitless and sometimes even dangerous.

The use of ear drops will be considered under individual disorders of the ear which can be helped by this method of treatment.

## INSTILLATION OF DROPS

1. Warm ear drops to approximately blood heat.
2. The head is turned so that the affected ear is uppermost.
3. Discharge is gently mopped away.
4. Two or three drops are instilled and the head is held in position for a minute or two.

## WAX IN THE EAR

Wax may become hard and impacted in the ear and may resist efforts to move it by syringing. A 5.0% solution of sodium bicarbonate or warm almond or olive oil instilled for a few days will usually soften it satisfactorily.

## OTITIS EXTERNA

Severe infection is best managed with expert guidance as regular aural cleansing and medication are required.

Ear drops will only be effective if the meatus is cleared of debris. The following agents may be used three times daily if bacterial infection is suspected:

- **clioquinol 1% with flumetasone 0.02%** (*Locorten-Vioform*) has a mild antibacterial and antifungal action, but stains the skin and clothes
- **gentamicin 0.3% with hydrocortisone 1%** is anti-inflammatory and antibacterial.

Other combinations of antibacterial drugs with steroids are available.

The following precautions should be observed:

- treatment with antibiotic ear drops should not be continued for longer than 1 week owing to the risks of drug sensitization and the development of fungal infection
- gentamicin or neomycin ear drops should not be used if the eardrum is perforated as deafness may result.

In eczema of the ear, local steroids should be used to reduce irritation and inflammation. Prednisolone 0.5% or betamethasone 0.1% are satisfactory.

## OTITIS MEDIA

If the drum is not perforated the instillation of antibiotics into the external ear is useless as it will not reach the site of infection. Many infections are viral and require only an analgesic. Bacterial infections, which are usually due to *Streptococcus pneumoniae* or *Haemophilus influenzae*, should be treated by systemic antibiotics. Amoxicillin is usually effective and erythromycin can be used for those who are sensitive to penicillin.

### Summary

- Prolonged use of non-medical grade lanolin can lead to sensitization to lanolin
- Pastes are particularly useful for localized lesions, e.g. psoriasis
- Dusting powders are particularly useful in the folds of the skin
- The choice of a topical corticosteroid should be the least potent preparation at the lowest strength which is effective
- No corticosteroid stronger than hydrocortisone ointment (0.5–1%) should ever be used in infants or on the face
- Aciclovir cream is the treatment of choice for herpes simplex of the skin and should be applied as early as possible
- With hyperkeratotic conditions the skin should be hydrated before applying emollients
- Nurses should wear gloves when applying any preparation to the patient's skin
- Patients should be taught the correct technique for applying skin preparations
- Steroids are best applied to hydrated skin
- The rule of nines is a recognized method for assessing the quantity of the steroid preparation to be applied
- Topical application of antibiotics, antihistamines and local anaesthetics should be avoided as they often cause sensitization rashes
- Make-up should always be removed at night
- Strong solutions of antibiotics or vasoconstrictors will paralyse the cilia of the nose and will impede the clearance of infected material from the nasal cavities
- Ephedrine nasal drops should not be used for more than 1 week
- Ephedrine nasal drops should not be used with MAOIs or within 2 weeks of stopping MAOIs.
- Treatment with antibiotic ear drops should not be continued for longer than 1 week owing to the risks of drug sensitization and the development of fungal infection

- Gentamicin or neomycin ear drops should not be used if the eardrum is perforated as deafness may result

- In otitis media, instillation of ear drops is useful if the eardrum is not perforated.

## Further reading

Ashcroft D M, Wan Po A L, Williams H C, Griffiths C E 1999 Clinical measures of disease severity and outcome in psoriasis: a critical appraisal of their quality. British Journal of Dermatology 141(2): 185

Cerio R, Jackson W F 1992 Photosensitivity and photoallergy. A colour atlas of allergic skin disorders. Wolfe Publishing, London

Charman C 2000 The treatment of atopic eczema in adults. Dermatology in Practice 8(4): 21

Dawkes K 1997 How to … treat scalp psoriasis. British Journal of Dermatology Nursing 1(1): 8

Douglas W S, Poulin Y, Decroix J et al 2002 A new calcipotriol/betamethasone formulation with rapid onset of action was superior to monotherapy with betamethasone diproprionate or calcipotriol in psoriasis vulgaris. Acta Dermato-Venereologica 82(2): 131

Editorial 1995 Management of acute otitis media and glue ear. Drug and Therapeutics Bulletin 33: 12

Ersser S J 1998 Annotated bibliography of the dermatology nursing literature. Oxford Centre for Health Care Research and Development, Oxford

Fincham-Gee C 1988 Safe use of topical steroids. Nursing 29(3): 1043

Findlay A Y, Edwards P H, Harding K G 1989 The fingertip unit: a new practical measure. The Lancet 2: 155

Greaves M W, Weinstein G D 1995 Treatment of psoriasis. New England Journal of Medicine 332: 581

Griffiths C E M, Cox N H 2001 Psoriasis 2000: the state-of-the-art today … and tomorrow. British Journal of Dermatology 144, Suppl 58

Gruber P C, Ratnavel R 2001 Childhood fungal infections. Dermatology in Practice 9(4): 6

Hughes E, Van Onselen J 2001 Dermatology nursing: a practical guide. Churchill Livingstone, Edinburgh

Jackson K 2002 Chronic psoriasis: an overview. Nursing Standard 16: 45

McClelland P B 1997 New treatment options for psoriasis. Dermatology Nursing 9(5): 295

Rolfe G 2002 Nursing role for acne in primary care. British Journal of Dermatology Nursing 6(3): 9

Roujeau J C, Stern R S 1994 Severe adverse cutaneous reactions to drugs. New England Journal of Medicine 331: 1272

Stone L A 2000 Medilan: a hypoallergenic lanolin for emollient therapy. British Journal of Nursing 9(1): 54

Stone L A, Lindfield E M, Robertson S 1989 A colour atlas of nursing procedures in skin disorders. Wolfe Medical, London

Symposium 1990 Ear, nose and throat disease. Prescribers Journal 30: 191

Turnbull R 1994 Use of wet wrap dressing in atopic eczema. Paediatric Nursing 6(2): 22

Weiner J M 1998 Intranasal corticosteroids versus oral H antagonists in allergic rhinitis. British Medical Journal 317: 1624

Chapter **30**

# Vitamins, iron and treatment of anaemia

## Learning objectives

At the end of this chapter, the reader should be able to:

- give an account of the sources, symptoms of deficiency and preparations for treatment for the vitamins
- describe the use of antioxidants
- describe the use of iron preparations for treatment of iron deficiency anaemia
- appreciate that anaemia is associated with vitamin B$_{12}$ deficiency and describe how it is treated

## VITAMINS

Vitamins are substances which are present in certain foods, but which humans cannot manufacture for themselves. They are necessary for the proper functioning of animal tissues, and a deficiency of vitamins in the diet leads to a number of diseases which are specific for each particular vitamin. Many of the vitamins exert their action by taking part in the complex chemical reactions which occur within the cell.

It is important to realize that provided a sufficiency of vitamins is taken, which should be provided by a good mixed diet, there is no advantage to be gained by taking further large doses of the various vitamins unless there is some form of malabsorption. In fact, the taking of excessive amounts of certain vitamins, for example vitamin A, can even be harmful. At present there is no firm evidence that extra vitamins protect against cancer and heart disease to any appreciable extent, and reports that supplementary vitamins given to children increase their IQ should be treated with scepticism until confirmed.

The vitamins may now be considered in detail:

- vitamin A (retinol) and retinoids
- vitamin B group
- vitamin C (ascorbic acid)
- vitamin D (calciferol)
- vitamin E (tocopherol)
- vitamin K (phytomenadione).

## VITAMIN A (RETINOL)

### Occurrence

Retinol is a fat-soluble, oily liquid. It is present in dairy products such as milk, butter and cream and in fish liver oils. Beta-carotene, a substance which is closely allied to retinol and can be converted to retinol by the body, is found in carrots, green vegetables and liver.

### Absorption and function

The absorption of retinol is helped by the presence of fat and bile salts in the intestine. Retinol is concerned with maintaining the health of the epithelium. Deficiency leads to keratinization of the epithelium of the nose and respiratory passage and to changes in the conjunctiva and in the cornea that may lead to blindness. Retinol is also concerned with the mechanism of dark adaptation by the retina and deficiency leads to night blindness.

### Therapeutic use

Retinol should be given in cases of deficiency causing night blindness or epithelial changes. The minimum human requirements in the adult are 2250 IU (international units) daily. The therapeutic dose is 50 000 IU.

### Toxicity

Overdosage with retinol can produce liver damage, headache and vomiting. Fatalities have been reported. Pregnant and breast-feeding women are advised to avoid vitamin A supplements or liver products as there is some evidence that excessive intake is associated with fetal defects.

## RETINOIDS

These substances are related to vitamin A, but are used for their effect on the skin.

### Therapeutic use of retinoids

**Safety note**

Retinoids have severe potential toxicity and teratogenicity and should be used under expert supervision.

Retinoids are used mainly in the treatment of psoriasis and acne. **Calcitriol** is an active form of vitamin A. **Acitretin** causes desquamation of the skin (the process in which the outer layer of the epidermis is removed by scaling). Its main indication is for psoriasis, although it is also prescribed for other keratinization disorders such as ichthyosis and Darier's disease (keratosis follicularis). **Isotretinoin** can be applied locally and taken systemically in the treatment of acne where it reduces the secretion of sebum. **Tazarotene** is an odourless retinoid that is effective for psoriasis. **Tretinoin** is the acid form of vitamin A and is used topically for the treatment of acne.

### Adverse effects, precautions and contraindications

**Topical application.**  Both isotretinoin and tretinoin may initially cause peeling of the skin and reddening when first used, but this effect usually disappears after a period of time. All retinoids for topical use should be used sparingly and applied thinly to the skin. They should not be smeared over large areas of skin, especially if the acne is severe. Contact with broken or sunburned skin, mucous membranes, mouth, nose and eyes should be avoided, and patients who apply these should protect their skin from direct sunlight and not use UV lamps.

**Oral use.**  Patients taking retinoids orally should have regular tests of liver function and blood lipid concentrations. Patients taking retinoids orally may experience effects on epithelial tissues such as sticky palms, cracked and dry lips, paronychia (whitlows), which is a painful swelling of the nail folds, and hair thinning. These are reversible effects.

## Contraindications

Retinoids alter cell division and are teratogenic (cause fetal malformations). They must not be used in pregnancy or during breast-feeding, especially when for oral use. The danger of possible teratogenicity can persist for years after stopping oral treatment with retinoids. With acitretin, for example, whose main indication is for psoriasis, it is recommended that patients with child-bearing potential should cease taking the drug for at least 2 years before a planned pregnancy.

## VITAMIN B GROUP

The vitamin B group comprises:

- thiamine (vitamin $B_1$)
- riboflavin (vitamin $B_2$)
- pyridoxine (vitamin $B_6$)
- nicotinic acid (niacin, nicotinamide, niacinamide)
- cyanacobalamin (vitamin $B_{12}$).

## Thiamine (vitamin $B_1$)

**Occurrence.** Vitamin $B_1$ is a white crystalline solid, soluble in water. It is obtained from wheat germ, yeast, egg yolk, liver and some vegetables.

**Function and deficiency.** Vitamin $B_1$ is essential for certain stages of carbohydrate metabolism. Deficiency of this vitamin leads to a nervous system disorder known as *beriberi*. This deficiency may not only result from an inadequate intake of vitamin $B_1$ but may also occur in disturbances of metabolism in which requirements of vitamin $B_1$ are higher than normal, a good example being chronic alcoholism. *Beriberi* is characterized by heart failure and polyneuritis.

**Therapeutic use.** *Beriberi* responds rapidly to vitamin $B_1$. Severe cases will require up to 100 mg daily by intramuscular injection; in milder cases oral administration is satisfactory. Vitamin $B_1$ is also used in high doses in the polyneuritis of chronic alcoholism and in Korsakov's psychosis and Wernicke's encephalopathy, which are also usually due to excess alcohol. The minimum human requirements for adults are 2 mg daily. The therapeutic dose is 50 mg orally or intravenous daily.

**Adverse effects.** Patients given parenteral thiamine should be observed afterwards in case of an anaphylactic reaction.

## Vitamin $B_2$ (riboflavin)

**Occurrence and deficiency.** This vitamin is found in high levels in fish, egg yolks, cheese, meat, milk, poultry and whole grains. Vitamin $B_2$ is necessary for antibody production, red cell formation, cell respiration and growth. Deficiency in humans causes several symptoms, including cracking and fissures at the corner of the mouth and a sore tongue and skin lesions. The syndrome is called *ariboflavinosis*.

**Therapeutic use.** Vitamin $B_2$ may be given in doses of 2 mg daily. Some sources recommend an increased intake of this vitamin when taking oral contraceptives or during periods of strenuous exercise. Vitamin $B_2$ is destroyed by light, alcohol and antibiotics.

## Nicotinic acid

**Occurrence and deficiency.** Nicotinic acid is also called niacin. Some sources refer to it as vitamin $B_3$. It is a derivative of pyridine, from which the pyridine nucleotides, building blocks of DNA and RNA, are derived. Nicotinamide is the amide of nicotinic acid and is a component of the ubiquitous coenzyme NAD (nicotinamide adenine dinucleotide). It is therefore vital for the proper functioning of a large number of enzymes in the body. It is important in the production of hydrochloric acid in the stomach and is involved in the normal secretion of gastric and bile fluids. It has been claimed to lower cholesterol and aid circulation. It is needed for proper synthesis of the sex hormones. It is important for normal operation of the nervous system.

Nicotinic acid is found in high concentrations in brewer's yeast, dairy products and beef liver. Deficiency of nicotinamide leads to a disorder known as pellagra which may occur in alcoholism and renal failure as well as with deficient diets. This disease is characterized by the '3Ds', namely diarrhoea, dermatitis and dementia.

**Therapeutic use.**  Nicotinamide is available in both a 50 mg tablet and in cream form. The cream is used topically in the treatment of *acne vulgaris* and the tablets are used to treat nicotinamide deficiency.

**Adverse effects.**  It is worthwhile remembering that nicotinamide is also a vasodilator. If it is taken in large doses flushing and tingling of the face may occur. High doses can cause liver damage if taken for prolonged periods. Pregnant women and those suffering from diabetes, liver disease, gout, glaucoma or peptic ulcers should use nicotinic acid with caution and in any event should take medical advice before taking it.

## Vitamin B$_6$ (pyridoxine)

**Occurrence and deficiency.**  Pyridoxine occurs in all foods. High levels are found in brewer's yeast, walnuts, carrots, poultry, eggs, fish, meat, peas (not well cooked), and wheat germ and sunflower seeds. Pyridoxine is involved in very many metabolic processes. It is required for normal functioning of the nervous system, including the brain. It is involved in red blood cell formation and for that of DNA and RNA. It is important in immune function and is part of the body's mechanisms to prevent atherosclerosis. It is required for healthy heart function since it blocks the formation of homocysteine, a toxic chemical that promotes the deposition of cholesterol around heart muscle.

**Deficiency of pyridoxine** causes:

- dry and flaking skin
- nausea and vomiting
- headache
- sore tongue
- CNS symptoms, e.g. convulsions, difficulty with concentration, weak memory.

Other symptoms sometimes seen include acne and oily skin, anorexia, fatigue, hyperirritability, depression and impaired wound healing. Deficiency may be caused by use of some antidepressants, oral contraceptives and other estrogen therapy. Some sources claim that dietary deficiency of vitamin B$_6$ causes anaemia, but this is not universally accepted.

**Therapeutic use.**  Pyridoxine tablets for oral use are available and the dose for pyridoxine deficiency is 20–50 mg up to three times daily. It is sometimes used in the treatment of vomiting of pregnancy or following radiation. It can be used in doses of 10–20 mg daily to prevent the polyneuritis which rarely complicates the use of high-dose isoniazid and it has been tried with varying success in the treatment of premenstrual syndrome.

**Adverse effects.**  There is some evidence that high doses of pyridoxine can damage peripheral nerves and such doses should be avoided, particularly when pyridoxine is being used as a food supplement and not for a specific medical purpose.

For vitamin B$_{12}$, see p. 394.

Although the deficiency of vitamins in the B group have been discussed separately, it is common to find that deficiencies are often mixed and in treating patients who show evidence of vitamin B deficiencies it is worth giving all the vitamins of the group. The vitamin B group are available in tablet form universally labelled as vitamin B complex. An inspection of the ingredients will reveal a much larger list than might be expected. Other ingredients include inositol, choline, para-aminobenzoic acid and pantothenic acid, called by some sources vitamin B$_5$. The value of these added supplements is still in the process of being resolved.

> **Safety note**
>
> Several of the supplements listed in many commercial preparations of vitamin B complex are freely available over the counter, and unsupervised use of some of these is not without risk. For example, folic acid should never be used alone for vitamin B$_{12}$ deficiency states such as pernicious anaemia. This could result in a subacute combined degeneration of the spinal cord.

## VITAMIN C (ASCORBIC ACID)

### Occurrence

Vitamin C is a crystalline solid, soluble in water. It is found in fresh fruits, particularly citrus fruit, blackcurrants, tomatoes and green vegetables. It is important to remember that vitamin C is relatively unstable and it is destroyed by boiling, especially in an alkaline solution. Thus green vegetables should be eaten raw if required for their vitamin C content. Vitamin C is necessary for the formation and maintenance of the connective tissue proteins, which literally hold the organs together. Deficiency leads to a disorder known as scurvy.

## Scurvy

Scurvy has been recognized for hundreds of years. It was particularly liable to attack mariners who in the days of sailing ships were away from land for long periods and were thus deprived of fresh food and vegetables. Infants and children are also susceptible.

Scurvy is rarely seen in England at the present time, although it is occasionally found in people who for medical reasons, or more often *supposed* medical reasons, have been living on a very restricted diet such as bread and weak tea.

Scurvy is characterized by a tendency to bleed due to increased capillary fragility. Haemorrhages occur into the skin and mucous membranes; sponginess and haemorrhage around the gums may be found in those with teeth. Bleeding also occurs under the periosteum of bones and into joints, producing great pain and tenderness; the patient is anaemic. If vitamin C is not given the disease will prove fatal.

## Therapeutic use

Scurvy is cured by giving vitamin C, the dose for adults being 500 mg daily. The bleeding is arrested and the anaemia, which is not entirely secondary to haemorrhage, is relieved. Vitamin C is also used in a number of other disorders where it is of doubtful value; it does appear, however, to be useful in promoting the healing of wounds in those who, although showing no evidence of scurvy, have a mild degree of deficiency.

Very high doses of vitamin C are sometimes taken to prevent colds and other forms of ill health. The efficacy of this medication is not proven, but it does not seem to do any harm. Requirements are increased with prolonged exercise and illness.

## Minimum human requirements

- Children 100 mg daily
- Adults 50 mg daily
- Pregnancy 200 mg daily
- Lactation 150 mg daily
- Therapeutic dose 500 mg daily.

## VITAMIN B AND C COMBINATION

The B vitamins and vitamin C have been combined into preparations to give emergency replacement after malabsorption due to, for example, alcohol poisoning, postoperatively, after acute infection or in certain psychiatric conditions.

*Pabrinex* contains high doses of B and C vitamins and is given intravenously or intramuscularly. Rarely, it can cause a severe allergic reaction and infusion should be over at least 10 minutes and facilities should be available for treating an acute allergic reaction.

## VITAMIN D (CHOLECALCIFEROL)

### Occurrence

This fat-soluble vitamin is found in fish liver oils and dairy produce and is also formed in the skin on exposure to sunlight. It is essentially concerned with calcium metabolism and bone formation. After absorption it is modified in the liver to form 25-hydroxycholecalciferol, and undergoes further change in the kidney to form 1,25-dihydroxycholecalciferol (Fig. 30.1). This substance is highly active in facilitating calcium absorption from the gut and the laying down of calcium and phosphate during bone formation.

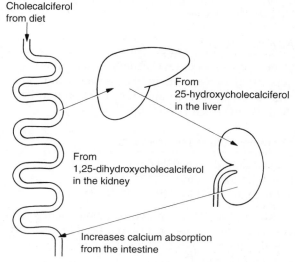

Figure 30.1    The changes undergone by cholecalciferol (vitamin D) in the body.

## Deficiency

A deficiency of vitamin D leads to inadequate calcification of the bones, resulting in their becoming soft and easily deformed. This disorder when it occurs in children is known as rickets and these children with their bowed legs and deformed chests were a familiar sight in former times. With the arrival of cheap milk, cod liver oil and better care of young children it has now become rare, although there has been a reappearance of the disease in some ethnic groups. In adults, prolonged deprivation of vitamin D gives rise to a disorder similar to rickets, but it is very rarely seen in this country, although certain groups, e.g. the elderly and vegetarians, are at some risk, as are those women who cover their bodies completely, thus barring light.

Vitamin D deficiency can also result from poor absorption from the intestine, as in coeliac disease, and from resistance to the action of vitamin D which is found in renal failure leading to stunting in children (renal rickets).

## Therapeutic use

Patients at risk of deficiency can be given one calcium and ergocalciferol tablet daily (400 units of vitamin D per tablet),* which should be crushed or chewed before swallowing: 5000 IU of vitamin D daily is adequate for the treatment of established rickets. In coeliac disease very large doses of vitamin D may be required at first, but these requirements diminish as the disease is controlled by diet. In chronic renal failure large doses of vitamin D or alfacalcidol are used.

## Adverse effects

Overdose with vitamin D is dangerous and leads to deposition of calcium in the kidneys and other organs. Patients receiving high doses should have their plasma calcium measured regularly.

## Minimum human requirements

- Young children 600 IU daily*
- Adults 400 IU daily
- Pregnancy and lactation 1000 IU daily.

Alfacalcidol (1-alpha-hydroxycholecalciferol) is closely related to vitamin D and is used to treat various disorders in which there is a resistance to the action of vitamin D.

*400 units of vitamin D ≡ 10 micrograms of ergocalciferol.

# VITAMIN E (TOCOPHEROL)

## Occurrence

Vitamin E is found in nuts, wheat germ, cold-pressed vegetable oils, dark green, leafy vegetables and brown rice. The daily requirements have not been fixed with certainty but are estimated to be in the region of 3–20 mg daily. It is an antioxidant, and on this basis it has been claimed by some sources that it may reduce the incidence of cancer and vascular disease, prevent cell damage by inhibiting the oxidation of fats and prevent the formation of free radicals. A number of other claims have been made and these are currently the subject of much investigation. There is no consensus at present as to whether vitamin E supplements in adults are of value and this question is being energetically debated at present (Brigelius-Flohe et al 2002). In children who have congenital cholestasis (a failure of normal amounts of bile to reach the gastrointestinal tract), there may be abnormally low levels of vitamin E associated with neuromuscular abnormalities.

### Safety note

The indiscriminate use of vitamin E is inadvisable. For example, diabetic or hyperthyroid patients, or those with rheumatic heart disease or on anticoagulant therapy should not take vitamin E without seeking advice.

# VITAMIN K (PHYTOMENADIONE)

## Occurrence

Vitamin K is a precursor of prothrombin, which is essential for the coagulation of blood. Vitamin K is fat soluble and requires bile salts for proper absorption from the intestine. It is also synthesized in the gut by bacteria. After absorption it is used by the liver for the synthesis of prothrombin.

## Deficiency

Deficiency of vitamin K will lead to bleeding and may result from insufficient uptake due to various intestinal diseases or to deficient utilization following liver disease or anticoagulant drugs. In the newborn there is a lack of vitamin K because it has not been synthesized by the gut bacteria and this may lead to bleeding (haemorrhagic disease of the new-born). It occurs at birth and, more seriously, about a week later when it is often intracranial. It can be prevented by giving vitamin K. There has been some anxiety that injected, but not oral, vitamin K may be associated with childhood cancers, but this fear appears to be unfounded.

## TRACE ELEMENTS

Certain elements, including zinc, manganese, boron, cobalt and copper, exist in very small amounts in the body. They are essential for some important metabolic processes and deficiency can cause or contribute to several disorders. Adequate amounts are present in a full, normal diet but insufficiency can arise in those whose diet is severely restricted, or with malabsorption. Patients who are on total parenteral nutrition are especially at risk of deficiency and trace elements may be added to their intravenous infusion.

Patients who are poorly nourished and are about to undergo surgery may be given dietary supplements before operation. Zinc and vitamin C are thought to be of particular importance in aiding wound healing and improving immunity to infection.

## ANTIOXIDANTS

Antioxidants (see also Chapter 8) include some vitamins and other compounds which are not usually classified as vitamins but are considered to be important constituents of the diet. Oxidation is a metabolic activity occurring in nearly all tissues and is necessary for life. It can, however, produce substances called free radicals which are chemically very active and can damage constituents of cells. They are believed to play a part in the development of vascular diseases, cancer and, possibly, some other diseases. Antioxidants suppress the formation of free radicals and might, therefore, be expected to protect against these conditions.

Although it has been shown that there is a relationship between the dietary intake of antioxidants and the development of certain diseases, there is, at present, little evidence that adding them to the diet has a prophylactic effect, other than a possible reduction of coronary artery disease by vitamin E (see above). Among those being used are vitamins C and E, beta-carotene and selenium. In addition, antioxidants are present in fruit and vegetables, which should form part of a healthy diet.

## IRON DEFICIENCY ANAEMIA

Iron is an essential constituent of haemoglobin, which is contained in the erythrocytes of the blood. Haemoglobin is concerned with the transport of oxygen from the lungs to the tissues. When the red cells break down, the iron is retained by the body and built up again into further haemoglobin molecules. There is very little iron held in storage depots, the major portion being constantly in use (Fig. 30.2). A little iron, probably about 2 mg a day or less, is lost by desquamation of cells by the skin and gut, but the chief drain of iron from the body occurs in the various forms of blood loss, either menstruation or parturition or due to chronic bleeding, usually from the gastrointestinal tract. In pregnancy the growing fetus requires a certain amount of iron, and during lactation iron is lost in the mother's milk.

It can be seen, therefore, that although the average diet which supplies about 25 mg of iron a day is sufficient for most people, if there is any prolonged iron loss, a deficiency will occur. The result is anaemia, since not enough haemoglobin is produced.

## ABSORPTION AND METABOLISM OF IRON

Iron, when taken by mouth, is converted into the ferrous form in the stomach. It is absorbed from the upper part of the small intestine, forming a loose compound with a protein in the intestinal wall which is called transferrin; in this form it is transported across to the bloodstream, where it is carried to the bone marrow for the synthesis of haemoglobin. The absorption of iron is carefully regulated so that just enough is absorbed to make good any deficiency. Iron is also stored in the liver in the form of ferritin.

**Iron deficiency anaemia** is sometimes associated with deficient secretion of hydrochloric acid by the stomach and this leads to a failure of release of ferrous iron from the diet. It can occur as a result of diseases of the intestine which interfere with iron absorption. If a deficiency of iron occurs, less haemoglobin is synthesized and the amount of haemoglobin in the erythrocytes decreases.

## IRON PREPARATIONS

Iron is given to correct a deficiency. It is usually given orally. The rise in blood haemoglobin level

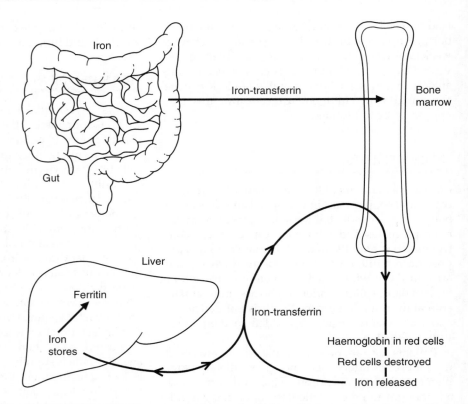

**Figure 30.2** Metabolism of iron.

should be at least 0.7 g/dl per week and treatment should be continued for 4 months after the blood haemoglobin level has returned to normal to replace depleted iron stores. It is also given during pregnancy when the iron requirements increase.

**Ferrous sulphate** tablets are a satisfactory way of giving iron to most people. Ferrous salts are rapidly changed to ferric salts in the air and thus ferrous salts are given as coated tablets. The therapeutic dose is 200 mg, three times a day. In sensitive subjects ferrous sulphate may cause gastric discomfort and nausea or diarrhoea or sometimes constipation. Ferrous sulphate tablets are usually coated with sugar; children are therefore very liable to take them and fatal poisoning by ferrous sulphate is not uncommon. Like all drugs they should therefore always be kept in a position of safety.

**Ferrous gluconate** is another ferrous salt. It is less irritating to the stomach than most ferrous salts. Ferrous glycine sulphate is a complex of ferrous sulphate and the amino acid glycine. It is perhaps less liable to cause gastrointestinal disturbances and is useful in sensitive subjects. Liquid preparations are also available.

**Sodium feredetate** (*Sytron*) and a **polysaccharide-iron complex** (*Niferex*) are satisfactory and do not stain the teeth. Although slow-release iron preparations are used they may be less effective as iron absorption takes place in the upper small intestine, but these preparations release it lower down the gut.

Iron can also be given by intramuscular injection in those who are not absorbing iron satisfactorily. Before injecting iron, oral iron should be stopped for at least 72 hours as this appears to reduce the chances of a reaction after injection.

**Iron sorbitol** is an iron preparation for intramuscular injection. It is rapidly absorbed from the injection site. It contains 50 mg of iron per ml of solution. Side-effects appear slight but shock-like reactions can occur and care must be taken when giving the injection to prevent leakage along the needle track and subsequent staining of the skin.

## DRUGS USED TO TREAT OTHER ANAEMIAS

### COBALAMINS (VITAMIN B$_{12}$)

#### Source

There are several factors required for the proper maturation of the red cells. The best known of these

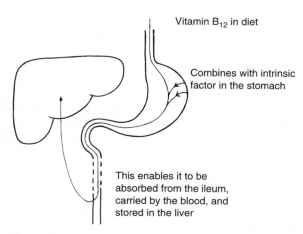

Vitamin B$_{12}$ in diet

Combines with intrinsic factor in the stomach

This enables it to be absorbed from the ileum, carried by the blood, and stored in the liver

**Figure 30.3**   Absorption of vitamin B$_{12}$.

is **cyanacobalamin** (vitamin B$_{12}$). It works together with folic acid to regulate the formation of red blood cells and promotes the utilization of iron. The principal dietary sources are milk, eggs, clams, herring, liver and kidney. Brewer's yeast is rich in vitamin B$_{12}$.

## Absorption of vitamin B$_{12}$

In the normal person, a factor (the intrinsic factor) is produced by the stomach and is necessary for the absorption of cobalamin in the intestine (Fig. 30.3).

## Deficiency of vitamin B$_{12}$

Deficiency of vitamin B$_{12}$ leads to a failure in production of erythrocytes. There is, therefore, a decrease in the number of circulating erythrocytes and those which do manage to mature appear abnormal, being large and irregular in shape and size. Primitive red blood cells may also appear in the blood.

In addition to the change in the blood, deficiency in cobalamin leads to glossitis (inflammation of the tongue) and degenerative changes in the nervous system. The syndrome produced by cyanocobalamin deficiency is known as **pernicious** or **Addison's anaemia**. This deficiency is believed to be due to a failure to absorb cobalamin from the intestine as a result of a lack of the intrinsic factor. Failure to absorb cobalamin can also result from diseases of the intestine, and in those who have had ileostomy.

## Treatment

Treatment is to give cobalamin by injection. There are two cobalamins available: **hydroxocobalamin**, which is stable and which is highly bound by the

plasma proteins so that it is excreted slowly and thus its action is prolonged; and **cyanocobalamin**, which is effective but more rapidly excreted.

## Therapeutic use

Treatment is started with hydroxocobalamin 1 mg three times weekly and then reduced to 1 mg every 6–8 weeks when a satisfactory remission has been produced. Maintenance doses of cyanocobalamin, however, should be given every 3–4 weeks.

The lesions in the nervous system also respond to cobalamin, but it may be many months before the full effect of treatment is seen.

Occasionally, vegans may develop vitamin B$_{12}$ deficiency due to a shortage in the diet. To prevent this 1 mg of cobalamin can be added weekly to their food.

## FOLIC ACID

### Sources

Folic acid is obtained from animal and vegetable sources and is also synthesized by gut bacteria. It is necessary for the maturation of red cells, and deficiency will produce changes in the blood similar to those found in pernicious anaemia.

### Deficiency

The common causes of deficiency in this country are: malabsorption syndromes such as coeliac disease and pregnancy.

Some women do not absorb folic acid in the later months of pregnancy and thus become anaemic. In addition, folic acid taken early in pregnancy reduces the incidence of neural tube defects. Iron deficiency is also common in pregnancy and it is usual to give both folic acid and iron supplements which are taken throughout pregnancy.

### Preparations

- **Folic acid tablets**
- **Ferrous fumarate + folic acid tablets**
  *(Pregaday)*

**Therapeutic use.**   Folic acid can be given orally in doses of 15 mg daily. Larger doses may be required in malabsorption states. Tablets containing both iron and folic acid are available for use in pregnancy. *Pregaday* contains ferrous fumarate equivalent to 100 mg of ferrous iron plus folic acid 350 micrograms, the dose being one tablet daily.

If possible, a woman considering pregnancy should start taking folic acid (400 micrograms daily) before conception and for the first 3 months of pregnancy, to minimize the risk of neural tube defects which occur very early in pregnancy. To prevent recurrence of a defect, a dose of 5 mg of folic acid daily should be used and continued for the first 3 months of pregnancy. There is also some evidence that the addition of folic acid to the diet reduces the incidence of cardiovascular disease. It is important not to treat pernicious anaemia with folic acid for, although it will improve the anaemia, it will worsen the neurological complications of pernicious anaemia.

## ERYTHROPOIETIN DEFICIENCY

Erythropoietin is a hormone manufactured by the kidney, which is necessary for erythrocyte formation. If the kidneys fail, the level of erythropoietin in the blood falls, with resulting anaemia.

### Patient education

Severe hypertension requires immediate treatment. Patients or relatives should be told to report headaches or confusion at once.

**Epoetin** is an analogue of erythropoietin. It is synthesized by recombinant DNA technology and two forms, alpha and beta, are available commercially. They are essentially the same. In patients with renal failure and anaemia, epoetin is given three times weekly by subcutaneous or intravenous injection until a satisfactory haemoglobin level is produced. Treatment then continues with maintenance doses.

**Darbepoetin** is a modified form of epoetin with a longer half-life, and less frequent dosages may be required than with **epoetin**.

**Adverse effects**. Hypertension is fairly common and may be severe. The blood pressure should be measured every week in the initial stages of treatment and then at 6-weekly intervals. Thrombosis and 'flu'-like symptoms occasionally occur.

## BLOOD GROWTH FACTORS

Factors which stimulate the growth of white blood cells are now available and are especially useful in patients whose white cells have been depressed by cancer chemotherapy, immunosuppression or treatments associated with the HIV virus:

**Human granulocyte-colony stimulating factor** (**filgrastim** and **lenograstim**), given by subcutaneous or intravenous injection, increases the production of neutrophils.

**Human granulocyte macrophage-colony stimulating factor** (**molgramostim**) also increases the white cells in the blood.

The use of these factors has considerably improved the treatment of a wide range of serious diseases in which it is necessary to suppress temporarily the white blood cell count to achieve a satisfactory therapeutic effect. They accelerate the recovery of the bone marrow and thereby decrease the risk of serious infection which accompanies leucopenia.

### Summary

- Vitamin A overdose can be toxic, and even fatal
- Retinoids are teratogenic and potentially toxic and should be used only under the supervision of a qualified person
- It is advisable to wait at least 2 years after taking retinoids such as acitretin before a planned pregnancy
- Pregnant women and those suffering from diabetes, liver disease, gout, glaucoma or peptic ulcers should use nicotinic acid with caution and in any event should take medical advice before taking it
- High doses of pyridoxine may cause damage to peripheral nerves
- Folic acid should never be used alone for vitamin $B_{12}$ deficiency states such as pernicious anaemia. This could result in a subacute combined degeneration of the spinal cord
- Vitamin C is destroyed by heat; vegetables, especially leafy vegetables, should be eaten raw or very lightly cooked
- *Pabrinex*, a mixture of vitamins B and C, is given intravenously or intramuscularly, and may cause a severe allergic reaction
- Overdose with vitamin D is dangerous and leads to deposition of calcium in the kidneys and other organs: patients receiving high doses should have their plasma calcium measured regularly
- The indiscriminate use of vitamin E is inadvisable: for example, diabetic or hyperthyroid patients, or those with rheumatic heart disease

or on anticoagulant therapy should not take vitamin E without seeking advice
- Ferrous sulphate is sugar-coated and looks like sweets; children may take them and fatalities have occurred, so they should be kept well away from children
- Iron sorbitol: shock-like reactions can occur when giving iron sorbitol citrate intramuscularly, and

care must be taken when giving the injection to prevent leakage along the needle track and subsequent staining of the skin
- Folic acid taken early in pregnancy reduces the incidence of neural tube defects

## Further reading

Bates C 1995 Vitamin A. Lancet 345: 31

Brigelius-Flohe R, Kelly F J, Salonen J T et al 2002 The European perspective on vitamin E: current knowledge and future research. American Journal of Clinical Nutrition 76: 703

Buttriss J, Hughes J 2002 A review of the MAFF Optimal Nutrition Status research programme: folate, iron and copper. Public Health Nutrition 5: 595

Editorial 1995 Vitamin A and birth defects. New England Journal of Medicine 333: 1414 31: 33

Editorial 1996 Dietary habits and mortality in 11 000 vegetarians and health-conscious people, results of 17 year follow up. British Medical Journal 313: 775

Editorial 1998 Which vitamin K preparations for the newborn? Drug and Therapeutics Bulletin 36: 317

Editorial 1998 Eat right and take a multivitamin. New England Journal of Medicine 338: 1060

Fraser D R 1995 Vitamin D. Lancet 345: 104

Hibbard B M, Horn E 1988 Iron and folate supplements during pregnancy. British Medical Journal 297: 1324

Kong C H, Brown S M 1991 Recombinant human erythropoietin in the management of anaemia. Professional Nurse 6(11): 650

# Chapter 31

# Drugs in pregnancy and at the extremes of age

## Learning objectives

At the end of this chapter, the reader should be able to:

- list the four stages of pregnancy when drugs may damage the fetus
- provide examples of drugs known to or be suspected of causing fetal abnormalities
- enumerate the general rules to be observed when thinking of treating pregnant women with drugs
- appreciate that dosages need to be altered in pregnancy and in babies, children and elderly people
- recognize some of the problems that the newborn infant has in dealing with drugs given to the mother during labour
- recognize that drugs do pass to the infant during breast-feeding
- appreciate that drug administration to children and older people sometimes needs to take into account problems such as swallowing tablets
- recognize that elderly people have impaired abilities to metabolize and excrete drugs, and this can cause toxicity
- explain how adverse reactions to drugs are more likely in elderly patients

## INTRODUCTION

Most facts about drugs are obtained from observations on young and middle-aged adults. Age, however, may modify the way drugs are handled by the body and also the way the body reacts to the actions of drugs. In recent years, increasing interest has led to studies of drugs given at the extremes of age and in pregnancy.

## DRUGS IN PREGNANCY

Drugs can affect the fetus either by interfering with some important function in the mother which indirectly damages the fetus or by passing across the placenta and acting directly on it. Most drugs cross the placenta.

## STAGES OF PREGNANCY

Damage can occur at four stages of pregnancy:

* **Implantation** (5–15 days). Drug toxicity at this stage usually results in abortion.
* **Embryo stage** (15–55 days). During this period the embryo is changing from a group of cells into a recognizable human being. The embryo is particularly susceptible to drug toxicity at this time, which leads to fetal malformation (teratogenesis) such as occurs with thalidomide.
* **Fetogenic stage** (55 days to birth). As the fetus continues to grow and develop, drug damage becomes less likely, but it is still possible.
* **Delivery**. Drugs at this stage may interfere with labour and modify the behaviour of the neonate immediately after birth.

In this country about 30% of women take some drug during pregnancy, although only 10% take one in the first trimester when the fetus is most vulnerable to damage. Those most commonly taken are mild analgesics and antibiotics.

It is important to discover which drugs can produce fetal damage and which are safe to use. This is difficult for two reasons:

* Fetal abnormalities can occur for various reasons even when no drugs are taken. About 2% of babies have some abnormality at birth, but only about 5% of these are believed to be drug-related.
* If the drug only rarely causes an abnormality, thousands of pregnant women need to be studied before a connection between a certain drug and fetal damage can be confirmed.

Experiments with pregnant animals have only a limited value.

## DRUGS AND FETAL ABNORMALITY

At present, drugs can be divided into three groups:

### A. Drugs known to produce fetal abnormalities

* Thalidomide
* Folic acid antagonists
* Tetracyclines
* Androgens
* Danazol
* Warfarin (during the first 4 months of pregnancy)
* Diethylstilbestrol
* Etretinate
* Lithium
* Some anticonvulsants.

### B. Drugs suspected of producing fetal abnormalities

* Oral hypoglycaemic agents cause neonatal hypoglycaemia
* Various cytotoxic drugs
* Anorexics (amfetamines)
* ACE inhibitors and thiazides should not be used for hypertension in pregnancy.

There are a number of other drugs which are under suspicion or for which information is not available.

### C. Drugs which probably do not harm the fetus
(see also *British National Formulary*, Appendix 4)

| | |
|---|---|
| • Simple analgesics | Paracetamol for minor pain. NSAIDs can be used if really necessary and ibuprofen, being mild and short-acting is preferred. |
| • Cough | Codeine. |
| • Powerful analgesics | Opioids can be used (but see below). |
| • Diabetes | Insulin. |
| • Drugs for dyspepsia | Antacids – advice on diet advisable. |
| • Drugs for constipation | Bulk purges, lactulose. |
| • Drugs for nausea | Avoid if possible and treat by modifying diet. |
| • Antibacterial drugs | Penicillins, cephalosporins, erythromycin; avoid trimethoprim in the first 3 months of pregnancy if possible. |

- Hypotensive
  agents

  Methyldopa; hydralazine
  for rapid lowering of blood
  pressure; β blockers may be
  used but retard fetal growth.

- Antimalarial
  drugs

  Chloroquine (low dose);
  proguanil.

- Anti-asthmatic
  drugs

  β₂ agonists; inhaled steroids;
  a short course of systemic
  steroids if absolutely
  necessary.

- Centrally acting
  drugs

  Benzodiazepines (but see
  below); neuroleptics and
  tricyclic antidepressants
  are probably safe;
  Antiepileptics – see p. 253.

- Hay fever

  Topical preparations; antihistamines – chlorphenamine
  (chlorpheniramine) and
  terfenadine.

When treating pregnant women some **general rules** should be observed:

- Avoid giving drugs if possible, especially in the first 3 months of pregnancy.
- Give drugs at the lowest effective dose for as short a time as possible.
- Avoid recently introduced drugs if possible.
- Drugs on lists A and B (see above) should be avoided if possible. The problem arises when there is no satisfactory substitute and treatment is vital. This is a matter of risk to the fetus against risk to the mother (and often therefore, the fetus as well).
- Ethanol and street drugs: alcohol taken by the mother during pregnancy can damage the fetus, resulting in an infant with a small head, facial abnormalities and of low intelligence. Although it may well be better to avoid alcohol altogether in pregnancy, there is no evidence that one glass of wine, or its equivalent, daily causes any harm. If the mother is dependent on opioids, the newborn infant may suffer acute withdrawal symptoms. Regular use of cocaine is associated with an increased risk of fetal abnormality.

## PREGNANCY AND DOSAGE

Pregnancy causes a number of changes in the way the drug is handled by the body:

- The volume of water in the body is increased so that the concentration of a given dose will be decreased, although this may be offset by a fall in protein binding which leaves freer active drug in the blood.
- Liver enzymes increase so that some drugs are broken down more rapidly and renal excretion may also be enhanced. Where dosage is not critical this does not matter, but for a few drugs (e.g. anticonvulsants and theophylline) adjustment of the dose may be necessary.

## DRUGS IN NEWBORN INFANTS

During the hours of labour, drugs may be given to the mother and some of these can pass via the placenta to the neonate. Among those which are important are the following drugs.

**Analgesics and hypnotics.**   Morphine and similar drugs affect the fetus and may lead to difficulties in establishing respiration immediately after birth.

**Barbiturates and benzodiazepines.**   Excessive dosing of the mother with barbiturates and benzodiazepines leads to accumulation of these drugs in the fetus and after birth the infant will be floppy with depressed breathing and failure to suck.

**β Blockers.**   These drugs pass to the fetus and produce a slow pulse rate.

**Chloramphenicol.**   Newborn infants are not able to break down drugs as effectively as older children or adults; thus accumulation may occur after repeated dosing. With chloramphenicol this can be dangerous, as accumulation of the drug produces the 'grey syndrome' which is due to collapse of the circulation.

**Oxygen.**   Treating a newborn, usually pre-term, infant with a high concentration of oxygen is known to cause blindness due to retrolental fibroplasia (abnormal proliferation of fibrous tissue behind the lens of the eye, causing blindness).

**Kernicterus and drugs.**   Certain drugs given to the mother late in pregnancy or to the infant in the first few days of life bind onto the plasma protein and displace bilirubin from the binding sites. This can be dangerous because too much uncombined bilirubin in the blood causes brain damage. Drugs that have been implicated are:

- sulphonamides
- tolbutamide
- aspirin.

**Kernicterus** is the staining of and subsequent damage to the newborn infant's brain by the bile pigment bilirubin, which may occur due to a haemolytic disease of the infant or through drugs displacing bilirubin from its binding sites on plasma proteins. Neurones in the basal ganglia are especially affected, and at about 6 months a form of cerebral palsy emerges with feeding difficulties, disturbed vision, deafness and uncoordinated movements. Speech, when it develops, is impaired.

## BREAST-FEEDING AND DRUGS

Most drugs will pass into the breast milk, but usually at very low and innocuous concentrations. However, this is not invariable, and a few drugs being taken by the mother can be a hazard to the baby. Generally, drugs should be avoided by nursing mothers, but if a drug is essential the baby should feed just before the mother takes her dose when blood levels will be low.

Certain drugs should not be used by nursing mothers and, if unavoidable, will require transfer to bottle feeding.

## DOSAGE OF DRUGS IN CHILDREN

Children should *not* be regarded as small adults when prescribing for them, particularly in the first few months of life.

They differ from adults in:

- body composition
- elimination of drugs.

In the first few weeks of life the breakdown of drugs by the liver is reduced, but thereafter, because of the relatively large size of a child's liver, the rate of breakdown is greater, weight for weight, than in adults. This discrepancy progressively disappears until adulthood.

Renal excretion is similarly reduced in the first few weeks of life, but reaches normal levels by about 6 weeks. It follows therefore that except for the first few weeks of life, weight-related doses of most drugs are higher in children than in adults. This means that dosage has to be carefully considered for each individual drug. Young children find it difficult to swallow tablets, so liquid preparations are preferable. However, they should not be mixed in the feeding bottle as milk may interfere with drug absorption. Older children respond to drugs more like adults but, even here, there may be differences.

There is no completely satisfactory way of calculating the correct dose of a drug for children. In practice three methods may be used:

1. $\text{Dose} = \text{Adult dose} \times \dfrac{\text{Patient's weight in kg}}{70}$

2. $\text{Dose} = \text{Adult dose}$
   $\times \dfrac{\text{Patient's body surface area (metres}^2)}{1.8}$

3.

| Age | Wt in kg | % of adult dose[a] |
|---|---|---|
| Newborn | 3.5 | 12.5 |
| 4 months | 6.5 | 20 |
| 1 year | 10 | 25 |
| 3 years | 15 | 33 |
| 7 years | 23 | 50 |

[a] This assumes that the child is 'average'.

Formula 1 is most satisfactory in deciding the initial loading dose but Formula 2, which takes into account the rate of breakdown of the drug, is to be preferred for maintenance dosage. These methods are only approximate and with certain drugs the dose in adults and children differs considerably.

Administration of drugs to children may present difficulties (see 'Giving drugs to children' section in Chapter 2). Children under 5 years of age cannot usually swallow tablets and will require liquid preparations. Volumes of less than 5.0 ml should be given via an oral syringe. These should be free of sucrose, which causes dental damage. For certain drugs (e.g. diazepam) the rectal route is useful.

Further information can be found in the *British National Formulary* or in various paediatric formularies.

## DRUGS IN ELDERLY PATIENTS

Elderly people are responsible for about one-third of the expenditure on drugs by the National Health Service and a high proportion of them receive regular drug treatment. It is therefore important to know whether the action of drugs is modified by old age and how advancing years may alter the handling of drugs by the body.

## ABSORPTION, DISTRIBUTION, METABOLISM AND EXCRETION

### Drug absorption

At present there is little evidence that the absorption of drugs after oral administration changes with age, provided there is no disease of the gastro-intestinal tract.

### Drug distribution

After absorption, drugs are carried round the body in the blood. They are to a greater or lesser extent bound to the plasma proteins, particularly albumin. Elderly people have less albumin in the blood; therefore with certain drugs less is protein-bound and more is free in the blood and tissue fluids and can therefore produce a greater pharmacological effect.

### Drug metabolism (breakdown)

Many drugs are broken down by enzymes in the liver, but with advancing age these enzymes become less active and, in addition, the blood supply to the liver decreases. Some drugs may therefore be more slowly broken down and their blood concentrations may rise to toxic levels. Those implicated include:

- lidocaine
- tricyclic antidepressants
- propranolol
- caffeine
- benzodiazepines.

### Drug excretion

Drugs are also excreted via the kidney. Old age, sometimes associated with kidney disease, leads to a decline in renal function, so that by the age of 80 years renal function is only half that at age 40. This again may cause drug accumulation. Among the most important drugs in this case are:

- digoxin
- aminoglycosides
- propranolol.

## ORGAN SENSITIVITY

This is more difficult to assess, but there is evidence that certain systems become more sensitive to drug action with advancing years. Brain function is easily disturbed in elderly people so that hypnotic and other centrally acting drugs can easily produce confusion and excessive drowsiness. The control of blood pressure is more easily disturbed, causing fainting, not only with hypotensive drugs but with tricyclic antidepressants and levodopa.

## COMPLIANCE

Complicated drug regimes may be impossible for elderly people to follow so they either give up taking their drugs or take the wrong doses at the wrong times, sometimes with disastrous results. Dispensing drugs for elderly and confused people is made easier through the supply of colour-coded, compartmentalized and labelled calendar packs in which the different medicines are placed.

## ADVERSE REACTIONS

Adverse reactions to a drug are two or three times more common in the elderly than in younger adults and there are several reasons for this:

- elderly patients often need several drugs at the same time and there is a close relationship between the number of drugs taken and the incidence of adverse reactions
- for reasons given above, the elimination of drugs may be impaired in elderly patients so that they are exposed to higher concentrations unless the dose is suitably adjusted
- elderly patients are often severely ill and this may interfere with elimination
- drugs which are associated with adverse reactions such as digoxin, diuretics, NSAIDs, hypotensives and various centrally acting agents are often prescribed for elderly patients.

All this does not mean that diseases should not be treated in elderly people, but drugs must be prescribed with care.

## SOME GENERAL PRINCIPLES

All these considerations have made it necessary to observe certain general principles when using drugs for elderly patients, and a **practical summary** is given below:

- **A full drug history** is important, as the patient may have experienced an adverse effect from a drug in the past. Medication already being taken (including over-the-counter preparations) may raise the possibility of an interaction. It will also enable the nurse to assess the patient's ability to manage the regime alone or whether help may be needed from relatives.

- **Keep the regime simple** and use as few drugs as possible.
- Prescribe the **smallest effective dose** and, if possible, use drugs which are short-acting.
- Do not continue to use a drug for longer than necessary.
- If an elderly person's condition deteriorates, remember that a drug may be responsible.
- **Ease of administration:** certain formulations such as elixirs may be easier than tablets for an elderly person to take, particularly if the tablets are very large or very small.
- **Clear and simple instructions** should be given to the patient and the container must be clearly labelled. Various types of calendar packs are available (see above), but it is important to ensure that the patient can use them.

## SPECIFIC THERAPEUTIC PROBLEMS

**Sleep.** Elderly people generally require less sleep than younger adults do, and broken sleep during the night is common. They do not usually require a hypnotic, but should avoid sleeping during the day and take more exercise. Alcohol, taken in the evening, may induce sleep, but often leads to waking in the night because its hypnotic effect wears off rapidly. If, however, the patient is used to a little alcohol before sleep it is usually best not to interfere. Various disorders can cause sleeplessness and they should be sought and treated if possible:

- pain
- depression
- urinary frequency
- heart failure
- constipation
- dementia
- caffeine taken in the evening.

The main problems for elderly people who are on hypnotic drugs are:

- **mental confusion** – drugs may cause mental confusion during the night
- **hangovers** – they may have hangover effects into the next day
- **sensitivity** – elderly people appear to be very sensitive to most centrally acting drugs.

Those most commonly used for insomnia are the benzodiazepines. Temazepam is short-acting and is preferred. Despite their relative safety, these drugs can produce excessive drowsiness, confusion and ataxia and the smallest possible dose must be used. If possible, they should only be given for short periods and a careful watch kept for adverse effects and falls.

**Tranquillizers.** Agitation with restlessness is common in elderly people, especially if they are demented. This can be controlled by phenothiazines such as thioridazine, but with all phenothiazines remember that postural hypotension and Parkinson-like symptoms and akathisia (restlessness and anxiety) can occur.

**Depression.** Tricyclic antidepressants are useful, but postural hypotension, urinary retention, dry mouth, exacerbation of glaucoma and a liability to fall can all be troublesome. The 5-HT re-uptake inhibitors are a considerable improvement as far as most adverse effects are concerned and are equally effective. However, they are much more expensive.

**Parkinson's disease (see p. 254).** Small doses of levodopa, combined with a dopa decarboxylase inhibitor, are useful. In the elderly, postural hypotension can be a problem. Anticholinergic drugs often cause troublesome side-effects, i.e. urinary retention and glaucoma and constipation should be avoided.

**Hypertension.** There is now considerable evidence that treating hypertension in older patients is worthwhile, and it is possible to reduce cardiovascular complications in this group. The cardiovascular systems of elderly people do not adapt to change as well as in younger patients; therefore a gentle approach is needed. A low-dose thiazide diuretic such as bendroflumethiazide (bendrofluazide) is often adequate. Calcium-channel blockers can be used, but must be avoided in heart failure. ACE inhibitors are also effective and well tolerated, but renal function must be monitored. β Blockers are rather less effective in elderly patients. The blood pressure should be taken standing and lying, as elderly patients may have a large postural fall.

**Chronic heart failure.** This condition is increasingly common and is usually, but not always, due to coronary artery disease. Treatment is along the same lines as in younger patients (see p. 59), but certain problems are more liable to arise in older people:

- **Diuretics**: sodium deficiency may develop with diuretics, causing postural hypotension and fainting on standing. With loop diuretics, the rapid diuresis can cause acute retention in men with enlarged prostates. With large doses, potassium deficiency occasionally occurs, requiring potassium supplements or the addition of a potassium-sparing diuretic.

- **ACE inhibitors** can cause hypotension, particularly with the first dose and in those already receiving diuretics. Renal failure can develop and renal function should be monitored.
- **Digoxin toxicity** may be a problem due to reduced renal elimination. Low doses should be given.
- **Oral hypoglycaemic agents**: diabetes in elderly people can be treated with these drugs. Tolbutamide or glipizide are to be preferred as they are rather short-acting and the risks of hypoglycaemia are less.

---

**Nursing point**

It is important not to confuse ankle oedema due to long periods of sitting with that due to heart failure.

---

**Epilepsy.** This results from cerebrovascular disease and is not uncommon in elderly patients. The most useful drugs are carbamazepine, sodium valproate and phenytoin. The same problems arise as in younger patients (see p. 246). The initial dose should be small and adverse effects are more easily provoked, mainly because of slower elimination. It is also important to remember that interference with cognitive function, which occurs with many centrally acting drugs, is more marked in elderly people.

**Antibiotics.** There is no particular contraindication to antibiotics in elderly patients as long as care is taken with aminoglycosides, as reduced renal function can lead to high blood levels and toxic effects.

**Analgesics.** Elderly patients are more sensitive to opioids and particular care is necessary if the patient has chronic obstructive airways disease. Co-codamol (codeine + paracetamol) can be used, but the resulting constipation may require a laxative. Paracetamol is preferred for minor pains because NSAIDs are especially liable to cause gastric bleeding in older people.

Further information about drugs and pregnancy can be obtained from:

- *British National Formulary*, Appendix 4
- National Teratology Information Service (Tel. 0191 232 1525)
- hospital drug information units.

## Further reading

Armour D, Cairns C 2002 Medicines in the elderly. Pharmaceutical Press, London

Cargill J 1992 Medication compliance in elderly people: interfering variables and interventions. Journal of Advanced Nursing 17: 422

Conn V C 1991 Older adults: factors that predict the use of over-the-counter medication. Journal of Advanced Nursing 16: 1190

Editorial 1996 Preconception, pregnancy and prescribing. Drug and Therapeutics Bulletin 34: 25

Glasper A, Oliver R W 1984 A simple guide to infant drug calculations. Nursing 2nd Series 22: 649

Grant E, Golightly P 1992 Drugs in breast feeding. Prescribers Journal 32: 90

Guy's, St. Thomas's and Lewisham Hospitals Paediatric Formulary 1999

Ito S 2000 Drug treatment in breast-feeding women. New England Journal of Medicine 343: 118

Klepping G 2000 Medication review in elderly care homes. Primary Care Pharmacy 1: 105

Koren C, Partuszak A, Ito S 1998 Drugs in pregnancy. New England Journal of Medicine 338: 1128

Rajaen-Dehkordi Z, MacPherson G 1997 Drug-related problems in older people. Nursing Times 93: 54

Rubin P 1998 Drug treatment during pregnancy. British Medical Journal 317: 5103

Rylance G 1998 Prescribing for infants and children. British Medical Journal 296: 984

Swift C G, Shapiro C M 1993 Sleep and sleep problems in elderly people. British Medical Journal 306: 1468

# Chapter 32

# Adverse reactions to drugs, testing of drugs and pharmacovigilance

## Learning objectives

At the end of this chapter, the reader should be able to:

- recognize that the nurse may be the first to notice a possible adverse reaction to a drug
- explain what is meant by type A and type B adverse reactions to drugs
- list the four causes of type B reactions
- explain what is meant by an acute anaphylactic reaction
- appreciate the possibility of drug interactions in patients on large numbers of drugs
- list the five main sites in the body where drug interactions can occur
- explain how certain types of drugs such as MAOIs are strongly associated with drug and food interactions
- list the important drug interactions listed on p. 412
- give an account of the processes involved in the introduction and testing of new drugs
- explain what is meant by phases 1, 2 and 3 clinical trials
- explain what is meant by a double-blind trial
- appreciate and describe the pivotal role of the nurse in the running of these trials
- explain what is meant by pharmacovigilance and pharmacoeconomics and how they affect the patient

## TYPES OF ADVERSE REACTIONS

During the last few years, adverse reactions to drugs have become increasingly common. They are responsible for about 5% of admissions to hospital and occur in 10–20% of hospital inpatients. This is probably due to the enormous increase in the range and number of drugs now in use. It is particularly important for nurses to be aware of the possibility of drug reactions as they may be the first to realize that something is wrong, and so the drug can be stopped before too much damage is done.

Drugs most commonly causing adverse reactions are:

- warfarin
- diuretics
- digoxin
- tranquillizers
- antibacterials
- steroids
- potassium
- antihypertensives.

The classification of adverse reactions to drugs has been simplified by Professors Rawlins and Thompson of the University of Newcastle. They have suggested that reactions can be divided into type A reactions and type B reactions.

**Type A reactions** are more common and are due to the normal pharmacological actions of the drug, which for various reasons are greater than would normally be expected. They are therefore predictable.

**Type B reactions** (idiosyncratic) are considerably less common and are unrelated to the drug's normal pharmacological action. They are therefore unpredictable and not related to the dose of the drug.

## TYPE A REACTIONS

They can be due to **incorrect dose** or excessive absorption, which is uncommon, **decreased elimination** of drugs or **undue sensitivity** of organs.

### Decreased elimination

This is due to slower breakdown or poor excretion by the kidneys. This in turn leads to accumulation of the drug in the body and adverse effects. Examples are the slow breaking down of morphine by the liver in patients with liver damage, causing undue sedation and even coma, and poor elimination of gentamicin by the kidneys in renal failure, causing accumulation of the antibiotic and damage to the ears.

### Undue sensitivity

Undue sensitivity to the action of a drug can produce symptoms of overdosage or abnormal responses. Examples include the increased sensitivity of the heart to digoxin, leading to toxicity in patients with potassium deficiency, and the undue sensitivity of the respiratory centre of the patient with chronic lung disease to opioids, so that normal therapeutic doses cause symptoms of overdose.

This type of reaction is usually related to the dose of the drug and can be relieved if a lower dose is given or the drug is stopped for a time.

## TYPE B REACTIONS

These are bizarre and unexpected reactions, and are not dose-related. In many cases the reason for and mechanism of this type of adverse reaction is not known: for example, chloramphenicol causes severe depression of the bone marrow in about 1:30 000 treatment courses. It is therefore very difficult to relate the adverse effect to the drug when it occurs in such a small proportion of patients.

Among the known causes of type B reactions are:

- genetic factors
- host factors
- environmental factors
- allergic reactions.

### Genetic factors

A tendency to certain reactions of this type is related to the genetic make-up of the individual. For example, subjects of tissue type HL-A D3 are more likely to suffer from gold toxicity.

Genetic factors may make the drug act in a completely abnormal way. For example, primaquine, an antimalarial agent, causes breakdown of red blood cells in a number of people of African and Indian descent. This has been shown to be due to a deficiency in the red blood cells of the enzyme glucose-6-phosphate dehydrogenase (G6PD). The same enzyme deficiency is responsible for favism, in which red blood cells break down as a result of eating beans.

### Host factors

Host disease may predispose to a certain adverse reaction. For example, patients with infectious mononucleosis (glandular fever) are liable to get a rash if given ampicillin.

### Environmental factors

These have been little studied, but it is possible in certain individuals that diet, tobacco or alcohol consumption and other, as yet unknown, factors may influence the response to a drug.

## Allergic reactions

Allergy plays an important part in unexpected drug reactions, although here the mechanism is only partially understood.

This type of reaction implies that the patient has been exposed to the drug on some previous occasion. This exposure has resulted in the production of an antibody against the drug. Antibodies are proteins which are formed in the body as the result of the introduction of some foreign substance (antigen). They often serve a useful purpose: for example, antibodies formed against bacteria combine with and destroy the bacteria. Several different types of antibodies are produced in response to drugs. Sometimes these antibodies combine with a drug in such a way as to cause damage to tissue and so produce the symptoms of an allergic reaction. Four types are described:

**Type I.**   The antibody (produced in response to a drug) may become attached to the surface of certain cells called mast cells which are scattered throughout the body. If the drug is given on a second occasion the drug (antigen) and antibody combine on the surface of the mast cells, which are destroyed, liberating substances such as histamine, which cause an acute anaphylactic reaction (see later).

**Type II.**   The antibody may become attached to the surface of red blood cells. On second exposure to the drug, the combination occurs on the surface of the red blood cells, which are destroyed, producing a haemolytic anaemia.

**Type III.**   Antigens and antibodies may combine in the bloodstream to form immune complexes. They may penetrate various organs where they are deposited, together with a further substance called complement, which is present in the blood. The antigen/antibody/complement combination stimulates inflammation, which may affect the skin, kidneys and other organs.

**Type IV.**   Drugs acting as antigens may sensitize lymphocytes, which, on further contact with the antigen, will cause tissue damage. This type of reaction usually causes rashes.

Although the exact mechanism of all allergic reactions is not understood, some form of drug/antibody combination is always involved.

## CLINICAL DISORDERS CAUSED BY ALLERGIC REACTIONS

Allergic reactions cause a number of clinical disorders:

- acute anaphylaxis
- serum sickness
- rashes
- renal disorders
- other allergies.

### Acute anaphylaxis

This may be caused by certain foods (especially nuts, eggs and fish), by drugs (notably penicillin), by wasp and bee stings, by injection of foreign serum and by contact with latex rubber. The onset is usually rapid.

Mild cases show urticaria, nausea and coughing. More severe attacks include bronchospasm, facial oedema, hypotension, substernal pain and collapse. Severe anaphylaxis can be fatal.

**Treatment.**   Acute anaphylaxis should be avoided if at all possible. Patients must always be questioned about previous reactions before they are given a drug or a vaccine, especially one such as a 'flu' vaccine, which is prepared in eggs. Particular care is required with sufferers from certain allergic disorders, notably asthma, hay fever and infantile eczema, as they are more prone to anaphylactic reactions.

The treatment depends on the severity of the reaction; if severe it consists of:

1. The patient should be recumbent.
2. Ensure a clear airway and give 100% oxygen.
3. Give epinephrine (adrenaline) 1 : 1000 solution 0.6 ml (600 micrograms) intramuscularly and repeat as required at 10-minute intervals.
4. Give hydrocortisone (as sodium succinate) 100 mg intravenously, and repeat as required, although its effect may be delayed.
5. Give chlorphenamine (chlorpheniramine) 10 mg intravenously or intramuscularly.
6. Give an intravenous infusion of 500–1000 ml of colloid, if circulatory collapse occurs.
7. Use a nebulized bronchodilator if bronchospasm is marked.
8. Nurses should never leave the patient alone.
9. Follow up to determine the cause of the reaction and to prevent a recurrence.

### Serum sickness

This develops about a week after the serum or drug has been administered. There is usually an urticarial rash with stiffness and swelling of joints, sometimes a mild nephritis and lymph node enlargement. Spontaneous recovery is usual, but calamine lotion applied to the rash and oral chlorphenamine (chlorpheniramine), together with prednisolone for a few days in more severe cases, will relieve the symptoms and speed recovery.

## Rashes

Rashes may occur as a result of drugs allergy, but not all rashes which occur when drugs are given are due to allergy. An example of a non-allergic drug rash is the typical erythematosus rash which often occurs when ampicillin is taken.

## Renal disorders

Damage to the glomerulus by several drugs, including penicillamine and gold, can cause gross proteinurea. NSAIDs and ACE inhibitors can cause renal failure and there are a number of other types of drug-induced renal disease.

## Other allergies

Other allergies have been implicated as the cause of various other disorders, including depression of the bone marrow leading to leucopenia, thrombocytopenia and anaemia, haemolysis (breakdown) of red blood cells, jaundice and renal damage. These drug reactions are not always caused by allergic mechanisms and in many cases the exact way in which a drug damages the tissues and organs is not known.

---

### Nursing points

Adverse reactions cannot be eliminated entirely, but they can be minimized by:

1. Taking a drug history to discover whether patients are already taking medicines and whether they have had adverse effects from a drug or drugs in the past.
2. Reducing prescribing to a reasonable minimum.
3. Remembering that certain patients (i.e. the elderly, those with liver or renal disease) may not handle drugs in the usual way and dose modifications may be required.
4. Always remembering that some unexpected change in a patient's condition may be due to an adverse drug reaction.

---

### Safety note

The Committee on Safety of Medicines and the Medicines Control Agency publish, at regular intervals, *Current Problems in Pharmacovigilance*, which provides up-to-date reports of adverse drug reactions.

---

## DRUG INTERACTIONS

If the prescription sheet of a patient in hospital is examined it will probably show that he is receiving perhaps half a dozen separate drugs. This treatment with multiple drugs, which has become a feature of medical practice, has brought with it the danger that certain drugs may interact, occasionally with disastrous consequences. Dangerous interactions are particularly liable to occur:

- in seriously ill patients because they will probably be taking several drugs at the same time
- in elderly patients because they may be very sensitive to relatively small changes in the blood concentration of certain drugs
- when there is only a small difference between the toxic and therapeutic dose of the drug.

Interactions may occur before the drugs enter the body. Intravenous infusions are commonly used, particularly in very ill patients, and a veritable cocktail of drugs may be mixed in the infusion bottle. Some of these drugs may be incompatible in solution, and precipitation or modification may occur. It is therefore very important that when drugs are given via an infusion, they should wherever possible be given as a bolus injected into the plastic tubing and flushed into the patient. If drugs have to be mixed in the infusion bottle, the advice of the pharmacist or doctor should be sought.

## SITES OF DRUG INTERACTIONS

After administration of drugs, interactions can occur at numerous sites (Fig. 32.1):

- in the gastrointestinal tract
- in the blood
- at the site of action of the drug
- at the sites of elimination of the drugs:
    liver
    kidney.

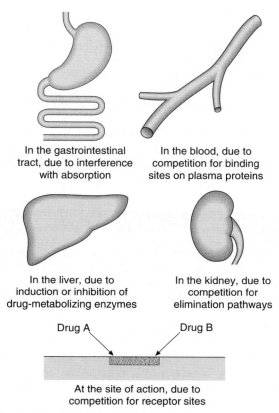

In the gastrointestinal tract, due to interference with absorption

In the blood, due to competition for binding sites on plasma proteins

In the liver, due to induction or inhibition of drug-metabolizing enzymes

In the kidney, due to competition for elimination pathways

Drug A          Drug B

At the site of action, due to competition for receptor sites

**Figure 32.1**    Main sites at which drug interactions can occur.

## The gastrointestinal tract

Most drugs are absorbed by diffusion through the gut wall. If a drug which is well absorbed becomes attached to a drug which is poorly absorbed, the well-absorbed drug will be held in the gastrointestinal tract and absorption will be decreased. For example, if tetracycline and iron are given together, the tetracycline is held in the gastrointestinal tract by the iron, which is poorly absorbed.

## The blood

Many drugs are transported partially attached to the plasma proteins and partially free in the blood. Only the free drugs have any pharmacological action. If two drugs A and B of this type are given together they may compete for sites of attachment to the carrier plasma protein. Drug A may be displaced from the carrier sites by drug B so that there is more drug A free, and thus drug A has an increased pharmacological action. For example, the anticoagulant warfarin is largely carried by the plasma proteins. If chloral hydrate is given to a patient taking warfarin,

the warfarin is displaced from the carrier protein and more of the free warfarin becomes available, resulting in increased pharmacological action and bleeding.

Drugs which will displace others from the plasma protein include NSAIDs, sulphonamides and tolbutamide.

## At the site of action

Drugs may antagonize or augment each other at their site of action: for example, the effect of a drug depressing the nervous system (e.g. a benzodiazepine) will be enhanced by another depressant (e.g. alcohol).

There may be antagonism at the receptors: for example, β agonists (e.g. salbutamol) and β blockers (e.g. propranolol) compete for receptors in the walls of the bronchi and thus produce bronchodilatation or bronchoconstriction, depending on their relative concentrations.

## At sites of elimination

Many drugs are broken down in the liver, where enzymes can be modified by drugs in two ways:

- They can be made more active (enzyme induction), so that other drugs are broken down more rapidly and their effect decreased. Phenytoin, rifampicin and erythromycin are powerful enzyme inducers.
- They can suppress enzyme activity. The antibiotic chloramphenicol is an enzyme suppressor.

**Monoamine oxidase inhibitors.**  One of the most important enzymes which breaks down drugs, and also some naturally occurring substances such as epinephrine and norepinephrine, is monoamine oxidase. It is possible to inhibit this enzyme with drugs called monoamine oxidase inhibitors (MAOIs), which are used to treat depression. If patients receiving MAOIs are given certain drugs or even foods containing amines, these substances will accumulate in the body and cause an abrupt and serious rise in blood pressure.

| *Such drugs are*: | *Such foods are*: |
|---|---|
| Epinephrine | Cheese |
| Norepinephrine | Broad beans |
| Amfetamine | Marmite and Bovril |

In addition, the effects of some drugs are potentiated, particularly those of:

- pethidine (meperidine)
- barbiturates
- anaesthetics.

Drugs may also be excreted via the kidney and in many cases they are passed through the renal tubule cell into the urine. At this site competition can occur. Perhaps the best known examples are probenecid and penicillin, both of which are excreted via the renal tubule cells. Probenecid blocks the excretion of penicillin and this fact is used when very high levels of penicillin are required. Similarly, thiazide diuretics block the renal excretion of lithium and small increases in blood levels of lithium lead to severe and dangerous toxicity.

## IMPORTANT INTERACTIONS

The number of drug reactions which have been described is now very large and many of them are of little or no clinical importance. In general those interactions which are important will occur when the dose of a drug is critical and a small change in the blood concentration or the patient's sensitivity to the drug results in toxicity or, conversely, a lack of therapeutic effect. It is impossible for the nurse or doctor to remember them all, but most of the important ones concern:

| | |
|---|---|
| ACE inhibitors | rifampicin |
| lithium | digoxin |
| anticoagulants | theophylline |
| oral contraceptives | erythromycin |
| β blockers | warfarin |
| phenytoin | hypoglycaemic agents. |
| cimetidine | |

When these drugs are being given to a patient, the possibility of interactions must be remembered if further drugs are added to the treatment regime.

### Nursing point

In outpatient prescribing it should be remembered that the patient may be taking over-the-counter drugs.

Many patients would not consider alcohol as a drug, but nevertheless it can cause serious interactions and should therefore be avoided when certain drugs are taken. For example:

- **disulfiram**, **griseofulvin**, **procarbazine**, **metronidazole** and **chlorpropamide** interfere with the metabolism of alcohol, causing flushing, headaches, sweating and nausea

- **hypnotics** and **sedatives** are potentiated by alcohol
- **warfarin's** anticoagulant action is enhanced with an acute overdose of alcohol
- **MAOIs** can precipitate a hypertensive crisis, particularly with Chianti
- **Metformin** carries a risk of lactic acidosis with alcohol
- **Aspirin and other NSAIDs** carry a risk of increased risk of gastric bleeding, although this risk is small and many people take alcohol and aspirin without disaster.

### Nursing point

Charts are available which show the most important interactions and it would be sensible to display such a chart in every ward and outpatients' department.

## BENEFICIAL INTERACTIONS

Not all interactions are harmful and some are used deliberately to enhance a therapeutic effect. For example, antibiotics may be combined to increase their efficacy and/or prevent the emergence of bacterial resistance, as in the combination of drugs used to treat tuberculosis. In hypertension, two agents acting in different ways (e.g. β blockers and diuretics) help to reduce blood pressure.

## THE INTRODUCTION AND TESTING OF NEW DRUGS

There are two ways in which newly introduced drugs can be licensed for use in the UK (Fig. 32.2).

The European Agency for the Evaluation of Medicinal Products (EMEA), which is based in London, covers all member states in the European Union, and is the only agency which can approve biotechnical products as well as other drugs.

Most countries also have their own licensing bodies. In the UK this is the Medicines Control Agency (MCA), which is a division of the Department of Health.

The Committee on Safety of Medicines (CSM) is an independent body composed of experts in relevant fields who advise the licensing authority on the safety and efficacy of drugs. The CSM is also responsible for monitoring adverse reactions.

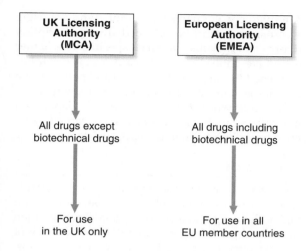

Figure 32.2   Procedures currently available for licensing drugs in the UK.

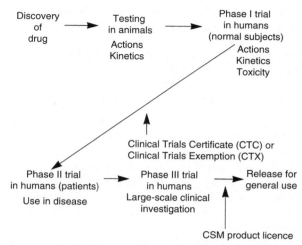

**Figure 32.3**   Stages in introducing a new drug, indicating when licences are required. A CTC requires full information about a drug.

The introduction of a new drug is a costly and protracted affair. It takes about 10–12 years from the time a chemical entity is discovered until its release for general use as a therapeutic agent, and the process costs about £300 million.

In the past, many substances were screened for an action which could be useful in treating disease. With greater understanding of the nature of drug action, it is now possible to design drugs which might be expected to have the desired effect. These are then synthesized in the laboratory. Certain proteins are very complex and difficult to synthesize, but this can be achieved by biotechnology. Genes responsible in human or animal cells for the manufacture of specific substances, such as hormones, can be introduced into bacteria or yeasts, which then produce these substances in large quantities. When harvested, they can be used therapeutically. Human insulin and growth hormone are produced in this way. The drugs are then tested in animals to ensure that they have the required pharmacological action.

A few drugs may appear promising and these have to be thoroughly tested for toxic effects. This is done in two stages. First, large doses of the drug are given to animals over a short period and their actions and toxicity determined. The drug is then given in smaller doses to animals over long periods to see whether there are any toxic effects from prolonged administration or whether histological changes are found after the animals are killed. At this stage the drug is also tested to see if it produces any fetal abnormalities in pregnant animals or cancer after long-term use. Only if this testing shows satisfactory results is the drug given to humans. Animal toxicology has a limited predictive value and even if a drug appears to be non-toxic in animals it may well cause an adverse reaction in humans. There are three phases of drug testing in humans:

**Phase I.**   The first time a new drug is used in humans it is given to young, healthy volunteers. Small doses are used at first and then increased. The subjects are kept under close observation either in hospital or in a special unit. Safety is evaluated and measurements are made of the various actions of the drug and estimation of blood levels will determine the rate and degree of absorption and elimination.

**Phase II.**   If the preliminary studies are satisfactory, permission must be obtained from the licensing authority for limited clinical trials of the new drug to find out whether, in fact, it is useful in treating disease (Fig. 32.3). About 250 patients are involved.

**Phase III.**   This is a larger trial involving about 2000 patients to confirm the safety and efficacy of the drug.

Only after this process will a product licence be given which allows the drug to be released for general use, although the licensing authority may still stipulate a limited period during which further information as to its effectiveness and possible dangers can be obtained.

This type of preliminary screening will usually discover serious and frequently occurring side-effects, but is of little use in picking up rare and unexpected adverse reactions. Other methods are being used to detect this type of adverse effect.

## POST-MARKETING SURVEILLANCE AND PHARMACOVIGILANCE

### Voluntary adverse reaction reporting

Practising nurses, doctors and dentists are asked to fill in a yellow card and send it to the CSM if they suspect an adverse reaction to a drug. For older drugs only severe or unusual reactions should be reported, but for recently introduced drugs designated by a black triangle in the *British National Formulary* doctors should report any unusual effect. This method is limited by under-reporting and probably only 5–10% of these untoward reactions are recorded on the yellow cards.

> ### Nursing point
>
> Nurses are now invited to use yellow cards to report adverse reactions to a drug.

### A study of the national statistics

Statistics such as causes of death may, rarely, give a clue to some adverse reactions, an example being the rise in sudden deaths in young people suffering from asthma which was probably due to overuse of pressurized inhalers. This method usually requires an unacceptable increase in morbidity or mortality before the adverse effect becomes apparent.

### Hospital–based systems

In a group of hospital patients all drugs given and their effects are carefully monitored, examples being the Medicine Monitoring Unit, Dundee and the Boston Collective Drug Surveillance Scheme. Such schemes provide valuable information, but are limited by the number of patients under surveillance. Nevertheless, large collaborative studies provide a great deal of useful information, not only about drug side-effects but also about other aspects of the use of drugs.

### Monitored release and prescription event monitoring

When a new drug is released for the first time for general use it may be limited to certain doctors who are asked to report any untoward reactions.

Alternatively, the names of doctors who are using a certain drug can be obtained from prescription returns and they may be asked specifically whether they have noticed any untoward event which has happened to the patient. This method may become popular as a means of following up a newly introduced drug when it is released. It does depend on the collaboration of the doctors concerned, who must be willing to fill in the appropriate reports.

### Cohort studies

This method involves a large number of patients who are divided (randomly, if possible) into a group taking the drug and a control group. They are then monitored for a long period and the frequency of adverse effects compared between the two groups. Although the results can be useful, it is very expensive and laborious.

### Case control studies

With this method the problem is approached in a different way. A watch is kept for a cluster of patients with similar symptoms which have occurred for no obvious reason; then the possible causes can be investigated. One problem with this technique is that even if taking a certain drug is a common factor, it does not prove that the drug actually caused the symptoms.

### Record linkage

This method involves studying the medical records of groups of patients over very long periods to ascertain whether delayed adverse effects emerge.

None of these methods is by any means perfect and, in spite of much effort, adverse effects still pose a difficult problem. One of the most important factors in their early detection is that those who look after patients, especially nurses and doctors, are always on the look-out for something unexpected happening to a patient.

## THERAPEUTIC TRIALS

In former times, opinion as to the usefulness of a drug depended on impression and anecdote. As a result, many drugs in common use were worthless, some of them having no therapeutic effect at all. One important advance in recent years has been the introduction of the clinical trial as a means of assessing the true value of a drug.

## Defining the question

First of all, the question to be answered by the trial should be defined. For example, it may be a simple one such as the prolongation of life or the cure of a disease, or it may be a more difficult question such as the relief of anxiety or improved quality of life.

## Trial design

It is not always easy to assess the efficacy of a drug in practice and its trial requires careful planning. Patients in the population to be studied are randomly allocated to one of two groups. One group receives the drug under trial and the other group, namely the control group, receives a placebo (a placebo being an inert substance which must be similar in appearance to the drug which is being tested), or possibly another active drug against which the trial drug is being compared. This is necessary because suggestion plays a considerable part in the relief of certain symptoms and may be responsible for some apparent therapeutic action of a drug.

The usefulness of the active drug is then compared with the placebo by noting the beneficial effect in both groups. It is also important that the nurses and doctors who are looking after the patients during the trial do not know who is receiving the active drug and who the placebo, as even they may bias the result by unconsciously communicating their hopes and fears to the patients. This is known as a double-blind trial.

The trial is designed so that the number of subjects involved is sufficient to give a clear answer as to the drug's efficacy. When completed, the results are subjected to statistical analysis, which will allow an estimation of the drug's therapeutic value.

## The placebo response

A placebo drug may be defined as a substance which has no pharmacological action but which, when used, produces a therapeutic effect.

There is now good evidence that in a wide variety of symptoms, including pain, cough, headache, etc., the administration of an inert substance (the placebo) will produce marked improvement in about 30% of subjects. It is important to realize that this does not mean that the patient's symptoms were imaginary. The mechanism whereby this improvement is produced is not known, but is obviously connected with the powers of suggestion.

The placebo effect has a number of important implications:

- It is possible in some patients to control symptoms without using active drugs
- In assessing the effectiveness of new drugs, the placebo response must be remembered and as far as possible excluded
- Further study of the placebo response might be useful in opening up new methods of treatment of symptoms by suggestion, thus making it possible to relieve symptoms without resorting to pharmacologically active drugs.

## Meta-analysis

Even with a well-designed controlled trial it is not always certain whether a particular new drug is more effective than those in current use. This is usually because the differences between the treated and control groups are small and the number of patients involved is not large enough to give a clear result.

To get round this difficulty the technique of meta-analysis has been introduced. This takes an overview of all properly controlled randomized trials of a particular drug or treatment. This technique has become very sophisticated and gives useful information and guidance as to the best treatment in certain clinical circumstances. For example, meta-analysis of the trials in the use of streptokinase in coronary thrombosis has firmly established that it reduces mortality and it is now standard treatment.

## Risk: benefit analysis

When a drug is licensed by the CSM or when it is used to treat a patient, it is important to consider the benefits which will result from its use and the possible risks involved.

When granting a product licence, the CSM needs to be convinced that the new drug is not only effective but also that the risks entailed in its use are acceptable in the context of the disease being treated (for example, greater risks are reasonable for an anti-cancer drug than for a hypnotic). It is essential that prescribers explain clearly to the patient the benefits and possible adverse effects of the drugs to be used.

It may not be easy for nurses to obtain up-to-date information about drugs, but prescribers should have a current edition of the *British National Formulary* available and should use (if possible) drugs which are frequently administered in the prescriber's clinical setting.

## ETHICS COMMITTEES

Experiments on human subjects, whether they be normal volunteers or patients, should be approved by an independent ethics committee before being started. This review is not statutory, but any investigator would be most unwise to proceed without it and no reputable journals will accept articles if the work has not been approved by an ethics committee.

These committees have now been set up by most major medical institutions such as medical schools, research bodies and pharmaceutical companies. They have no approved constitution but should contain a wide medical representation and, in addition, nursing and lay members. Their main task is to protect the subject of research from unnecessary risk and to ensure every safeguard is provided. They should also see that the subject will receive proper compensation if something goes wrong and some ethics committees take upon themselves the duty of criticizing, if necessary, the design of the experiment and ascertaining that the work is worth doing.

## GENERIC PRESCRIBING

When a new drug is introduced it is given two names – a generic (approved) name and a brand name applied by the pharmaceutical manufacturer. If a drug is prescribed by its brand name the pharmacist must dispense that brand.

On introduction there is usually only a single brand of a drug so that the generic and brand names apply to the same product. However, when the patent expires (after 20 years) several manufacturers may produce a particular drug, each giving it a different brand name.

For many years there has been a move to use generic names only and to abolish brand names. This would eliminate the confusion due to a drug having several different names and would reduce the cost, particularly after the patent has expired. Against this it is argued that different brands may differ in quality and the doctor should know which brand is being dispensed. Also, it would reduce the profitability of the drug to the company which had introduced it and had spent many millions of pounds on its development.

## FORMULARIES

Formularies and pharmacopoeias were originally introduced as reference books and were mainly

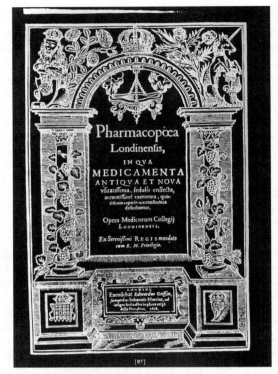

**Figure 32.4** Cover of the first formulary in England published by the Royal College of Physicians in 1618.

concerned with the preparation and composition of drugs in an attempt to achieve some uniformity of composition. The first formulary in England was published by the Royal College of Physicians in 1618 (Fig. 32.4). Since then, formularies have become more concerned with which drugs are available or approved and with their actions and uses.

## THE *BRITISH NATIONAL FORMULARY* (BNF)

The BNF lists the drugs and pharmacological preparations available in the UK together with indications for their use, dosage, adverse effects and cost. It also includes notes on the treatment of many conditions and useful guidance on a variety of problems encountered when using drugs. A copy should be available in every ward, outpatient department and doctor's surgery.

The BNF is updated twice a year. The BNF, however, is not selective: for example, the current edition lists at least 10 β blockers, and it is obviously wasteful and extravagant for a hospital pharmacy to stock all of these. A number of trusts and a few general practices have constructed their own formularies which list the drugs available in the pharmacy and chosen on the basis of efficacy and cost; these may also contain background information. Local formularies do seem to have reduced prescribing costs and have had some educational benefits by stimulating interest in rational and sensible prescribing.

## PHARMACOECONOMICS

In recent years there has been concern over the rising cost of health care. This has to some extent been caused by an increase in the number of elderly people, the introduction of new and more costly methods of treatment and the increased expectations from medical care.

In the UK the drug bill, at approximately 10% of the NHS budget, is the third largest area of NHS expenditure. The available resources are insufficient to meet all needs and so various attempts are being made to control this expenditure. Methods used include increasing the patient's contribution to the drug costs (i.e. raising prescription charges); introducing restrictive formularies which evaluate drugs and indicate which are considered most useful in patient care, i.e. 'best value for money'; limiting the drugs prescribable on the NHS; appointing pharmaceutical advisers who help general practitioners to prescribe in a cost-effective manner; and through the work of the National Institute for Clinical Excellence (NICE).

Pharmacoeconomics has emerged as a branch of health economics relating specifically to the area of drug usage. It is a tool which allows the comparative assessment of the costs and consequences of various uses for the available resources. Choices have to be made as resources used for one treatment cannot be used for another; pharmacoeconomics provides a framework to aid the decision-making process. Resource allocation does not only limit costs, but should maximize the benefit received from the use of these resources.

All health care workers, administrators and the pharmaceutical industry will increasingly need to participate in the practical application of pharmacoeconomics. This will be important as audit and the development of treatment protocols begin to define what should be used, how it should be used and who should receive it. This will move the emphasis of drug decision making away from acquisition costs and therapeutic efficacy towards the total effect of drug treatment on the life of the patient. Nurses by

**Table 32.1**    Four types of pharmacoeconomic evaluation

| Type of analysis | Definition |
|---|---|
| Cost-minimization | Determines the least costly of two interventions that produce clinically identical outcomes |
| Cost-effectiveness | Costs* are compared with outcomes measured in natural units; for example, per life saved, per symptom-free day |
| Cost-utility | Costs* are compared with outcomes measured in 'utility based' units – that is, quality adjusted life years |
| Cost-benefit | Places monetary values on both costs and outcomes |

*All relevant costs are measured in monetary terms.

virtue of a special relationship with patients, both in and out of hospital, are in an ideal position to be involved in this process.

The four main types of pharmacoeconomic evaluation, differing in how the consequences (outcomes) are measured, are (Table 32.1):

- **cost-minimization**
- **cost-effectiveness**
- **cost-utility**
- **cost-benefit analysis**.

Each of these methods involves the systematic identification, measurement and, where appropriate, valuation of all relevant costs and consequences of the treatment options under review. The costs and benefits will vary according to the viewpoint used in the analysis: for example, the patient or the hospital, the broadest viewpoint is that of 'society in general'.

Pharmacoeconomics may seem at first to readers to be an interesting if somewhat academic concept until the implications for the patient are experienced in the clinical situation, and this is best exemplified by an actual case history (Case History 32.1). The decision to approve infliximab involved not only the patient's history but also the cost of the treatment, which is probably in excess of £8000 per annum. This excludes the costs to the hospital for providing the bed, labour and resources made available. The doctor's decision was in line with the NICE guidance for the use of infliximab (see the BNF).

## Case History 32.1

Mr H had suffered from rheumatoid arthritis for over 20 years. He had had operations on both his hands and both feet to insert artificial knuckles. His doctor had recommended knee replacements for both knees, but Mr H demurred. He was on methotrexate injections (15 mg subcutaneously per week), folic acid and low-dose prednisolone (5 mg three times a week) and Celebrex (celecoxib) when needed. He had been switched to methotrexate after he no longer responded to other standard treatments such as ciclosporin and gold. The arthritis was clearly not in control and he had frequent flares. His consultant rheumatologist decided to apply to the local health authority to use infliximab and, after receiving his history, it was agreed that he should be given a course of infliximab. He came in as an outpatient for infusion and after routine urine tests and blood pressure was given a bed and cleared for I.V infusion of infliximab, which took 2 hours. He was kept in hospital for a further 2 hours and then allowed to go home. After the first infusion of infliximab Mr H reported a remarkable effect and said he had not felt so free from stiffness and pain for years. He has infliximab infusions every 2 months and to date has suffered no ill effects.

This is an example of pharmacoeconomics in action. Clearly the dramatic effects of drugs such as infliximab will produce an intense demand for the drug and decisions will be made on the basis both of need and of economic realities until the price of newer 'biologic' drugs such as infliximab comes down. The long-term effects of these drugs still need to be discovered, and that will also be factorized into the decision once these effects are known. The needs of the patient should come first, and this principle should be put before all other considerations. Unfortunately the practice of 'postcode' prescribing has dictated the drugs the patient gets depend on where that patient happens to be. Decisions about whether to provide expensive treatments have been taken locally by regional or district health authorities, and patients in one part of the country might get a particular drug that patients in another might not. This, understandably, has generated a great deal of anguish and anger.

Given the increasing cost of modern medicines, it is not surprising that disciplines such as pharmacoeconomics have come into being.

## Further reading

Brodie M J, Feely J 1988 Therapeutic drug monitoring and clinical trials. British Medical Journal 296: 1110

Brodie M J, Feely J 1988 Adverse drug reaction. British Medical Journal 296: 845

Davies D M, Ferner R E, de Glanville H 1998 Textbook of adverse drug reactions, 5th edn. Chapman and Hall Medical, London

Editorial 1992 Systemic analysis of controlled trials (meta-analysis). Drug and Therapeutic Bulletin 30: 25

Editorial 1992 Clinical trials and meta-analysis. New England Journal of Medicine 327: 273

Editorial 1994 European Medicine Evaluation Agency and the new licensing arrangement. Drug and Therapeutics Bulletin 32: 89

Editorial 1995: Risk/benefit analysis of drugs in practice. Drug and Therapeutics Bulletin 33: 33

Ewing D W 1998 Anaphylaxis. British Medical Journal 316: 1442

Ioannides-Demos L L, Ibrahim J E, McNeil J J 2002 Reference-based pricing schemes: effect on pharmaceutical expenditure, resource utilisation and health outcomes. Pharmacoeconomics 20: 577

Morrison-Griffiths S, Pirmohamed M, Walley T 1998 Adverse drug reactions: practice in the UK. Nursing Times 94:52

Naylor C P 1997 Meta-analysis and the meta epidemiology of clinical research. British Medical Journal 315: 617

Pirmohamed M, Breckenridge A M, Kitteringham N R et al 1998 Adverse drug reactions. British Medical Journal 316: 1295

Rawlings M D 1995 Pharmacovigilance. Journal of the Royal College of Physicians 29: 41

Robinson R 1993 Economic evaluation of health care: what does it mean? British Medical Journal 307: 670

Simon L S 2002 Pharmacovigilance: towards a better understanding of the benefit to risk ratio. Annals of Rheumatic Disease 61(Suppl 2): 88

Symposium 1991 Drug development and clinical trials. Prescribers Journal 32: 219

Walley T, Davey P 1995 Pharmacoeconomics: a challenge for clinical pharmacologists. British Journal of Clinical Pharmacology 40: 199

# Chapter **33**

# Disinfectants and insecticides

## Learning objectives

At the end of this chapter, the reader should be able to:

- explain what is meant by disinfection and the main types
- list which disinfectants are used on the skin and mucous membranes
- explain how to decontaminate the hands
- describe the disinfection of equipment such as bedpans
- identify the agents that are used for wound cleaning
- list the precautions for disinfecting when working with patients with HIV and hepatitis
- list the different types of insecticides and their medical uses
- distinguish between the terms 'cleaning' and 'disinfection'
- state the commonly used environmental disinfectants and antiseptics
- state the insecticides in common use and name the conditions which they are used to treat

## DISINFECTANTS

Disinfection is the destruction of vegetative bacteria, but not necessarily their spores. Sterilization processes (e.g. autoclaving, gamma irradiation) destroy both vegetative bacteria and spores. However, in most circumstances (e.g. standard ward cleaning procedures, cleaning of bedpans and urinals), a reduction in the total number of bacteria is sufficient to remove the threat of infection to the average patient and disinfection is the appropriate procedure. An exception to this rule is the severely immunocompromised patient nursed in protective isolation. Hospitals have their own protocols for the care of these very vulnerable patients. A good disinfectant is not necessarily a good cleaning agent and the two should not be interchanged.

There are two main types of disinfectant:

- **environmental disinfectants**, which are used on equipment such as bedpans and urinal bottles
- **antiseptics** – disinfectants used on living surfaces such as skin and mucous membranes

These two groups are not substitutes for one another. Environmental disinfectants are often potent chemicals which damage tissue, whereas antiseptics, which have been developed to prevent such damage, are not only too expensive for environmental use, but also tend to destroy a narrower range of organisms.

## ENVIRONMENTAL DISINFECTANTS

### Phenolic derivatives

Phenol was one of the first disinfectants used and it kills bacteria by destroying their proteins. It has now been replaced because it is not very effective, rapidly losing efficiency with dilution. It is very toxic, causing local corrosion of the mouth, throat and stomach if swallowed, followed by kidney damage.

Commercially available derivatives include *Hycolin*, which is used as a 2% or 1.5% solution, and *Clearsol*, which is supplied in sachets to be diluted before use. They are active against a wide range of bacteria, but are unable to destroy most spores and are inactive against some viruses. Phenolics can damage the skin and should be used with protective gloves. They should not be used on food preparation surfaces.

### Hypochlorite disinfectants

These disinfectants act by releasing chlorine, the amount released being measured in parts per million of available chlorine. They can be used as environmental disinfectants.

Sodium hypochlorite solution is available in sachet form (*Chlorasol*) and diluted as required.

A 1% solution (10 000 parts per million) is used as an environmental disinfectant:

- hypochlorite disinfectants destroy hepatitis B and HIV in a 1% solution
- diluted solutions decay rapidly and must be made up freshly before use.

### Glutaraldehyde

Glutaraldehyde solution is used for sterilizing certain heat-sensitive instruments. It is allergenic, toxic and irritant and its use has now been superseded by newer, less toxic chemicals. A freshly prepared 2% solution destroys HIV, but is much more expensive than hypochlorites.

> **Nursing point**
>
> Wear gloves when using environmental disinfectants.

## DISINFECTANTS USED ON THE SKIN AND MUCOUS MEMBRANES (ANTISEPTICS)

### Iodine

Iodine is an effective disinfectant which destroys spores as well as vegetative bacteria, but is rapidly inactivated by the tissues. It can also cause skin sensitization. It is now used mainly in the form of **povidone–iodine**, a non-staining and less irritant complex available as:

- povidone–iodine 10% alcoholic solution
- povidone–iodine 10% (aqueous) antiseptic solution, used for preoperative skin preparation
- 7.5% surgical scrub as a hand disinfectant.

### Chlorhexidine

Chlorhexidine is an expensive skin disinfectant and is most unsuitable for environmental use because it is effective mainly against Gram-positive bacteria (e.g. staphylococci and streptococci). It has little action against Gram-negative rods (e.g. *Pseudomonas*, *Klebsiella* and *Escherichia coli*) and will destroy few spores or viruses.

It is used as:

- a 0.5% alcohol solution as a skin disinfectant
- a 0.2% solution of chlorhexidine gluconate as a mouthwash
- a 4% solution as a preoperative scrub and hand hygiene agent
- a 0.015% solution with cetrimide (*Tisept*, see below) for wound cleaning.

### Hexachlorophene

Hexachlorophene is similar and is available in several forms, including a 3% cream used for surface disinfecting.

It can penetrate the skin, particularly if it is excoriated (damaged by scraping destruction of the skin surface) and the application is not followed by rinsing. It should therefore be used with special care in newborn infants.

## Hydrogen peroxide ($H_2O_2$)

Hydrogen peroxide is used for irrigating infected wounds. It is not a very powerful disinfectant, but when it comes into contact with damaged tissues, enzymes which are present release oxygen which bubbles up from the wound and helps to loosen debris, thus cleaning the contaminated area.

## Surface–active agents

These lower surface tension and allow fats to be more easily emulsified. They are also bactericidal. This combined action is useful in that it cleans the contaminated area and allows the disinfectant to penetrate widely, thus extending its range of antibacterial activity. One of the most widely used is cetrimide, which is available as a cream or as a solution and may be combined with another disinfectant such as chlorhexidine (*Tisept*).

## Isopropyl alcohol

Isopropyl alcohol is used as a skin disinfectant and is most effective as a 70% solution, but it may also be used as a vehicle for other disinfectants such as chlorhexidine, marketed as *Hibisol*, used as a hand disinfectant. It is now also used in the newer alcohol gels and wipes. In gels it is combined with emollients without loss of its disinfectant activity.

## HAND DECONTAMINATION

Hands can be decontaminated with soap from a wall container, an aqueous medicated product or an alcoholic hand-rub. Trials have repeatedly shown the superiority of products such as chlorhexidine over ordinary soap, but such trials are difficult to reproduce under ward conditions where nurses hurry between patients and from clean to dirty tasks. Any hand hygiene product will only be efficient if it is used frequently and appropriately, even between such manoeuvres as mouth care and patient feeding. Hands should also be washed when plastic gloves are removed, as bacteria multiply in the warm, moist environment inside them.

Whichever product is used, all hand and interdigital surfaces must be decontaminated and dried thoroughly, as damp hands transfer bacteria more readily than dry ones. Although a thorough handwashing technique may take longer, this is of value, particularly with medicated agents which need a minimum contact time with bacteria to be effective. When soap is used, evidence shows that the bacterial count is adequately reduced by the mechanical action of washing and thorough drying. The soreness which medicated products are said to induce can be reduced by wetting the hands before application and rinsing and drying thoroughly. Incorporation of emollients and the use of hand-rubs and gels is producing soreness and the risk of occupational dermatitis in health professionals.

## USE OF DISINFECTANTS IN VARIOUS CIRCUMSTANCES

The following recommendations are necessarily incomplete and most hospitals will have their own procedures:

| | |
|---|---|
| Ampoules | Swab neck with 70% alcohol or use a *Mediswab*. |
| Bed pans | Washer Disinfector – NB these do not sterilize. |
| Bladder washouts | 1. Normal saline or 2. Chlorhexidine 1:5000 aqueous solution. |
| Wound cleaning | 0.9% Sodium chloride |
| Cleaning cuts and abrasion | Chlorhexidine 0.015% with cetrimide (*Tisept*). |
| Hand-washing | Liquid soap and water (ward staff) from a wall dispenser. In special circumstances, povidone–iodine surgical scrub. |
| Surgical scrubbing: | Povidone–iodine surgical (surgeon) scrub or chlorhexidine scrub if iodine-sensitive. |
| Operating theatres (walls, floors, etc.) | 1. Neutral detergent. 2. Infected material – *Hycolin* 1.5% or hypochlorite (0.1%) with detergent. |
| Skin preparation (injection) | 70% isopropyl alcohol or 0.5% chlorhexidine in 70% alcohol. |
| Skin preparation (preoperative) | Povidone–iodine 10% in alcohol solution or chlorhexidine 0.5% in |

alcohol solution. Care is necessary if diathermy is used with alcoholic solutions. Surgeons have their preferences and may require a coloured solution to delineate the disinfected area.

Thermometers (clinical)
Individual – wipe with 70% alcohol swab after each use and store dry. After discharge – wash with detergent and soak in fresh 70% alcohol for 10 minutes and store dry.

## HIV AND HEPATITIS B AND C

These virus-carried diseases now present a special problem and local guidelines will be available in most districts and are also available from the Royal College of Nursing. All blood and body fluids should be regarded as potentially infectious. Contamination should be immediately treated with 1% hypochlorite solution or, in the community, 1 part of bleach in 10 parts of water, freshly made. Gloves should be worn whenever handling blood or body fluids and the hands washed afterwards.

## INSECTICIDES

### TYPES OF INSECTICIDES

Some knowledge of insecticides is important to the nurse, for these substances are widely used in the treatment of patients' bedding and houses, and some of them are highly poisonous substances which produce side-effects unless used properly.

### Anticholinesterases

**Malathion** is commonly used. It paralyses the nervous system of the parasite. Used correctly it is not toxic, but the alcoholic solution should be avoided in patients with asthma and very young children.

### Carbamates

**Carbaryl** is similar to the above. There is slight evidence that it may be carcinogenic and is now only available on prescription. It has been in use for many years and, so far, it has never been known to cause cancer in humans when applied locally.

### Pyrethroids

This group of insecticides is obtained from the pyrethrum flowers which belong to the chrysanthemum family. They are quick-acting insecticides used in many insecticidal sprays. They are effective and, if used properly, are safe, although sensitization can occur.

---

**Nursing point**

Patients often ask the nurse about the use of topical preparations such as skin disinfectants and medical insecticides. With the advent of nurse prescribing the nurse will not only be expected to provide practical help and reassurance but also to assess the circumstances in which such preparations are needed.

---

## MEDICAL USES OF INSECTICIDES

Scabies and pediculosis (lice) are the two most common clinical uses for insecticides.

### Scabies

Scabies is due to a mite *Sarcoptes scabiei*, the female of which burrows into the skin at certain sites, namely between the fingers, wrists, hands, buttocks and skin folds.

**Therapeutic use.** A number of substances have been used in the treatment of scabies. **Malathion** 0.5% aqueous solution (*Derbac-M*) is very effective. The solution is applied to the entire body from the neck downwards. It is very rare for the face or hair to be affected in adults. If the solution is applied to the face, avoid the eyes and around the mouth. It is left on for 24 hours. All close contacts are treated whether they have symptoms or not. The mite dies very quickly away from the skin, but it is worth laundering sheets and clothes. Itching takes about a month to subside and calamine lotion or 1% hydrocortisone ointment are useful for symptomatic treatment.

**Permethrin** (a pyrethroid) is available as a cream (*Lyclear*), which is applied over the whole body except the head. The body should be washed 12 hours later. It appears to be effective, but occasionally causes itching and erythema.

Benzyl benzoate has now been largely superseded.

## Pediculosis (lice)

It is necessary to prevent the development of strains of lice which are resistant to treatment; therefore the preparations used should be rotated every 3 years. Effective preparations include:

- **Carbaryl** 0.5% in alcohol (*Carylderm*).
- **Malathion** 0.5% in alcohol (*Prioderm*) for head pediculosis.
- Malathion 0.5% in aqueous solution (*Derbac-M*) for pubic pediculosis or for those with abrasions or sensitive skin.
- The pyrethroids, **permethrin** cream and **phenothrin** 0.2% lotion in alcohol are used for head lice. In patients with asthma and very young children alcoholic solutions should not be used.

There is no clearly preferred preparation. Shampoos containing insecticides are not very effective and should not be used. Preparations are rubbed into dry hair, scalp or other affected areas. They are allowed to dry naturally; direct sunlight or heating should be avoided as they break down the drug and could ignite the alcohol. After 12 hours the hair is washed in the normal way. Special medicated shampoos are unnecessary as the lice are already dead. The hair can be combed with a Secker comb to remove nits and treatment should be repeated after 1 week to kill lice emerging from the eggs.

Only those contacts who are infected need to be treated.

## Further reading

Butler M 1998 A guide to nurse prescribing of insecticides and anthelmintics. Nursing Times 94(22): 55

Editorial 1998 Treating head louse infections. Drug and Therapeutics Bulletin 36(6): 45

Elliot R, Torrance C 1998 Zoo-otic diseases. Nursing Times 94(12): 52

Gould D 1991 Skin bacteria. What is normal? Nursing Standard 5(52): 26

Gould D 1991 Hygienic hand decontamination. Nursing Standard 6(32): 33

Mayhall C G (editor) 2000 Hospital epidemiology and infection control. Lippincott, Williams and Wilkins, Philadelphia

Smith F, Ross F 1992 Prescribing topical agents. Community Outlook 2(7): 29

# Chapter 34

# Poisoning and its treatment

## Learning objectives

At the end of the chapter the reader should be able to:

- list and discuss circumstances that can result in accidental poisoning in adults and children
- name the three criteria on which the severity of poisoning is based
- describe the non-specific measures for treatment of poisoning
- describe the strategies for treating poisoning for the drug examples given in this chapter

## INTRODUCTION

The treatment of acute poisoning has of recent years become increasingly important. About 10% of acute medical admissions to hospital are due to an overdose, but 80% of these require only observation until the effects of the poison wear off. Most of the section on general treatment in this chapter applies to the more severely poisoned patient. This may be due to attempted suicide, less often to accidental poisoning and very rarely to homicide. Perhaps the commonest cause of overdosage is an attempt by the patient to draw attention to or modify some intolerable situation. In these circumstances he or she is not seeking death, but merely trying to shock relatives or friends into realization of his or her problems.

In children, poisoning occurs most commonly in the 1–5 year age group as the child becomes mobile and is inclined to put everything in his mouth. Drugs and other harmful substances must be kept not only out of reach, but also out of sight as children are adept at reaching 'impossible' places. Occasionally, poisoning may be due to accidental overdose of a drug.

The most frequently used suicide agents are centrally acting drugs such as sedatives, hypnotics and antidepressants, analgesics such as aspirin, paracetamol and opioids and a mixed bag which includes cardiovascular drugs. Coal gas, although still used, is less common than formerly as methane has replaced it for domestic use. In addition, poisoning can occur, particularly in children, from various chemicals used domestically or in the garden and from a number of berries.

## GENERAL MANAGEMENT

When a patient is admitted to hospital suffering from poisoning the first step is to decide if life is at immediate risk from airway obstruction or respiratory arrest. If so, the appropriate measures should be taken at once.

The next steps are to assess the severity of the poisoning, the nature of the poison used (overdose by more than one drug is common) and to institute appropriate treatment.

### SEVERITY OF POISONING

The severity of the poisoning will be based largely on three criteria:

- level of consciousness
- circulation
- respiration.

### Level of consciousness

This is usually classified in four grades:

- **Grade I**: drowsy, but responds to light stimulation
- **Grade II**: unconscious, but responds to light stimulation
- **Grade III**: unconscious, but responds to severe stimulation
- **Grade IV**: unconscious, with no response to stimulation.

### Circulation

Many drugs cause circulatory failure. The nurse is frequently asked to measure the blood pressure at intervals and a low blood pressure is indicative of failing circulation. However, it must be realized that what really matters is the perfusion of vital organs such as the brain and kidney. It is possible to have a reasonable blood pressure maintained by intense constriction of blood vessels, but organ perfusion will be poor. In such a situation the hands and feet will be cold and blue and this may be a useful sign. In addition, certain drugs (particularly antidepressants) can cause cardiac arrhythmias so that ECG monitoring is necessary.

### Respiration

Depression of respiration so that less oxygen reaches the lungs is a common cause of death in overdosage. Respiratory rate should be charted at regular intervals. Cyanosis is a useful sign of under-ventilation of the lungs, and the respiratory minute volume and blood gases must be measured.

### NATURE OF POISON USED

The identification of the poison used will depend on history and circumstantial evidence, on clinical signs and on analysis of gastric aspirate, blood and urine. Samples should be collected, carefully labelled and analysed as soon as possible. The results may not only be useful in the management of the patient but also they may have medicolegal implications.

## TREATMENT

The treatment of poisoning can be divided into:

- non-specific measures
- specific measures, which are considered under individual poisons.

### NON-SPECIFIC MEASURES

Non-specific measures comprise procedures A–F, which are described below.

### A. Maintenance of ventilation

In the unconscious patient the reflexes which protect the airways may be lost, so there is a danger of respiratory obstruction by the tongue and the aspiration of vomit. These patients should be nursed in the coma position with an airway in place until it is possible to insert a cuffed endotracheal tube which can be kept in place for up to 72 hours. Secretions should be aspirated regularly.

With severe respiratory depression, oxygen and/or assisted ventilation will be required.

## B. Reducing absorption of poisons

It is obviously desirable to minimize the absorption of poison from the gut and this can be achieved in two ways:

- emptying the stomach by emesis or washouts
- giving substances which bind to the poison in the gut and thus prevent its absorption.

**Emptying the stomach.** If the patient is conscious, vomiting can be induced by stimulation of the posterior pharyngeal wall.

**Lavage.** In the unconscious patient lavage may be used:

- **When dangerous amounts of poison have been taken within the previous hour**; a longer period is reasonable with certain drugs, e.g.

  | | |
  |---|---|
  | salicylates | 4 hours |
  | tricyclic antidepressants | 4 hours |
  | opioids | 4 hours |

- **After a cuffed endotracheal tube has been inserted**, as there is considerable risk of inhalation of vomit in these patients.

Lavage is carried out via a 30 English gauge Jaques catheter lubricated with *Vaseline*, and a 50 cm length should be adequate.

> **Nursing point**
>
> Great care is needed to ensure that the tube is in the stomach and not the trachea.

A 300–500 ml volume of warm water should be used for each wash, which is repeated three or four times. At the end the stomach should be empty. Although gastric lavage and emetics have been used for many years in the treatment of poisoning, they do not empty the stomach completely and their efficacy is under critical review. It seems probable that, except when very large amounts have been taken, they have little effect on the prognosis unless carried out within an hour of ingestion.

**Activated charcoal.** Absorption can also be reduced by giving activated charcoal by mouth. The dose is 50 g and it is usually given via a nasogastric tube. It prevents the absorption of many poisons throughout the gut and often is more effective than gastric lavage, which in many circumstances it should replace.

## C. Maintenance of blood pressure

Some patients will have a low blood pressure and failing circulation. Adequate ventilation (see earlier) will often improve matters. Raising the foot of the bed is simple and is usually successful in mild poisoning. With severe hypotension the infusion of volume expanders such as dextran may be required.

## D. Increasing elimination of poisons

This can be achieved by increasing elimination via the kidneys or by haemoperfusion. *Renal elimination* of some drugs can be increased by altering the pH of the urine and an example is in the treatment of salicylate poisoning (see p. 428).

**Haemoperfusion.** In haemoperfusion the blood is passed through a column of charcoal or some other substance which removes the poison. This method undoubtedly removes poisons, but there is a risk of damaging platelets and blood cells so it is rarely used.

A similar effect can be more easily achieved by giving repeated oral doses of activated charcoal; the poison passes from the gut wall and binds to the charcoal in the lumen.

## E. Nutrition, hydration and electrolyte disturbances

In comatose patients the problems of nutrition, hydration and electrolyte disturbances will require consideration, although intravenous infusion will not usually be necessary unless the coma is prolonged.

## F. Follow-up

When the patient has recovered it is important that the social and psychiatric background to a suicide attempt is investigated and most of these patients will require continued supportive treatment.

## INDIVIDUAL POISONS (Table 34.1)

### BENZODIAZEPINES

These drugs are widely used so it is not surprising that overdose is common. They produce coma without any specific features and cardiorespiratory depression is usually minimal. However, death can

Table 34.1   Individual poisons

| | Plasma concentration producing severe overdose | Upper limit of therapeutic plasma level |
|---|---|---|
| *Hypnotics* | | |
| Barbiturates | 50 mg/l | 5 mg/l |
| Diazepam | 5 mg/l | 1 mg/l |
| *Anticonvulsants* | | |
| Phenobarbital | 100 mg/l | 30 mg/l |
| Phenytoin | 35 mg/l | 20 mg/l |
| *Analgesics* | | |
| Salicylates | 600 mg/l | 250 mg/l |
| Paracetamol | 200 mg/l (4 h after ingestion) 30 mg/l (15 h after ingestion) | 20 mg/l |
| *Miscellaneous* | | |
| Amitriptyline | 1 mg/l | 0.2 mg/l |
| Ethanol | 3 g/l | 0.8 g/l is the legal limit for driving |

occur from respiratory depression and/or the aspiration of stomach contents, particularly if they have been combined with other more sinister agents. There is some evidence that death from temazepam overdose is more frequent. Some of this group of drugs have long half-lives and/or active metabolites and full recovery may take several days.

## Treatment

It is usually sufficient to maintain a clear airway and give general nursing care. Flumazenil is a specific antidote which reverses the actions of this group of drugs, but it is only rarely required in severe overdose.

## SALICYLATES (ASPIRIN)

Aspirin has long been a common cause of poisoning, although in recent years its place has been partially taken by paracetamol. In addition to suicide attempts, it is particularly dangerous as a cause of accidental overdosage in children who are more sensitive to its toxic effects than adults.

## Symptoms

Symptoms are mainly nausea, vomiting, tinnitus, increased respiration and with severe overdose confusion, convulsions and coma.

Aspirin also produces complicated changes in the acid–base state of the body. Early on it causes increased respiration and thus washes carbon dioxide out through the lungs and causes an alkalosis. Aspirin is an acid and tends to produce an acidosis after some hours.

## Treatment

- Wash out the stomach with water. This is worth doing up to 4 hours after ingestion of the drug.
- If the patient is conscious, give 5% sodium hydrogen carbonate solution by mouth together with a high fluid intake.
- In severely ill and unconscious patients (serum salicylate >500 mg/litre for adults and >300 mg/litre for children) intravenous fluid and electrolyte replacement is essential. Elimination of salicylate by the kidneys can be enhanced by infusing sodium hydrogen carbonate solution to make the urine alkaline (forced alkaline diuresis) or haemodialysis should be considered. Equally effective is oral charcoal 50 g followed by 50 g every 4 hours, although vomiting may make this difficult. It not only prevents absorption but also enhances elimination.

## PARACETAMOL

Over dosage with paracetamol produces liver damage which may be fatal. This is due to abnormal breakdown products which do not occur with normal dosage, but only when excess has been taken. As little as 7.5 g (15 of the usual tablets) can be dangerous. Early symptoms, usually nausea and vomiting, are minimal and it is only after 2 or 3 days that jaundice with hepatic failure and/or, more rarely, renal failure develop. Patients in whom the blood level of paracetamol is above 200 mg/litre 4 hours after ingestion, or 30 mg/litre 15 hours after ingestion of the drug, are likely to develop severe liver damage.

## Treatment

Activated charcoal (50 g) should be given if a large dose of paracetamol has been taken in the previous hour. There are several drugs available which alter metabolism of the drug and prevent liver damage:

- **methionine** 2.5 g every 4 hours orally for 4 doses, or
- *N*-acetylcysteine 150 mg/kg in 200 ml of 5% dextrose over 15 minutes followed by 50 mg/kg infused over 4 hours, and finally 100 mg/kg infused over the next 16 hours.

Methionine is effective; absorption is slower, however, and may be nullified by vomiting; therefore N-acetylcysteine is preferred.

**Need for rapid treatment.** These treatments are very effective if given within 10 hours of ingestion of paracetamol; after this their efficacy declines. They should therefore be given immediately to all patients in whom there is good evidence of overdose without waiting for the results of a blood level estimation. When this information becomes available treatment can be modified if necessary.

Otherwise, treatment is symptomatic.

## OPIOIDS

Opioids include:

- **morphine**
- **heroin**
- **dihydrocodeine**
- **dextropropoxyphene.**

Morphine and related substances are common causes of poisoning. This may occur as a suicide attempt or because an addict has misjudged his 'fix'. Although morphine and heroin are the best known of this group, serious overdosage can occur with so-called weak narcotics such as codeine, dihydrocodeine and dextropropoxyphene (see later), provided a large enough dose is taken.

### Symptoms

The classic symptoms are coma, depressed respiration and pinpoint pupils. The patient sweats and is liable to develop hypothermia. The pulse is slow. Pulmonary oedema may develop rapidly and is often fatal.

### Treatment

Respiratory depression is reversed by **naloxone** (see also p. 140) 800 micrograms to 2.0 mg given intravenously. It is, however, short-acting and repeated doses may be required. Respiratory arrest will require full resuscitation with assisted ventilation. Hypothermia should be treated in the usual way.

**Dextropropoxyphene** requires special mention. In the UK it is usually taken combined with paracetamol as co-proxamol (*Distalgesic*) tablets and this combination is one of the commonest causes of fatal poisoning. In relatively small doses, i.e. more than 20 tablets, it can produce marked respiratory depression and circulatory collapse. If the patient survives this there is a danger of paracetamol liver damage. The effects of dextropropoxyphene, but not paracetamol, are reversed by naloxone.

The central effects of all opioids are increased by concurrent consumption of alcohol.

## TRICYCLIC ANTIDEPRESSANTS

Tricyclic antidepressants include:

- **imipramine**
- **amitriptyline**

The older tricyclic antidepressants are very dangerous in overdose, largely because of their effects on the heart. Some of the more recently introduced drugs, however, are less toxic.

### Symptoms

With small overdosage the patient is flushed, agitated with some blunting of consciousness and has a rapid pulse. The pupils are dilated and accommodation paralysed. The QRS interval on the ECG becomes progressively longer with increasing severity of poisoning. Larger doses cause fits, coma, depression of respiration and blood pressure and various cardiac arrhythmias.

### Treatment

There is no specific remedy, and diuresis and dialysis are no help. Wash out the stomach up to 4 hours after ingestion and leave 50 g of activated charcoal in the stomach. Further doses of charcoal, 50 g every 4 hours, should be given orally to minimize absorption. Cardiac arrhythmias are treated along the usual lines. Hypotension can be reversed by raising the cardiac output with dopamine and fits controlled by diazepam. Systemic acidosis may require correction by infusion of sodium hydrogen carbonate.

## ALCOHOL

The patient may be conscious but mentally disorientated or may be unconscious. There is a smell of alcohol on the breath.

### Treatment

Most patients will recover if kept warm and allowed to sleep it off. In severe cases the stomach should be washed out if the alcohol has been taken recently and treatment continued as in barbiturate poisoning.

It is very important to remember that patients who are drunk may have received injuries of which they are not aware. It should also be remembered that patients may have taken other drugs in addition to alcohol.

## BARBITURATES

These are no longer the commonest cause of fatal poisoning in Great Britain.

### Symptoms

The patient is confused or in a coma. The respirations are depressed and the blood pressure is low. Skin blistering is a fairly common feature.

### Treatment

In barbiturate poisoning death is usually due to respiratory depression, circulatory failure, or pneumonia at a later date.

**Points.** Please note:

- **the airway** must be kept clear and if the cough reflex is absent an endotracheal tube should be inserted, particularly for gastric lavage in the unconscious patient
- **gastric lavage** is only justified if the drug has been taken within the previous 2 hours
- **ventilation** is important and if there is respiratory depression some form of mechanical ventilation is required
- **fluid and calories** must be given intravenously
- the appropriate **antibiotic** should be given if pulmonary infection develops.

## CARBON MONOXIDE

Carbon monoxide is the most frequent cause of fatal poisoning. It may be accidental or a suicide attempt, although the use of North Sea gas (which does not contain carbon monoxide) makes this less common. It may be due to the escape of gas from faulty heating or lighting installations, to car exhaust fumes or to combustion stoves in poorly ventilated rooms.

### Symptoms

Confusion or coma usually combined with cyanosis or pallor. The classical bright red colour of the skin and mucous membranes due to carboxyhaemoglobin

is rare. After recovery a few subjects may develop symptoms similar to Parkinson's disease.

### Treatment

1. Get the patient out of the poisonous atmosphere.
2. Ensure a clear airway.
3. Give 100% oxygen (not oxygen and $CO_2$).
4. Artificial respiration may be necessary.

## PHENOTHIAZINES

### Symptoms

Phenothiazines such as chlorpromazine produce coma, with hypotension and sometimes hypothermia. Chronic intoxication causes a Parkinson-like state.

### Treatment

Treatment is largely symptomatic, although it is worth trying gastric lavage up to 6 hours after ingestion. Parkinson-like states and other forms of dystonia respond to orphenadrine (see p. 256).

## IRON COMPOUNDS

These substances, particularly ferrous sulphate, are sometimes taken by children because of their colour and sugar coating.

### Symptoms

Vomiting with haematemesis; pallor, collapse and tachycardia. Fatal collapse sometimes occurs after apparent recovery. Iron overdose in children must always be taken very seriously.

### Treatment

- Wash out the stomach with 5% sodium hydrogen carbonate solution (1 oz per pint, 50 g per litre).
- The iron chelating agent **desferrioxamine**, which combines with iron and prevents absorption, should be used in severe cases. Desferrioxamine can be given intravenously to a maximum dose of 80 mg/kg of body weight in 24 hours.

## PARAQUAT

*Paraquat* is a weed killer. The granules available for domestic use contain only 5% of the substance and are not lethal. However, the pure substance used in agriculture is very dangerous: 30 mg may be fatal. Death usually occurs after 1–2 weeks and is due to progressive lung failure, sometimes combined with kidney and liver damage. Treatment is nearly always ineffective, although, if administered soon after ingestion, an oral suspension of Fuller's earth has proved valuable in preventing the absorption of *Paraquat*.

## CHELATING AGENTS

Chelating agents combine with metals and thus render them inactive. They are used for the treatment of heavy metal poisoning.

## DIMERCAPROL (BAL)

Some heavy metals produce their toxic effects by combining with a chemical grouping found in living tissues and called SH groups. Their toxic effects can be prevented by giving dimercaprol, which also contains SH groups and thus combines with and inactivates heavy metals.

### Therapeutic use

Dimercaprol is useful in poisoning by arsenic, mercury and gold.

## PENICILLAMINE

Penicillamine is used in treating Wilson's disease, which is due to the excessive deposition of copper in the brain and liver. It chelates the copper, which is then excreted. It can be given orally daily. It is also used in treating rheumatoid arthritis.

## INFORMATION

There are Poisons Information Centres in the UK and in the Republic of Ireland. They can be contacted by day or night by telephone and will give information about poisoning and its treatment. Telephone numbers of these centres can be found in the *British National Formulary*. The UK National Poisons Information Service (NPIS) is available to health care professionals 24 hours a day. The NPIS has now uploaded a database called TOXBASE (URL at time of writing http://www.spib.axl.co.uk/)

### Further reading

Buckley N A, Dawson A H, Whyte I M et al 1995 Relative toxicity of benzodiazepines in overdose. British Medical Journal 310: 219

Davis J E 1991 Activated charcoal in acute drug overdosage. Professional Nurse 6(12): 710

Editorial 1998 Paracetamol (acetaminophen) poisoning. British Medical Journal 317: 1609

Perry J 1994 Nurse care following overdose. Nursing Times 90(38): 33

Thorsby S 1997 Methods of gastric decontamination. Nursing Times 93(21): 49

Vale J A, Proudfoot A T 1995 Paracetamol (acetaminophen) poisoning. Lancet 346: 547

# Chapter 35

# Herbal medicines (phytotherapy) and homoeopathy

## CHAPTER CONTENTS

## Learning objectives

At the end of this chapter, the reader should be able to:

- recognize the huge increase in self-medication with herbal and other alternative treatments and appreciate the need to find out from the patient whether they are self-medicating
- recognize that many herbal remedies are in fact potent drugs that can poison and interact with other drugs and be able to give examples
- describe how some herbal remedies may actually exacerbate problems rather than cure
- be familiar with the names of commonly used herbal remedies and what they are used for
- respect the decision of the patient to seek alternative therapies, but be prepared to research and advise

## HERBAL MEDICINES

### INTRODUCTION

The use of herbal remedies worldwide is growing at an immense rate. In the UK it has been estimated that at least £72 million was spent in 1996 on alternative therapies (defined as licensed herbal medicines, homoeopathic remedies and essential oils used for aromatherapy). In the USA, perhaps 40% of the annual expenditure on medicines can be attributed to sales of herbal medicines directly to the public and other naturopathic treatments. This runs into billions of dollars. Clearly there is a widespread disaffection with conventional medicine and more and more people are seeking alternative forms of healing.

Most of this is virtually unregulated, although efforts are being made to ensure that standards of quality and integrity among suppliers can be put in place, as well as efforts to educate the public and health professionals about the uses, effects, adverse effects and drug interactions of this bewildering array of medicines.

Many medical schools, particularly in the USA, are now instituting training courses in alternative forms of therapy, both at the undergraduate and postgraduate level. An example is the recent institution of the Program of Integrative Medicine at the College of Medicine at the University of Arizona, directed by Dr Andrew Weil.

Nurses, particularly if working in the community, will quickly realize that many people use various types of alternative or complementary medicines. This chapter is not intended to discuss their merits or demerits; for this nurses are referred to specialist publications. However, some knowledge of herbal medicines is important for several reasons:

- herbal medicines may have pharmacological actions which affect the patient
- not all herbal medicines are free from adverse effects
- herbal medicines may interact with orthodox medicines if they are taken concurrently
- patients may be more likely to tell a nurse rather than a doctor that they are taking herbal remedies; therefore a good drug history is essential.

## HISTORY OF HERBAL MEDICINE

Medicines derived from plants have been used for centuries. The pragmatic and most definitive classics on Oriental medicine are *Shang Han Lung* (*Treatise on Febrile Disease*) and *Chin Kuei Yao Lueh* (*Summaries of Household Treatments*) described in southern China by Chang Chung-ching in the eastern Han dynasty (AD 25–220). This empirical system has been followed for the past 2000 years and many of the formulae in these two books are still used today.

Many herbs have found their way into the pharmacopoeias of orthodox medicine, sometimes as the isolated and chemically standardized active ingredient. Drugs such as cocaine, coumarin, curare, digoxin, ephedrine, morphine, quinine and quinidine, reserpine, senna and the ergot and vinca alkaloids entered orthodox medicinal use by this route.

Many other herbal substances are freely available to the public, and in the UK only a small proportion comes under the direct control of the Medicines Act. Individual unprocessed traditional herbs are not considered as medicines and, therefore, do not require product licences in the UK. In Britain alone it has been estimated that 6000–7000 tons of herbs are extracted annually for use as ingredients of herbal remedies.

## CATEGORIES OF TRADITIONAL HERBS

Traditional herbs (including Chinese herbs) can be divided into three categories:

- licensed herbal products
- dried herbs which are exempt from licensing requirements
- herbal products sold as food supplements with no medical claims.

### Licensed herbal products

Licensed herbal products are those which are sold or supplied with claims for use as medicines (currently over 500 products are licensed). Almost all the licensed herbal medicines on the UK market have been available for some time and most originally held a Product Licence of Right (PLR). The Medicines Control Agency (MCA) has, since 1995, applied new regulations as a result of EC legislation and the Medicines Act of 1968, and, prior to marketing, all new licensed herbal products are assessed for quality, safety and efficacy.

### Dried herbs which are exempt from licensing requirements

Dried herbs are those which are exempt from licensing requirements under Section 12 of the Medicines Act and are not sold or supplied with medicinal claims on the labelling. These products, often sold as 'teas', are prepared from dried, crushed or comminuted (reduced to small fragments) plants, and sold under their botanical names. The exemptions under the Act give herbal practitioners the flexibility to prepare their own remedies for individual patients and will not have to prove quality, safety and efficacy.

## Herbal products sold as food supplements with no medical claims

This category includes herbal products sold as food supplements with no medical claims, although some therapeutic value may be implied.

## THE PRACTICE OF HERBAL MEDICINE

Medical practitioners rarely prescribe herbal remedies and medical herbalists, who constitute only a small professional body, are not consulted by most people who purchase herbal products. Consequently, the principal outlets are health food stores or mail order firms advertising in health magazines and brochures. Now herbal products are available at community pharmacies and are stocked by some supermarkets.

In some areas of the UK certain immigrant races have brought their own medical traditions. Oriental medicine in particular has remained the most widely used traditional medicine. Oriental drugs are alleged to have specific characters such as the 'four properties' ('chill' and 'cool' of yin and 'lukewarm' and 'heat' of yang with 'intermediate') and the 'five flavours' ('acrid', 'sour', 'sweet', 'bitter' and 'salty'). Drugs are dispensed according to their character (e.g. diseases with fever are treated with chill and cool drugs). Over 500 herbal remedies are used in Chinese medicine and there are about 600 or more varieties of crude drugs.

Asian medicine has also been brought to the UK with the traditional practices of Unani and Ayurvedic medicine. The traditional healer is termed hakim if he practices the Unani system or vaid if he practices the Ayurvedic. Unlike Oriental medicine which follows traditional formulae, the philosophy behind the Asian system is that preparations are not uniform from country to country, i.e. a preparation sold in India under a certain name will differ from the nominally identical product prepared for sale in Britain. The addition or omission of certain herbs is usually explained by reference to different climates or temperaments of the person being treated.

In general, herbal medicines aim to use the patient's natural resistance and to restore the balance of health. They are commonly used in treating chronic disorders which respond poorly to orthodox remedies, such as the common cold, arthritis, back pain, mental and stress problems and, sometimes, malignant disease. They are being increasingly used to treat intractable diseases such as dementias in the elderly and diseases of obscure aetiology and poor prognosis, such as multiple sclerosis.

## SAFETY AND EFFICACY

Many of the plants used in herbal medicine contain principles whose effects can be demonstrated pharmacologically, and the action of the whole plant extract can usually be related to that of the isolated constituents. However, for some herbal remedies it is not possible to demonstrate or evaluate their pharmacological activity and the situation is further complicated by the concurrent use of a number of drugs, the supposed active ingredients of which have not been identified.

It seems to be a commonly held belief that, by and large, herbal remedies, being natural products, are inherently safer than the potent synthetic drugs of orthodox medicine which sometimes produce undesirable side-effects. However, toxicity from herbal medicines does occur, although it is rarely an acute episode due to accidental consumption of an overdose. Herbal remedies are often taken over long periods and the appearance of toxicity may be considerably delayed and may even appear after the remedy has been discontinued. The quality of the product can be affected by environmental factors, such as climate and growing conditions before harvesting, and toxicity may vary with the part of the plant used, time of harvesting, post-harvest factors and method of preparation.

Concern over the uncontrolled supply and administration of these products has led the Committee on the Safety of Medicines (CSM) to remind doctors that the yellow card scheme applies as much to these products as it does to conventional medicines. However, the CSM can take little action as these medicines do not have a product licence.

## HERBAL EXTRACTS OF PROVED OR SUSPECTED TOXICITY

### Herbal teas

Traditionally, **comfrey** has been used as a demulcent in chronic catarrhs, as a treatment for gastrointestinal disorders and less specifically as a tonic. In the UK it is used by herbalists as a demulcent, an antihaemorrhagic and antirheumatic agent and as an anti-inflammatory agent. Safety concerns over comfrey centre on its content of pyrrolizidine alkaloids; their toxic effects are due to activation in the liver, leading to liver cell necrosis. Human hepato-toxicity of comfrey has been illustrated by characteristic veno-occlusive lesions with hepatomegaly and inhibition of mitosis. Hepatotoxicity has also occurred with other herbal teas containing pyrrolizidine.

A 'babchi' herbal tea has been associated with photosensitivity. The seeds of this plant contain psoralen, isopsoralen and psoralidin, known to cause photosensitivity reactions.

## Contamination

Herbal medicines may be contaminated with pesticides, mycotoxins (fungi) or substituted herbs, e.g. herbs containing podophyllum or substances with anticholinergic effects. Sometimes an orthodox drug such as aspirin or paracetamol may be added to enhance efficacy. The MCA has detected microorganisms in some solid dosage forms.

## Metals in herbal mixtures

Metals may be added to Asian and Oriental medicines in varying amounts, but in sufficient quantities to cause toxicity. Asian and East African preparations called 'Kushtay', used as tonics and aphrodisiacs, contain oxidized heavy metals such as arsenic, mercury, tin, zinc and lead. A typical Kushtay may contain 10–12% of each of several of these metals.

## Other herbal preparations

Table 35.1 summarizes some reported adverse effects of herbal medicines. There are also problems with the apparently widespread use of khat or ghat and betel nut. Concern has been expressed about the incidence of carcinoma of the oral cavity when these are chewed for their stimulant properties.

Aconitine, the poisonous alkaloid in the plant aconite is cardiotoxic and can induce life-threatening arrhythmia. *Aconitum* is used predominantly in Chinese medicine and is well reported in Chinese literature.

### Safety note

All kava-containing medicinal products have now been banned in Britain (Editorial 2002). Kava root has been recommended for many years as a treatment for anxiety, insomnia and mental tension. It also acts as a diuretic and a genitourinary antiseptic. The substance can be toxic to liver; the incidence is relatively rare but appears to be idiosyncratic, i.e. it is impossible to predict under which circumstances and in which patients this is more likely to happen.

## Interactions between herbal medicines and drugs used in orthodox treatment

In view of the large amounts of medicine consumed, both prescribed and over the counter, it is not surprising that interactions (some dangerous) are possible. As well as interactions between orthodox drugs (see p. 410) interactions may also occur with herbal remedies, some of which are shown in Table 35.2

**Table 35.1**   Possible adverse effects of herbal medicines

| Herbal preparation | Indication | Adverse effect |
|---|---|---|
| Alfalfa seeds | Lowers cholesterol | Pancytopenia, reactivation of systemic lupus erythematosus |
| Aristolochic acid (tincture/infusion) | Anti-inflammatory | Carcinogenic, renal damage |
| Coffee enemas | Anti-cancer | Hypokalaemia |
| Ginseng | Anti-fatigue, anti-stress | Estrogen-like effects, hypertension |
| Honey (rhododendron) | Food supplement | Intoxication, nausea, vomiting, hypotension, bradycardia, reduced consciousness |
| Margosa oil (Neem tree extract) | Insecticide, spermicide | Hepatotoxicity |
| Mistletoe | Antispasmodic, diuretic, hypotensive | Hepatotoxicity (hepatitis), diarrhoea |
| Zemaphyte (Chinese herbs) | Eczema | Hepatotoxicity (hepatitis) |

Adapted from D'Arcy (1991) Adverse reactions and interactions with herbal medicines. Part 1. Adverse Drug Reactions Toxicological Review 10(4): 189–208. Published by permission of Adis International.

# USE OF SOME COMMON HERBAL REMEDIES

There are numerous herbal drugs and just a few of those most commonly used, together with their suggested therapeutic effects, are described here. There is no doubt that many people obtain benefits from herbal remedies and they should not be disregarded. However, some contain active substances and their use should be attended with some caution. There is a body of opinion that believes that some licensing agency is required for herbal medicine to ensure quality and to monitor any adverse effects. The scheme which is now operated in Australia would serve as a good model.

**Valerian** contains volatile oils and alkaloids. Its main use is as a tranquillizer, but it is also recommended for a variety of other disorders.

**Ginseng** (Asiatic) contains saponins, glycosides and sterols. It is claimed to have a wide variety of actions, including improvement in adrenal, muscular and cerebral function. It is used for debility and as an antidote to stress. There are constraints applied to its use which may result in increased tension and sleeplessness. In healthy adults it is advised not to take ginseng for long periods.

**Echinacea** root contains a mixture of high molecular weight branched polysaccharide and caffeic acid derivatives. It produces a non-specific stimulation to

**Table 35.2** Possible interactions between herbal medicines and drugs used in orthodox medicine

| Herbal preparation | Orthodox medicine | Interaction |
|---|---|---|
| **Cardiovascular** | | |
| Cardiac glycoside containing prep. | Digoxin | Potentiation, digitalis toxicity |
| Diuretic | Digoxin/digitoxin anti-hypertensives | Increased loss of $K^+$, loss of hypertensive control |
| Kyushin | Digoxin | Interferes with plasma digoxin assay, false high levels |
| Linn prep. (Ayurvedic medicine) | Amiloride + hydrochlorothiazide | Haemolysis, hypertension, fever |
| Liquorice | Antihypertensives | Hypokalaemia, hypernatraemia, oedema |
| **Sedatives** | | |
| Sedative preps. | Alcohol/antihistamines, hypnotics | Potentiation |
| Tropane alkaloids | Alcohol/antihistamines, hypnotics | Potentiation |
| **Anticoagulants** | | |
| Vitamin K containing preps. | Anticoagulants | Antagonism, loss of anticoagulant control |
| **Endocrine** | | |
| Antidiabetic preps. e.g. Damsissa, Karela | Antidiabetic agents, insulin | Loss of diabetic control |
| Guar gum | Penicillin | Reduced bioavailability of antibiotic |
| Rauwolfia, ginseng | Drugs causing gynaecomastia, phenothiazines | Potentiation of gynaecomastia, galactorrhoea |
| **Antidepressant** | | |
| Ginseng | Phenelzine | Headaches, insomnia, visual hallucinations |
| **Hallucinogens** | | |
| Cassia bark (cinnamon) | Tetracycline | Reduced bioavailability of antibiotic (theoretical) |
| Hallucinogenic preps. 'magic mushroom' (*Psilocybe semilanceata*) | Propranolol, alcohol | Enhanced hallucinogenic effect, schizophrenic states |
| **Miscellaneous** | | |
| Ispagula husk | Lithium | Reduced bioavailability of lithium |
| Kelp | Thyroid hormones/anti-thyroid agents/iodine preps. | Reduced thyroid control (hyper/hypothyroid) |
| Germander | Hepatotoxic agents | Hepatitis |
| Ink cap | Alcohol | Disulfiram-like reaction |
| Eucalyptus oil | Drugs metabolized via liver | Hepatic microsomal enzyme induction |
| Shankhapushpi (Ayurvedic origin) | Phenytoin | Reduced seizure control |

Adapted from D'Arcy (1993) Adverse reactions and interactions with herbal medicines. Part 2. Adverse Drug Reactions Toxicological Review 12(3): 147–162. Published by permission of Adis International.

the immune system and may be useful both as a prophylactic and a treatment in common infectious diseases. It is available as an alcoholic extract in a liquid form or in the dry state as capsules or tablets. The tincture is now licensed and will be marketed for the relief of colds, influenza and other respiratory infections. Dosage of 50 drops twice daily for 5 days a week, to examine its use in the prevention of upper respiratory tract infections, has not proved effective.

---

### Safety note

Some rheumatologists are very concerned about the use of echinacea in patients with autoimmune diseases such as rheumatoid arthritis, lupus and psoriatic arthritis. Echinacea, being an immune stimulant, may cause flares, and this highlights the need for the doctor to know what the patient is taking. Unfortunately, from experiences of doctors both in the UK and elsewhere, patients are often unwilling to admit to doctors that they are seeking medical help on their own. They may perhaps be more willing to talk to the nurse or pharmacist.

---

**Agnus castus** contains volatile oils, castine and alkaloids. It is used to treat the symptoms of hormonal imbalance associated with menstruation and the menopause and is said to improve the function of the corpus luteum. The powdered fruit can be incorporated into tablets or used as a liquid extract or tincture.

**Feverfew** has active ingredients called sesquiterpene lactones from the aerial parts of the plant, and is recommended for the prophylaxis of migraine. The sesquiterpene lactones are spasmolytic and render smooth muscle less responsive to norepinephrine, acetylcholine, bradykinin, histamine, prostaglandins and serotonin. Feverfew's activity in migraine is thought to be due to its inhibition of (a) the production of the inflammatory, platelet-aggregating prostaglandins and (b) serotonin release from the platelets.

**Chamomiles** contain aliphatic esters of angelic and tiglic acids and other oils extracted from the flowers. Roman chamomile promotes digestion, increases appetite and is anti-emetic, antispasmodic and mildly sedative when taken orally. German chamomile or matricaria is used most extensively as a panacea. Preparations of warm and cold infusions of both chamomile and matricaria serve as medicinal agents and as health-related drinks. Teas, made by steeping loose fresh or dried flowers in water or teabags, are used both orally and externally.

**Herbal diuretics** include bearberry, celery and dandelion. These herbal diuretics are used traditionally by herbalists in the treatment of microbial infections and chronic inflammatory disorders. In more recent years they have been incorporated in over-the-counter products used for other applications, such as the symptomatic relief of premenstrual syndrome, and as slimming aids. Dandelion is probably the preferred diuretic as it is unlikely to result in toxicity and the roots and leaves contain high quantities of potassium, which reduces the likelihood of hypokalaemia. Bearberry is primarily of use as a urinary antiseptic and is effective only if the urine is alkaline. Celery may cause allergic reactions or photodermatitis in some subjects.

**Garlic** contains various volatile oils including allicin, which is believed to form other sulphur-containing compounds responsible for its cholesterol-lowering effects. Studies have used doses of 600–900 mg of garlic powder a day or one half to one garlic clove a day to produce reductions in cholesterol of 9–12% compared with placebo in patients with hyperlipidaemia. Interest has been shown in using garlic as an antihypertensive, but clinical trials have not shown significant results. Traditionally, it has been used to treat a wide range of conditions, including chronic bronchitis, coughs, colds and influenza, and it is believed to have expectorant, antiviral, bacteriostatic and anthelmintic properties.

**St John's wort** (*Hypericum perforatum*) is used extensively in both homoeopathic and herbal preparations traditionally as a sedative and for wound healing. However, more recently, interesting clinical trials have been conducted with extracts of St John's wort using doses of 350–900 mg daily for 4–8 weeks to treat mild or moderately severe depressive disorders. Similar responses have been noted when compared with drugs such as amitriptyline in mild-to-moderate depression and with imipramine in severe depression. The greater tolerability demonstrated by hypericum warrants further study.

A known side-effect of St John's wort is photosensitivity and so patients should be advised of this when taking it. Most extracts of hypericum are standardized on their hypericin content, although it is considered that the effects of hypericum may be due to a variety of constituents. In-vitro studies have reported that hypericin inhibits monoamine oxidase (MAO), but these studies have not been replicated and the precise mechanism of hypericin's antidepressant effect is unclear.

**Ginkgo biloba** (maidenhair tree) has been used medicinally for thousands of years. Traditionally, it has been used as a tea for the treatment of asthma and bronchitis. It is widely used in France and Germany in licensed herbal remedies for the treatment of circulatory insufficiencies (peripheral and cerebral). Many clinical studies of varying quality have examined its use in cerebral insufficiency employing doses of 120 mg daily for 4–6 weeks or 50 mg three times a day for up to 52 weeks. Further study is required but clinically significant effects have been found for improving cognitive impairment and daily living/social behaviour.

**Coltsfoot** (*Tussilago farfara*) – the leaves and flowers from this common wild plant have long been used in the form of tea as a popular remedy for coughs and bronchial congestion. The mucilage produced from the leaves is thought to produce a throat soothing effect. The preparations available often contain complex mixtures of different medicinal plants. Safety concerns have been expressed about its long-term use and use in pregnancy due to its content of pyrrolizidine alkaloids which could be potentially tumour-inducing.

## ESSENTIAL OILS

Essential oil constituents are found in conventional medicinal products, e.g. peppermint oil for the relief of abdominal colic and distension. However, the practice of aromatherapy for the palliative care of patients with cancer and for hospice patients has brought the use of essential oils into a different area for the nurse. Some midwives are using aromatherapy for pregnancy and childbirth and for both the mother and infant after birth.

Essential oils are obtained from plant material, e.g. root, leaves, flowers, seeds, usually by distillation, although physical expression is used to obtain some essential oils, mainly those from citrus fruit. It should be noted that there are no controls on the quality of the product sold to the consumer. The concentration of constituents can vary between plant sources and adulteration and contamination is known to occur with pesticides, synthetic oils and other oils. The chemistry of essential oils is complex. A typical essential oil will contain about 100 or more chemical constituents, but most will be

**Table 35.3**    Constituents found in essential oils

| Constituent | Source |
|---|---|
| Limonene | Citrus oils, e.g. bergamot |
| Thymol | Thyme oil |
| Cineole | Eucalyptus oil |
| Citral | Lemongrass |
| Linalyl acetate | Lavender oil |

present in concentrations below 1%. In aromatherapy it is the constituents of the oils that are thought to provide the 'relaxant' or 'stimulant' effect. Examples of constituents found in some essential oils are given in Table 35.3.

Essential oils are believed to act in two ways:

- by exerting pharmacological effects following absorption into the circulation
- via the effects of their odour on the olfactory system.

Topical application (i.e. massage) and inhalation have been shown to result in constituents absorbed into the circulation. However, some oils can cause skin irritation or contact dermatitis even when highly diluted in a bath, and some, particularly citrus fruit (with the exception of mandarin), have resulted in photosensitvity. Tea tree oil has been used for the treatment of certain skin infections and clinical trials have shown its potential for use in treating acne.

Patients wishing to consult an aromatherapist should be advised to choose one who has undertaken relevant training, is registered with an appropriate professional body and who has adequate professional indemnity.

## HOMOEOPATHY

Homoeopathy is perhaps one of the most controversial complementary therapies, but at the same time appears to be one of the most popular in the UK. There is a lack of conclusive evidence that the clinical effects of homoeopathy are completely due to placebo, but at the same time there is insufficient evidence that homoeopathy is clearly efficacious for any single clinical condition.

### HISTORY AND PHILOSOPHY OF HOMOEOPATHY

The basic principle of homoeopathy has been known since the time of the Ancient Greeks.

Devised from the Greek word *homios* meaning 'like', homoeopathy is the medical practice of treating like with like. In modern parlance, homoeopathy has been described as akin to the healing philosophy underpinned by the expression taking 'a little of the hair of the dog that bit you.'

In the 18th century Dr Samuel Hahnemann (1755–1843), a German-born physician, appalled by the medical practices of the day, sought a method of healing which would be safe, gentle and effective. He believed that human beings have a capacity for healing themselves and that the symptoms of disease reflect the struggle of individuals to overcome their illness. He reasoned that instead of suppressing symptoms he could seek to stimulate them and so encourage and assist the body's natural healing process.

Hahnemann discovered that when he self-administered an infusion of cinchona bark (quinine) it produced the symptoms of malaria. When given to a patient suffering from the disease it alleviated the symptoms. He used this procedure with numerous active substances from animal, vegetable and mineral sources in healthy volunteers to determine the 'symptom picture' of each substance. This approach came to be known as 'proving'. He then went on to establish the smallest effective dose to reduce the toxicity of the substance. He diluted his medicines and subjected them to vigorous shaking ('succussion') at each dilution step. He claimed that the more dilute the remedies were, the more potent they became; this process of serial dilution and succussion became known as 'potentization'.

Homoeopathy became extremely popular in Europe, especially in France and Europe, and all but dominated medicine in the USA, not least because it offered another, gentler route than the drastic and damaging treatments such as bleeding, purging and violent emesis that were all that conventional medicine had to offer for many of the diseases that contemporary doctors did not understand.

Homoeopathy's run of popularity came to an abrupt end with the discovery of the antibiotics, whose dramatic, fast and life-saving actions swept it away for much of the 20th century. It was still taught and practised, and retained much respectability. Now, however, there is a great resurgence in the use of homoeopathy, due perhaps to a combination of an accumulation of knowledge of the adverse effects of many of our modern drugs, coupled with the rapidly expanding cost of modern treatments and the growing list of antibiotics which modern bacteria are resistant to. Whatever the case, homoeopathy is enjoying a new wave of popularity in many countries.

## FEATURES OF HOMOEOPATHY

Classical homoeopathy has the following characteristics:

- medicines are chosen on the basis of the similarity between the symptoms they produce in healthy people and the symptoms from which the patient is suffering
- the medicines are given singly
- the medicines are given in very minute doses
- medicines are not repeated routinely, but only when the patient's symptoms demand it.

In practice there are wide variations in how these principles are applied; a good deal depends on the orientation of the particular homoeopath with respect to the symptoms they consider important (physical and psychological), the type of illness and whether the illness is acute or chronic. Many homoeopaths ignore the 'single remedy' rule, preferring to adopt a multiple prescribing approach, e.g. remedies for hay fever.

## DIAGNOSIS AND TREATMENT

In addition to the basic principles of classical homoeopathy there are other basic tenets of homoeopathy. Homoeopaths believe that illness results from the body's inability to cope with challenging factors, such as poor diet and environmental conditions, and that the signs and symptoms of disease represent the body's attempt to restore order. Homoeopathic remedies are believed not to act directly on the disease process but to stimulate the body's own healing activity known as the 'vital force'. As homoeopaths believe that the 'vital force' is expressed differently in each individual, their choice of treatment is based on each individual's unique set of symptoms. It is usual for a homoeopath during a first consultation to take a very detailed history to determine the patient's physical, mental and emotional symptoms. A homoeopath may then use a homoeopathic repertory to choose a remedy that most closely fits a patient's symptom picture. Computerized repertories are now available which greatly facilitate this process.

Having chosen the remedy the homoeopath must select the potency and the form, e.g. tablets, pills or powders. The method of preparing a homoeopathic medicine usually commences with the 'mother tincture', which is usually a concentrated alcoholic extract. One drop of this is mixed with 99 (or sometimes 9) drops of water and shaken hard to give the first potency, i.e. 1c the first centesimal dilution. One drop of this preparation is then mixed with 99 drops of water and shaken to give the second potency (2c), and this process is repeated for as many times as required. Insoluble substances, such as metals, are ground up in a mortar and mixed with lactose. Some commonly used potencies are the 6c, 12c and 30c.

Modern molecular theory suggests that the 12th centesimal potency is the limit beyond which no molecules of the original substance would be present. This is therefore taken as the boundary between 'low' and 'high' potencies. In practice the high potencies are considered more powerful than the low ones despite the absence of any of the original substance. This claim is justified by suggesting that the medicine has been 'dynamized' to a greater extent. The 'seriousness' of the symptoms determines how frequently the remedy is administered and the number of total doses.

## MECHANISM OF ACTION

The lack of a plausible mechanism of action continues to be one of the arguments against homoeopathy. Numerous hypotheses of the mechanism of action of homoeopathic potencies exist. How the solution 'remembers' information from the original substance is speculative. Results from rigorous placebo-controlled trials do not support the hypothesis that it is a placebo effect and further studies are required to investigate any positive benefit these remedies may have (Sturgess 2002).

## THE PLACEBO RESPONSE

The placebo response is a beneficial effect of a preparation that has no medicine in it, and contains only vehicle (e.g. lactose in pills). No health professional these days dismisses the placebo response out of hand; too many have seen dramatic cures and improvements in symptoms from patients who have taken treatments such as homoeopathy, faith healing or who have taken part in clinical trials. This is not to say that homoeopathy works through the placebo response. No one knows. A popular response among some health professionals is that if something is completely safe and works then use it. It has been pointed out that many modern drugs are used despite any clear indication about how they work. Aspirin was used for over a century before its effects on the prostaglandins was discovered about 35 years ago.

## SAFETY

Homoeopathic remedies are often claimed to be entirely free from adverse effects. However, there are isolated reports in the literature of suspected adverse effects, usually allergic reactions, following the use of homoeopathic remedies. It is difficult to assess these claims without a detailed chemical analysis of the preparation used, which might have contained impurities (see also below). Also, it is often stated that a patient may experience an 'aggravation' (a temporary worsening of symptoms) within a few days of starting treatment. Homoeopaths claim that this is a sign that the correct remedy has been chosen and that it is working.

There have been reports of homoeopathic remedies adulterated with corticosteroids and reports of homoeopathic preparations that contained unusually high levels of arsenic. The CSM accepts yellow card reports for any licensed homoeopathic medicines.

Certain homoeopaths (usually lay practitioners) have been criticized in the past for advocating the use of homoeopathic remedies as an alternative for immunization in childhood. Under UK law anyone can set themselves as a homoeopath, regardless of whether or not they have had any training. Patients seeking a consultation should be advised to check that the homoeopath has recognized qualifications, is registered with a relevant professional body, e.g. Faculty of Homoeopathy, Society of Homoeopaths of UK Homoeopathic Medical Association, and has adequate professional indemnity. There is also a plethora of remedies available for self-administration. Choosing the right remedy is not always easy.

It is often claimed that the use of caffeine, aromatic substances (e.g. peppermint, essential oils) or certain orthodox drugs (e.g. corticosteroids) can inactivate homoeopathic remedies if used concurrently. However, there does not appear to be any reliable evidence to support this and there is no evidence that homoeopathic remedies interact with

**Table 35.4** Source of some homoeopathic remedies

| Homoeopathic remedy | Source |
|---|---|
| Arsenicum album | Chemical |
| Arnica (*Arnica montana*) | Plant (all parts) |
| *Apis mellifera* (honey bee) | Insect (bee sting) |
| *Calcarea fluorica* | Chemical |
| *Hamamelis virginiana* (witch hazel) | Plant (bark) |
| Nux vomica | Plant (seeds) |
| Sulphur | Chemical |

conventional medicines, although homoeopaths may claim that a patient's symptoms may be 'masked' by conventional medicines, therefore making an accurate choice of homoeopathic remedy more difficult.

## HOMOEOPATHIC REMEDIES

In the UK, the majority of homoeopathic remedies can be bought in pharmacies, health stores and other retail outlets. Some low-potency (i.e. high-concentration) homoeopathic remedies are however classified as prescription-only medicines. About 65% of homoeopathic remedies are prepared from extracts of plant materials. The remainder may be of animal, insect, biological, chemical or other origin, with over 1600 substances routinely in use today (Table 35.4).

The *British Homoeopathic Pharmacopoeia* was first published in 1870; a new edition, published by the British Homoeopathic Manufacturers Association, became available in 1993 and is designed to be used in conjunction with the *German Homoeopathic Pharmacopoeia*.

The remedies are usually prescribed as tablets or pills with the following advice:

- Do not take remedies within 30 minutes of eating, drinking, smoking or using toothpaste
- Avoid touching the remedies (tip tablets and pills onto the bottle cap and then onto the tongue)
- Hold remedies in your mouth for a few seconds before swallowing
- Store remedies away from strong smelling substances
- Do not stop taking conventional medicines unless told to do so by the doctor who prescribed them

Each remedy is thought to be of benefit for a range of symptoms (Box 35.1).

---

**Box 35.1    Uses of *Arnica***

Use after any injury
Bruises
Sprains
Physical exhaustion following sustained exercise, e.g. a day's gardening or a long walk
Insomnia due to over-tiredness
Muscle-ache all over
Bed feels too hard – constant desire to move to a soft part
Cannot bear to be touched
Great sensitivity to pain
Gout, rheumatism, with a fear of being touched
Use when symptoms are worse: from touch; from motion; in damp, cold conditions
Use when symptoms are better: when lying down; with head low

---

## References

*Herbal medicines*
Editorial 2002: Kava products banned from 13 January 2003. Pharmaceutical Journal 270: 3

*Homoeopathy*
Sturgess R 2002 Is it possible to move towards a consensus on homoeopathy? Pharmaceutical Journal 269: 138

## Further reading

*Herbal medicines*
Barnes J 2002 Herbal therapeutics (1). An introduction to herbal medicinal products. Pharmaceutical Journal 268: 803
Barnes J 2002 Herbal therapeutics (7). Colds. Pharmaceutical Journal 269: 716
British Medical Association Report 1986 Alternative therapy. British Medical Association, London

Chan T Y K et al 1995 Poisoning due to Chinese proprietary medicines. Human and Experimental Toxicology 14: 434
D'Arcy P E 1991 Adverse reactions and interactions with herbal medicines. Adverse drug reactions. Toxicological Reviews 10(4): 189
De Smet P 1992 Adverse effects of herbal drugs. Springer-Verlag, Berlin

Editorial 1994 Herbal medicines. Pharmaceutical Journal 253

Editorial 1995 Should herbal medicine-like products be licensed as medicines? British Medical Journal 310: 1023

Editorial 1998 Alternative medicine – the risks of untested and unregulated remedies. New England Journal of Medicine 339: 839

Ernst E 1998 Health food shops, risks of complementary medicine and ethical standards of research. Journal of the Royal College of Physicians London 32: 399

Fulder S 1989 The handbook of complementary medicine, 2nd edn. Coronet Books, London

MacGregor F B 1989 Hepatotoxicity of herbal remedies. British Medical Journal 299: 1156

Mills S 1989 The complete guide to modern herbalism. Thorsons, London

Ministry of Agriculture, Fisheries and Food, Department of Health 1991 Dietary supplements and health foods

Newall C A, Anderson L A, Phillipson J D 1996 Herbal medicines. A guide for health care professionals. Pharmaceutical Press, London

Penn R G 1983 Adverse Reactions Bulletin No. 102

*Homoeopathy*

Castro M 1990 The complete homoeopathy handbook. A guide to everyday health care. Macmillan, London

Ernst E, Hahn E 1998 Homoeopathy. A critical appraisal. Butterworth-Heinemann, Oxford

Kayne S B 1997 Homoeopathic pharmacy. An introduction and handbook. Churchill Livingstone, Edinburgh

Linde K, Clausius N, Ramirez G et al 1997 Are the clinical effects of homoeopathy placebo effects? A meta-analysis of placebo controlled trials. Lancet 350: 834.

Schiff M 1994 The memory of water. Thorsons, London

# Appendix

# Weights and measures

## WEIGHTS AND MEASURES

### WEIGHT

| | |
|---|---|
| 1 kilogram (kg) | = 1000 grams (g) |
| 1 gram (g) | = 1000 milligrams (mg) |
| 1 milligram (mg) | = 1000 micrograms (mcg) |
| 1 microgram (mcg) | = 1000 nanograms (ng) |

### CAPACITY

| | |
|---|---|
| 1 litre (l) | = 1000 millilitres (ml) |
| 1 decilitre (dl) | = 100 millilitres (ml) |
| 1 litre of water at 4°C weighs 1 kilogram | |

### QUANTITY

| | |
|---|---|
| 1 mole (mol) | = 1000 millimoles (mmol) |
| 1 millimole (mmol) | = 1000 micromoles (mcmol) |

### PERCENTAGE SOLUTIONS

| | |
|---|---|
| 0.1% solution | = 100 mg in 100 ml (1 mg/ml) |
| 1% solution | = 1 g in 100 ml (10 mg/ml) |
| 10% solution | = 10 g in 100 ml (100 mg/ml) |

### DOMESTIC MEASURES

| | |
|---|---|
| 1 teaspoonful | = about 5 ml |
| 1 dessertspoonful | = about 7.5 ml |
| 1 tablespoonful | = about 15 ml |
| 1 tumblerful | = about 250 ml |

### INFUSION SETS

#### Standard giving set

20 drops (15 for blood) deliver 1 ml

#### Microdrop set

60 drops deliver 1 ml

# Index